a LANGE medical book

Behavioral Medicine in Primary Care

A Practical Guide

First Edition

Edited by

Mitchell D. Feldman, MD, MPhil
Department of Medicine
University of California, San Francisco

John F. Christensen, PhD
Department of Medicine
Legacy Portland Hospital
Portland, Oregon

Lange Medical Books/McGraw-Hill
Medical Publishing Division

New York St. Louis San Francisco Auckland Bogotá Caracas Lisbon London
Madrid Mexico City Milan Montreal New Delhi San Juan
Singapore Sydney Tokyo Toronto

McGraw-Hill

*A Division of The **McGraw·Hill** Companies*

Behavioral Medicine in Primary Care: A Practical Guide

5 6 7 8 9 0   HPC/HPC   0 9 8 7 6 5 4 3 2 1

ISBN: 0-8385-0636-4
ISSN: 1093-3468

Notice

Medicine is an ever-changing science. As new research and clinical experience broaden our knowledge, changes in treatment and drug therapy are required. The authors and the publisher of this work have checked with sources believed to be reliable in their efforts to provide information that is complete and generally in accord with the standards accepted at the time of publication. However, in view of the possibility of human error or changes in medical sciences, neither the authors nor the publisher nor any other party who has been involved in the preparation or publication of this work warrants that the information contained herein is in every respect accurate or complete, and they disclaim all responsibility for any errors or omissions or for the results obtained from use of the information contained in this work. Readers are encouraged to confirm the information contained herein with other sources. For example and in particular, readers are advised to check the product information sheet included in the package of each drug they plan to administer to be certain that the information contained in this work is accurate and that changes have not been made in the recommended dose or in the contraindications for administration. This recommendation is of particular importance in connection with new or infrequently used drugs.

Acquisitions Editor: Shelley Reinhardt
Development Editor: Cara Lyn Coffey
Production Editor: Chris Langan
Senior Art Manager: Eve Siegel
Designer: Libby Schmitz

Table of Contents

The Authors

Robert B. Baron, MD, MS
Professor of Clinical Medicine; Vice Chief, Division of General Internal Medicine; Director, Primary Care Internal Medicine Residency Program; Director, Continuing Medical Education, Department of Medicine, University of California, San Francisco, San Francisco, California
Internet: Bobby_Baron@ucsfdgim.ucsf.edu
Obesity

Howard B. Beckman, MD
Professor of Medicine and Family Medicine, University of Rochester School of Medicine and Dentistry, Rochester; Chief of Internal Medicine, Highland Hospital, Rochester, New York
Internet: hbeckman@highland.rochester.edu
Difficult Patients

Douglas K. Beers, MD
Assistant Chief of Medicine, Legacy Portland Hospitals, Portland, Oregon
Pain

Alicia Boccellari, PhD
Associate Clinical Professor of Psychology, University of California, San Francisco; Director, Division of Psychosocial Medicine, San Francisco General Hospital, San Francisco, California
Internet: Alicia_Boccellari@sfgh.org
Dementia

Jeffrey L. Boone, MD, MS
Assistant Clinical Professor of Medicine, University of Colorado College of Medicine, Denver, Colorado; Director of Stress Medicine and Hypertension, The Cooper Clinic at the Cooper Aerobics Center, Dallas, Texas
Internet: www.cooperinst.org
Stress & Disease

Gail F. Brenner, PhD
Assistant Clinical Professor, Department of Medicine, University of California, San Francisco, San Francisco, California
Chronic Illness

David G. Bullard, PhD
Clinical Professor of Medicine and Medical Psychology (Psychiatry), University of California, San Francisco; Psychotherapist in private practice, San Francisco, California
Internet: llubd@aol.com
Sexual Problems

Jeffrey H. Burack, MD, MPP, BPhil
Assistant Professor of Medicine, University of California, San Francisco; Adjunct Assistant Professor of Public Health, University of California, Berkeley, Berkeley, California
Internet: jeff_burack@ucsfdgim.ucsf.edu
HIV/AIDS

Harvey W. Caplan, MD
Former Co-Director of Clinical Training, Human Sexuality Program, University of California, San Francisco, San Francisco, California
Internet: hcaplan@ix.netcom.com
Sexual Problems

John F. Christensen, PhD
Clinical Assistant Professor, Oregon Health Sciences University, Portland; Director of Behavioral Medicine Curriculum, Internal Medicine Residency, Legacy Portland Hospitals, Portland; Faculty, Northwest Center for Physician-Patient Communication, Lake Oswego, Oregon
Internet: christej@ohsu.edu
Suggestion & Hypnosis; Depression; Stress & Disease; Mistakes in Medical Practice

Thomas J. Coates, PhD
Professor of Medicine and Epidemiology, University of California, San Francisco; Director, Center for AIDS Prevention Studies; Director, University of California, San Francisco, AIDS Research Institute, San Francisco, California
Internet: Tom_Coats@quickmail.ucsf.edu
HIV/AIDS

Steven A. Cole, MD
Professor of Psychiatry, Albert Einstein College of Medicine of Yeshiva University, Bronx; Director of Managed Care and Service System Development, Department of Psychiatry, Long Island Jewish Medical Center, Glen Oaks, New York
Internet: cole@LIJ.edu
Depression

M. Robin DiMatteo, PhD
Professor and Chair, Department of Psychology, University of California, Riverside, Riverside, California
Internet: Robin@Citrus.ucr.edu
Adherence

Barry Egener, MD
Assistant Clinical Professor, Oregon Health Sciences University School of Medicine, Portland; Medical Director, Northwest Center for Physician-Patient Communication, Lake Oswego; Faculty, Portland Program in Internal Medicine, Portland, Oregon
Internet: begener@lhs.org
Empathy

Michael Eisman, MD
Internist, Schuyler Hospital, Montour Falls, New York
Death & Dying

Charles C. Engel, Jr, MD, MPH
Assistant Professor of Psychiatry, Uniformed Services University of the Health Sciences, Bethesda, Maryland
Internet: cengel@pobox.com
Anxiety

Adriana Feder, MD
Assistant Clinical Professor of Psychiatry, University of California, San Francisco, San Francisco, California
Internet: feder@itsa.ucsf.edu
Personality Disorders

Mitchell D. Feldman, MD, MPhil
Assistant Professor of Medicine; Director, Behavioral Medicine Training; Director, Faculty Development Program; Faculty, Center for AIDS Prevention Studies, Division of General Internal Medicine, Department of Medicine, University of California, San Francisco, San Francisco, California
Internet: mitchell_feldman@ucsfdgim.ucsf.edu
Cross-cultural Communication; Depression; HIV/AIDS; Domestic Violence

Michael F. Fleming, MD, MPH
Associate Professor of Family Medicine, University of Wisconsin, Madison, Wisconsin
Internet: mfleming@fammed.wisc.edu
Alcohol & Substance Use

Richard M. Frankel, PhD
Professor of Medicine, University of Rochester School of Medicine and Dentistry, Rochester, New York
Internet: Frkl@db1.cc.rochester.edu
Sexuality & Professionalism

Lawrence S. Friedman, MD
Associate Professor of Pediatrics; Chief, Division of Primary Care Pediatrics and Adolescent Medicine, University of California, San Diego, School of Medicine, La Jolla, California
Internet: LSFriedman@ucsd.edu
Adolescents

Linda Ganzini, MD
Associate Professor of Psychiatry, Oregon Health Services University, Portland; Director of Geriatric Psychiatry, Portland Veterans Affairs Medical Center, Portland, Oregon
Internet: ganzinil@ohsu.edu
Older Patients

Geoffrey H. Gordon, MD
Associate Professor of Medicine and Psychiatry, Oregon Health Sciences University, Portland; Staff Physician, Portland Veterans Affairs Medical Center, Portland; Faculty, Northwest Center for Physician-Patient Communication, Lake Oswego, Oregon
Internet: Gordon.Geoffrey_H@portland.va.gov
Giving Bad News; Managed Care

Steven R. Hahn, MD
Associate Professor of Medicine and Instructor in Psychiatry, Albert Einstein College of Medicine of Yeshiva University, Bronx, New York
Internet: shahn@aecom.yu.edu
Families

Katherine A. Halmi, MD
Professor of Psychiatry; Director, Eating Disorders Program, Cornell Medical Center-Westchester Division, White Plains, New York
Eating Disorders

Stephen R. Jones, MD
Professor of Medicine, Oregon Health Sciences University, Portland; Chief, Department of Medicine, Legacy Portland Hospitals, Portland, Oregon
Internet: sjones@lhs.org
Older Patients

Craig B. Kaplan, MD, MA
Director, Primary Care Program, University of Rochester School of Medicine and Dentistry, Rochester, New York
Internet: ckaplan@rghnet.edu
Somatization

Wendy Levinson, MD
Professor of Medicine and Chief, Section of General Internal Medicine, Department of Medicine, University of Chicago, Chicago, Illinois; Founding Medical Director, Northwest Center for Physician-Patient Communication, Lake Oswego, Oregon

Internet: wendy@medicine.bsd.uchicago.edu
Anxiety

Mack Lipkin, Jr, MD
President, American Academy on Physician and Patient; Professor of Medicine and Director, Primary Care, New York University Medical Center, New York, New York
The Medical Interview

Stephen J. McPhee, MD
Professor of Medicine, Division of General Internal Medicine, Department of Medicine, University of California, San Francisco, San Francisco, California
Internet: Steve_McPhee@ucsfdgim.ucsf.edu
Mistakes in Medical Practice

E. Montez Mutzig, MD
Assistant Professor of Medicine, University of Oklahoma College of Medicine, Tulsa, Oklahoma
Internet: montez_mutzig@uokhsc.edu
Women

Daniel O'Connell, PhD
Clinical Instructor, Department of Psychiatry and Human Behavior, University of Washington School of Medicine, Seattle; Clinical psychologist in private practice, Seattle, Washington; Faculty, Northwest Center for Physician-Patient Communication, Lake Oswego, Oregon
Internet: danoconn@u.washington.edu
Behavior Change

David M. Pope, PhD
Assistant Clinical Professor, Department of Psychiatry, University of California, San Francisco, School of Medicine; Neuropsychology Service, San Francisco General Hospital, San Francisco, California
Internet: pope@itsa.ucsf.edu
Dementia

Timothy E. Quill, MD
Professor of Medicine and Psychiatry, University of Rochester School of Medicine and Dentistry, Rochester, New York
Internet: TQuill46@aol.com
Death & Dying

Mary A. Raju, RN, MSN
Formerly Project Director, MacArthur Foundation Depression Education Project; Presently, Editor, *The Nursing Spectrum,* Staten Island, New York
Internet: mrajucole@aol.com
Depression

Gita Ramamurthy, MD
Instructor and Fellow in Medicine, University of Rochester School of Medicine and Dentistry, Primary Care Institute, Highland Hospital, Rochester, New York
Physician Well-being

Nancy A. Rigotti, MD
Assistant Professor of Medicine and Ambulatory Care and Prevention, Harvard Medical School, Boston; Director, Tobacco Research and Treatment Center, Massachusetts General Hospital, Boston, Massachusetts
Internet: nrigotti@sol.mgh.harvard.edu
Smoking

Seth Wigdor Robbins, MD, MPH
Clinical Instructor, Department of Psychiatry, University of California, San Francisco, San Francisco, California
Personality Disorders

Steven J. Romano, MD
Formerly Assistant Professor of Psychiatry, Director of Eating Disorders Outpatient Clinic, Cornell Medical Center-Westchester Division, White Plains, New York
Eating Disorders

Robert L. Sack, MD
Professor of Psychiatry; Medical Director, Sleep Disorders Clinic and Sleep and Mood Disorders Laboratory, Oregon Health Sciences University, Portland, Oregon
Internet: sackr@ohsu.edu
Sleep Disorders

Clifford Singer, MD
Associate Professor of Psychiatry; Clinical Director of Geriatric Psychiatry; Geriatric Sleep Researcher, Sleep and Mood Disorders Laboratory, Oregon Health Sciences University, Portland, Oregon
Internet: singerc@OHSU.edu
Older Patients; Sleep Disorders

Gregory T. Smith, PhD
Director, Progressive Rehabilitation Associates, Portland, Oregon
Internet: pragreg@aol.com
Pain

Anthony L. Suchman, MD
Associate Professor of Medicine and Psychiatry, University of Rochester School of Medicine and Dentistry, Primary Care Institute, Highland Hospital, Rochester, New York
Internet: ASUC@db1.cc.rochester.edu
Physician Well-being

Howard L. Taras, MD
Associate Professor, University of California, San Diego, La Jolla, California
Internet: htaras@ucsd.edu
Children

Melissa Welch, MD, MPH
Assistant Clinical Professor of Medicine, University of California, San Francisco, San Francisco, California
Internet: melissa_welch@ucsfdgim.ucsf.edu
Cross-cultural Communication

Jocelyn C. White, MD
Assistant Professor of Medicine, Oregon Health Sciences University, Portland; Faculty, Department of Medicine, Legacy Good Samaritan Hospital, Portland; Faculty, Northwest Center for Physician-Patient Communication, Lake Oswego, Oregon
Internet: whitejo@ohsu.edu
Lesbian & Gay Patients

Sarah Williams, MD
Instructor, Department of Psychiatry, New York University Medical Center; Liaison Psychiatrist, Gouverneur Hospital, New York, New York
Sexuality & Professionalism

Albert W. Wu, MD, MPH
Associate Professor of Medicine, School of Medicine; Associate Professor of Health Policy and Management, School of Hygiene and Public Health, The Johns Hopkins University, Baltimore, Maryland
Internet: awu@phnet.sph.jhu.edu
Mistakes in Medical Practice

Foreword

Not the least of the many important changes that have occurred in medical care over the past 10 years is the heightened emphasis on primary care and its practitioners. The resulting new prominence has been accompanied by high expectations and expanded responsibilities—for greater productivity, for increased cost-effectiveness, for gatekeeping, and for integrating all aspects of patient care. In a sense, primary care has come to be seen as a solution for many of the problems in our medical system.

High expectations are of course burdensome. But in this setting they are more so because of the ways in which many primary care practitioners view themselves—as victims rather than beneficiaries of all this attention, expected to do more with less, with greater responsibility but no greater resources, and with a scope that is broader than what their expertise may permit.

Behavioral medicine offers help. While not a panacea, behavioral medicine can enrich primary care practice by providing a new perspective and the tools to implement it. For behavioral medicine holds the promise that greater attention to the mind/body connection—and to the effect of emotions on physical health and on the way patients seek medical care—can enhance physician and patient satisfaction, produce better treatment outcomes, and reduce inappropriate use of medical care. A behavioral medicine orientation can also help physicians look at themselves and better understand the ways in which their own behavior affects the patient. The ways physicians relate to their patients—what they say, how they say it, and nonverbal messages—have an important effect on the course and outcome of treatment and on compliance. Skillful communication is, of course, not a substitute for biomedical competence; both are necessary.

Behavioral medicine is both simple and profound, traditional and new, commonsensical and scientific. New research in psychoneuroimmunology, for example, suggests that the way people feel can affect, perhaps significantly, the immune system. Also, researchers using new brain scanning techniques, such as positron emission tomography (PET), are demonstrating the plasticity of the brain, the susceptibility to changes in its physical properties as a result of life experiences. Less esoteric is the good evidence that supportive group counseling with cancer patients can enhance compliance with treatment and prolong life.

Above all, a behavioral medicine orientation instructs but also reminds physicians of much of what they already know but often fail to incorporate into practice—the symbiosis between psyche and soma, the inseparability of psychological well-being from general physical health, and the importance of being alert to signs of psychological distress, such as depression.

Doctors Feldman and Christensen have done primary care practice a good and important service with the publication of their book. It remains for clinicians and teachers to open their minds and practices to the ideas within it.

Steven A. Schroeder, MD
President, The Robert Wood Johnson Foundation
Princeton, New Jersey
Clinical Professor of Medicine
The Robert Wood Johnson Medical School
New Brunswick, New Jersey

Preface

Behavioral Medicine in Primary Care is a comprehensive text for clinicians, students, and teachers. This first edition cohesively brings together the broad spectrum of psychosocial problems commonly seen in the practice of primary care medicine and provides practical, clinically relevant solutions.

Although the term "behavioral medicine" is used widely in both medical and social science literature, there is little agreement as to its exact definition. We broadly define it as an interdisciplinary field that aims to integrate the biological and psychosocial perspectives on human behavior and apply them to the practice of medicine. Our perspective includes a behavioral approach to somatic disease, the mental disorders as they commonly appear in medical practice, issues in the relationship between physician and patient, and other important topics that affect the delivery of medical care, such as adherence to medical treatment and care of the dying.

It is our hope that general internists, family practitioners, nurse practitioners, and other primary care providers will find that this book helps them better understand and care for persons with a wide variety of mental and behavioral problems. For residents and students in primary care settings, *Behavioral Medicine in Primary Care* can function as a valuable resource for understanding the psychosocial dimensions of medicine in much the same way that *Current Medical Diagnosis & Treatment* (36th edition, Appleton & Lange, 1997) helps them to understand the biomedical domain.

We also hope that this book will serve as a clinically relevant text for the increasing number of primary care residency programs, schools of nursing, and medical schools that are adding behavioral medicine to their required curricula. For faculty and students who wish to explore a topic in greater depth, the suggestions for further reading provided at the end of each chapter will be helpful.

Most chapters include case illustrations of behavioral strategies that can be used in the context of primary care. Many of these cases include sample dialogues to help illustrate—and, it is hoped, enhance—clinician-patient communication.

The impact managed care has had in medicine (eg, emphasis on cost-effectiveness and time pressures on busy clinicians) is an important issue that, when relevant, has been considered by several of the authors. It is our belief that the incorporation of behavioral medicine principles and techniques into practice can help clinicians work more effectively with the requirements of managed care. Behavioral approaches can also help clinicians obtain greater satisfaction from patient care.

This first edition of *Behavioral Medicine in Primary Care* is divided into five sections. Section I, "The Doctor & Patient," focuses on topics that influence the development and maintenance of the doctor-patient relationship. Chapter 1, "The Medical Interview," lays the groundwork for how to communicate with patients effectively and efficiently. Chapter 2 explores a key element in doctor-patient communication, empathy, and suggests ways in which primary care clinicians can use empathy therapeutically. Chapters 3 and 4 focus on some specific challenges to doctor-patient communication, such as giving bad news and dealing with "difficult" patients. In Chapter 5, "Sexuality & Professionalism," the authors draw on material gathered from primary care providers at numerous workshops to explore the important but rarely acknowledged issue of how sexuality affects interactions with both patients and colleagues. Chapter 6 reviews ways in which busy primary care clinicians can use suggestion and hypnosis as part of their ongoing care of patients. The impact of managed care on the doctor-patient relationship is discussed in Chapter 7, and the final chapter in this section focuses on physician well-being. Effective doctor-patient communication requires that physicians (and all clinicians) learn ways to enhance their own well-being and remain professionally and personally fulfilled.

Section II, "Working With Specific Populations," takes a broader perspective yet provides an in-depth review of some specific groups of patients cared for in the primary care setting. In Chapter 9, "Families," the author draws on an extensive case discussion to illustrate the importance of a family systems approach in caring for patients. Chapters 10, 11, and 12 focus on the developmental cycle from childhood to adolescence to old age, touching on the key developmental and emotional problems the primary care provider is likely to encounter in each patient group. The emphasis in these chapters, as it is throughout the book, is on both recognition and treatment of common disorders. The next three chapters, "Cross-Cultural Communication," "Lesbian & Gay Patients," and "Women," offer suggestions for enhancing the diagnosis and treatment of primary care patients who often have specific needs and concerns.

Section III focuses on health-related behavior in the primary care context. The framework for this section is provided in Chapter 16, "Behavior Change," in which the theory of stages of change is applied to the primary care setting, and in Chapter 17, "Adherence." Chapters 18, 19, 20, and 21 address specific health-related behaviors most commonly encountered in the primary care setting—smoking, obesity, eating disorders, and alcohol and substance use.

Section IV, "Mental & Behavioral Disorders," is a guide to diagnosis and treatment of several problems often seen in primary care. The chapters on depression and anxiety offer clinical guidelines for patient management, in which both pharmacotherapy and counseling are provided by the primary care practitioner. Chapters 24 and 25 address the challenges of working with patients with somatization and personality disorders; included are practical, clinically relevant suggestions to aid clinicians in the management of these patients. Primary care approaches to working with patients with dementia, sleep disorders, and sexual problems (Chapters 26, 27, and 28, respectively) are also covered in this section. Guidelines for when to refer patients to a mental health specialist are included.

Section V, "Special Topics," examines a variety of additional behavioral issues seen in primary care medicine. Chapter 29, "Stress & Disease," presents a model of the complex interaction between stress and somatic illness that can guide clinicians in diagnosis, prevention, and treatment. Chapters on pain (30) and HIV/AIDS (31) offer a behavioral perspective on managing patients with these problems. Mistakes in medical practice can be devastating for both clinicians and patients; Chapter 32 addresses this issue and provides methods for clinicians to discuss mistakes with patients and families and to cope with their own emotions. Domestic violence (Chapter 33), a public as well as personal health issue, is often first detected by the primary care provider. This chapter describes its clinical presentation and offers practical interventions. Section V concludes with chapters on chronic illness and death and dying, which offer behavioral and relational perspectives on these challenging areas of patient care.

Acknowledgments

This book would not have been possible without the support and mentorship of a number of people. We are indebted to Stephen McPhee, MD, for recognizing the need for a book such as this and for continually providing encouragement and advice. We thank Shelley Reinhardt, our senior editor at Appleton & Lange, for skillfully shepherding this book through its many iterations, and we also appreciate the helpful comments of the editors, Greg Huth, Cara Lyn Coffey, Muriel Solar, and Linda Davoli. We have benefited from the professional administrative support of Mark Sargent and Michelle Hittner. We are very grateful to our contributing authors who, despite busy schedules as clinicians and teachers, have been generous and conscientious in going the distance with us.

Jane Kramer and Julie Burns Christensen and our children, Jake and Hank Christensen and Nina and Jonathan Kramer-Feldman, have had to cope with frequent incursions into our family life during preparation of this book; they have done so with good humor and abundant patience. This book would not have been possible without their love and support.

Mitchell D. Feldman, MD, MPhil
San Francisco, California
John F. Christensen, PhD
Portland, Oregon

San Francisco
March 1997

Section I.
The Doctor & Patient

The Medical Interview

1

Mack Lipkin, Jr., MD

INTRODUCTION

The medical interview is the medium—the vehicle—of patient care and is therefore of central importance to practitioners from both a professional and a personal perspective. The interview is a principal determinant of the accuracy and completeness of data elicited from the patient. It is the most important factor in determining patient adherence to the plans agreed on—whether to take a medication, take a test, or change a life style. The interview is also the keystone of patient satisfaction: More than 80% of diagnosis derives from the interview. The interview is therefore a major determinant of professional success, yet fewer than 10% of medical practitioners have spent any time since graduation working on their interviewing skills.

The interview, which is also centrally important to practitioners' sense of well-being in their work, is the major factor in practitioner satisfaction with each individual encounter. Physicians who cite reasons for career dissatisfaction place unsatisfactory relationships with patients very high on their lists. Physicians with high job satisfaction are those who have a significant interest in the psychosocial aspects of care, who relate effectively with patients, and who are capable of managing difficult patient situations.

The Ubiquitous Interview

The central importance of the interview derives from its epidemiology. For most physicians (exceptions are radiologists, pathologists, and some surgeons), it is more prevalent than any other activity in their work. For example, the average internist works at the rate of 15-minute visits, the average family practitioner at about 12 minutes per visit, and pediatricians at about 8 minutes; physicians overall work at about 6 minutes per visit (some groups are obviously moving very quickly). Making conservative assumptions about how many hours a practitioner will work over a 40-year professional lifetime, a generalist will

have somewhere between 160,000 and 300,000 patient encounters. Each interview can be the source of satisfaction or distress, of learning or numbing, of efficiency or wasted effort (Table 1–1). Too few physicians, however, think systematically—or at all—about how to achieve the desirable goals of satisfaction, learning, and efficiency for themselves.

Each discipline or special interest, such as psychiatry, occupational health, women's health, or domestic violence, asserts that a special set of questions must be asked of every patient in order to be complete and to elicit that patient's particular set of problems. (If an interviewer were to ask all the questions recommended by all the disparate interests, the interview would go on for hours.) In most cases, these question sets have not been validated or shown to be sensitive or specific; a notable exception is the CAGE questionnaire (Table 1–2), which is highly specific, sensitive, and efficient as a screening test for alcoholism (see Chapter 21).

Rather than using a series of overdetermined questions, the most efficient approach is to be patient-centered, starting with eliciting the patient's complete set of concerns and questions and using open to closed cones of questions to encourage elaboration on the information and complete the needed data about each concern. Open-ended questions elicit information more efficiently than do lists of closed-ended questions. A patient-centered approach also ensures that the patient's concerns are understood and agreed on—a predictor of increased compliance.

This approach is most efficient for several reasons. First, patients usually have a sense of what is relevant and will include information and data most interviewers might not think of. If the physician is thinking of the next question rather than listening to what is being said, the ability to attend and hear at multiple levels is compromised. If the interviewer is talking, the patient is not speaking and is not providing data. The physician can always refer later to specific items and ask other questions to round out the data once the patient's

Table 1–1. Gains from improved interviewing techniques.

- Increased efficiency in use of time
- Increased accuracy and completeness of data
- Improved diagnosis
- Fewer tests and procedures
- Increased compliance
- Increased physician satisfaction
- Increased patient satisfaction
- Decreased dissatisfaction
- Increased mutual learning from each encounter

story is told. In addition, if the same basic format is used for each interview, variations in responses are caused by the patient and themselves provide significant information.

The evidence favoring a patient-centered approach goes beyond its practical advantages in the interview; outcomes are also favorably affected. More complete and higher quality information—with the attendant reduction in procedures and tests—reduces cost, needless side effects, and complications. Increased patient adherence to diagnostic and therapeutic plans leads to greater clinical efficiency and effectiveness. Patients take a more active role in their own care.

Active Listening and Efficiency

A number of factors enhance the interview's efficiency. This is currently of special concern as managed care—what some call the "corporatization" of care—leads to shorter visits in primary care. This trend will undoubtedly prove short-sighted: When the visit is cut in length, the psychosocial discussion is the first thing omitted, which can lead to unnecessary testing, patient dissatisfaction, and hazardous and needless procedures and treatments. This direction is exacerbated when behavioral medicine is removed from the benefits provided by the clinician and is provided instead by an external company. Then both sides compete not to care for the patient, and—as might be expected—the relationship deteriorates.

Nonetheless, when cost-effectiveness and time-efficiency are paramount, certain techniques can be helpful. Open-ended questions, as noted earlier, allow patients to elaborate on their responses and thus provide additional information. Active listening refers to listening to all that is being said, at multiple levels, how it is being said, what is included and what is left out, and how what is said reflects the person's culture, personality, mental status, conscious and unconscious motivation, cognitive style, and so on. A skilled active listener acquires such information and other data quickly and continuously. The experienced listener

Table 1–2. The CAGE questionnaire.

C: Have you ever tried to **C**ut down on your drinking?
A: Do you feel **A**nnoyed when asked about your drinking?
G: Do you feel **G**uilty about your drinking?
E: Do you ever take an **E**ye opener in the morning?

gives these observations their appropriate weight—as clear data, hypotheses, or biases. This enables the efficient creation of a complex and textured portrait of the patient that can be used in crafting replies, giving information, relating behaviors, and further questioning to test the hypotheses generated.

THE STRUCTURE OF THE INTERVIEW

The recent literature on the interview runs to roughly 7000 articles, chapters, and books. Although only a modest portion of these derive from empirical bases, sufficient work has been done to describe the interview's conceptual framework as having **structure** and **function.** Behavioral observations and analyses of interviews have related specific behaviors and skills to both structural elements and functions; performance of these behaviors and skills improves clinical outcomes. The following description of essential structural elements and their associated behaviors, or techniques, while comprehensive, is not so exhaustive as to be impractical. Key behaviors are summarized in Table 1–3.

Preparing the Physical Environment

Just as some architects and designers believe that form follows function, so the way in which practitioners organize their physical environment reveals characteristics of their practice: how they view the importance of the patient's comfort and ease; how they themselves want to be regarded; how they as practitioners control their own environment. This last is a key point, since providers often exhort patients to control their own environment. Does the patient have a choice of seating? Are both patient and provider seated at a comparable eye level? Is the room easily accessible? Quiet? Private?

Preparing Oneself

Humans can process seven bits of information simultaneously (plus or minus two). How many of these bits are consumed by distractions or trivia in a clinical encounter? The hypnotic concept of *focus* or the recently accepted psychological concepts of centering or flow apply to the clinical encounter (see Chapter 6). If thoughts about the last or next patient, yesterday's mistake, last night's argument or passion or movie intrude, concentration lapses—and information and opportunity are lost. In contrast, if one is focused, without external or internal distractions, and expects the interview to be a challenging, fascinating, and unique experience, chances are it will be.

How to achieve such a state of mind is a somewhat personal process that is related to each situation. Nevertheless, a few things are common to successful centering: eliminating outside intrusion by having someone else answer the beeper and take phone calls;

Table 1–3. Structural elements of the medical interview.

Element	Technique or Behavior
Prepare the environment	Create a private area. Eliminate noise and distractions. Provide comfortable seating at equal eye level. Provide easy physical access.
Prepare oneself	Eliminate distractions and interruptions. Focus: ■ Self-hypnosis ■ Meditation ■ Constructive imaging Let intrusive thoughts pass.
Observe the patient	Create a personal list of categories of observation. Practice in a variety of settings. Notice physical signs. Notice patient's presentation and affect. Notice what is said and not said.
Greet the patient	Create a flexible personal opening. Introduce oneself. Check the patient's name and how it is pronounced. Create a positive social setting.
Begin the interview	Explain one's role and purpose. Check patient's expectations. Negotiate about differences in perspective. Be sure expectations are congruent with patient's.
Detect and overcome barriers to communication	Be aware of and look for potential barriers: ■ Language. ■ Physical impediments such as deafness, delirium. ■ Cultural differences. ■ Psychologic obstacles such as shame, fear, and paranoia.
Survey problems	Develop personal methods to elicit an accounting of problems. Ask "what else" until problems are described.
Negotiate priorities	Ask patient for his or her priorities. State own priorities. Establish mutual interests. Reach agreement on the order of addressing issues.
Develop a narrative thread	Develop personal ways of asking patients to tell their story: ■ When did patient last feel healthy? ■ Describe entire course of illness. ■ Describe recent episode or typical episode.
Establish the life context of the patient	Use first opportunity to inquire about personal and social details. Flesh out developmental history. Learn about patient's support system. Learn about home, work, neighborhood, and safety issues.
Establish a safety net	Memorize complete review of systems. Review issues as appropriate to specific problem.
Present findings and options	Be succinct. Ascertain patient's level of understanding and cognitive style. Ask patient to review and state understanding. Summarize and check. Tape interview and give copy of tape to patient. Ask patient's perspectives.
Negotiate plans	Involve patient actively. Agree on what is feasible. Respect patient's choices whenever possible.
Close the interview	Ask patient to review plans and arrangements. Clarify what patient should do in the interim. Schedule next encounter. Say good-bye.

tuning out other sounds; eliminating internal distractions and intrusive thoughts by resolving not to work on other matters and letting disturbing thoughts simply pass through and out of consciousness for the moment; and controlling distracting reactions to what is occurring in the interview by noting them, thinking about their origins, and putting them aside if they are not helpful.

Observing the Patient

A great deal can be learned by simply observing the patient's behavior and body language both before and during the conversation. While the physician's initial behavioral observations are purely heuristic—used to generate testable hypotheses about the patient—nonverbal behavior can sometimes reveal as much about the patient's state of mind as the patient's verbal responses do. Clinicians who are unaware of being influenced by initial reactions and observations in the patient interview may note that when they themselves get on a bus or an airplane, they—like other people—instantly recognize whom they would prefer—or prefer not—to sit next to. Such responses result from integrating a considerable number of nonverbal cues. Similar input about patients can relate to their overall state of health, vital signs, cardiac and pulmonary compensation, liver function, and more. Observations about grooming, state of rest, alertness, and style of presentation can reveal much about the patient's self-confidence, depression or anxiety, or the presence of psychosis; the physician may also detect signs of possible alcohol or drug use. Escorting patients from the waiting area, letting them walk slightly ahead into the office, allows the practitioner to observe how patients have used their waiting time, to note their gait, check on who accompanies them, and look for clues to the relationship with these escorts.

Developing the ability to make and use such clinical observations starts with the intention to do so. A decision to systematically retain and integrate initial observations will provide the physician with important data that have been easily available, but typically overlooked. Asking oneself pertinent questions about behavioral cues, keeping in mind the kinds of observations that are possible, and refining these skills through practice will increase the speed and comprehensiveness of observing. By practicing in crowds, at rounds or in lectures, on the airplane or at parties, it is possible to train oneself to become a more astute observer.

Greeting the Patient

The greeting serves to identify each party to the interaction, to set the social tone, to telegraph one's intentions concerning equality or dominance, and to avoid mistaken identity. It also allows the practitioner to establish immediately with patients that they are entrusting themselves to a confident, compassionate professional. It enables the physician to learn how patients assert their own identity—and how to pronounce their names. Using a standard greeting—saying virtually the same thing each time—provides a basis for evaluating a variety of patient responses.

Beginning the Interview

The introductory phase of a medical encounter is the opportunity for both parties to express their understanding of the purposes and conditions of the encounter, to check each one's expectations against the other's, and to negotiate the differences. For example: The patient expects the physician to be the head of the clinic—but the physician is only a year out of residency. Or the practitioner expects that the consultation will lead to cardiac catheterization, while the patient thinks the cardiologist's opinions are to be sent to his primary care physician for her decision. Perhaps the physician can spare only 15 minutes, but the patient feels he needs a full hour.

Since one of the best predictors of the outcome of a dyadic relationship is the expectations of each person, clarifying and reconciling these is extremely important before beginning the main part of the interview.

Detecting & Overcoming Barriers to Communication

Many factors can interfere with communication between people—and still more place barriers between doctor and patient. There are tangible barriers in patient care: delirium, dementia, deafness, aphasia, intoxication on the part of patient or physician, and ambient noise. Psychological barriers can include depression, anxiety, psychosis, paranoia, and distrust; and social barriers often involve language, cultural differences, fears about immigration status, or legal problems. It is essential to detect such barriers early in an encounter; failure to do so not only wastes time but can seriously and sometimes dangerously mislead the physician. In addition, detecting a barrier is the first step toward its correction, whether by waiting until delirium or intoxication has cleared; finding a professional interpreter or signer; moving to a quiet, private place; or waiting to deal with the difficult issues until trust is established.

Surveying Problems

Because patients come into medical encounters with multiple problems and may not lead with the most pressing issue, and because physicians typically interrupt very quickly (within 18 seconds on average, according to one study), it is vitally important not to jump in at the first important-sounding problem but to survey all problems first. For example, the clinician might ask, "What problems are you having?" or "What issues would you like to work on first?" After getting the initial answer or series of answers, the clinician can then ask what else is bothering the patient until the list of problems ends.

Negotiating Priorities

Once the physician and the patient clearly understand the full list of problems, the patient should then be asked, "Which of these would you like to work on first?" If the physician considers something else to be more important, there should be negotiation about this difference: "Our time is short today, and I think your shortness of breath is potentially more dangerous than your back pain. Suppose we deal with that first and, if we have time, go on to your back pain? If not, we'll take that up on your next visit."

Failure to ascertain and acknowledge patients' priorities will cause them to feel, appropriately, that the physician is not sensitive to their concerns. This can lead to failure to comply with treatment—or failure to return to the office.

Developing a Narrative Thread

Once the physician and the patient have decided which problem has priority, exploration of that problem can begin. The most efficient method to use in exploring a problem is to ask the patient to tell the story of the problem. While many persons will begin at an appropriate point and move toward the present, some patients may need or wish to be guided as to where to start: The physician may have to ask when the patient last felt healthy, when the current episode began, or when he or she thinks the problem started. The patient may not have a feel for the desired level of detail and may be either too inclusive or too quick and superficial. It may therefore be necessary for the physician to interrupt and indicate to the patient that he or she wishes to hear more—or less—about the problem. Clarifying questions will show the patient what is needed, and most persons will thereafter provide the appropriate level of detail.

Establishing the Life Context of the Patient

Once the narrative thread is in place, the physician can take the opportunity, when it arises, to inquire about specific points. Such inquiries help the physician learn about and understand the context of the patient's life—spouse, family, neighborhood, job, culture—in more detail. When enough information has been supplied, simply saying, "You were saying . . . ; what happened next?" can return the patient to the narrative.

Creating a Safety Net

Once the problems the patient wishes to discuss have been explored, there may be remaining areas or questions that have not been covered. For these, the physician may choose to ask a series of specific questions or to use a review of systems not already covered. These questions may take the form of the seven dimensions of symptoms described as the location, duration, severity, quality, associations, radiation, and exacerbants and ameliorants or a subset of these dimensions. The final closed-ended questions tie up the loose ends and provide the safety of completeness.

Presenting Findings & Options

After the history-taking and physical examination have been completed, it is time for the physician and patient to discuss what the problems appear to be, related findings, the physician's hypotheses or conclusions, and possible approaches to further diagnostic evaluation and treatment. This should be done in a fashion that the patient can understand. First, it is very valuable to foreshadow any bad or potentially upsetting news (see Chapter 3). This preparation helps the patient hear and retain the information better. When bad news is a certainty, it is useful to record the doctor's explanation and any discussion so the patient can review it later, when out of shock. It has been documented that this reconsideration leads to better outcomes of care. It is essential not to underestimate the potential impact of both positive and negative findings on the patient; after presenting each item the physician should explore the patient's understanding and reactions. The presentation itself should be problem-oriented and systematic—and as simple and succinct as possible. Although the dictum is to be brief, content and empathy should not be sacrificed to brevity.

Negotiating a Plan

Once the patient has been factually informed of the diagnosis and prognosis, it is crucial in developing diagnostic and therapeutic plans to involve the patient actively in making choices. Such "activation" of the patient has been shown to increase adherence to the plans and improve both the medical outcome and the patient's quality of life.

Where the physician and patient disagree in emphasis or choice, negotiation is necessary. The principle of negotiation can be summarized as finding the areas of mutual interest, emphasizing them, and avoiding the adoption of inflexible positions that can only lead to conflict and defeat. If the physician takes the time to understand the patient's position and respect his or her concerns, the issues can usually be worked out, for example, by agreeing to do a procedure after a grandchild's graduation or performance or agreeing to do noninvasive tests first in the hope they will suffice.

Closing the Interview

Issues to be managed in the closing are reviewing the principal findings, plans, and agreements; making arrangements for the next visit and giving the patient instructions for the intervening time; making sure outstanding issues have been covered; and saying good-bye.

THE FUNCTIONS OF THE INTERVIEW

The three functions of the interview (initially described by Bird and Cohen-Cole and subsequently refined and rationalized by Lazare, Putnam, and Lipkin) describe the major purposes of the interview and the associated skills and behaviors that improve the interview process and outcomes. The functions—gathering information and monitoring progress; developing, maintaining, and concluding the therapeutic relationship; and educating the patient and implementing treatment plans—are interdependent. For example, patients cannot be expected to reveal personal or humiliating information unless they have developed considerable trust in their physicians. The physician cannot educate a patient effectively without knowing what level of language and which concepts to use, how to frame things for clarity, which formulations will interpose needless barriers to acceptance—all data derived during information-gathering. Therefore, the three functions cannot be pursued sequentially but must be integrated.

Gathering Information & Monitoring Progress

These are medical activities thought of by many physicians as the dominant function of the interview. The tasks associated with this first function are to acquire a knowledge base of diseases and disorders and of psychosocial issues and illness behavior; to elicit the data relevant to each problem; to perceive the relevant data; and to generate and test relevant hypotheses to the elicited data. Skills useful in these tasks include starting with open questions such as "Tell me about it" and gradually narrowing the queries down to more specific questions; use of minimal encouragers (eg, "Uh huh," "Hmmm") to facilitate flow; gentle use of direction to steer without dominating; and summarizing and checking ("I think you have said point *a,* point *b,* point *c;* is that right?").

Developing, Maintaining, & Concluding the Therapeutic Relationship

This second function of the interview includes defining the nature of the relationship (short- or long-term, consultation, primary care, disease-episode-oriented); communicating professional expertise; communicating interest, respect, empathy, and support; recognizing and resolving relational barriers to communication; and eliciting the patient's perspective. This is a pivotal function because its success is necessary for success in the first and third functions.

Although there are those who feel that relationships cannot be improved, worked on, or manipulated, the vast literature in psychotherapy disproves these skeptics. It is clear that use of appropriate relationship-building skills significantly improves interview outcomes in terms of satisfaction, compliance, data disclosure, quality of life, biological outcomes, and personal growth.

These issues are particularly germane in cases involving mental disorders, where skill in managing the patient in a way compatible with the disorder is essential. In general, naming feelings, communicating unconditional positive regard, expressing empathy and understanding, and being emotionally congruent (having what one says be actually what one means and feels), produce the best outcomes. Other skills include reflection, legitimization, partnership, the nonverbal skills of touch and eye contact, and the avoidance of shame or humiliation (see Chapter 2).

Educating the Patient

Patient education and implementation of treatment plans require being aware of the patient's current level of knowledge and understanding, the patient's cognitive style and level, having a receptive patient who is neither in shock nor in disagreement, and using plain language that avoids jargon or undue complexity. The tasks associated with this third function include communicating the diagnostic significance of the problem(s); negotiating and recommending appropriate diagnostic and treatment options; negotiating and recommending appropriate prevention and life-style changes; and enhancing the patient's ability to cope by understanding and communicating the psychological and social impacts of the illness. Involving the patient in making choices, clarifying uncertainties, and expressing fears and concerns markedly improves outcomes. Having the patient actively review what has been discussed and decided is critical to check for understanding and to reinforce memory (see Chapter 17).

SPECIAL CIRCUMSTANCES & INTERVIEW MODIFICATIONS

While the preceding principles are applicable to most situations, many circumstances require a modified approach to maximize the usefulness and durability of the interview and relationship. Early detection of special situations is crucial so that the appropriate modifications in technique can be made as soon as possible. In most special situations, meticulous attention to the particular relationship needs of the patient is paramount, as, for example, with the paranoid or psychotic patient.

Aids to Diagnosing Mental Disorders

Physicians currently have a variety of aids to use in diagnosing and monitoring mental disorders. The simplest aids have relatively high sensitivity (they detect most of the real cases) but lower specificity (they register as positive cases those that do not meet the diagnostic criteria). Among the screening devices for depression are the Beck, Zung, and Hamilton scales. Some physicians administer these as part of a packet of materials to be filled out prior to the initial visit. As with other such questionnaires, however, these create the additional problem of having to deal with a large number of false-positives, which can be extremely time-consuming.

Two recently developed devices (with pharmaceutical company support) can screen for several common mental disorders at the same time. Prime-MD (Primary Care Screen for Mental Disorders) and SDDS-PC (Symptom-Driven Diagnostic System for Primary Care) both have preliminary endorsement as reasonably sensitive and specific instruments, and both are being modified now for telephone use and for computerized administration. The problem many empathic physicians have with their use, however, is that the programs ask about feelings but cannot respond to their expression. The role of these devices is still evolving.

SUGGESTED READINGS

Bird J, Cohen-Cole SA: Teaching psychiatry to non-psychiatrists: 1. The application of educational methodology. Gen Hosp Psychiatry 1983;5:247.

Bird J, Cohen-Cole SA: The three-function model of the medical interview: An educational device. In: Hall M (editor): *Models of Consultation-Liaison Psychiatry.* Kaizer AG, 1990.

Clark W: Effective interviewing and intervention for alcohol problems. In: Lipkin M Jr, Putnam SM, Lazare A (editors): *The Medical Interview: Clinical Care, Education, Research.* Springer-Verlag, 1995.

Csikszentmihalyi M: *Flow.* Harper, 1990.

Erickson MH: *Life Reframing in Hypnosis: The Seminars, Workshops, and Lectures of Milton H. Erickson,* Vol 2. Irvington, 1985.

Hogbin B, Fallowfield LJ: Getting it taped. Br J Hosp Med 1989;41:330.

Lazare A: The interview as negotiation. In: Lipkin M Jr, Putnam SM, Lazare A: *The Medical Interview: Clinical Care, Education, Research.* Springer-Verlag, 1995.

Lazare A, Putnam SM, Lipkin M Jr: Three functions of the medical interview. In: Lipkin M Jr, Putnam SM, Lazare A: *The Medical Interview: Clinical Care, Education, Research.* Springer-Verlag, 1995.

Lipkin M Jr: The medical interview. In: Branch WT Jr (editor): *Office Practice of Medicine,,* 2nd ed. Saunders, 1987.

Lipkin M Jr et al: Performing the interview. In: Lipkin M Jr, Putnam SM, Lazare A: *The Medical Interview: Clinical Care, Education, Research.* Springer-Verlag, 1995.

Mulrow DC et al: Case-finding instruments for depression in primary care settings. Ann Intern Med 1995;122:913.

Quill TE: Barriers to effective communication. In: Lipkin M Jr, Putnam SM, Lazare A: *The Medical Interview: Clinical Care, Education, Research.* Springer-Verlag, 1995.

Roter DL, Hall JA: Physicians' interviewing styles and medical information obtained from patients. J Gen Intern Med. 1987;2:325.

Roter D et al: Personal communication, 1996.

Spitzer Rl et al: Utility of a new procedure for diagnosing mental disorders in primary care: The PRIME-MD 1,000 study. JAMA 1994;272:1749.

Starfield B et al: The influence of patient-practitioner agreement on the outcome of care. Am J Public Health 1981;71:127.

Stoeckle JD: Patients and their lives: Psychosocial and behavioral aspects. In: Lipkin M Jr, Putnam SM, Lazare A: *The Medical Interview: Clinical Care, Education, Research.* Springer-Verlag, 1995.

2

Empathy

Barry Egener, MD

INTRODUCTION

The concept of empathy dates from the early years of this century, when discussions of the topic were restricted to psychotherapists' analyses of their interactions with patients. More recently, the concept has received renewed attention from a wide spectrum of health practitioners and educators. They believe that empathy can positively affect communication with patients and thus lead to improved therapeutic outcomes. Many of the lay public regard empathy as an avenue to the restoration of compassion and humanism to a doctor-patient relationship that has been corrupted by cold technology. Studies, in fact, have shown that patients are more satisfied when their physicians attend to their emotional needs.

Why such grand expectations of empathy? The answer lies in its definition as an intellectual identification with, or vicarious experiencing of, the feelings, thoughts, or attitudes of another. Thus empathy allows the physician and patient to escape the constraints of their respective roles and be simply two humans sharing the patient's experience of illness. Illness is more than the accumulated symptoms of disease—it includes the disruption of normal healthy relationships with family, friends, community, and work as well as the psychologic reactions to those disruptions. The patient yearns for the healer to incorporate an understanding of those ramifications of disease into a prescription for health. Empathy alone does not mandate a biopsychosocial approach; but once the patient's perspective is glimpsed, the physician finds focusing solely on disease mechanisms to be inadequate.

Some have described empathy as a momentary identification with the patient in which the doctor's human capacity to feel what another feels erodes the boundaries of self. If the interviewer in fact temporarily loses awareness of self, the process might better be termed "sympathy," or "feeling with" the patient. Empathy has also been described as being cognitively aware of this process of emotional identification; such cognitive self-awareness prevents total dissolution of ego boundaries.

The question arises as to whether empathy can be taught. Research suggests that it can, and certainly doctors can learn to pay more attention to their patients' emotions. There are numerous barriers to discussing emotions with patients, from the impersonal office setting to the disinclination of both physician and patient to address particularly sensitive topics. Nonetheless, appropriate skilled communication can break through these barriers.

OVERCOMING BARRIERS TO EMPATHY

Understanding the feelings, attitudes, and experience of the patient is the first step toward a more potent therapeutic alliance. Many patients, however, may not be skilled in revealing their feelings to their providers. They need to be led to an awareness that their doctor is interested in their feelings, values them, and that feelings are a legitimate topic for discussion in a medical interview.

Emotions can be difficult for both doctors and patients (Table 2–1), and the doctor particularly may prefer the certainty of science. From the patient's point of view, if difficult emotional issues are transformed into a somatic complaint, denial might be the first reaction to a psychologic interpretation of his symptoms. The physician must appreciate and mirror the terms in which a patient will speak about illness. In many cultures, emotions are simply not discussed. In the United States, where the biomedical model of disease still predominates over the biopsychosocial model, patients may feel that it is more acceptable to have physical rather than emotional complaints. Because this expectation is often reinforced by their physicians, it behooves the physician to establish a climate conducive to the expression of emotional material and a language useful to that end. Some of the

Table 2–1. Barriers to discussing emotions.

Doctor
Takes too much time
Is too draining
Will lose control of interview
Can't fix patient's distress
Not my job
Managed care is not conducive

Patient
Cultural taboo about discussing emotions
Preference for a physical rather than an emotional source for the problem
Somatization disorder
Desire to meet doctor's expectations
Worry about being emotionally overwhelmed
Fear of the physician or of being seriously ill

barriers physicians raise to having a discussion about emotions with patients follow.

1. It takes too much time. In a busy practice, concerns about time are legitimate. Given an organized framework, however, it takes only a few minutes to deal effectively with emotion, and the strategies discussed later in this chapter can prove time-efficient for the physician. In fact, it may be far more time-consuming to deal with the indirect effects of unaddressed emotions during the rest of the interview. To this end, it may be useful to distinguish between "acute efficiency" and "chronic efficiency." "Efficiency" should take into consideration not only the duration of a particular visit, but the total amount of time required to address the patient's concerns. Even if it takes a few extra minutes to address emotions, that time is more than compensated for by fewer phone calls and unscheduled visits.

2. It's too draining. It is unrealistic to expect all providers to be emotionally available at all times to all their patients. A physician who has been awake all night or is emotionally needy herself may be justified in putting off a discussion of emotions that should otherwise occur. If the physician chooses to defer, it would be wise to return to the topic at another time. Primary care providers sometimes exert a tremendous amount of energy avoiding emotions in the belief that dealing directly with them will be draining. To the contrary, it can be far more efficient to make an emotional connection, since so much energy goes into resisting it.

In addition, patients may inadvertently raise issues that are emotionally difficult for their providers. Sometimes the difficulty can be discussed with friends, family, or colleagues; at other times it may be most fruitfully addressed in the physician's own therapy. (A longer discussion of this area is beyond the scope of this chapter, but difficult encounters with patients offer physicians an opportunity for personal growth; see Chapter 4.)

3. The interview will get out of control. Although many doctors worry that addressing emotions will cause feelings to escalate, the opposite is often true: Naming emotions helps diffuse them. Learning a language to handle emotions creates a comfortable distance from the emotions themselves, so that neither the doctor nor the patient becomes overwhelmed.

4. I can't fix it for the patient. Primary care providers are used to "fixing" things. Feelings, however, simply exist—and can't be "fixed." Patients do not expect that their feelings will be eliminated; they just want them to be understood.

5. It's not my job. Some doctors feel it's their job to address disease and the psychotherapist's job to address mental illness. There are several problems with this attitude. Although it is certainly true that collaboration with mental health practitioners may at times be useful, about 65% of mental illnesses are cared for exclusively by primary care physicians. About 26% of primary care patients have mental health diagnoses, and even a higher percentage have important psychiatric comorbidities. Physicians who insist on interpreting the physical symptoms of psychiatric disease such as panic disorder or depression in purely biomedical terms miss the point—and their patients will not get better. Telling a patient who develops chest pain on the anniversary of his father's death (see "Therapeutic Language of Empathy") that there is nothing wrong with him will help the patient only briefly. Moreover, many physical illnesses have psychosocial sequelae that must also be addressed.

When a patient keeps returning with the same complaint, unimproved by a physician's interventions, the patient is trying to communicate a message. Physicians are often frustrated by these patients; this frustration can be relieved and doctor satisfaction markedly improved by the progress that comes with addressing the underlying problem.

6. I can't be empathic in a managed-care setting. The national movement toward more tightly managed health care delivery systems presents special challenges to the doctor-patient relationship. There is an inherent conflict of interest introduced when the physician has to balance the patient's needs against the financial resources of the plan (or against the physician's income under some arrangements). One can see that the consequent erosion of trust may jeopardize the kind of empathic relationship that this chapter advocates (see Chapter 7).

At a time when patients and physicians are feeling distanced by the interposition of managed care, empathic skills can help preserve trust. Both doctor and patient may resent having their health care choices constrained by a third party. But if physicians also feel obligated to represent the insurer's position to the patient, they are likely to act defensively if the patient attacks the arrangement. Acknowledging and supporting the patient's feelings offers an alternative that makes the physician a partner again and removes an unwanted burden. This does not, however, compromise the physicians' other roles of that may place them in conflict with the patient (see "The Therapeutic Language of Empathy," "Legitimization").

Another relevant effect of managed care is the pressure for doctors to see more patients in less time. Predictably, physicians are reluctant to enter into discussions with patients that have the potential to destroy their schedules. As mentioned earlier, however, a little energy invested—at a time chosen by the physician—can prevent emotional material from resurfacing at an inconvenient time. Efficient and clear doctor-patient communication (as described in this chapter) can maintain the connection between patient and doctor despite the constraints imposed by the managed-care environment.

THE ROLE OF EMPATHY IN DIAGNOSIS

Feelings that arise in the provider during an encounter may be useful in forming a diagnostic hypothesis about the patient. For example, if during an interview a doctor becomes aware of feeling burdened, heavy, or "down," she might consider the possibility that the patient is depressed.

All clinicians have had the experience of trying to help a patient with a behavior change, such as weight loss, only to have each suggestion rejected by the patient: "I've already tried that, Doc; it doesn't work." The physician's own feelings of frustration and powerlessness in trying to motivate the patient are often mirrored by the patient's sense of frustration and powerlessness in attempting to accomplish the behavior change. Confirming the hypothesis that the patient is frustrated is accomplished, just like any other diagnosis, by testing: "I'm feeling frustrated with this problem, and I'm wondering if you're feeling the same way."

Some patients consistently elicit dislike and rejection from their providers. It may seem to the provider that the patient is intentionally trying to manipulate her into becoming angry with him. This may in fact be true. When the provider becomes aware of these feelings, she should consider the possibility that her own impulses to punish the patient may be playing into the patient's self-image as deserving of punishment. This pattern may be consistent with a borderline personality disorder (see Chapter 25).

The physician's experience does not invariably reflect the patient's experience. Rather, the physician should notice his feelings and ask, "Does the way I feel tell me something about the patient or something about myself?" For example, if the physician has recently seen a number of drug-seeking patients and begins to feel angry and defensive on noticing that the nurse has recorded "low back pain" as the next patient's chief complaint, these feelings say a lot about his recent experiences and nothing about the next patient. Feelings are primary data about the person in whom they arise and indirect data about others. The next section clarifies how to test the hypothesis that a patient is feeling a particular emotion and outlines how to respond.

The Therapeutic Language of Empathy

Although empathy is not generally considered a therapeutic tool, discussion of emotional issues can be therapeutic. An empathic relationship is crucial in psychotherapy and enhances the power of all therapeutic relationships. The following sections show how to talk about emotions using specific skills. A premise of this discussion is that biomedical aspects of disease cannot be effectively addressed without considering their emotional consequences. Emotions, whether related to physiologic dysfunction or psychosocial issues, color the discussion in the examining room and may be so distracting that the patient cannot fully concentrate on other issues until the emotions are addressed.

A clinical scenario helps to illustrate the usefulness of the emotion-handling skills described here.

Case illustration 1: A 35-year-old man presents with a 2-week history of sharp substernal chest pain that occurs at rest, when working in the yard and while trying to fall asleep at night. He does not smoke but has a positive family history of heart disease. On examination he appears anxious, he has borderline blood pressure, and he is 5% over ideal body weight. The rest of his examination, lab tests, ECG, and chest x-ray are normal, except for his cholesterol, which is 210 mg/dL.

The doctor reenters the room to review the data.

PATIENT: Well, Doctor, what did you find?

DOCTOR: Only some minor abnormalities. I think you need to lose a little weight and perhaps change your diet slightly.

PATIENT: Is the pain coming from my heart?

DOCTOR: I don't think so.

PATIENT: But you're not sure?

DOCTOR: Nothing in medicine is certain, but your age, the character of your pains, and the fact that antacids help somewhat reassure me that the problem is most likely acid indigestion or muscular pain.

PATIENT: Don't you think we should do more tests to be sure?

DOCTOR: With your managed care policy, we need to be very careful about doing unnecessary tests. I think you should resume your normal activities. I'll see you in a month, and we'll see if there's been any change.

PATIENT: I'm still worried.

DOCTOR: Don't be. You'll be all right.

PATIENT: Well, okay, if you say so.

Comment: Despite a probably accurate diagnosis of noncardiac chest pain, giving good information, and attempts to reassure the patient, something goes awry in this interaction. The patient still doesn't seem satisfied. Let's look at the effect empathic skills might have.

The techniques discussed in the following sections are adapted from a three-function model of the medical interview developed by Bird and Cole. The goals of the interview are described as gathering medical data, building a relationship with the patient, and educating and motivating the patient. (see Chapter 1) The following emotion-handling skills are related to the second function, building relationships with patients (Table 2–2).

Reflection: This refers to naming the emotion the doctor sees and reflecting it back to the patient. Reflection communicates the physician's understanding of the patient's experience. It also has the effect of making the feelings behind the patient's behavior or words explicit, where they can be dealt with directly.

For example, when a patient greets a doctor who is 20 minutes late with, "My time is as valuable as yours," the doctor might say, "I'm sorry I'm late. You seem pretty angry with me." The patient might then ventilate about the doctor's lateness or his treatment at the hands of doctors. He might even deny his anger, since many patients might view the expression of anger at their physicians as unacceptable. In any case, the doctor has a chance to deal with the emotion directly and then proceed with the interview, rather than trying to work with a patient who is angry and has not had a chance to express his anger.

After reflecting an emotion, the doctor should stop talking and see how the patient responds. Although the patient will usually elaborate, if the physician keeps talking, the exploration may be prematurely ended.

Sometimes it is clear that a patient is feeling a strong emotion, but it is not clear what that emotion is. It is perfectly acceptable (and perhaps preferable) to treat the emotion as having a differential diagnosis and test out a hypothesis as one would for any other medical entity: "I'm wondering if you're upset," or, more tentatively, "It seems that you're feeling something strongly, but I'm not sure what it is. Can you help me out?"

Table 2–2. The empathic skills.

Skill	Example
Reflection	*You seem upset.*
Legitimization	*I can understand your anger with the callous way you were treated.*
Support	*You're doing very well handling your grief.*
Partnership	*Perhaps we can work together to make you feel better.*
Respect	*Obviously you have tremendous compassion for your siblings.*

Legitimization or Validation: This skill informs the patient that you understand the reason for the emotion. This has the effect of normalizing the emotion and making the patient feel less isolated. For example, to a somatizing patient who has been to several doctors who have been unable to find a cause for her abdominal pain, you might say, "I can understand how frustrating it's been, to be no better after seeking so much help." Some physicians are reluctant to validate emotions in difficult patients for fear of adding fuel to the fire. But you don't have to agree with patients to express understanding of their feelings. For example, to a patient with chronic low back pain who has responded angrily to your informing him that you will not prescribe narcotics, you might say, "Even though I see it differently, I can understand why you would be angry with me." Such a statement allows you to support the patient while disagreeing with him and enhances your chances of continuing a therapeutic relationship. Validation of feelings emphasizes that the patient and doctor are equals in the human condition, although they have different roles in the therapeutic relationship.

Support: An expression of support tells patients that the physician cares about them and is willing to be present to their emotion. The expression can be verbal or nonverbal. Examples of nonverbal expression are handing the tearful patient a tissue or touching the patient. In judging whether touching a patient will be perceived as supportive, invasive, or inappropriate, the physician should consider such factors as culture, age, gender, sexual orientation, previous experience of abuse, and the presence or absence of psychiatric symptoms, such as paranoia. In general, putting a hand on the patient's hand or arm will not be misinterpreted. Many physicians prefer to take the lead from the patient by matching the patient's nonverbal behavior.

Some verbal expressions of support are "It's pretty normal to get angry with children when they act out," and "A spouse's death is one of the most difficult life transitions." Again, these responses are not an attempt to suppress, eliminate, or fix the emotion, but rather an offer to help patients, to reassure them that they are not alone with an uncomfortable emotion. These three skills—reflection, legitimization, and support—are the most important of the emotion-handling skills and will be involved in most of the work physicians do in this area.

Partnership: Partnership implies a team approach, in which the patient and doctor work together toward the same goal. Doctors support and are partners with patients in many ways, but in the context of this chapter, the word *partnership* makes it explicit that you would like to help the patient with the troubling emotion. An advantage of partnership is that it may help motivate patients to take an active role in their improvement and may lay the foundation for a contract for behavior change. This is consistent with the notion, especially important when illness results from patient behaviors, that physicians facilitate the patient's healing rather than curing disease in the passive patient. The physician's use of the pronouns *we* and *us* to expresses partnership, as in "Perhaps we can make a plan to help you feel better," or "Let's figure out a way to help you deal with this difficult diagnosis."

Respect: This skill honors the emotional resources within a patient. The doctor might say "You've been through a lot," or "I'm impressed with how well you're holding up under the circumstances."

Sometimes it is not credible that the physician could know what it would be like to be the patient. The physician can acknowledge the patient's experience nonetheless: "I'm not a parent, so I can only imagine what it would be like to lose a child. I can see you're feeling the loss quite deeply." On a happier occasion, she might say "What a joy it must be for you to see your grandchild's birth!"

Although it often makes sense to use reflection or legitimization first when addressing emotion, these skills can be used in any order, and it may be best to go through the sequence several times at different points in an interview.

> *Case illustration 1 (Contd.):* Let us return now to the scenario of the 35-year-old man with chest pain to see how that interaction might be improved with a physician who uses empathic skills. The empathic skills used are listed to the right of the text.
>
> PATIENT: Well, what did you find?
>
> DOCTOR: Only some minor abnormalities that I don't think are significant.
>
> PATIENT: Then why do I have this pain?
>
> DOCTOR: You seem pretty anxious. (*reflection*)
>
> PATIENT: Wouldn't you be anxious if you thought you were working up to a heart attack?
>
> DOCTOR: I certainly would be. Are you worried you're going to have a heart attack? (*validation*)
>
> PATIENT: That's what happened to my father. He was raking leaves and just keeled over. I'm the one who found him.
>
> DOCTOR: That must have been horrible. (*support*)
>
> PATIENT: You can't imagine how awful it was. Every time I think of it I get upset. Sometimes it even brings on this chest pain. I've been thinking about him more and more lately, especially when I go to sleep at night. It makes me afraid to fall asleep. I'm afraid I'm not going to wake up.
>
> DOCTOR: Is there a reason why you've been thinking about him more lately?
>
> PATIENT: Yeah. I thought I got over his death. But this is the time of year he died. Just raking leaves, which I do every weekend, makes me think of him. Then I get this chest pain and worry about myself. Heart disease runs in families, I don't have to tell you.

> DOCTOR: I'm sorry about your father. It sounds as though there's a pretty strong connection between thinking about your father and the chest pain. (*support*)
>
> PATIENT: Yeah. I thought maybe being upset stressed my heart. Do you think maybe this is all in my head?
>
> DOCTOR: I'm sure you really feel the pain, and I suspect your heart still aches for your father—even if only figuratively. It's pretty hard to lose a father. Now, you know there's a pretty strong connection between the body and the mind, and if you've been worrying about your own health, this could be your way of making sure you take care of yourself. (*respect*)
>
> PATIENT: I never thought of it that way. What you say makes a lot of sense, and I think you're probably right. But I still have this nagging worry in the back of my mind.
>
> DOCTOR: That's understandable. How about this?
>
> (*legitimization*) Let's work together to reduce whatever risk factors you do have for heart disease to make sure you don't have a problem down the line.
>
> (*partnership*) Let me see you again in a month so we can check you over physically to make sure everything's still okay. Right now you're having some pretty strong feelings about your father, and I think that may be the source of your chest pain. See what happens in the next few weeks; if you're still having problems next month, we can talk some more about it.
>
> PATIENT: That seems reasonable to me. I appreciate your listening to me.
>
> DOCTOR: Okay, then, I'll see you next month. And if you have severe chest pains, call me immediately; don't wait till the next day.
>
> PATIENT: Thanks, Doc. See you next month.

Comment: Patient satisfaction, as indicated by the patient's responses toward the end of the interview, seems much greater than in the first scenario. Although this scenario is longer than the first, using empathic skills added only approximately one minute to the interview, and if that additional minute prevents unnecessary visits by allaying the patient's concerns, the time is well spent. Early in the interview, the doctor does very little talking, and what he does say primarily addresses the patient's charged emotional state. He initially resists the patient's invitation to confirm conclusively that this is all in his head and instead allows the patient to continue to explore his feeling state. There is uncertainty at the end of the medical interview, but it seems to be an uncertainty that both the doctor and patient can accept comfortably, with a sense of partnership.

IMPLICATIONS FOR PROFESSIONAL DEVELOPMENT

Suppose the content of what the patient reveals is upsetting, distasteful, or even abhorrent to the physician. Suppose in the previous example of the patient with chest pain that the doctor's mother has just died and his father is scheduled for triple-bypass surgery; the mere contemplation of losing his father is so threatening that the physician withdraws into himself. Psychologic defense mechanisms may cause the physician to become distracted from the patient's visit and think about his own concerns.

Suppose, on the other hand, that the patient describes a situation that is emotionally charged, but so alien to the physician's experience that he cannot empathize. If, for example, a homosexual patient reveals that his partner has become HIV-positive, the heterosexual physician may pity (feel sorry *for*) the patient but be unable to relate to his grief and fears. On the other hand, the physician may be so repelled by the concept of homosexuality that his body language betrays his rejection of the patient. The patient, feeling judged and embarrassed, is likely to withhold relevant information. Or suppose the physician must present to a patient indicated treatments that he considers disgusting or repulsive. Her own obvious feeling may influence the patient so that he cannot make a truly informed decision.

Finding just the right therapeutic stance is essential; it may be partly intuitive and partly learned, and it may vary from patient to patient—or even with the same patient over time—depending on the patient's needs. Opportunities may be lost when the physician is unable to empathize with the patient, or when the loss of ego boundaries makes a therapeutic stance impossible. The most effective physicians are those whose repertoire permits a rapid interplay of objectivity and emotion.

Empathy in Medical Training

Viewing empathy in this way may have special applications to medical training. It is remarkable how the fresh enthusiasm and caring of medical students can quickly devolve into the wry cynicism of residents. What accounts for this withdrawal? The usual explanation is that insulating oneself in this way is an act of self-preservation in the face of overwhelming demands. It can be torturous to feel another's pain, and if the self is already marginally maintained because of long hours and the other exigencies of training, it may be more difficult to sustain an open posture.

The ways in which doctors withdraw depend on both their personalities and their environment. Especially if the culture around the resident tolerates derogatory labels for patients, it can be easy to see patients as *other,* as not sharing some element of humanity with *us.* Even if such labels are not tolerated and caring for patients is a highly preserved value, dark humor may surface as a means of insulation. In order to take care of others, one must first take care of oneself. Finding the right balance is a major develop-

mental task of the health-care professions. Perhaps by attending to the well-being of trainees, we will make them better doctors (see Chapter 8). Training programs can demonstrate that caring for others is valuable. Experienced physicians can attend to trainees' growth, help them develop effective and healthy working styles, model those styles, and draw attention to the importance of being aware of one's own development. There is a huge contrast between the concept of residency training as nurturing or mentoring and the concept of residency as "trial by fire." And fire, we know, steels metal, making it harder.

Empathy in the Practice of Medicine

What happens after training? For some practitioners, the pressure becomes less, healthy coping styles develop, and the caring physician reemerges. Far too many, however, are casualties of the training process—or their families are. Gabbard and Menninger have observed that physicians' compulsive personality styles are susceptible to a pattern of delayed gratification. Constantly nurturing others, physicians may have no time left for themselves. Family relationships may atrophy. The most effective physicians may be those who attend to their own needs as well as those of their patients, who understand their own unique struggles, so that these struggles—by making physicians aware of their own humanity—can enhance, rather than detract from, their relationships with patients.

Since the culture of an institution strongly influences the practice of medicine within its purview, physicians who practice together have a unique opportunity to enhance each other's empathic skills. Patient-care conferences can incorporate psychosocial issues into the discussions of difficult cases. When a physician notices a certain type of patient who is uniquely challenging, discussions with colleagues may provide useful suggestions about strategies for success in treating that patient. Videotaped interviews with difficult patients are a powerful tool that allows physicians to examine their own contributions to the difficulty of such interactions.

Regular videotaped conferences, in which physicians take turns presenting cases, allow physicians to feel at ease in front of the camera, demonstrate collaboration and mutual support, and reinforce the importance and value of empathy to the group. Balint groups or other types of support groups, which may include nonphysician office staff, can help health practitioners cope with collegial interactions or family relationships that have become stressed by practice. Such groups also show that a psychosocial perspective can benefit both physicians and their patients.

Understanding the interaction between illness and emotion helps us become more effective physicians. Familiarity and practice with the skills in this chapter can make us more comfortable discussing this interaction with our patients. Becoming aware of our own personal response to patients promotes personal growth as well. The emotional demands of the medical profession can be enriching or impoverishing.

Using skills of empathy we may become more satisfied and effective clinicians; our patients may become more satisfied and healthier.

SUGGESTED READINGS

Brothers L: Biological perspective on empathy. Am J Psychiatry 1989;146:10.

Cohen-Cole S, Bird J: Building rapport and responding to the patient's emotions (relationship skills). In Cohen-Cole S: *The Medical Interview: The Three Function Approach.* Mosby Year Book, 1991.

Gabbard G, Menninger R: The psychology of postponement in the medical marriage. JAMA 1989;261:2378.

Jordan JV: Empathy and self boundaries. In *A Developmental Perspective.* Wellesley College, No. 16, 1984.

Mengel M, Mauksch L: Disarming the family ghost: A family of origin experience. Fam Med 1989;21:45.

Spiro H: What is empathy and can it be taught? An Intern Med 1992;116:843.

Wilmer HA: The doctor-patient relationship and the issues of pity, sympathy, and empathy. Br J Med Psychol 1968;41:243.

Zinn W: The empathic physician. Arch Intern Med 1993;153:306.

Giving Bad News

3

Geoffrey H. Gordon, MD

INTRODUCTION

A debilitating or terminal illness, a catastrophic injury, death—these are situations both patients and physicians face, and they are all situations in which the physician must break the news to patients, partners, and family members. The following sections of this chapter use a diagnosis of cancer to illustrate some general principles that can help physicians in this task. Despite these suggestions, however, there is no one right—or easy—way to present bad news.

Most physicians now inform cancer patients of their diagnosis. This trend to near-universal disclosure is the result, in part, of greater public awareness of advances in cancer diagnosis and treatment, greater patient autonomy and self-determination, and greater physician collaboration with patients to decrease their isolation and fear and to mobilize their resources and coping skills. Self-report surveys of cancer patients since 1950 suggest that physicians have always underestimated patients' desires to know their cancer diagnosis and prognosis.

One might expect that the content of the bad news is overwhelmingly more important than the process with which it is delivered. This does not appear to be the case. Patients usually have vivid recall of the physician's manner and style but need repeated explanations of the facts. For example, the way that parents are told that their child has a developmental disability or mental retardation affects the emotional state and attitudes of both child and parents. These parents can distinguish the message from the messenger, and one-third to one-half are dissatisfied with how they were given the news.

TECHNIQUES FOR GIVING BAD NEWS

A systematic approach to giving bad news (Table 3–1) can make the process more predictable and less emotionally draining for the physician. The process of giving bad news can be divided into six categories: preparation, setting, delivering the news, offering emotional support, providing information, and closing the interview.

Terminal or Catastrophic Illness
Preparation: When cancer is a strong diagnostic possibility, consider discussing it with the patient early in the work-up:

> DOCTOR: That shadow on your x-ray worries me. It could be an old scar, a patch of pneumonia, or even a cancer. I think we should do some more tests to find out exactly what it is. That way, we'll be able to plan the best treatment.

Plan ahead with the patient about how he or she would like to receive the news:

> DOCTOR: Whatever the biopsy shows, I'll want to explain it carefully—is there someone you'd like to have with you when I go over this?

Knowledge of the patient's prior reactions to bad news can be useful—but not necessarily predictive of the patient's response. Ideally, primary and specialist physicians should decide in advance who will give bad news and arrange follow-up.

Setting: Although it is always best to give bad news in person, if the patient is unable to come to the office and asks for the diagnosis over the phone, it is best not to lie. Instead, begin a dialogue that provides basic information:

> DOCTOR: The biopsy showed a type of lung cancer.

The dialogue should conclude with a request to come to the office soon for further discussion:

> DOCTOR: As soon as you can come in, I'll be able to tell you more about what we need to do next.

Always take responsibility for delivering bad news yourself. Find a private place to talk with patients.

Table 3–1. Techniques for giving bad news.

Category	Technique
Preparation	Forecast possibility of bad news. Clarify who should attend the bad news visit. Clarify who should give the bad news.
Setting	Give bad news in person. Give bad news in private. Sit down and make eye contact.
Delivery	Identify what the patient already knows. Give the news clearly and unambiguously. Identify important feelings and concerns.
Emotional Support	Remain with the patient and listen. Use empathic statements. Invite further dialogue.
Information	Use simple, clear words and concepts. Summarize and check patient's understanding. Use handouts and other resources.
Closure	Make a plan for the immediate future. Ask about immediate needs. Schedule a follow-up appointment.

Patients in examination gowns should have the opportunity to dress before receiving bad news. Sit down at eye level and give them your full attention and concern.

Delivering the News: The next step is test the patient's readiness to hear the news. Review the workup to date:

> DOCTOR: You know we saw that shadow on your chest x-ray. When we did the CT scan of your chest, we saw a mass in your lung, and then we looked down your windpipe and took a small sample of your lung. We have the results of that biopsy now.

Remember that most patients will have consulted an informal health advisor (a family member, book, or neighbor) at some point during the illness and will have already developed an "illness model" or "cognitive map" of what is wrong, what it means, and what can be done. It is useful to elicit this model because the clinician can correct the patient's misconceptions and also put the explanations into a context with which the patient is already familiar. To elicit the model, ask about the patient's understanding and concerns:

> DOCTOR: What do you already know about this? What concerns you the most about it?

Allow for silence during the conversation, especially as emotions set in. Avoid lecturing about the disease, workup, and treatment. While detailed information is familiar territory for physicians and helps reduce their own anxiety, it is rarely helpful for patients who are hearing bad news for the first time.

Some patients will immediately ask if the diagnosis is cancer and want to be told promptly and directly. Others will tell the physician, verbally or nonverbally, to go more slowly. There are at least two ways to slow down the message: To grade the exposure and to present the hopeful news first.

1. Grade the exposure. Begin with an introductory phrase that prepares the patient for the bad news:

> DOCTOR: I'm afraid I have bad news for you. . . . This is more serious than we thought. . . . There were some cancer cells in the biopsy.

The main challenge with this approach is to finish with a clear, unambiguous statement that the patient has cancer.

2. Present the hopeful message first. This technique is based on the fact that patients remember little of what they are told after the bad news is given:

> DOCTOR: Whatever I tell you in a moment, I want you to remember that the situation is serious, but there's plenty we can do. It's important that we work closely together over the next several months. I'm sorry, but your tests were positive for a type of lung cancer.

Once the news sinks in, the patient will typically react with a mixture of emotions, concerns, and requests for information and guidance. Spend a few moments on feelings and concerns before giving more information, or patients may be unable to hear and assimilate it. Explore the origins of these feelings and concerns, because they may arise from misconceptions based on experiences with friends or family.

Offering Emotional Support: Getting bad news is primarily an emotional rather than a cognitive event. Common, immediate emotional reactions are fear, anger, grief, and shock or emotional numbness. An important challenge for many providers is to remain present with patients having strong emotional reactions and to tolerate their distress. There are no magic words or right thing to say. Sit near the patient and use empathic statements:

> DOCTOR: I can see this is a terrible blow for you. I can't imagine what it must be like. I want you to know that I'll continue to be your doctor and work with you on this.

Many patients find a touch on the hand or shoulder to be supportive and reassuring. It is also helpful to ask unaccompanied patients if there is anyone who should be called after they receive the news.

Some patients direct anger at the physician:

> PATIENT: You'd better check again—you doctors are always making mistakes!

or

> PATIENT: I've always come in for check-ups; why didn't you find this sooner?

Rather than becoming defensive, the physician should acknowledge that many people in this situation feel cheated and angry. It is important to emphasize that the disease, not the doctor, is the enemy and that doctor and patient must work together to fight it.

Patients who are very businesslike or too stunned to communicate their feelings are hard to evaluate because the degree of distress is not always obvious. They may express their grief alone or want to be with others, such as a friend or minister, before sharing their feelings with a doctor. The physician can acknowledge the difficult nature of the news and legitimize future expression of feelings:

> DOCTOR: I know this is hard to believe. You may have some feelings about it later that you'd like to talk with me about—I'm always ready to listen.

Providing Information: Patients often want to know whether they really have cancer, if it has spread, if it is treatable or curable, and what treatment will involve. Some patients also want to know whether they are going to die and, if so, how much time they have left. Even with careful explanations, many patients are unable to assimilate much information at the time the bad news is given. Effective educational strategies include using simple, clear words; providing information in small, digestible chunks; summarizing and checking the patient's understanding of what has been said; and using handouts or other resources. Questions should be answered directly and honestly:

> DOCTOR: There are statistics on how long people with this condition are likely to live, and I can share them with you, but they are just averages. No one can say for sure how long you will live.

Closing the Interview: Most patients, even when initially distraught, compose themselves quickly with support and direction. The most effective way to reach closure is to provide a plan for the immediate future. This includes asking patients who else needs to know the news and if they want help sharing it. It is important to reassure patients that the physician will still be their doctor even though they will need to see consultants and have further testing. A follow-up appointment should be scheduled within the next several weeks, and patients should be asked to write down questions and concerns that they or their families have between visits. Ask about immediate problems such as anxiety, depression, or insomnia. While some physicians like to prescribe a short course of medication for sleeplessness or anxiety, patients should also be told that it is normal to feel upset or to have trouble sleeping after receiving bad news.

Death

Some additional considerations apply when notifying family members of the death of a loved one (see Chapter 35). Unexpected or traumatic deaths are often the most difficult because survivors are unprepared and rarely have a prior relationship with the notifying physician. Physicians should begin by identifying themselves and their role in the deceased's care. Survivors who must be reached by telephone should be told to come to the hospital prior to the actual death notification, unless they specifically ask about death.

Once given the news, survivors may want to view the body. This is an important part of the grieving process and should not be discouraged. Survivors are often concerned about whether their loved one suffered or was alone at the time of death and whether they could have done anything to prevent it. They can often be told truthfully that the patient was unconscious prior to death, there was no evidence of suffering, and that maximal efforts were made to help. People also may need to be reassured that none of their actions hastened the patient's death.

Depending on the cause of death and comorbid conditions, the deceased may be a candidate for organ donation. Although some families object, many others find comfort in making an anatomic gift. Many states inquire about and record anatomic donor permission on drivers' licenses, and families may discover that the deceased did, in fact, give such consent. Permission for autopsy can also be requested at this time. Once the notifying physician has brought up these topics, many hospitals have specially trained staff to work further with families. Some hospitals and physicians routinely send sympathy cards or make follow-up calls to recently bereaved survivors.

PROBLEM AREAS

Acceptance
Don't Tell Me if It's Cancer: Some patients specifically request not to be told that they have cancer. The physician should ask these patients what bad news would mean to them, or what they are afraid might happen if they were given bad news.

When patients ask not to be given bad news, it is important to explain the rationale for their knowing the diagnosis:

> DOCTOR: Your job is to create the best environment for our medicines and treatments to work. This includes working with us to plan your treatment, finding which parts of you are healthy and strong, and which areas still need some work. Your attitude and interest are important parts of your treatment; they may help you feel better, and in some cases, the treatment may work better. We want you to ask questions about what is happening—remember that there are no stupid questions. If it would help you to talk with someone who has been through this, please let me know.

Don't Tell Him or Her It's Cancer: Family members may ask that patients not be told the diagnosis of cancer. Families should be thanked for their concern and reassured that information will not be forced on the patient. They should also be told that patients' questions will be answered truthfully. Explain the rationale for patients' knowing the diagnosis, and help families find ways to provide emotional support. Some families will find this difficult because of prior experiences with bad news. Consider eliciting the family's concerns about what might happen if the patient knows. It may help to approach patients with the dilemma:

> DOCTOR: Your family has told me that you'd prefer not to be informed about some important aspects of your care—what are your thoughts about this?

Such an approach can facilitate further discussion with the patient and family.

I Don't Believe It's Cancer: Some patients are unable to accept the diagnosis, offering such statements as "I just know it isn't cancer. If I can get some rest I'll be fine." This is most frustrating when it delays the early implementation of potentially curative treatment. Physicians often use logical arguments and dire predictions to persuade patients to agree to workup and treatment. Paradoxically, this approach makes many patients more resistant. Instead, the physician should try to depict denial as a sometimes useful, but currently maladaptive, way of coping. This can be done by explaining that patients are often of two minds:

> DOCTOR: Many patients find this kind of diagnosis hard to believe. I can see that part of you wants to look on the bright side and stay hopeful, but I wonder if you don't also have times when you realize that problems might arise. Let's think about how to proceed if the diagnosis is more serious.

The physician should offer to answer any future questions the patient might have and expect day-to-day variation in the patient's ability to acknowledge the accuracy of the diagnosis. Conversations should be documented in the patient's chart to notify others of the patient's reaction. Sometimes anticipating future needs helps patients accept the reality of the diagnosis:

> DOCTOR: Let's take a few minutes to think about your plans if your condition worsens. You may want to make decisions and plans now, in case you're unable to handle them in the future.

Different Cultural Values

Attitudes and beliefs about bad news, death, and the expression of grief are determined in part by cultural norms (see Chapter 13). For example, in some Asian cultural groups, bad news about health-related matters is routinely withheld from patients. In some Ethiopian cultural groups, the delivery of bad news to patients is a process that involves the whole family. There are also cultural differences in responding to death; such rituals surrounding patient death as opening windows and burning candles may be difficult to accommodate in an acute care setting. Cultural differences between physicians and patients and their families become problematic when they are not recognized as such and are attributed to patient or family uncooperativeness or psychopathology. Physicians who were born and raised in a cultural group with behavioral norms that differ from those in the system in which they are training or working may find such differences hard to reconcile and may experience role conflicts in caring for patients and families from their own culture. In this case, consultation with a colleague whose background is outside the subculture may lend some objectivity.

HOPE & REASSURANCE

Patients and families are fearful of losing hope. Unfortunately, many physicians have never learned how to offer hope and reassurance along with bad news. To physicians, hope and reassurance bring to mind cure, prolonged survival or, at the very least, tumor response. To patients and families, hope may initially mean cure but later can mean reconciliation with friends or family who have been estranged, or the opportunity to finish projects, find new sources of self-esteem, see a next birthday or family event, live without pain, or spend valuable time with loved ones.

There are several ways physicians can provide hope and reassurance at the time of bad news:

- Use positive words. Recognize the difference between the uncertain perception of "Your scan is negative" and the clarity of "The test showed your liver is normal and healthy."
- Encourage the patient to think of illness as a challenge. Most patients will have faced one or more severe challenges in their lives. Invoke their past successes in coping or mention those of other patients, saying, for example, "I'm always surprised at how well patients do. . . ."
- Work to improve patients' function and participation in their health care. Help them understand that their thoughts, attitudes, and activities affect how they feel, and stress the importance of learning to relax, identifying new sources of pleasure and self-esteem, and learning coping skills from other patients.
- Help patients learn how to face and deal with their illness realistically. Patients who focus exclusively on positive approaches may delay and inhibit their own grieving or feel guilty if they can't laugh or love their cancer away. These patients, and their families, may need permission to accept and grieve their losses. Other patients cope best by consis-

tently fighting the disease and maintaining a positive focus, in the face of all odds, to the very end.

THE HEALTH-CARE TEAM

Although the physician's role is to deliver the bad news, other health-care team members also play important roles.

Nurses can be present for the giving of bad news, interpret it if necessary, help patients verbalize their feelings and questions, and provide emotional support. Nurses are trained to evaluate patients' emotional and physical responses to treatment, their levels of comfort and activity, and their progress toward expected goals. Some nurses are also skilled at ensuring that treatment decisions are congruent with the overall direction and goals of care.

Social workers are skilled at identifying resources, enhancing coping skills, and working with patients' families. Chaplains can help in identifying and meeting patients' spiritual and emotional needs.

Nutritionists, physical therapists, and clinical pharmacists specializing in palliative care can also make important contributions to the management of seriously ill patients.

Occasionally patients and families will need referral for counseling or other mental health services. Indications for referral include prolonged or atypical grief, particularly when it interferes with daily activities or medical care; concern about a patient's suicide potential if given bad news; difficulty communicating within the family or with health-care providers; and assistance in maximizing coping skills. Mental health referrals are most successful when the referring physician explains the goals of the referral to the patient and tells the patient what to expect:

> DOCTOR: This physician may find ways in which you and I can work together more effectively. Dr. Pierce will talk to you and then call me to make a care plan.

It is important to ensure follow-up care:

> DOCTOR: I'd like you to make an appointment to see me after you've seen Dr. Pierce so we can make some plans together.

For a physician, checking in with one's own feelings is an invaluable skill. Dissociating from painful feelings protects physicians' psychological equilibrium and allows them to conduct the tasks of medical care objectively. Experiencing and expressing feelings that arise in the course of professional activities, however, are an important component of physician well-being. Patients nearly always sense what their physicians are feeling. They often value demonstrations of personal caring and express their appreciation: "I knew the doctor really cared about Jimmy when I saw tears in his eyes when he was talking to us." In some cases, physicians may need to identify and talk about their own grief with a trusted colleague before—and after—giving the bad news to the patient (see Chapter 8).

SUGGESTED READINGS

Brewin TB: Three ways of giving bad news. Lancet 1991;337:1207.
Buckman R: *How to Break Bad News: A Guide for Health Care Professionals.* Johns Hopkins University Press, 1992.
Butow PN et al: When the diagnosis is cancer: Patient communication experiences and preferences. Cancer 1996;77:2630.
Charlton RC: Breaking bad news. Med J Aust 1992; 157:615.
Creagan ET. How to break bad news—and not devastate the patient. Mayo Clin Proc 1994;69:1015.
Fallowfield L: Giving sad and bad news. Lancet 1993;341:476.
Girgis A, Sanson-Fisher RW: Breaking bad news: Consensus guidelines for medical practitioners. J Clin Oncol 1995;13:2449.

Krahn GL, Hallum A, Kime C: Are there good ways to give bad news? Pediatrics 1993;91:578.
Maguire P, Faulkner A: Communicate with cancer patients: Handling bad news and difficult questions. Br Med J 1988;41:330.
Muller JH, Desmond B: Ethical dilemmas in a cross-cultural context: A Chinese example. West J Med 1992;157:323.
Ptacek JT, Eberhardt TL: Breaking bad news: A review of the literature. JAMA 1996;276:496.
Quill TE, Townsend P: Bad news: Delivery, dialogue, dilemmas. Ann Intern Med 1991;151:463.
Tolle SW, Elliot DL, Girard DE. How to manage patient death and care for the bereaved. Postgrad Med 1985;78:87.

4

Difficult Patients

Howard B. Beckman, MD, FACP

INTRODUCTION

Whenever and wherever health professionals congregate, it doesn't take long for the topic of difficult patients to surface. Patients and families we experience as difficult increase the personal frustration of delivering care, decrease our satisfaction with work, and make it almost impossible to deliver the person-centered care that is at the heart of high-quality, satisfying, effective health care. Why, we ask, would someone choose to come to the office or hospital and harass, abuse, ignore, or lie to us?

Fortunately, most difficult interactions are both diagnosable and repairable. Aside from the unusual individual who is determined to be difficult, many problematic situations are created by unsatisfactory communication between provider and patient or by personal issues the provider unknowingly brings into these important interactions. These issues can include reminders of similar problems within the provider's own world or negative reactions to the patient's physical condition, sexual orientation, or personality.

Medical educators are increasingly finding that practitioners consider patients difficult based on their similarity to others, often family members, with whom they have had interpersonal problems. For example, a physician whose uncle used anger to control her may now have problems with older men who similarly express anger. Another common situation is the practitioner who becomes very angry with patients who don't stop smoking. Possibly the physician in this case had a close relative whom he could not convince to stop smoking and who, as a result, developed lung cancer. Separating one's own past experience from a patient's current behavior can moderate the physician's aversive response.

The key to dealing with such situations is to examine them with a critical eye and a more flexible style of communication that includes considerable room for negotiation. Greater self-awareness about their own feelings, experiences, and beliefs can help practitioners offer more nonjudgmental care to their patients. The case illustrations that follow focus on the situations practitioners most frequently find difficult and discuss specific approaches to these challenging patients and situations. Table 4–1 summarizes some general guidelines for working with difficult patients. Table 4–2 recommends techniques for approaching specific situations.

THE ANGRY PATIENT

Case illustration 1: When the doctor enters the room to see the fourth of the dozen patients scheduled for his Thursday morning session, his patient, Ms. B., a 35-year-old social worker, is sitting with arms crossed, refusing to make eye contact. The doctor greets the patient by asking, "Ms. B., how are you?" She responds, "I've been waiting 35 minutes! This is no way to run an office." The doctor, who is emotionally drained after spending the last 50 minutes working with a patient newly diagnosed with breast cancer, wonders why he's chosen medicine as a career.

Diagnosis

Even without this straightforward verbal response, an angry patient is not difficult to recognize. Harsh nonverbal communication such as stony silence, piercing stare, abrupt movements, a refusal to shake hands, gritting the teeth, and confrontational or occasionally abusive language provide unmistakable evidence. More subtle behaviors include the patient refusing to answer questions; failing to make eye contact; or constructing nonverbal barriers to communication such as crossed arms, turning away from the provider, or increasing the physical distance between them.

Table 4–1. General guidelines for working with difficult patients.

- Seek broader possibilities for the patient's emotion or problems.
- Respond directly to the patient's emotions.
- Solicit the patient's perspective on why there is a problem.
- Avoid being defensive.
- Seek to discover a common goal for the visit.

Differential Diagnosis: All too often, practitioners assume that the patient is angry with *them,* and, as a result, feel blamed for something they must have done or forgot to do. Although that is one possibility, other important reasons must be considered as the cause for anger. These include, but are not limited to the following (Table 4–3).

- Difficulty in getting to the office
- Problems with the office staff
- Anger directed toward the illness from which the person suffers
- Anger at the cost of health care
- Problems with consultants to whom the practitioner referred the patient
- Unanticipated problems from a procedure or medication recommended by the practitioner
- Previous unsupportive or condescending treatment by a physician
- Anger directed at family members' response—whether inadequate or overemotional—to the patient's illness

- Other significant news or problems unrelated to medical service, such as work- or family-related stress.

Psychological Mechanisms: Many patients view medical practitioners as "special" individuals who are supposed to be interested in the problems their patients experience. Patients expect to have their concerns investigated with compassion and interest. For many, this special relationship is among the safest they experience in their lives, and it is therefore quite common for patients to express emotions they would never consider revealing—let alone discussing—in other relationships. Any suggestion that the patients' concerns are not taken seriously or that they are not cared for—that the doctor sees them as an aggregation of symptoms—may diminish that feeling of safety and replace it with anger.

Patients have lofty expectations of medical practitioners. They expect timely service, relevant information about evaluations and treatments offered, and advice on how to cope with their illness. Interactions that fall short can result in feelings of humiliation and rejection that can quickly turn to anger.

From the provider's point of view, the patient's expression of anger may trigger feelings as diverse as somehow having failed the patient or of being treated disrespectfully. In either case, common response is are defensiveness, expressed as anger returned to the patient, withdrawal from the relationship, or defense of the behavior that the practitioner *assumes* prompted

Table 4–2. Tips for approaching difficult situations or patient behaviors.

Situation	Recommended Techniques
Angry patients	Elicit the patient's reason for being angry: *You seem angry; tell me more about it.* Empathize with the patient's experience: *I can understand why you would be angry.* Solicit the patient's perspective: *What can we do to improve the situation?* If appropriate, apologize: *I'm sorry you had to wait so long.*
Silent patients	Point out the problem: *You're being very quiet.* Elicit the patient's reason for silence: *Why are you being so quiet?* Explain the need for collaboration: *In order for me to help you, I really need you to talk to me more about your problem.* Respond to cues of hearing impairment or language barriers: *Are you having trouble hearing or understanding me?*
Demanding patients	Take a step back from the demand: *You seem adamant about the MRI. Why do you think it's so important?* Solicit the goal of the demand: *Is there a particular problem you think the MRI will help us diagnose?* Acknowledge emotions unexpressed at the time of the demand: *It must be very frustrating that your back still hurts.* Solicit the patient's perspective: *What do you think is causing your problem?* *In what way had you hoped I could help you?*

Table 4–3. Possible causes of patient anger.

Cause	Discussion
Difficulty in getting to the office	*Take a second and relax; the construction on Highway 6 is a nightmare. . . .*
Problems with the office staff	*What happened? How could our people have been more respectful?*
Anger directed toward the illness from which the person suffers	*It must seem unfair. . . .* *I can understand how angry this makes you. . . .*
Anger at the cost of health care	*Empathize, then brainstorm alternative approaches.*
Problems with consultants to whom the practitioner referred the patient	*What was the problem—from your point of view?* *I appreciate knowing this.*
Anger at being unable to see a specialist	*Negotiate: How about your seeing a specialist if my treatment plan doesn't relieve your symptoms in 2 weeks?*
Misdiagnosis or dismissive treatment from prior physician	*I see. I hope you'll let me know if I do anything like that!*
Unanticipated problems from a procedure or medication recommended by the practitioner	*This is disappointing. Let's see if we can get a better response. . . .*
Anger directed at family members' response—whether inadequate or overemotional—to the patient's illness	*Would you like me to explain the situation to your mother? She may not understand the problem.*
Other significant news or problems unrelated to medical service, such as work- or family-related stress	*Acknowledge appropriately.*

the anger. The problems are magnified if the expression of anger is problematic in the practitioner's own family. After recognizing the contributions of one's own experiences, openly encouraging and confronting a patient's feelings creates and honest and open relationship, defines the problem explicitly, and permits an accurate and timely response.

Management

In most situations involving anger, evaluation and understanding should also begin the therapeutic process. Responding calmly, without judgment or projection, with "You seem angry" tests whether the doctor has correctly identified the emotion. Failing to confront anger early keeps the interaction at a superficial level, informs the patient that the provider is impervious to or unsettled by emotion, and discourages any meaningful sharing of feelings. On the other hand, confronting anger is both efficient and medically appropriate.

Although many patients in this situation respond with, "You bet I'm angry," some patients deny their anger. Nonetheless, their body language or tone of voice betrays the emotion. In this case, the physician can address the denial: "Maybe 'angry' is too strong a word. It seems to me that you're upset by something; if you'd like to tell me about it, I might be able to help." The practitioner's invitation to explain offers the patient the chance to express his or her feelings, often leading to a discussion about the reasons for the patient's anger. As a result, the practitioner develops a more complete understanding of the causes and implications of the patient's experience of the health-care process. Armed with the patient's point of view and an accurate account of the patient's experience, the prac-

titioner and the patient can agree to focus on the problem. This point in the encounter is usually marked by a reduction in the patient's anger, relief on the part of the provider, and the re-creation of patient-doctor collaboration with the mutual goal of solving the identified problem. The subsequent management of the problem depends on the particular cause of the anger.

Case illustration 1 (Contd.): In response to the question, "Why are you angry?" Ms. B. responds, "The surgeon you sent me to wasn't prepared when I saw her and said that she hadn't received your letter. I had to take half a day off from work—which I could not afford—I drove 2 hours to get there, and all I did was waste my time. And now *you* keep me waiting when I'm due in court in an hour."

In response, the doctor apologizes, saying that the letter had been dictated but apparently not mailed in time and that the practice is purchasing a fax machine to allow more efficient communication. He also tells the patient that this morning's delay was unavoidable because of another patient's needs. Ms. B. feels better understood, accepts the apology, and ends by saying, "I hope this doesn't happen again; I have enough stress at work as it is." The doctor says, "I should have asked the receptionist to tell you that I was running late—I'm sorry about that. We're really trying hard to make sure that we communicate more effectively with our patients and our consultants." The total exchange takes 50 seconds—a time cost that is certainly worthwhile.

Patient Education

Sometimes, patients need to learn that it is not only permissible but important for them and their families to express their feelings. By encouraging the expression of anger, the practitioner helps identify unresolved conflicts that can interfere with the process of delivering appropriate care or can, if ignored, cause far more serious problems later. Encouraging patients and their families to express concerns or disappointments actually offers the practitioner the opportunity to become more efficient by removing significant barriers to effective, honest collaboration. The use of this approach by the office and nursing staff extends the environment in which patients feel respected, further increasing their willingness to share thoughts, concerns, and ideas.

Summary

Too often we assume that angry patients are simply angry with the practitioner. Sometimes this is so, but there is usually a much broader and more complex range of reasons for anger that must be explored prior to responding emotionally, offering an explanation, or creating a treatment plan. By working hard to avoid becoming defensive, practitioners can acknowledge and then constructively resolve the cause of the anger. Confronted with such a responsive approach, most angry people become quite satisfied and resume effective collaboration in their care.

THE SILENT PATIENT

> *Case illustration 2:* The doctor begins her afternoon office hours scheduled to see Mr. K., a 47-year-old man who has recently relocated to the area. On entering the room, the doctor is aware that Mr. K. fails to make eye contact and fiddles with a piece of paper folded over many times. In response to "Good afternoon; I'm Dr. W.," Mr. K. quietly says, "Good afternoon." When asked what problems he is having, Mr. K. answers, "I've been really tired." After waiting a few seconds, Dr. W. encourages the patient to speak by asking him to tell her more. The patient responds, "I don't know what to say."

Diagnosis

By definition, the silent patient offers little verbal interaction in the interview. In addition to the lack of communication, however, there are a number of important nonverbal cues that deserve attention. The patient may seem withdrawn, as indicated by sitting a greater distance from the physician than usual, failing to make eye contact, avoiding the physician's gaze, seeming distracted, or not acknowledging the physician's attempts at interaction. Alternatively, the patient may seem anxious, evidenced by nervous or repetitive habits such as nail-biting, pacing, or folding and refolding papers. Finally, the patient may seem sad with deep sighs, red eyes, or tears.

Differential Diagnosis: Based on the observation of the patient and the responses to questions, one might consider the following bases for the silence (Table 4–4):

- Anger
- Fear of the physician's authority

- Fear of serious disease causing the presenting problem
- Depression, dysthymia, or adjustment disorder with depressed mood
- Adverse affects of psychoactive medications
- Preoccupation with auditory or visual hallucinations
- Hearing impairment
- Passive personality
- Cultural or language barriers
- Forced by third party (rehabilitation program, court, spouse, nursing home) to be at the visit.

Psychological Mechanisms: In many families, individuals in positions of authority may demand "silence unless spoken to," a demand whose effects frequently carry over into other situations. This deference of silence may also be found in interactions in which a significant difference in gender or social class exists (whether real or perceived) or a previous history of mistreatment in medical cross-cultural encounters occurred.

When a patient has a serious or potentially life-threatening basis for concern, silence may indicate denial or serve as a protective behavior. For example, a patient can avoid confronting her fears about breast cancer if she does not mention feeling a breast lump while in the shower.

Silence may also be a common behavior in individuals who are described as having passive personalities. These individuals want the partner in the interview to take control and direct the flow of the visit (see Chapter 25). Finally, silence may be a profound indicator of a depressed mood with psychomotor retardation or an adverse effect from a psychoactive medication. Those struggling with depression or dysthymia may find it difficult to express their concerns or even initiate conversation.

Management

It is often helpful, when confronted with a patient who finds it difficult to speak, to address the behavior by saying, "You seem very quiet." This offers the patient the opportunity to acknowledge the behavior and express the reason. It is valuable to provide a significant amount of time, at least 3–5 seconds, for the person to respond to this reflection. When a patient seems passive, it is appropriate to explain the need for the patient to collaborate in the visit: "In order for me to help you, I really need you to tell me about this problem in more detail."

If the person seems actively distracted, it is fair to ask, "Are you hearing voices or seeing things you think might not be real?" If the patient gives evidence of anger, reflecting the emotion would be appropriate (as described earlier). Especially with older patients, if the patient responds with "What?" one has most likely diagnosed a hearing impairment and need only speak louder face-to-face. One of the most common complaints by older patients is that their providers don't speak clearly or loudly enough.

Table 4–4. Possible causes of silence in patients.

Cause	Discussion
Adverse reaction to prescription medication (eg, sedation)	*Check for overdose or drug interactions.*
Alcohol or other drug intoxication	*Screen with CAGE questionnaire and elicit history of substance abuse.*
Alzheimer's or other dementia	*Age-dependent; although some dementias strike as early as the mid-40s, most occur in the 66+ age group. Silence is usually a sign of advanced disease associated with withdrawal from the environment.*
Anger	*The patient is feeling wronged or slighted and is trying to elicit an emotional reaction. . . . (see Table 4–3).*
Cultural or language barrier	*Ask whether patient can understand; use interpreter or bilingual staff member, if available.*
Depression, dysthymia, or adjustment disorder with depressed mood	*Name the feelings; request elaboration.*
Distraction secondary to depression	*Associated with drawn features, sad affect, lack of eye contact.*
Fear of being told that serious disease is causing the presenting problem	*State clearly that, regardless of the outcome, the practitioner will be there to help.*
Fear of physician authority	*Family background, other experience with domineering authority figures may have demanded submissiveness; a gentle demeanor, reassurance, and an explicit request for collaboration can help win the patient's confidence.*
Hearing impairment	*Use whisper test.*
Passive or shy personality	*Change to a more direct, closed-ended pattern of questions; encourage descriptions and elaboration.*
Preoccupation with auditory or visual hallucinations	*Request additional information from family or attendant.*
Quiet person	*Usually responds to encouragement, offers to elaborate.*
Stroke, TIA (transient ischemic attack), mass lesion	*Conduct thorough neurologic examination for focal findings.*

Case illustration 2 (Contd.): In response to "You seem quiet," Mr. K. responds, "Today is 3 months since my favorite aunt died." When the provider says, "I'm sorry to hear that; would you like to reschedule the visit?" the patient thanks her for the offer, adding that he's concerned about the fatigue and would like to talk about it. With that, the patient becomes more animated and engages in the discussion about his fatigue, which is subsequently diagnosed as being a symptom related to depression.

Patient Education

By explaining to patients that their silence creates additional barriers to the delivery of effective care, barriers that must be overcome, physicians can invite patients to collaborate and to make decisions about their own care. Emphasizing the importance of the patient's or family member's role in evaluating and treating problems underscores the value of participation. It also discourages the patient from making the practitioner solely—and inappropriately—responsible for evaluation or treatment.

Summary

Obviously, there are many reasons why individuals might be silent in the office. Acknow-ledging, in an open-ended way, the problems silence creates, and then

asking for an explanation offers the patient the chance to express a feeling state, an extenuating circumstance, fear of an outcome, or fear of the projected role of the practitioner. Further questioning can also result in the diagnosis of a physical disability like acoustic neuroma or a psychiatric condition that causes hallucinations or delusions that make a response impossible. Premature hypothesis testing runs the risk of insulting patients or driving them further from the relationship.

Silent patients are always distressing, particularly for individuals who particularly value the social dynamic and satisfactions of medical practice. Learning to encourage a more mutual collaboration is usually beneficial and rewarding when specific causes for unusual degrees of silence are discovered and overcome. It is interesting that sometimes the reason for struggling with particular types of patients is that they remind us of others from previous experiences who evoke strong negative responses. For example, someone easily frustrated by silent patients may be reminded of a parent who died because he didn't let anyone know he was having chest tightness. Recognizing the sources of our personal intense responses can be most helpful in assisting practitioners to remain focused on a patient's problem or response and avoid unproductive replays of unsettling experiences from the past. Acknowledging the power of these prior experiences allows the practitioner to decide how to confront or address these important personal issues.

THE DEMANDING PATIENT

Case illustration 3: The doctor is seeing Mr. G., a 48-year-old bricklayer, her fifth patient of the afternoon, for follow-up of his back pain that began after a day of particularly heavy work on the job. In the initial visit, after excluding historical points suggestive of an underlying cancer or spinal cord injury, the doctor prescribed limited activity, exercise as tolerated, analgesics, and the application of heat. Two weeks later, Mr. G. returns, and when asked how things have gone in the last 2 weeks, responds, "I'm no better and I want an MRI today." The doctor leans back in her chair, anticipating an extremely frustrating encounter.

Diagnosis

When a demand is made, the practitioner may quickly identify the signs of anger. Alternatively, the patient's actions—nail-biting, repetitive movements, or poor attention—might suggest frustration or anxiety. A grimacing facial expression, an inability to move, or obvious pain with movement suggests greater-than-anticipated pain. A focus on a seemingly unrelated article—a medical device like a cane or brace, a magazine article, or an advertisement—can reveal a concern directly or indirectly related to the item on which attention is focused.

Differential Diagnosis: Although a patient's demand is usually tied to dissatisfaction with the current plan for evaluation or treatment, there are many possible causes of the dissatisfaction. As a rule, if there is disagreement about treatment, the problem results from a concern about the accuracy of the diagnosis. If the problem involves a diagnostic test, the problem often arises either in the prior evaluation or a failure to solicit important aspects of the history. On the other hand, a recommended test or treatment may remind the patient of a similar and unpleasant experience among family or friends, causing the patient to anticipate a similar undesirable outcome.

Sometimes the reason for an unexpected demand involves secondary gain, such as a workers' compen-

sation claim, a lawsuit, or disability insurance income. Another possibility is that the patient has read something in the press, listened to a friend, or seen something on television that suggests a simplistic or "right" way to solve the problem while attacking other approaches. More and more often in a managed-care settings, the patient also may be concerned that the practitioner is withholding a more expensive test or treatment in order to limit cost—at the expense of quality medical care. The demand then becomes part of the anticipated struggle to wrestle needed services from the gatekeeper practitioner (see Chapter 7). Finally, it must be remembered that the patient may be frustrated with the lack of relief because additional treatment is actually indicated. The patient's dissatisfaction can prompt the practitioner to rethink the diagnosis and seek appropriate alternatives to the current treatment plan. An example would be the patient, presumed to have a sprained wrist, who returns with unremitting pain. The increased severity of symptom-reporting prompts a search for a fracture—which is subsequently diagnosed by x-ray.

Psychological Mechanisms: The demand for additional intervention can be triggered by any of the following feelings (Table 4–5):

- Anger
- Fear
- Frustration
- Doubt

Individuals are often isolated from family and friends during times of illness. The isolated person may begin to doubt that the practitioner is sufficiently interested in the problem to ensure the best possible outcome. As distrust of the physician grows, the patient feels increasingly responsible for the outcome of his or her care and, therefore, becomes both more fearful and more demanding. On the other hand, if secondary gains are connected with the illness, the patient may demand testing to demonstrate levels of disability or prove that the problem is as severe as claimed. This is especially true in pain syndromes in which testing is generally unrevealing, and the patient, the family, or the employer begins to feel that

Table 4–5. Possible reasons for demanding additional interventions.

Feeling	Discussion
Anger	*The patient is feeling wronged or is reexperiencing a previous bad outcome (see Table 4–3).*
Fear	*The patient may be afraid that the illness is terminal, serious, horrible, disfiguring, etc., if not attacked quickly.*
Frustration	*The patient may feel that no—or insufficient—progress has been made.*
Personal responsibility for health outcome	*Previous experience may have convinced the patient that physicians are not trustworthy, competent, or interested.*
Doubt	*The patient may wonder if economic reasons are driving decision making or if the practitioner is skilled enough or up-to-date with current evaluation and treatment technologies.*

the problem is "all in the patient's head." As a result, the patient seeks evidence of a severe condition capable of causing such problematic symptoms.

A demanding patient often provokes feelings in the practitioner of rejection, distrust, blame, or humiliation. As a result, the practitioner is often defensive, assuming reasons for the demand that may not be accurate. By assuming a defensive posture, the practitioner loses the opportunity to recognize the patient's subtle clues to the reasons for a demand. For example, casual asides; postural shifts in response to a topic; and expressions of fear, agitation, and grief are easily ignored.

Management

Rather than respond to a presumed cause for the demand, the first step in evaluating or reevaluating the demand is to appropriately identify and explore the patient's affect. Let us consider case illustration 3. Because Mr. G. seems frustrated, the doctor reflects the feeling: "You seem frustrated." The patient responds, "I am frustrated. My father had a similar condition, and 2 years later they found he had a herniated disk. I don't want to wait that long to find out what I have."

In response to an acknowledgment of affect, the patient usually confirms or denies the practitioner's hypothesis. If the patient responds affirmatively (eg, "I am angry, frustrated, sad, nervous"), the practitioner would ask, "Why are you. . . ." This permits the patient to explain and share the experience that surrounds the emotion. Often, this prompts a story or a piece of information that is instrumental in allowing the physician to ask and the patient to answer pertinent questions. In Mr. G.'s case, hearing what the patient fears better prepares the practitioner to understand what prompted the request for an MRI and determine to what extent education, a redescription of the results of evaluation or treatment, another examination, or confrontation about possible secondary gain might be most appropriate. In this way, all aspects of a demand are explored and an appropriate response initiated.

When this approach is less successful, a number of probing questions are useful. One is to ask patients what they think is causing their problem; often patients do not offer their opinions without being asked. Given the opportunity, patients frequently say that after an evaluation they were told the test results were all negative, but the cause of the problem they perceived was not addressed. This point cannot be stressed enough: *In order to provide meaningful reassurance, the patient's attribution for the symptom must be elicited and confronted.*

Another useful question is: "How had you hoped I could help you?" This gives the patient the opportunity to express dissatisfaction with the extent of evaluation, treatment, or commitment by the practitioner; it often lightens the practitioner's burden, since the patient's request may be significantly less difficult than what the practitioner anticipated. A typical example might be the arthritic patient who complains bitterly about the pain in his hip. When the physician asks, "How had you hoped I could help you?" the patients responds, "I'd like a prescription for a cane." The physician had anticipated a request for a hip replacement.

> ***Case illustration 3 (Contd.):*** In response to the doctor's question, Mr. G. says, "I want to know how I can find out exactly what I have and make sure I don't have any problems with my disk." The doctor then describes the recently developed guidelines that support the use of MRI testing only for determining operability in patients with defined neurologic syndromes, such as radiculopathy and cauda equina syndrome.
>
> By offering alternatives to the demand that would accomplish the same goal—while taking into account the patient's reason for the demand—the practitioner has begun the process of negotiation. Respect for the patient's point of view generally provides the basis for construction of a mutually satisfactory plan.
>
> The doctor further explains to Mr. G.: "I've examined you again and I find no evidence of nerve root involvement. From what you've said about your father's symptoms, his back problem was quite different from what you're experiencing. Let's put off doing any tests for now. What I would like to do is continue our present course of treatment, since in 90% of cases the symptoms you describe resolve within 12 weeks. If at the end of that time you're still having these symptoms, I'll refer you to a neurologist for another opinion on what we might do. I appreciate your telling me about your dad because it's obviously causing you some distress and making you wonder whether I was doing the right thing. Looking at things from your perspective helps me do a better job." The time cost of this explanation is 33 seconds; the reexamination adds only 2 minutes.

It may appear to the practitioner that the demand is related to secondary gain (for example, a desire to remain away from work for an extended period). In that case, the practitioner can confront the patient and offer a plan that provides ample time for recovery, within a timeframe that is also acceptable to the practitioner and that sets reasonable boundaries for the practitioner's agreement to the demand.

Patient Education

Patients respond to instruction when they believe it will be helpful in solving their problem. Until there is an agreement on the need for education by practitioner and patient, the patient might perceive education as the practitioner's way to control the visit, ignoring or masking a failure of collaboration. The patient's usual response in such an encounter is either to tune out the information or to construct mental barriers to implementing the practitioner's recommendations. On the other hand, once the patient's concerns have been addressed and the alliance has been formed, the patient often asks for and benefits from the information supporting the practitioner's point of view. In case illustration 3, recent guidelines that support the doctor's plan serve to educate and reassure the patient that the plan is consistent with his best interests.

Summary

A patient's demands can serve as a focal point for understanding when an interaction has been unsuccessful. Exploring the cause of the demand in a non-judgmental fashion allows most demands to be both understood and addressed. A plan that is mutually agreeable to practitioner and patient can then be negotiated. When it becomes clear that such a negotiation is not possible, the patient should be informed of realistic limits on what the practitioner can offer. The patient can then decide whether he or she is willing to accept the practitioner's boundaries or needs to seek the services of another practitioner.

THE "YES, BUT . . ." PATIENT

Case illustration 4: Mrs. M. is a 58-year-old woman who is being followed for obesity and poorly controlled high blood pressure. Her doctor is frustrated because his continued attempts to get Mrs. M. to lose weight have been unsuccessful. As a result, he is frustrated and pessimistic about their ability to work together to treat her hypertension, which he feels is a clear risk to her health. When the doctor notes that Mrs. M.'s blood pressure is still elevated, he asks whether she is still taking her medication.

She responds, "Oh, I'm sorry doctor, I ran out of my medicine 3 days ago and didn't want to bother you for a refill." Later in the visit the doctor asks, "Did you join that exercise program you said you would last time?" Mrs. M. replies, "I've been so busy. I'll do it next week." The doctor pulls back in his chair, thinking to himself, "This will never go anywhere."

Diagnosis

When problems are being discussed, the nonverbal behavior of patients in this group usually involves an active posture: leaning forward, bright affect, and dynamic gestures. As recommendations for evaluation and treatment are made, however, the patient typically becomes withdrawn, eye contact diminishes, and language becomes significantly less animated. Verbally, during the discussion of evaluation and treatment, the patient becomes quiet, volunteers little, and characteristically offers no solutions to problems. In fact, as the practitioner makes recommendations, the patient often responds with the classic, "I'd like to do that but. . . ."

Differential Diagnosis: Frequently, this behavior indicates a passive-aggressive personality. The practitioner initially feels encouraged to explore and offer suggestions to the patient—who then invariably rejects the offer or agrees to the plan but does not carry it out.

There are other possibilities, however, that are often not explored. Probably most important is that the

practitioner's plan has not taken the patient's perspective into account and is therefore unrealistic or is economically or logistically impossible. Another consideration is that the patient comes from a highly controlling family and is attempting to follow the recommendations but is unable to for psychosocial reasons. Another, similar possibility is that the patient's previous experiences with practitioners may have been so hierarchical and paternalistic that the thought of disagreeing or negotiating a position with a practitioner does not come to mind.

Psychological Mechanisms: Passive–aggressive behavior is often a form of control used by persons who do not feel capable of asserting themselves directly. They may become skilled in positioning themselves so that others feel they want to—or must—save them, frequently on a long-term basis. The practitioner's attempt to solve the problem is invariably followed by the patient's frustrating failure to collaborate. Continued failure results in the need for repeated visits, thus offering the desired outcome of frequent ongoing attention (secondary gain rather than healing).

Other patients who are unable to offer an opinion may have been emotionally, verbally, or physically abused earlier in life or may have had family or other personal experiences that taught unquestioning submission to authority.

Most people who enter the healing professions have a desire, even a need, to be of help. The solicitation by passive-aggressive patients for the practitioner to save them can be extremely seductive, luring practitioners into believing that these patients will singularly benefit from their expertise. The extent to which practitioners use a patient's recovery to validate their competence or professional value may determine how frustrated and angry they will become when treatment is unsuccessful. Rather than focusing initially on outcomes, the physician is better served answering the questions "Am I encouraging patients to take a more active role in their care?" and "Am I giving patients the chance to say why they're not using the treatments I thought we agreed on?"

Management

In working with individuals who apparently need to have the practitioner solve their health problems, it is important to remember (and to remind the patients) that ultimately only they themselves can do so. To help differentiate patients who are dependent and unable to carry out plans from those with a definable personality disorder, the physician can confront the patient and offer, "I'm frustrated with how things are going. Let's start again and see if what I see as a problem is really a problem for you."

Agreement on the diagnosis of the problem initiates the sequence for treatment. If there is disagreement, such questions as "What do you think the problem is?" or "What do you think should be done?" should be asked explicitly. If agreement is not reached, practitioner and patient must work to resolve the conflict.

If the patient agrees with the problem statement, the next step is to ask what he or she thinks would be helpful in solving the problem. Again, to distinguish patients who are unable to collaborate successfully from those who have a personality disorder, one can ask, "Do you think you can really do this?" If the question is asked in a supportive fashion, many patients who initially agreed to an unrealistic plan (perhaps to please the practitioner), respond more honestly, acknowledging that they are unable to participate. If asked respectfully, they generally explain their reasons. Once the patient has been truthful, the practitioner can encourage collaboration by saying, "Let's explore what we can do to solve this problem together. It will certainly help if you tell me what's possible for you and what's not." The approach to patients with personality disorders, which is beyond the scope of this chapter, is covered in Chapter 25.

If the patient displays passive-aggressive behavior, the practitioner can seek agreement on the nature of the problem and then make very specific contracts for what the patient will do. They can be as simple as "So, until our next visit, you will remain abstinent from alcohol," or "Between now and our next visit, you'll keep a diary and record when, and under what conditions, your headaches occur." The physician's support and enthusiasm can be directly tied to the degree to which both parties carry out the requirements of the contract. In this way, the physician can promote the patient's autonomy and offer support, without taking full responsibility for the patient's behavior. Over time, patients learn to respond to the support offered and begin to take a more active role in their care. Of course, there is the risk that a passive-aggressive individual attempting to control the relationship will seek another practitioner who can be more easily controlled.

Patient Education

Patients who are unfamiliar with a collaborative model can be given specific information about the practitioner's understanding and particular style of collaborating. Explicit requests for patients' opinions about doctor-patient collaboration can be extremely useful. Over time, given the opportunity to state opinions and formulate plans, most individuals find such an approach satisfying and engaging. Indeed, there is convincing evidence that patients taught to be more assertive improve their health outcomes, such as lowering blood pressure and controlling diabetes.

Educating patients who exhibit passive-aggressive behavior about such behavior can begin a process of introspection and self-awareness. Encouraging individuals to explore the origins of these behaviors and also to consider a therapeutic relationship to facilitate the process can be rewarding for both patient and practitioner. Descriptions of behavior that hit home can

provoke emotional responses in patients, but penetrating long-held psychologic defenses can spur growth. The physician might say, for example, "You say your mother was overbearing and controlling and withheld praise. Isn't that what your children are telling you?" In most instances, the benefits outweigh the risks.

> **Case illustration 4 (Contd.):** The doctor leans forward and says, "Mrs. M., your actions tell me I'm pushing you to do something you don't want to do. I'm concerned about your weight—what are your thoughts on this?" Mrs. M.'s eyes moisten and she responds, "I want to lose weight, but I can't do it. I've tried for years, and it's so frustrating." The doctor nods and says, "Let's hold off on the weight control for now. How about taking one thing at a time and focusing on your blood pressure?"
>
> Mrs. M. agrees to take her medication and to return for a blood pressure check in 2 weeks. The doctor gives her a card so that she can record her own blood pressure when she checks it at the drug store or the mall.

Summary

Setting limits and providing explicit feedback can teach patients to collaborate more effectively in their care. Being aware of yes-but patterns can help the practitioner initiate a strategy to develop shared responsibilities that prevent the ultimately unhelpful rescuing behaviors that leave all parties frustrated and dissatisfied and that interfere with successful treatment.

INDICATIONS FOR REFERRAL

Indications for referral of individuals whose interactions are difficult include the practitioner's inability to make a diagnosis, negative personal feelings that create a barrier to a therapeutic relationship, an objective assessment that the patient is not benefiting from evaluation or treatment, or the practitioner's feeling of being threatened or in danger.

With particular reference to a practitioner's negative feelings, when an inability to work together significantly impairs the provision of effective care, outside assistance and advice are not only desirable but may also be cost-effective. Since the negative feelings can relate to a practitioner's previous family and life experiences, a patient who is difficult for one physician may not be difficult for another.

Once the decision to refer is made, framing the referral in a positive way is particularly valuable. One strategy is to acknowledge the need for assistance in managing difficult situations or problems. The dialogue might take the following form:

> DOCTOR: Mrs. S., for the last 2 months I've been trying to figure out how to make your headaches better. I think it would help us if you could be evaluated by a psychologist; we might be able to get a better handle on what else we could do to deal with the problems.

Mrs. S.: Are you saying that I'm imagining this? Do you think it's all in my head?

DOCTOR: No, not at all. But nothing we've tried has stopped your headaches. It often helps me to have another person listen to the story and maybe find a new direction to take. Dr. F. has helped me with a number of people in the past, and I'm hopeful she can help us here as well.

Mrs. S.: What do I have to do? I really do want these headaches to end.

DOCTOR: Great. In addition to the referral, I'll schedule you for three visits with me over the next 12 weeks to see how things are going and help answer any questions you or Dr. F. may have.

Proposing a positive outcome from the referral can be remarkably useful. In addition, scheduling a visit for the person to return after the referral reassures the patient that the referring physician is truly seeking assistance rather than simply "dumping" the problem on someone else.

Learning to understand the person's perspective, negotiating for realistic plans of evaluation and treatment, and being aware of and responsive to verbal and nonverbal evidence that a recommendation was misunderstood or rejected creates a collaboration that can be remarkably satisfying for both participants.

Underused skills such as soliciting the patient's attribution for a problem, offering praise and support, listening carefully to the patient's description of a problem, and explicitly confronting problematic or confusing behavior inform the patient that a serious attempt is underway to understand and work with the patient's concerns.

By exploring their own expectations and feelings, practitioners become more self-aware and recognize who else is in the room. Clearly, to the extent practitioners improve their self-awareness and learn to confront their feelings, their effectiveness as physicians will improve.

SUGGESTED READINGS

Beckman HB et al: The doctor-patient relationship and malpractice: Lessons from plaintiff depositions. Arch Intern Med 1994;154:1365.

Beckman HB et al: Getting the most from a twenty minute visit. Am J Gastroent 1994;89(5):662.

Branch WT, Malik TK: Using "windows of opportunities" in brief interviews to understand patients' concerns. JAMA 1993;260:1667.

Burack RC et al: The challenging case conference: An integrated approach to resident education and support. J Gen Intern Med 1991;6:355.

Drossman DA: The problem patient: Evaluation and care of medical patients with psychosocial disturbances. Ann Intern Med 1978;88:366.

Groves JE: Taking care of the hateful patient. N Engl J Med 1978;298:883.

Kaplan SH, Greenfield S, Ware JE Jr: Assessing the effects of physician-patient interactions on the outcome of chronic disease. Med Care 1989;27(3):S110.

Lazare A: Shame and humiliation in the medical encounter. Arch Intern Med 1987;147:1653.

Lazare A, Eisenthal L, Wasserman L: The customer approach to patienthood: Attending to patient requests in a walk-in clinic. Arch Gen Psychiatry 1975;32:553.

Quill TE: Partnerships in patient care: A contractual approach. Ann Intern Med 1983;98:228.

5

Sexuality & Professionalism

Richard M. Frankel, PhD, & Sarah Williams, MD

INTRODUCTION

Case illustration 1: One of my patients, a young, attractive, buxom blonde woman has been incredibly suggestive toward me. I honestly don't think I did anything to provoke her sexually, but I haven't been as firm as I should be in discouraging her behavior. Each time she comes (to the office) wearing low-cut outfits that cling to her body. She speaks in a soft, seductive voice and makes completely inappropriate suggestions like: "Can't we go someplace and be alone?" I always tell her no, but I haven't really clamped down and confronted her with how inappropriate this is and how uncomfortable this makes me. The problem is that I kind of enjoy it.

Sexuality and sexual feelings are omnipresent parts of life. They do not magically disappear (although sometimes we wish they would!) just because we become doctors, nurses, or therapists, or because we are interacting with patients or professional colleagues. Despite the importance and complexity of this aspect of medicine, most of us enter practice quite unprepared to deal with these issues.

Not surprisingly, education about sexuality in medical practice remains woefully inadequate. Furthermore, when these issues are addressed, discussion tends to focus on issues of excess, abuse, and harassment, thereby precluding a fuller and fairer exploration of the role of sexuality in professional relationships with patients, colleagues, and trainees.

For the past 4 years, the authors have conducted a small group workshop designed to explore sexuality and professionalism with practicing physicians, faculty, and trainees. We have done workshops with more than 75 doctors and other health professionals at various levels of training about sexual issues in pro-

fessional life. Their stories make up the raw data for this chapter.

From listening to and studying these stories, we have learned that sexual feelings and conflicts inform many aspects of providers' interactions with patients and colleagues. When these issues are recognized and accepted (and worked through as needed), they need not be harmful and may, in fact, enhance work satisfaction and effectiveness. On the other hand, when providers are uncomfortable with their sexual feelings or conflicts, and try to avoid or ignore them, negative consequences for patient care, and perhaps for the providers themselves, are much more likely.

Specific negative consequences include:

- Not performing indicated examinations, particularly genital, breast, and rectal examinations due to embarrassment or avoidance.
- Avoidance of the patient generally, or not performing important services such as sexual histories or risk counseling, an especially egregious omission in an age of widespread HIV infection.
- Inability to effectively manage patients' sexual advances or sexual attractions between doctor and patient. As many of the case illustrations in this chapter reveal, this leads to tensions and confusion in the encounter, preventing the development of an appropriate and therapeutic doctor-patient relationship and may cause the patient to terminate care prematurely.
- Increased risk of boundary confusion or violation. Strong emotions (sexual or otherwise) are much more likely to distort our perceptions or behaviors when they are unacknowledged or ambiguous. The provider who is unaware or feels clouded about his or her sexual feelings is less able to separate feelings from actions, and more likely to engage in inappropriate behaviors that allow professional boundaries to become blurred.
- An erosion of professional satisfaction and well-being because of unresolved sexual issues. Sexuality in its broadest sense is an integral part of our

The authors gratefully acknowledge critical reading and comment on this manuscript by Ronald Epstein, MD, and Cecile Carson, MD. The authors also acknowledge Dawn Masetta for her help in manuscript preparation.

personal and professional identity, our energy and engagement in work, and our relationships. Hence, we cannot ignore issues of sexuality without risking cutting off parts of our selves and our vitality.

Methods & Materials

Since 1991, the authors have led several workshops entitled, "Sexual Issues in the Workplace," designed for physicians and other health-care professionals to explore issues of sexuality in professional life. At these workshops, participants are invited "to write a 5-minute narrative about sexual issues in the work-place." Of the 75 physicians and other health-care providers who have attended the workshops, 55 (73%) have volunteered stories for inclusion in a re-search database. These 55 narratives form the basis of our chapter in this book.

These stories are a rich source of qualitative data that can be used to explore the intriguing and rela-tively unexplored territory of sexuality and profes-sionalism, and suggest guidelines for personal and professional development and teaching.

Personal & Relational Boundaries

The concepts of "boundaries" and boundary confu-sions/crossings/violations are integral to this chapter and thus merit some explanation. Personal boundaries refer to the individual's physical and emotional "space," which provides separateness from others. Relational boundaries enclose the set of behaviors that are felt to be safe and appropriate within a specific re-lationship, or class of relationships. Certain behaviors (eg, lending money, accompanying one another to so-cial events) fall easily within the boundaries of per-sonal friendship, but not the doctor-patient relation-ship. Conversely, certain actions commonly performed by doctors (such as rectal examinations and sexual his-tories) fall well outside the bounds of normal social re-lations! Falling between these extremes are behaviors that are more difficult to classify in terms of their ap-propriateness in a doctor-patient relationship.

THE PHYSICIAN'S SEXUALITY: IDENTITY, TRAINING, & DEVELOPMENTAL EXPERIENCES

The Doctor as Sexual Being

Sexuality, defined narrowly, means engaging in sexual activity with another person. Sexuality of this sort has been widely discussed and is generally con-sidered to be inappropriate in the medical workplace; as such it is not explored further in this chapter.

There has been far less discussion, however, of a more comprehensive understanding of sexuality, one that includes thoughts and feelings about sex, or—even more broadly—sees sexuality as part of our identity, our desire and capacity for intimacy, and an integral part of our physical and emotional vitality.

This subtler but no less important aspect of our pro-fessional lives is the topic of the following section, in which we look at the physician's sexuality in terms of identity and connectedness, medical training, and de-velopmental experiences.

Sexuality, Identity, & Work

For some participants, sexuality and "connected-ness," or energy, at work were related. The presence or, more characteristically, the absence of sexual feelings at work was found to be related to work satisfaction and broader questions of identity. One physician writes:

Case illustration 2: This year I lost the joy of living for a time. I know myself by this quality—it is the core of me to wake up excited about a new day or know that I *could* be [excited]. It had to do with feeling paralyzed to change. The work is incredibly important to me as are the people with whom I've connected in the process, and so even the thought of leaving stopped me cold and stopped me inside—including sexually. I didn't desire or hope. Ultimately I felt that no work, no matter how "meaningful," is more important than the capacity to hope, to feel joy, and to feel sexual and alive, and [so] I have left the job that I was in.

Another participant describes the experience of los-ing her identity as a sexual woman, which was neces-sary—as she noted in the group discussion that fol-lowed—for her to feel energy and enthusiasm for work.

Case illustration 3: For the first time in my life since I was a teenager, I am without a sexual partner. All my life I've felt good about my sexuality—figured it would stay this way forever (I know the positive literature on con-tinuing sexual activity into old age). Now, with my hus-band gone, I find I am very visible as a person, but in-visible as a woman. Somewhere I crossed the line from desirable to undesirable. Maybe not that, maybe just "not considered." All my colleagues are much younger. I'm currently cut off from what I'd always thought would be mine—my femaleness!

Sexuality in Medical Training

Learning to be a doctor involves intense contacts and physical intimacy, which can heighten sexual feelings and tensions. Often the setting becomes so routine for practicing professionals and teachers that its effect on trainees may be overlooked. One partici-pant, a clinical teacher, describes an experience that brought this issue vividly to the fore.

Case illustration 4: I was precepting two male medical students. They were sitting in with me while I saw a young female patient. . . . I asked her to sit on the table because I wanted to examine her spleen, which had been enlarged. I was excited because it was such a "good" exam . . . One of [the students, however,] couldn't "ap-preciate" the spleen, so I took his hand and placed it over the [splenic] area and we spent a few seconds in this po-sition. Then we stepped out in the hallway to "discuss the case." Within a second the med student was swaying and then dropped to the floor, hitting his head . . . he had fainted! I was so frightened and impressed by the enormity of what happened and with how intimate the physical examination is . . . and how little we acknowledge the sexual issue . . . (Note: the student recovered quickly.)

Clinical care is often intensely intimate as patients share their innermost feelings, fears, and secrets. It is generally assumed and taught that most of the needs and vulnerabilities expressed in these interactions are the patient's (and this inequality of power and vulnerability is an important issue when sexual relationships develop between patient and doctor). Doctors, however, may also have their own unmet needs, particularly during training, or at other times when their personal life is "on hold" or is unfulfilling for some reason. At such times the physician who is lonely, or without satisfying intimate relationships outside the hospital, may turn for intimacy and comfort to those closest at hand, namely patients and colleagues. Such a tendency may be further heightened by the stress and emotional intensity of medical work, particularly with critically ill patients. One participant writes about his internship year.

> *Case illustration 5:* I was sitting with my resident in a call room at 2:00 AM. Another resident entered for a second to say that she was going to the ER to do a pelvic exam. She jokingly said she was going to "tickle the vagina" of this patient, then she left (leaving me, a single male, with my female resident). My resident then looked over at me and said, "Gosh, I wish someone would tickle my vagina . . . that hasn't happened in so long." I chuckled wondering if this was a solicitation/proposal or what? Since we were all alone in a room with a bed, I excused myself to go get some coffee.

The intern maintained the relationship within professional boundaries by finding a diplomatic way to terminate a sexually charged encounter. In the following story, a woman physician describes how a relationship, fueled by the emotional needs of both members, slowly grew beyond the boundaries of resident camaraderie.

> *Case illustration 6:* It was March of my junior residency year. I was running the ward team—the height of power in my program. The team was "tight"; we spent from 7:30 AM to 11:00 PM on the wards, in our back room, eating takeout food at night, running codes together and laughing.

She then goes on to describe the close relationship that developed between herself and the intern who eventually disclosed that she was gay and had never had a romantic relationship.

> *Case illustration 6 (Contd.):* . . . we immediately developed an intense bond with an intense edge and secrecy not unlike that of a new romantic relationship. She came over to my apartment, as I was still playing the role

of a confidant/resident/therapist. We talked into the early morning and at one point I held her and she cried. She declared her love for me.

The unexpectedly rapid and intense escalation from boundary confusion to boundary crossing described in this story was very frightening to the storyteller and caused her to abruptly sever the relationship by avoiding her intern. As will be seen in subsequent doctor-patient case illustrations, this is a common outcome of boundary confusions.

Developmental Experiences & Workplace Sexual Issues

How individuals handle the sexual tensions of collegial and provider-patient relations is often influenced by their personal history, including development issues, past sexual experiences, and sexual attitudes and beliefs. In this narrative, one participant describes her struggle to define the role of sexuality in her work life.

> *Case illustration 7:* When I was younger, I was a very seductive person and I had a lot of sexually charged interactions with colleagues and teachers. In some ways I valued these because I felt—especially during medical school and training—that they humanized what was otherwise an incredibly repressed and interpersonally barren environment. At the same time, I think my abilities to be seductive were bad for me because they reflected and reinforced my sense that [they were] the only valuable part of me. As I began to change and feel more self-confident about other parts of me, I began to see my sexuality as a bad thing and to feel ashamed about it. As a result I began to keep this aspect of myself totally out of my workplace self. After a while, I realized that this sort of "repression" was making me feel bad about my sexuality in general, and also it took away an important part of my pleasure and energy at work. So, more recently my struggle has been to let these feelings back into my sense of myself, including my professional self. I have also realized that I really like feeling sexy and feeling sexual attractions, but at the same time . . . the nice part is that I don't feel any pressure to act on those feelings.

Another participant, a 49-year-old medical educator, describes how his adolescent experience of being sexually molested by a teacher sensitized him to the importance of these issues for his residents.

> *Case illustration 8:* When I was in the ninth grade, I was invited by a popular science teacher on an overnight camping trip. It was just the two of us and when I woke up in the morning, I found his hand on my penis trying to arouse me. I told him to take his hands off me and to drive me home, which he did, but I never said anything to my parents, friends, or the school authorities. I was too embarrassed and ashamed. Five years later at a reunion of some high school friends, the subject of this science teacher came up and it turned out that all of us had the same experience and that none of us had done or said anything to bring the situation to light. It has now

been 32 years since my victimization and I have a wonderful 5-year-old son. It troubles me that in my own silence I may inadvertently be making him more vulnerable to being victimized as I was. As a result of this experience, I take an active interest and role in working with medical students and residents around issues of sexuality, professionalism, and the workplace.

Finally, a woman resident describes the effects of early "boundary violations" on her professional life:

Case illustration 9: I feared being physically violated by my stepfather and was so fiercely determined to keep this from happening that it affected the way I present myself to the world. Only once did he come close: I was wrapped in a towel after bathing and he was "showing" me how to rub alcohol on my chest above my towel. At that time I thought "I just dare you to do something, I'll finally have real evidence against you and get you thrown out of here." He did not pursue to active violation although I was scared, angry, and determined. As a result I . . . go to what might be extremes (ie, rarely wear skirts) to avoid appearing vulnerable. I've taken karate to . . . marshall my sense of confidence to "potential" violators . . . I attribute the fact that I have no memorable encounters of inappropriateness with patients to the fact that I give *no room* for these things to happen.

BOUNDARY CONFUSIONS, CROSSINGS, & VIOLATIONS

Ethical codes of conduct for physicians have existed for thousands of years. In the modern era the doctor-patient relationship has been viewed as a type of contract with both legal and ethical standards against which behavior may be judged. Ethical standards of behavior based on contract are an important and much discussed aspect of providing medical care. Less well-described is the *relational* basis of ethical or appropriate behavior. Such a description is particularly needed by physicians, who must balance legal and ethical concerns with caring and compassion; when, for example, is a caring hand on a patient's shoulder a welcome gesture of comfort, and when is it an unappreciated boundary crossing? Each doctor-patient relationship must, therefore, develop its own appropriate boundaries, which is often difficult, as the following narratives will show.

For this discussion we use the concepts of personal and professional boundaries, as previously described, and as further defined by Petersen as:

the limits that allow for safe connection based on the client's needs. When these limits are altered, what is allowed in the relationship becomes ambiguous. Such ambiguity is often experienced as an intrusion into the sphere of safety.

We have observed in our participants' narratives a range of ambiguities that lead to boundary confusion

and boundary crossings and that place participants at risk for actual violations.

Boundary Confusions

Boundary confusions occur when one or more elements of the doctor-patient relationship become ambiguous. The majority of our case examples are of this sort, in which the physician becomes aware that something about a patient or an encounter is different or unusual in terms of sexuality. One physician describes her awareness of a sexual ambiguity in her relationship with a male patient and her response.

Case illustration 10: I had a 65-year-old male patient who was wonderful to take care of. He was funny, charming and had led an interesting life. He was also alone—I couldn't imagine why. I enjoyed spending a few minutes after dealing with the complaint talking with him. Usually, he left with a warm handshake. One Christmas he hugged me, and that was fine. Come the New Year, he kept hugging me when he left the office—no more handshakes. I was confused. I was attracted to him but not intensely. I also loved his company. I just wasn't convinced these hugs were appropriate, but I did nothing, afraid of confronting him.

Often when boundary confusion occurs, the provider masks his or her awareness of its effect. A male resident describes the arousing effect taking a sexual history had on him.

Case illustration 11: I was working at the adolescent clinic where I had been told that it was my obligation to talk about sex with my patients. There was this young, attractive black teenager who came to see me and the discussion got very detailed and explicit about sexual positions and arousal and things. And I couldn't help it. I was trying to be very professional about my questions but the more she talked, the more aroused I felt myself become. It was embarrassing sitting there with an erection, but I just couldn't help it.

Note that, despite having an erection and feeling embarrassed (confused), the physician inappropriately continued to elicit additional sexual history from the patient; had he had more awareness and training for dealing with these issues, he might have been able to redirect the interview more effectively.

In some cases boundary confusion around sexual issues may create enough tension to inhibit or prevent a physician from providing appropriate care, as is illustrated in the following case illustration.

Case illustration 12: I was working in the emergency department and here comes an attractive 20–21-year-old lady with a complaint of severe abdominal pain. She has a history of pancreatitis in the past. I know that I have to do a pelvic/rectal on her in order to be complete and not to miss any other etiologies for her abdominal pain. But I opted not to, hoping that her amylase and lipase would come back positive, so I wouldn't have to do them.

Boundary Crossings

Boundary confusions arise because the physician or patient becomes aware of ambiguous feelings around sexual issues in the relationship. Boundary crossings occur when the physician or patient begins acting on these feelings. Some boundary crossings are brief, episodic, and unilateral as described in the following case illustration.

> *Case illustration 13:* I recall an elderly gentleman who was homeless and indigent that I saw in the emergency room as a medical student. After he received his care, he asked if he could have a kiss and pulled me down to kiss me (not sexual, but more intimate than I wanted to be with this patient).

More characteristically the boundary crossings described in our case illustrations developed over time and followed a certain developmental "trajectory" in which both the physician and patient (and sometimes the staff) are aware that something other than an appropriate doctor-patient relationship is emerging. Characteristic in these illustrations is an abrupt "cut off" of the relationship at the point at which a suggestion (such as having sex) would move the relationship from a boundary crossing to a violation of the physician's ethical code.

> *Case illustration 14:* A young, attractive woman presented to the emergency room for evaluation of asthma. After initial treatment by me, she was given an appointment for follow-up in my general medicine clinic. Over the course of the next several months she presented to clinic unexpectedly several times with complaints of breast problems, genitourinary symptoms, requesting breast and pelvic exams. During the course of these she regularly made seductive comments. These episodes progressed to the point of frequent calls to me during office and nonoffice hours. I obviously enjoyed the encounters—yet when, finally, I was explicitly solicited, I declined sexual participation, after which the patient was never heard from.

The characteristic feature of sexual boundary crossings is ambiguity: The relationship appears to become increasingly sexualized, but nothing explicit has been said or done. As each person's perceptions become clouded by his or her own desires and fears, it becomes increasingly difficult to "read" the other's behavior or understand its meaning.

In the next case illustration, a resident physician describes a growing awareness of his own attraction to a female patient and his perception or assumption of reciprocation on her part. At the point at which he brings explicit attention to the sexual dimension of their relation-ship, the patient responds with anger and terminates the relationship. Was it the resident's fantasies and mistaken interpretation of the patient's behavior that characterized their relationship or mutual sexual attraction?

> *Case illustration 15:* There was a patient that I saw recently. She's 19 and came in with complaints of irregular periods wanting a pregnancy test and pelvic exam. I went ahead and did a pelvic exam . . . I did a thorough exam, but maybe I was a little too thorough. Sometimes I don't do a breast exam when I do a pelvic exam, but in this case I did and it was extra thorough. And I thought to myself, "Am I toying with this patient?" because she was kind of . . . very flirtatious and I knew I had this position of power and I was kind of struggling with that in the long run but I didn't resolve it, I didn't step outside and try to collect my thoughts and stuff. It made me feel really clouded, you know.
>
> I gave her my card and told her to call me at my regular clinic . . . and she's been here twice and she made several phone calls. And initially I was kind of friendly, you know, maybe a little too friendly. You know, there was probably some mutual flirtation going on here . . . she came to me another time for a rash. When I asked her to show me the rash she took off her sweatshirt and jeans and underneath it all she was wearing this sexy "teddy." Well, the next time she came back, about a week later, she had a different teddy on and I said in a flippant sort of way, "That's an interesting way of dressing to come to see the doctor." Well, she got really angry and basically walked out of my clinic and hasn't been back since. I know I wasn't completely blameless in this situation, but still I was surprised that she got so angry and never came back.

These kinds of situations, which were common in the residents' stories, show how interpersonal confusion and lack of self-awareness prevent physicians from effectively "reading" and dealing with the patients' behavior. The therapeutic relationship was often the casualty, as abrupt termination of the relationship by the patient was a frequent outcome.

Boundary Violations

As the sexual dimension of a doctor-patient relationship becomes more explicit, understood, and acted upon, it becomes a boundary violation. Gutheil and Gabbard suggest that the most serious form of boundary violation, sexual misconduct, usually begins with relatively minor boundary crossings, ". . . which often show a crescendo pattern of increasing intrusion into the patient's space that culminates in sexual contact. A direct shift from talking to intercourse is quite rare." And Peterson suggests that, "In every story of a (boundary) violation, however, four motifs surface: a reversal of roles (the patient takes care of the doctor), a secret (shared intimate feelings), a double bind (it is impossible to stay in or get out of the relationship), and an indulgence in professional privilege (the doctor prevails upon the patient to meet a personal need)." Interestingly, in the 55 narratives we studied, we did not find any examples of significant boundary violations, although several participants did report developmental experiences that involved boundary violations, and one participant reported boundary violations in the context of sexual harassment by her supervisor. It is hard to know whether the absence of reported violations in our sample reflects participants' discomfort in reporting such events or whether their frequency is low compared with boundary confusions and crossings. This is obviously a difficult area to study; however, the few anonymous physician surveys that have been conducted have found a prevalence of physician-patient sexual contact ranging from 3–12% for male physicians and 1–4% for female physicians.

Sexual Relationships Between Colleagues

In workshop sessions with residents and students, stories of boundary issues tended to focus on patients and the sexual tensions surrounding the care delivery process. In sessions with more senior physicians, stories were increasingly likely to address sexual attractions and relationships between colleagues. Several of these stories focused on sexual needs outside of work affecting relationships in the workplace. The following narrative is illustrative.

Case illustration 16: While in a prior relationship, I had sexual feelings for a couple of women with whom I worked, which I proceeded to act upon. In neither case did I feel guilty. In both cases everyone involved was under a lot of stress and seeking outside comfort. In both cases, the relationships ended amicably and at mutually agreeable times. Subsequently, my primary relationship dissolved, and it was clear that the relationship had been lacking sufficient sensuality and sexuality, among other problems, which led to my acting upon these prior feelings.

Another story conveys the intensity of sexual feeling that can arise between colleagues. Note that the physicians involved were away from their normal work routine, a situation that often creates boundary confusion.

Case illustration 17: I was taking a trip to the theater district in New York with my new boss. We were there to attend some meetings but mostly to write a grant that was due shortly after we got back. I know I was attracted to him and hadn't thought about the feelings being reciprocated until we were on our way to a Broadway show and I realized he had his arm around me the way boys used to do when I'd go out on a date as a teenager. When we walked up to join a group of people he knew, he quickly jerked his arm away. I was surprised and amazed. Later when we each went back to our respective hotel rooms which happened to be next door [to each other], fantasies kept crowding into my concentrated efforts to write a portion of the grant. I did a lot of yoga just to cool down but recognized that if he had made a move, I would have said yes willingly and lived with the negative consequences for my marriage later. He never asked.

Although we are all aware of situations in which physicians meet in training or professional work and develop long-term love relationships, we did not hear any stories of this kind in our groups.

Boundary Crossings & Power

Although the preceding incident occurred between a faculty member and her boss, the power differential between them does not seem to have played much of a role. Often, however, when boundary crossings occur between people of unequal power, the consequences are intensified and potentially more dangerous (with sexual harassment representing the extreme case).

Power differences can be explicit, as in the formal hierarchies of medical teaching institutions, or implicit, based on differences in age, gender, social status, access to knowledge and resources, and the like. The doctor-patient relationship is often a good example of an implicit power differential. Adult learner-teacher relationships can involve formal or informal power relationships, depending on the situation (for a more extended discussion of this point, see Gordon, Labby, and Levinson). The following story written by a woman attending physician, describes the complex interaction of sexuality in a semiformal teacher-learner relationship.

Case illustration 18: Several years ago at a seminar, I had a facilitator with whom I had very charged interactions throughout the week. I saw us as being very similar in style and personality; we were both somewhat dramatic, a bit flamboyant and flirtatious, and expressive about our reactions and feelings. Initially, the experience was positive and added energy to the process; but as the week wore on, we began to clash and irritate one another . . . Ultimately, he, in front of the group in which we both participated, accused me of being seductive and "sucking him up." I felt shamed, humiliated, and angry. Sometime later we discussed the incident and he apologized. Our relationship remains amicable but still strained when we've interacted since in various professional ways and subsequent courses.

Note the similarity of this type of colleague relationship, based on an asymmetry of power, to boundary confusions in the doctor-patient relationship, in which the provider denies any role in encouraging or at least not discouraging increasing sexual tension in the relationship.

Sexual Harassment

Reported to be fairly common in medical settings, particularly in training, narratives of sexual harassment were rarely reported in our sessions. The only sexual harassment story reported in our data illustrates how power in an academic medical hierarchy allowed a department chairman to personally and professionally devastate a junior faculty member.

Case illustration 19: First job out of residency, at a teaching hospital. My direct supervisor was also the chairperson of the department. He began keeping me late after hours to discuss new directions in the department which he wanted me to be involved in. Then it was multiple phone calls to my office almost every day for after-hours dinners which I refused for 3 months. Day after day he still would call. I explained that I would meet him over lunch to discuss pertinent issues, but he refused these counteroffers. He began to "question my loyalty to the department." He spontaneously began to relate stories of his past career—talking without bridges to inappropriate issues—for example, how he could "sky-write with his penis." He next wanted me to join him in coffee houses to meet Friday–Sunday every week to do intensive "group" work.

When I refused all these advances he began to write memos of my "uncooperativeness." I felt forced out of the workplace by his threats to fire me.

SHAME & HUMILIATION

These two themes run through many of the narratives we studied. As described by Lazare, there is a high, and generally unrecognized, potential for shame and humiliation in medical encounters. Some of these feelings may be potentiated by the nature of medical care—particularly the physical examination—and the inability of many physicians to deal with sexual issues; a tendency reinforced by years of ignoring or denying sexual feelings in medical education. The following narrative illustrates the extent to which lack of sexual awareness on the provider's part can cause shame and humiliation in the patient.

Case illustration 20: The only really uncomfortable experience I had was a rectal exam I did on a young man about 17 or 18 . . . I was just going through my list, it was very mechanical. And I told him what I was going to do and he [replied with a sense of dread], "Oh, wow!" And it just didn't click, you know. I just should have backed off and instead I just said, "Okay, well just go ahead, bend over and we'll get this done." And afterward, just the look on his face of horror and embarrassment and humiliation and tears almost in his eyes just made me feel awful. And he just said, "I don't believe you did that." He left and I thought that [going through with the examination after all] probably was not the best thing I could have done. I felt really bad after that.

Similarly, as one participant's narrative illustrates, feelings of shame and humiliation can occur where professional boundaries are crossed.

Case illustration 21: I was a third-year medical student on a surgery rotation scrubbed in the OR. My resident came up behind me and reached around my waist and untied my scrub pants. Because I could not leave the sterile field I stood holding my pants with my elbows until a nurse took pity on me and helped me out—I was very humiliated.

Note that this "shaming" of the student by the resident could also be considered harassment, irrespective of gender.

Finally, shame and embarrassment may accompany encounters in which cultural differences in values and orientations exist. The narratives that touch on this theme include one from a Pakistani physician who describes the embarrassment of being kissed and hugged by a grateful nurse. Although the behavior described would seem innocuous in an American or Western context, it caused significant embarrassment for the resident in whose own cultural context such behavior is considered highly inappropriate.

DISCUSSION

From reviewing the 55 narratives collected during our workshops, we have learned that sexuality and sexual feelings are present in many types of workplace interactions in medicine including training, patient care, and peer relationships. The majority of narratives in our sample (29 of 55) focused on a type of sexual issue that we have defined as boundary confusion. The most salient feature of these cases is the awareness or perception of another's behavior (patient, supervisor, or peer) toward the doctor as being potentially sexual in nature, creating an ambiguous or "clouded" interactional field. There were many fewer examples of boundary crossings where more explicit behavior is initiated by one or the other party. Finally, we saw no examples in our data of true boundary violations in which the provider deliberately exploited a patient's vulnerability and indulged in professional privilege.

Ours is not a representative sample, but we believe that the vast majority of sexual boundary issues in the medical workplace involve confusion around personal and professional identity and role, particularly for residents. Learning about appropriate personal and professional boundaries is one of the most important and challenging developmental tasks for young physicians, one which relates to all aspects of emotional involvement with patients. Residents struggle with such difficult questions as: How close should I get to patients I like or identify with? How much can I be personally affected when patients do not do well, or die?

A related task is learning to identify and meet one's own emotional needs without adversely affecting patient care. In our resident narratives we see these boundary struggles playing out in the sexual realm. What we find most striking about these narratives is the sense of confusion; about the other's intentions, about the residents' own feelings and behavior, and about how to deal with these emotionally charged interactions.

Unfortunately, there seems to be little opportunity in undergraduate medical training or residency to discuss these important issues. As a consequence, students and residents are often left to their own devices in terms of developing healthy approaches to boundaries. In addition to preventing some physicians from providing necessary care (as previously discussed), the lack of opportunity to discuss sexually confusing situations may have other negative effects, such as encouraging boundary crossings and violations.

Opportunities for students and residents to discuss personal feelings and role play difficult or challenging situations on a regular basis can help in the development of healthy approaches to sexuality in the medical workplace.

We were impressed by the apparent lack of reflection given by physicians to the reasons patients may attempt to test or cross sexual boundaries in a medical encounter. We find it useful to explore with physicians (and especially residents) a range of possible reasons that patients "come on" to physicians. These include the physician's own needs and communication patterns, patients' needs to control, anxiety, and psychiatric impairment. Again, facilitated opportunities for self-reflection and discussion are useful in improving awareness of the complex nature of these interactions.

Some physicians do acknowledge enjoying their sexually charged interactions with patients, at least initially. Others express discomfort or anxiety with patients' boundary crossings, but don't know how to set limits in a caring way. This may reflect the confusion noted earlier about caring and personal involvement. Little guidance is available to help physicians in training to acquire appropriate limit setting skills. Workshops, clinical demonstrations, and observed interviews with "difficult" patients over time are useful in teaching limit setting.

Boundary confusions and crossings in patient care dominated resident sessions, but seemed to be less common with increasing experience. Perhaps as physicians become more confident and comfortable with professional identity, and have opportunities for more fulfilling personal lives, they project a clearer sense of boundaries. They may also have learned to relate to patients within the boundaries of a caring but professional relationship. They do not need, for example, "to be the patient's friend," a typical medical student conflict.

In sessions with more senior physicians, the focus was more on relationships between colleagues. Several revealed clear parallels between the physician's personal issues regarding intimacy, loneliness, and behavior at work. We are not entirely certain about why collegial stories dominate among more senior physicians. Perhaps as physicians mature, marry and begin their own families, they focus more on peer relationships and experiences. For academic physicians there may be less intense exposure to patients and more emphasis on interactions with colleagues. Whatever the reasons, workplace issues involving sexuality seem to correspond with different levels of training and expertise. Continuing medical education programs should reflect these differences.

Finally, shame and humiliation seem to accompany a significant number of the interactions reported in participants' narratives. Of particular relevance is the fact that much of the potential for shame and humiliation appears to go unrecognized. Physical examination skills and cross-cultural aspects of care are two areas where increased attention and awareness would be useful. Support groups and targeted clinical exercises are useful in bringing to light the potential for shame and humiliation in medical work, as well as providing the requisite skills to deal with this problem.

CONCLUSIONS & RECOMMENDATIONS

- It is important for physicians in training, as well as practicing physicians, to recognize and talk about the importance of sexual feelings in all aspects of medical work. Acceptance of one's own sexual feelings is a subset of acceptance of feelings in general.
- It is also important to be able to separate sexual feelings from sexual actions and to work through issues of guilt, shame, and personal needs.
- Most sexual issues in patient care involve confusion over appropriate ways to demonstrate caring, or confusion between physician and patient needs.
- True boundary violations are more likely to relate to power and vulnerability, than to sex per se.
- For medical providers, rigid boundaries based on legal and ethical codes alone are insufficient as guides to behavior. A relational and developmental approach is more helpful in understanding appropriate boundaries in any particular relationship.
- Such an approach requires awareness of the physician's own feelings and needs as well as those of the patient.

We recommend and encourage the use of facilitated discussion groups, workshops, support groups, and personal awareness groups as well as individual and group therapy to encourage open discussions of sexual issues in the workplace. These approaches can increase self-awareness, prevent unconscious acting out of sexual needs, help distinguish feelings from actions, and help trainees and practitioners develop appropriate personal and professional boundaries.

We close with the following story, which eloquently embodies the basic principles of dealing with sexual tensions (and many other emotionally laden issues) in the doctor-patient relationship. Being aware of one's feelings and accepting them, distinguishing one's own feelings or needs from the patient's, and separating feelings from actions.

Case illustration 22: Some years ago, as a fellow, I had a patient referred to me by another patient. She was my age, stunningly dressed, with all the physical characteristics I have found to be beautiful. I was unmarried and, at the time, searching for a mate.

When I met her in my office, there was an unforgettable moment of heightened tension. She was the paradigm of physical beauty to me, I was the doctor who her closest friend had spoken so highly of. I wondered if I could get through the session while maintaining my professionalism—and without compromising my ability to care for this person.

My questions were the same ones I ask every new patient. They included inquiries about education, work, professional aspirations, significant relationships, principal stressors, past use of, or desire for, professional counseling . . . and what one does for fun. As my questions were asked, her attraction for me seemed to meet my initial attraction for her. Fortunately, in yet another fateful moment, I realized that this was a terribly sad, lonely, needy, albeit beautiful woman. She needed counseling more than a boyfriend. The last thing she needed was an intimate relationship with her new doctor.

My composure regained, I sighed a sigh of relief and mustered enough courage to proceed with the physical exam.

SUGGESTED READINGS

Council on Ethical and Judicial Affairs, American Medical Association: Sexual misconduct in the practice of medicine. JAMA 1991;266(19):2741.

Gabbard GO, Nadelson C: Professional boundaries in the physician-patient relationship. JAMA 1995;273(18):1445.

Gordon G, Labby D, Levinson W: Sex and the teacher-learner relationship in medicine. J Gen Intern Med 1992;7:443.

Gutheil TG, Gabbard GO: The concept of boundaries in clinical practice: Theoretical and risk-management dimensions. Am J Psychiatry 1993;150(2):188.

Kilborn PT: In a rare move, agency acts swiftly in a sexual harassment case. New York Times, January 10, 1995. A–16.

Lazare A. Shame and humiliation in the medical encounter. Arch Int Med 1987;147:1653.

McDaniel S, Campbell T, Seaburn D: *Family Oriented Primary Care.* Springer-Verlag, 1990.

Peterson MR: *At Personal Risk: Boundary Violations in Professional-Client Relationships.* Norton, 1992.

Sheehan KH et al: A pilot study of medical student abuse: A student perceptions of mistreatment and misconduct in medical school. JAMA 1990;263(4):533.

Sherman C: Behind closed doors: Therapist-client sex. Psychol Today. May/June 1993:64.

Silver HK, Glicken AD: Medical student abuse: Incidence, severity, and significance. JAMA 1990;263(4):527.

Suggestion & Hypnosis

6

John F. Christensen, PhD

INTRODUCTION

Over the last two centuries, the history of hypnosis as a healing art has varied from acceptance as a treatment modality to dismissal as a parlor trick. Discredited in 1784 by a French royal commission appointed to investigate the healing techniques of Mesmer (although commission chairman Benjamin Franklin did note that belief might influence bodily effects), in more recent decades, hypnosis has regained respectability as a medical procedure. Hypnosis appears to be a special manifestation of the mind-body system's ability to process information by transducing it from a semantic to a somatic modality. Its therapeutic effectiveness is supported by both research and clinical experience. Today, hypnosis is widely used as an adjunctive or primary treatment for a variety of conditions—from pain, airway restriction, skin lesions, burns, anxiety, and preparation for surgical procedures to habit change (such as smoking cessation or dieting).

Trance and suggestion occur naturally throughout human experience and are a function of how the mind works. Being absorbed in a novel and ignoring surrounding sounds or daydreaming while driving and not remembering the last few miles are common experiences that illustrate the ubiquitous nature of trance. Responding to subliminal messages in advertising by thinking about purchasing a product—or actually doing so—represents ordinary reactions to suggestions made in a carefully crafted trance. These common human experiences of trance and suggestion also occur with patients in health care. The power of certain somatic sensations (eg, abdominal pain) to evoke a trance (a restriction of the field of the patient's awareness to the abdominal region), coupled with autosuggestion as to the meaning of the symptom (eg, "I wonder if that could be cancer"), increases attention to the sensation and may prompt a visit to the doctor.

The medical encounter can be considered a trance phenomenon; there is a natural absorption of patients in their somatic symptoms, and the clinical environment concentrates the focus of awareness on some aspects of experience. Because patients in this naturally occurring trance may be in a hypersuggestible state, it is important to avoid making negative suggestions and to be alert to opportunities for making positive, health-promoting suggestions. Because clinicians, too, can be induced into a complementary trance that maintains the focus on pathology, they must be alert to their own trances and find ways of shifting their awareness.

DEFINITIONS

Derived from a Greek word meaning "sleep," hypnosis is in fact a therapeutic procedure that requires active cooperation on the part of the patient. The following definitions, which will be used in the course of this chapter, describe the states and processes involved:

Trance: A state of focused attention, in which a person becomes uncritically absorbed in some phenomenon and defocused on other aspects of reality. Trance states can be positive or negative.

Suggestion: A communication that occurs in trance, with special power to elicit a particular attentional, emotional, cognitive, or behavioral sequence of events.

Hypnosis: A communicative interaction that elicits a trance in which other-than-conscious processes effect therapeutic changes in the subject's mind-body system. Hypnosis can be other- or self-induced.

Induction: The process by which a trance is initiated. This can occur naturally or as the first phase of hypnosis.

Utilization: The therapeutic use of trance to achieve desired outcomes and the phase of hypnosis following induction in which this occurs.

TRANCE & SUGGESTION IN THE MEDICAL ENCOUNTER

Both patient and clinician undergo a mutual trance induction that, depending on the self-awareness of the participants, can leave either more susceptible to suggestion. This state is neither pathologic nor unwarranted, but part of the natural pattern of human awareness in this environment. Generally, because of the power imbalance inherent in help-seeking situations, the patient is more vulnerable to suggestion. Being cognizant of trance and suggestion can give clinicians greater flexibility and influence in leading their patients to more positive outcomes.

Many patients waiting in an examining room are in a trance that has developed through a series of events that started with the onset of the symptom. The patient's awareness of this stimulus then leads to an internal search for meaning. Prior beliefs, personal experience, or the prompting of family or friends may lead the patient to attribute a particular meaning to the symptom. This attribution constitutes the initial suggestion, which in turn increases awareness of the sensation and further restricts the patient's attentional field. Increased absorption in the symptom and decreased awareness of other sensations are the essence of the trance.

The decision to see the doctor further deepens the trance, and this process continues as the patient rehearses how to describe the symptom and discuss it with the doctor. As noted earlier, this process of trance-induction around a symptom is not pathologic, but part of the natural unfolding of awareness surrounding a medical visit. Further trance induction occurs in the doctor's office with the experience of waiting in the waiting room, absorbing the sights and sounds of the clinic, encountering the nurse and, finally, waiting in the examining room for the doctor to open the door.

By the time the physician enters the room, the patient is in a trance and consequently in a hypersuggestible state. Whatever the provider says or does not say in the course of the interview can, because of the power generated by the patient's suggestibility, further develop the patient's trance, shift its focus, augment or diminish the patient's somatic awareness, and influence ongoing patient emotions, cognitions, and behaviors surrounding the symptom.

It is not only the patient, but the provider as well, who is susceptible to trance. Patients can sometimes unwittingly induce a trance in the provider through a combination of verbal and nonverbal techniques. The initial verbalization of the problem, hand gestures, grimacing, changes in voice tone and tempo, all contribute to focusing the attention of the provider on the problem or on what hurts. This narrowing of the physician's focus (even while a differential diagnosis is being developed) precludes other internal images, such as the future good health of the patient or a positive

doctor-patient relationship, that could otherwise give rise to helpful discussions. A too-rapid response by the physician results in premature closure on the nature of the patient's problem and solidifies the provider's initial trance. Attending to and eliciting the whole story from the patient (see Chapters 1 and 2), on the other hand, keeps that focus fluid. Sometimes patients induce a recurrent negative trance in the provider, leading to antagonism or aversion for the patient or to feelings of powerlessness in the face of the patient's problem (Chapter 4).

> *Case illustration:* A 55-year-old single woman was being followed by her primary care physician for chronic chest pain after a thoracotomy. Pain complaints, which became the patient's sole basis for her visits, continued for several months. The physician discovered that the pain restricted the patient's life by causing her to withdraw from social activities. Continued complaints appeared inconsistent with the progress of healing around the surgical wound, however. Various pain-management strategies that the physician proposed, including physical therapy, acetaminophen, and a tricyclic antidepressant, had little effect on the complaints. Both patient and doctor became frustrated with the visits. The patient would leave, dissatisfied that nothing new was being done for her pain; the physician felt powerless to affect the patient's suffering.
>
> Eventually, when the physician saw the patient's name on the appointment schedule, he would have a sinking feeling and tightness in his stomach, and his breathing would become more shallow. As he walked into the examining room and observed the patient's slumped posture and grim facial expression, he could predict how the discussion would go:
>
> DOCTOR: How have you been doing since our last visit?
>
> PATIENT: (*pointing to her chest, and responding with slow speech and long latencies*) This pain really has hold of me, and I can't escape it.
>
> DOCTOR: (*anticipating a negative answer*) Did you try any of the exercises the physical therapist recommended?
>
> PATIENT: (*grimacing, shifting position, looking down and then back at doctor*) I've tried that before, and it only makes the pain worse. (*eyes filling with tears*) Can't you do something for me?

This case illustrates several components of trance in both patient and doctor. The patient's recurring chest pain induces a trance of suffering and disability; her attention is withdrawn from the field of all possible objects and becomes narrowly focused on her somatic awareness. Anticipation of a visit to her doctor further restricts her focus, and her rehearsal of how she can convince the doctor of how bad it really is further heightens the trance. She has learned to associate the image of her doctor's face and the sound of his voice with frustrating discussions about the intractable nature of her pain. Her continued presence at these appointments corresponds with a belief that the power to alleviate her suffering lies outside of her-self—if only this doctor knew everything there was to know about her pain, he would be able to help. This expectation keeps her in a hypersuggestible state.

The doctor, too, has shifted into a negative trance by the time he enters the examining room. The induction began as he saw the patient's name on the schedule. His accompanying somatic responses shifted his focus to his own powerlessness to effect change—and away from his habitual openness to the field of possibilities. His trance is deepened by the patient's non-verbal and verbal communications about continuing pain. The doctor is more vulnerable to suggestion, and the patient's plea to do something for her builds in him the expectation that he must indeed do something. This expectation, in the face of the patient's persistent pain, deepens his sense of powerlessness.

Therapeutic Uses of Trance & Suggestion in the Medical Encounter

The clinician can use the patient's trance to make specific suggestions that enhance therapeutic outcomes. It is worth noting that the language used in medical encounters can lead to unintended patient beliefs and behaviors that influence both illness and healing. For example, the prediction of continued problems for a patient with a weak knee—"You'll probably always be bothered by some pain in that joint"—in the first postsurgical visit has enhanced power to influence the patient's future awareness of and belief in the knee's integrity. The warning becomes a self-fulfilling prophecy as the patient unwittingly guards the knee and develops a compensatory gait. A positive suggestion—"Whatever residual discomfort you feel, in time you will notice more freedom of motion and activity"—can create expectations that are more likely to enhance healing and the resumption of activity.

A more subtle consideration is the use of positive images and avoidance of negative modifiers. Consider the following statement to a patient after surgery:

DOCTOR: Your ankle ought to hurt less in a few weeks.

The unconscious mind tends to delete negative modifiers, in this case "less." The embedded suggestion becomes: "Ankle . . . hurt . . . in a few weeks." A positive suggestion would be:

DOCTOR: You will notice much more freedom from pain within a few weeks.

Because the primary words of the sentence are positive, the suggestion might be incorporated as:

DOCTOR: You will notice . . . freedom . . . within a few weeks.

In the context of discussing sleep hygiene with an insomniac patient, the well-intended suggestion,

"When you go to bed, try not to worry about staying awake," might contain several unintended messages leading to disturbed sleep. The word "try" connotes effort; it becomes associated with "bed"; the negative modifier "not" is deleted by the unconscious mind, leaving the additional message to "worry about staying awake." The suggestion could be positively restated:

DOCTOR: After you get into bed, I want you to enjoy a few minutes of deep relaxation before falling soundly asleep.

Clinicians can also use temporal clauses to embed suggestions that lead to positive patient expectations. For example, linking pain with expectations for healing can be accomplished by the following statement:

DOCTOR: When you first experience postoperative pain, it is important to realize that the healing has already begun.

Predicting positive change that precedes the patient's awareness of it can build positive expectations—even if the discomfort continues. For example, the physician might predict the course of recovery as a patient responds to antidepressant medication:

DOCTOR: Your spouse and others close to you will notice the changes in you long before you begin to feel better.

The implied suggestion is that you will begin to feel better, and when you do, positive changes will already have occurred.

The provider can also reframe uncomfortable side effects of some medications as an indicator of their potency, thus enhancing the placebo effect. In prescribing an antidepressant, the physician could disclose the anticipated side effects:

DOCTOR: If you notice this kind of discomfort as you begin to adjust to the medication, keep in mind that this is a potent drug that has the capability of achieving the results you and I want.

The message contains two positive associations with the side effects: adjustment to the medication, and movement toward the desired outcome.

The clinician who appreciates the trance nature of the medical encounter can use the patient's openness to suggestion not only to present positive suggestions and avoid those that are negative, but also to promote healing. This is true both for the clinician's own trance and that of the patient.

Shifting from a Negative to Positive Trance

When clinicians become aware that they or their patients are in a dysfunctional trance that runs counter to the goals of healing, several options can shift the trance in a more open direction.

Changing Body Position: This works directly with the somatic configuration that maintains a trance state. A depressed patient may hold that state somatically by means of a frozen, slumped posture, downcast eyes, and shallow breathing. This frozen posture amplifies negative self-images and self-statements and inhibits any focus on possibilities for change. The physician can comment on this posture and suggest modifications, such as looking up frequently; raising the eyes to observe cloud formations, birds, or airplanes; and shifting breathing to the abdomen. The physician might also suggest that the patient occasionally put on some music and dance—even alone—at home. Clinicians, too, can use a shift of physical position to break an unwanted trance in themselves. A physician who feels ineffectual in the face of an inordinately blaming or demanding patient and reacts physically with chest tightness and throat constriction can stand up, say, "Excuse me while I adjust the light," walk to the window, adjust the blinds or shade, move the chair to a slightly different location, and then sit down. During this activity, the physician can shift breathing to the abdomen and prepare to open a new line of discourse with the patient:

> DOCTOR: It's quite obvious how frustrated you are with the way things are going. Let's refocus for a moment on our goals and how things will look for you then.

Confusion: Confusion can be helpful for breaking a pattern that locks patient and clinician into repeatedly acting out a script whose negative outcome both can predict:

> PATIENT: Fix me.
>
> DOCTOR: Try this.
>
> PATIENT: That won't work.
>
> DOCTOR: What do you think will work?
>
> PATIENT: I don't know. You're the doctor.

When the clinician becomes aware of such a pattern, it is helpful to ask oneself, "What is the patient predicting I will say or do next?" If at this point the clinician can do something unpredictable, the result will be temporary confusion, which can be used to shift the patient's trance in a more resourceful direction. The unpredictable action might be something that can be called the "Columbo technique" (named for the television detective). In this technique, the physician suddenly and dramatically remembers some minor personal problem (eg, forgetting a spouse's birthday gift), asks the patient's forgiveness for the distraction, and requests the patient's aid. The momentary confusion that ensues (whether or not the patient is able to offer any help) breaks the previous trance and allows formation of a new one. This temporary role reversal is only one example of the use of unpredictable behavior to induce confusion, interrupting the pattern, and allowing greater rapport or more effective communication.

Mining for Gold: This phrase refers to a technique that shifts the focus of discussion away from distress and toward an exploration of the patient's resources. Useful at any time, this is especially helpful when the tone of meetings with the patient is persistently hopeless, when the patient appears to legitimize the visit by focusing exclusively on somatic complaints, or when the patient's continuing complaints make the clinician feel ineffective or frustrated. In mining for gold, the physician may inquire about things the patient is proud of—past successes, hobbies, travels, relationships, and obstacles overcome. The clinician observes when the patient becomes animated or otherwise shifts from the negative trance and notes the topic in the chart, returning to this topic briefly in subsequent sessions. Sometimes the change in the patient's state leads to a change in behavior, emotions, or outlook that had been precluded by the "what's wrong with me" trance. Similarly, the clinician's feeling about the patient may change; renewed interest and curiosity about the patient's personal resources may transform the previously difficult relationship.

Eliciting Target States: Here the clinician engages the patient in thinking and talking about a future well state, asking the patient to describe what things will be like when the medical problem is resolved or no longer interferes with the patient's life. It is important that the patient be able not only to name the target state ("I want to feel good again" or "I want to be free of pain"), but also to generate visual, auditory, and kinesthetic images of activities associated with that state. This discussion helps physician and patient establish criteria for knowing when the problem is resolved; it also engages the patient in imagining a well state unrelated to and incompatible with present suffering. This trance shift may be accompanied by positive physiologic changes and increased animation and hope.

> *Case illustration (Contd.):* In the case cited of the woman with post-thoracotomy pain, the physician tried using the technique of eliciting a target state to alter the patient's trance.
>
> PATIENT: (*grimacing*) I feel trapped. I never imagined it would hurt this bad.
>
> DOCTOR: How do you imagine it will be when you've completely recovered from your surgery?
>
> PATIENT: Well, I hope I'll feel better.
>
> DOCTOR: Well, let's think about what that would be like for you. Once you're feeling better, what do you see yourself doing differently?
>
> PATIENT: Fly fishing.
>
> DOCTOR: (*smiles; eyebrows raised, voice more animated*) You like to fish? (*the doctor is himself is a fly fisherman and has shifted automatically into a state of high interest*)
>
> PATIENT: (*looks at doctor, smiles*) I used to enjoy being out on the river in my waders, fishing for steelhead and Chinook salmon.

The interview proceeded for the next 3 minutes with a discussion between doctor and patient of various rivers they had fished. The patient had momentarily shifted her mental imagery and her kinesthetic state away from the pain trance toward future health. This created the context in which she could construct a full sensory image of that future well state, to which she could attach her hope and orient her activities. Her image of herself fishing was incompatible with the pain behaviors she had displayed. The doctor was no longer associated exclusively with her pain awareness, and in subsequent visits he became associated with recovery images. The doctor's impression of the patient also changed, so that he looked forward to their meetings instead of dreading them.

MEDICAL APPLICATIONS OF HYPNOSIS

As an alternative or ancillary mode of treatment, hypnosis can be an effective therapeutic option for a variety of problems. The neurophysiologic processes by which hypnosis can effect change in such a wide range of complaints are still open to debate. One current theory uses information processing as a heuristic model, regarding the body, brain, cells, and organs as an information-processing system. In the brain, semantic information (encoded in language) is transduced into molecular information that uses neurochemical and neurohormonal channels to cause changes in diverse organ systems.

In deciding whether to use hypnotic procedures with patients (or to refer them to a hypnotherapist), it is important to consider patients' beliefs about hypnosis, their openness to other therapeutic modalities, and their locus of control. Some religious groups (eg, Jehovah's Witnesses) forbid use of hypnosis, and some patients may fear that they will surrender control to a powerful "other," who can then control their minds. Brief education by the physician about the nature of hypnosis and its usefulness as a tool to help patients increase control over their symptoms may correct these beliefs. If the patients are not convinced, they are probably not good candidates for hypnosis.

Furthermore, some patients may resist hypnosis because they infer that the physician thinks the problem "is all in their head." For such patents, anything other than a biomedical intervention may be viewed with suspicion. Assuring them that hypnosis is simply part of a comprehensive medical management of their problem may increase their openness.

Locus of control—internal or external—is also a significant factor. Patients with an internal locus of control expect that they can influence many of life's rewards or punishments, and they may be better candidates for hypnosis than those with an external locus of control. This latter group may respond better to biofeedback, which relies on equipment that is external to the patient.

In the following brief descriptions of clinical situations, hypnosis can be considered as an adjunctive or, in some cases, primary treatment.

Relaxation & Stress Management: One of the physiologic effects of therapeutic hypnosis is stimulation of the parasympathetic nervous system. Several stress-related conditions have been attributed to hyperstimulation of the sympathetic nervous system, which is modulated by the parasympathetic in a dynamic interrelationship. Sympathetic activation can be part of the fight-or-flight response to perceived threats. Given the plethora of real or perceived threats in today's world, stress-related illnesses may be a common primary care presentation of patients' habitual levels of sympathetic arousal (see Chapter 29). Sympathetic responses include tachycardia, muscle tension, adrenaline release, pupil dilation, inhibited intestinal mobility, shortness of breath, and sweating. This autonomic activation is reversed during hypnosis, and with parasympathetic stimulation the individual becomes relaxed, leading to energy restoration, conservation, and renewal.

Anxiety: Hypnosis, or self-hypnosis, can be quite effective as a primary or adjunctive treatment for anxiety. Patients with an internal locus of control will find self-hypnosis an especially satisfying alternative to anxiolytic medication. When introducing this as an alternative treatment, the physician can say:

> DOCTOR: You have a powerful pharmacy in your brain that can produce significant healing effects. Through hypnosis you can learn to mobilize that pharmacy and let it work cooperatively with the other approaches we use.

The provider can devote 15–20 minutes to inducing a trance, suggesting that the patient imagine being in a relaxing place. If the session is audiotaped, patients can take the tape home for daily practice, learning to self-induce trances and regulate their own levels of autonomic nervous system arousal.

Pain Management: Since cortical elaboration of nociception is a component of pain, hypnosis can be used to shift the focus of attention away from pain sensations. In some surgical or dental procedures, hypnosis can be used as an adjunct to, or instead of, anesthesia. In addition, patients with chronic pain can be taught to relax the muscles they tense around areas of pain as part of their "guarding" or bracing efforts. This hypnotic relaxation reduces the component of the pain that is due to muscle contraction. Patients with migraine headaches can be taught to dilate blood vessels in their hands and feet through hand- and foot-warming imagery—sitting in front of a campfire, for example. In the early prodromal stage of migraine, this procedure can sometimes reverse the progress of the headache. Temporomandibular disorders and tension headaches have also been treated effectively with hypnosis.

Cancer: There is strong evidence that hypnosis is effective in alleviating the chronic pain associated with cancer. In addition, hypnosis can control symptoms such as nausea, anticipatory emesis, and learned food aversion; it is also helpful in managing anxiety and other emotions associated with cancer. There are indications that some patients can use hypnotic imagery to retard the progression of cancer tumors and, in some cases, achieve remission; controlled studies, however, have not yet demonstrated this.

Skin Problems: Certain dermatologic conditions, such as warts and alopecia, have been treated successfully with hypnosis. While in trance, patients are given the suggestion to experience tingling or flushing in the affected area. Warts may respond to these suggestions by shrinking in size or—in some cases—disappearing. Burns have also responded to hypnotherapeutic suggestion, both in lessening the degree of the burn and in controlling pain.

Immune System Function: Hypnosis has been used successfully to treat genital herpes, both in reducing the number of flare-ups and in decreasing the duration of flare-ups. Hypnosis has been shown to decrease blood levels of herpes simplex virus, increase T-cell effectiveness, and increase NK-cell activity.

Respiratory Problems: Asthmatic patients have been taught to use self-hypnosis to expand airways and minimize stress-induced attacks. Some patients are able to decrease their bronchodilator use with daily self-hypnosis.

Hypertension: Hypnosis for relaxation can be a useful adjunct to other therapies for hypertension. Daily practice, perhaps using an audio tape made in the doctor's office, can help patients reduce their blood pressure.

Gastrointestinal Problems: Problems such as irritable bowel and peptic ulcer that can be stress-related are amenable to adjunctive treatment with hypnosis. In one study on the use of hypnosis with irritable bowel syndrome, 85% of patients showed significant reduction or elimination of symptoms of abdominal pain, abdominal distention, diarrhea, and constipation. The primary approach is to reduce anxiety, induce relaxation, incorporate abdominal breathing, and suggest warmth in the abdomen and proper functioning in the bowels. Preoperative suggestions have been used successfully to promote an early return of gastrointestinal motility following intra-abdominal surgery, leading to shorter hospital stays.

Sleep Problems: Sleep-onset insomnia—associated with anxiety, obsessive worrying, or sympathetic arousal conditioned to the cue of getting into bed—can be treated with hypnotherapy. By making an audiotaped recording of an induction in which the patient is led into a relaxed state and invited to form positive associations with lying in bed before falling asleep, the clinician can give the patient a new nightly ritual that will enhance relaxation. A relaxing trance can also help the patient return to sleep more quickly after waking up.

Preparing for Surgical and Other Difficult Procedures: Patient expectations appear to play a role in the degree of pain and distress felt with surgery and such procedures as colonoscopy. Hypnosis has been used to anesthetize patients who are allergic to anesthetic drugs and to decrease the use of postoperative pain medication. Usually hypnotic anesthesia requires a deep level of trance, which calls for advanced skill on the part of the hypnotist along with the patient's ability to be hypnotized. Using the naturally occurring trance of patients anticipating surgery, physicians can make simple suggestions to enhance surgical wound healing and reduce postoperative pain. Referring to pain as "discomfort" or an "unusual sensation," the physician can offer a patient a statement such as:

> DOCTOR: No matter what you've been thinking about the time after surgery, you'll be pleasantly surprised at how little discomfort you have.

Table 6–1. Hypnotic smoking-cessation interview.

The following questions are designed not only to gather information about the patient's smoking behavior and its parameters, but also to raise the patient's awareness about behaviors that are usually automatic and unconscious. The interview presupposes that the patient has already expressed a desire to stop smoking.

- Have you ever quit smoking before? How long were you successful at curtailing your smoking? What allowed you to succeed at not smoking for that long?
- What other habits have you overcome? How have you done that?
- What brand of tobacco have you been using?
- What motivates you to continue smoking?
- Where do you have your first cigarette of the day?
- Where do you have your second cigarette?
- What is the sequence of activities that precede the first cigarette of the day?
- Describe the different situations in which you are likely to smoke.
- Describe the mood or emotional state that usually precedes smoking.
- Please describe the urge to smoke in detail.
- Describe how you light a cigarette (if the response is vague, offer the following prompts):
  - Which hand do you use to reach for the pack?
  - Which hand do you use to pull the cigarette out of the pack?
  - Which hand do you use to put it in your mouth?
  - Which hand do you use to light it?
  - Which hand do you use to continue smoking?
- Will you describe in detail all of the reasons that you can think of for not taking a first puff after you have stopped smoking?
- How long will you have to stop before you realize that you are permanently free of smoking?
- How will you tell people that you have stopped smoking?

Presurgical hypnosis can also decrease disorientation and confusion following surgery.

Habit Change: For patients in the **determination** or **action** stage of readiness to stop smoking or to change eating behavior (Chapter 16), hypnosis can be a useful ally. The ritual pattern of patient behavior around smoking can be viewed as a trance phenomenon. There is an automatic, other-than-conscious sequence of kinesthetic (tactile, visceral, emotional, and postural) awarenesses and behavior usually set in motion by contextual cues (eg, finishing a meal, drinking coffee or alcohol, talking on the telephone). Hypnosis can be described to patients in the determination stage as a useful tool "to help you come out of the smoker's trance and into a more satisfying, health-promoting trance." The clinician can call patients' attention to the automatic behavioral sequence while taking a hypnotic smoking history (Table 6–1). Asking patients to describe in detail which hand they use to pick up the cigarette pack, which hand they use to take the cigarette out of the pack, which to hold the lighter or strike the match, and so on will call their attention to the automatic, trance-like nature of their behavior. After inducing a hypnotic trance, the clinician can suggest that patients visualize in slow motion the entire sequence prior to lighting each cigarette. When the previously automatic behavior is raised to the level of awareness, patients are able to break the previous pattern and approach each episode of smoking with increased deliberation. Once patients are in the action stage of cessation, the parasympathetic effects of self-hypnosis can be used as an alternative stress-reducing activity.

SELF-HYPNOSIS

With proper training, patients who respond well to hypnotic trances can learn to self-induce hypnosis to achieve both relaxation and specific therapeutic effects. A useful transition to confidence in self-hypnosis is the patient's regular use of a taped hypnotic induction made by the clinician (primary care provider or referral specialist) in the office, thereby extending the clinician's presence into the patient's milieu. As the patient gains experience going into therapeutic trance by listening to the tape, the clinician can teach the patient one of several self-induction protocols, such as the one shown in Table 6–2 (this can also serve as a handout). Some patients are able to develop their skill at self-hypnosis and retain it as a life-long health resource.

REFERRAL FOR TREATMENT WITH HYPNOSIS

The various medical applications of hypnosis described above require one or more sessions with a trained hypnotherapist. Skilled hypnotherapists spend time with patients prior to hypnosis discussing their understanding and expectations of the hypnotic experience and addressing their anxieties and misconceptions. The aim here is to establish rapport and raise positive expectations in the patient's mind. When this preliminary discussion is completed, the clinician proceeds to the induction of a trance, using one of several approaches. (The specifics of these inductions are too numerous and complex to be discussed properly here, and special training is required to use them appropriately and with flexibility to the patient's responses.) Once the patient exhibits signs of a trance, the clinician proceeds to the utilization of that trance for the specific benefit desired. This involves offering suggestions for the patient to imagine changes in somatic sensations, emotions, or future behaviors. The clinician then concludes by alerting and reorienting the patient to the external surroundings. After the procedure, the hypnotherapist can discuss the patient's subjective experiences and answer questions.

As noted earlier, some primary care providers become trained in hypnosis (see the section titled "Training in Hypnosis,") so they can integrate this treatment seamlessly into their medical practices. Others may choose to refer to a specialist (psychiatrist, psychologist, clinical social worker, or psychiatric nurse practitioner) trained in hypnosis and familiar with its medical applications. In order to maximize the therapeutic outcome, it is essential that the referring

Table 6–2. Eyeroll technique for self-hypnosis.

1. Find a relaxed, quiet place to sit or lie down.
2. Open yourself to a few minutes of inner renewal and refreshment.
3. Use a one-two-three count:
   - One: Roll your eyes up to the top of your head.
   - Two: Slowly close your eyelids over raised eyes. Inhale deeply.
   - Three: Slowly exhale while you relax your eyes.
4. Continue breathing in a relaxed way from your abdomen.
5. Imagine yourself in some pleasant scene or experience for a few minutes.
6. Imagine the sights, sounds, feelings, and smells.
7. While imagining this scene, focus on the desired outcome of this trance (relaxation, pain reduction, etc).
8. To alert yourself, use a three-two-one-zero count:
   - Three: Tell yourself, "I'm ready to be alert."
   - Two: Roll your eyes up under your closed eyelids.
   - One: Slowly open your eyes and make a fist.
   - Zero: Relax your eyes and your hand. Enjoy reorienting yourself to your surroundings.

practitioner communicate with the specialist—before the visit—about the nature of the medical problem, the desired clinical outcome, and the patient's expectations about treatment. It is also important to prepare the patient by explaining the nature of therapeutic hypnosis and that its intent is to increase the patient's control over both symptoms and their impact.

TRAINING IN HYPNOSIS

Clinicians who are interested in developing their own skills in hypnosis are encouraged to receive formal training from an accredited training program or receive supervision from a licensed health professional with formal training in hypnosis. Three organizations that provide such training in the United States are the following:

■ The American Society of Clinical Hypnosis
(ASCH)
2200 East Devon Ave., Suite 291
Des Plaines, IL 60018-4534
Phone: (847) 297-3317
Fax: (847) 297-7309

The ASCH has chapters in many cities that provide introductory training for physicians, dentists, psychologists, and social workers. The organization certifies practitioners who have completed its training program. It holds annual regional and national meetings.

■ The Milton H. Erickson Foundation
3606 North 24th Street
Phoenix, AZ 85016-6500
Phone: (602) 956-6196
Fax: (602) 956-0519
e-mail: mhef103479@aol.com
Web site: http://www.erickson-foundation.org

The Erickson Foundation carries on the teaching, research, and clinical applications of hypnosis initiated by Milton H. Erickson, MD. It offers comprehensive international programs every two years and publishes a newsletter and lists of continuing education offerings.

■ O.T.C.C., Inc.
P.O. Box 697
Friday Harbor, WA 98250
Phone: (206) 378-4999
Fax: (206) 378-7266
e-mail: drdobson@otcc.com
Web site: http://www.otcc.com

O.T.C.C. (Other Than Conscious Communication), founded by David R. Dobson, PhD, offers seminars that run from a few days to a few weeks in length.

SUGGESTED READINGS

Bowen DE: Ventilator weaning through hypnosis. Psychosomatics 1989;30:449.

Cadranel JF et al: Hypnotic relaxation: A new sedative tool for colonoscopy? J Clin Gastroenterol 1994;18:127.

Christensen JF, Levinson W, Grinder M: Applications of neurolinguistic programming to medicine. J Gen Intern Med 1990;5:522.

Crasilneck HB: The use of hypnosis in the treatment of impotence. Psychiatr Med 1992;10:67.

Disbrow EA, Bennett HL, Owings JT: Effect of preoperative suggestion on postoperative gastrointestinal motility. West J Med 1993;158:488.

Gilligan S: Therapeutic Trances. Brunner/Mazel, 1987.

Haanen HC et al: Controlled trial of hypnotherapy in the treatment of refractory fibromyalgia. J Rheumatol 1991;18:72.

Kirsch I, Lynn SJ: The altered state of hypnosis: Changes in the theoretical landscape. Am Psychol 1995;50:846.

Levinson W: Reflections: Mining for gold. J Gen Intern Med 1993;8:172.

Levitan AA: The use of hypnosis with cancer patients. Psychiatr Med 1992;10:119.

NIH Technology Assessment Panel on Integration of Behavioral and Relaxation Approaches into the Treatment of Chronic Pain and Insomnia. JAMA 1996;276:313.

Patterson DR: Practical applications of psychological techniques in controlling burn pain. J Burn Care Rehabil 1992;13:13.

Rapkin DA, Straubing M, Holroyd JC: Guided imagery, hypnosis and recovery from head and neck cancer surgery: An exploratory study. Int J Clin Exp Hypn 1991;39:215.

Rossi E: The Collected Papers of Milton H. Erickson on Hypnosis, Vols I-IV. Irvington, 1980.

Rossi E: The Psychobiology of Mind-Body Healing. Norton, 1986.

Rossi E, Cheek D: Mind-Body Therapy: Ideodynamic Healing in Hypnosis. Norton, 1988.

Spiegel D et al: Predictors of smoking abstinence following a single-session restructuring intervention with self-hypnosis. Am J Psychiatry 1993;150:1090.

Syrjala KL, Cummings C, Donaldson GW: Hypnosis or cognitive behavioral training for the reduction of pain and nausea during cancer treatment: A controlled clinical trial. Pain 1992;48:137.

Whorwell PJ: Use of hypnotherapy in gastrointestinal disease. Br J Hosp Med 1991;45:27.

Whorwell PJ, Prior A, Faragher EB: Controlled trial of hypnotherapy in the treatment of severe refractory irritable bowel syndrome. Lancet 1984;2:1232.

Whorwell PJ et al: Physiological effects of emotion: Assessment via hypnosis. Lancet 1992;340:69.

Wyler-Harper J et al: Hypnosis and the allergic response. Schweiz Med Wochenschr Suppl 1994;62:67.

Zilbergeld B, Edelstein MG, Araoz DL: Hypnosis: Questions and Answers. Norton, 1986.

Managed Care

7

Geoffrey H. Gordon, MD

INTRODUCTION

The doctor-patient relationship is an integral part of medical care. Good doctor-patient communication improves health care outcomes and enhances patient satisfaction. Breakdown in communication is cited by patients as a frequent reason to change physicians, disenroll from managed care plans, or initiate malpractice litigation.

Managed care can present a variety of challenges to effective doctor-patient relationships and communication. First, long-standing relationships may be disrupted as patient and physician groups "change hands" in the managed care market. Second, physicians may have less time to spend with patients, limiting opportunities for effective communication. Third, patients joining health care plans may have unrealistic expectations or a sense of entitlement about their medical care. When their expectations collide with the charge to physicians to limit cost and use of medical care , both parties may lose trust in each other and seek administrative rather than clinical solutions to medical problems.

The following are brief statements by patients to their doctors. Each case illustration portrays a common dilemma in doctor-patient communication that is especially problematic in managed care (Table 7–1). Following each case illustration is a brief description of corrective techniques and procedures suggested by recent medical literature on doctor-patient communication.

Case illustration 1:

PATIENT: Oh, by the way, Doctor, I still have a few other things bothering me. You're not going to rush out the door again, are you? Can't we talk for more than 10 minutes?

This chapter is reprinted by permission of *The Western Journal of Medicine* (Gordon GH, Baker L, Levinson W: Physician-patient communication in managed care. 1995 [December];163:43:47)

This patient expects to talk with the doctor for more than the usual time allotted for a return visit in many managed care settings. The physician's goal in this situation is to help the patient feel "heard" without sacrificing efficiency. Sitting down and making eye contact is a simple but powerful facilitator of rapport. Allowing patients to finish their opening statements without interruption usually takes 2 minutes or less and establishes the importance of their concerns and participation in care. Matching patients' breathing and tempo of speech, followed by "pacing" them into a more efficient pattern, is a more sophisticated but potentially useful technique. Allowing brief pauses before each time you speak can increase the patients' estimation of the time spent in the visit.

Invite patients to voice all of their concerns early in the visit. This may avoid the problem of patients saving the most serious or difficult problems for last. Once all of the patient's concerns and requests are revealed, a consensual agenda for the present visit can be negotiated.

Ready-made lists of requests and problems that some patients compile and bring to the consultation are often seen as burdensome by doctors. Instead, physicians should recognize the usefulness of having all the items on the patient's agenda presented "up front" for negotiation. Consider acknowledging the patient's efforts.

DOCTOR: You've done a great job outlining your various concerns, and I appreciate the work you've put into this.

Then put the list into the chart. It is also important, however, to draw attention to the time constraints of the visit. This can be done in such a way as to emphasize the positive.

DOCTOR: The things you've brought up deserve more time than we have today, and fortunately we'll be able to cover them in detail over the next several visits. You can help me decide now which one is the most important to cover today.

Table 7–1. Suggested approaches to overcoming potential barriers to physician-patient communication in managed care settings.

Potential Barrier	Approach
The physician must care for too many patients in too little time.	Allow patients to offer and finish opening statements. Negotiate a consensual prioritized agenda for the visit. Respond to patients' reactions and concerns with empathy. Orient patients to the events of the visit.
The patient makes misguided or unreasonable requests of the physician.	Ascertain patient's beliefs about diagnosis and treatment. Acknowledge that doctors and patients may disagree. Empathize with patient's frustration arising from disagreement. Clarify ways in which you can and cannot help.
The patient demands referral to a specialist.	Empathize with the patient's feelings of concern or frustration. Frame the discussion in terms of the quality of the patient's health care, not administrative rules. Explain the use of specialty consultations in your managed care system. Counter feelings of distrust by creating a partnership with the patient.
The physician is confronted with managed care directives or restrictions that run counter to his or her clinical judgment as to what is best for the patient.	Identify what treatment the managed care plan does and does not cover. Differentiate between clinical, administrative, and ethical aspects of the problem. Clarify in your own mind your role and what you wish to communicate to the patient. Clarify your obligations regarding uncovered care needs.

For patients with emotionally distressing problems, empathy can be therapeutic without sacrificing efficiency. Cohen-Cole describes five elements of empathic communication: reflection, legitimization, respect, support, and partnership (Table 7–2). Patient expressions of emotion are often brief, self-limited, and responsive to direction by the physician. The best way to decrease the intensity of patients' emotions is simply to acknowledge the emotions rather than attempt to "remedy" the patient's emotional distress or discomfort. Visits that include discussion of patients' emotions are not significantly longer than visits without such discussions, and although such visits may seem more challenging to the physician, they are associated with greater patient satisfaction and compliance.

Finally, some patients truly do not know what to expect from a visit with a physician. They may need an initial orientation and subsequent redirection to the events of the visit. For example:

Table 7–2. Elements of empathic communication and corresponding statements by physician.

Element	Statement
Reflection	You're really feeling overwhelmed by these symptoms.
Legitimization	I can imagine how upsetting it is.
Respect	I can see you're doing your best to cope.
Support	I'd like to help.
Partnership	Maybe we can work on these together.

Source: Adapted, with permission, from Cohen-Cole SA: *The Medical Interview: The Three-Function Approach.* Mosby-Year Book, 1991.

DOCTOR: I can help you most if I can hear from you for a few minutes about what is bothering you. Then I'll ask you some short-answer questions. I may also want to examine you today. After we do those things I'll be able to discuss what we should do next. You might feel frustrated that we don't have more time, but I'm confident that we can use our time wisely to help you.

A brochure or handout in the waiting room explaining the organization of a routine office visit may be helpful.

Interruptions, repetitions, and premature assumptions are early signs of communication breakdown. If they occur, consider acknowledging that a communication problem exists and invite the patient's input:

DOCTOR: I think we both want to understand each other, but we're having trouble doing it. How can we get back on track?

MISGUIDED REQUESTS

Case illustration 2:

PATIENT: I always need antibiotics to get over these colds. I can't miss any more time at work, and the wife says "Don't come home without the pills." That's why we signed up for this health plan.

Some patients make specific requests that are medically unjustifiable. Most patients have beliefs or concerns about the meaning of their symptoms, based on lay literature, folk knowledge, or prior experiences with others' illnesses. Often a friend or family member is an informal health "advisor" who suggests diagnoses and treatments. Asking about these ideas and concerns is important, because patients may be unable to listen until they feel they have been heard and understood. Ask patients what they think is wrong with themselves. (Most patients already have some ideas about what is causing their medical problems: "What thoughts or concerns have you had?") Many patients will say, "I don't know, you're the doctor, that's why I'm here." Respond to this with, "Yes, I'll tell you what I think, but it's often helpful for me to know what you've already learned or worried about." Patients may reveal new data ("My brother thought he had a cold, but it was really pneumonia. He ended up on a breathing machine."). Before examining patients, ask "As I go about your physical examination, is there anything that you'd like me to pay particular attention to? " Ask patients what they think should be done for them ("What have you already tried? What else do you need to get better? "). Asking patients what others have said about the problem can also help reveal hidden concerns.

Misguided patient requests can also be driven by technologic advances, coupled with a sense of entitlement.

In addition to eliciting and discussing the patient's concerns (for example, worry about a brain tumor), physicians should be prepared to constructively discuss entitlement with patients.

Case illustration 3:

PATIENT: Doctor, I'm still getting those headaches. I brought in this article about MRI scans. I'm covered for that, aren't I?

DOCTOR: I can see you feel entitled to this test as part of your health care coverage. I want to confirm your entitlement to the very best medical opinions and services we have. In chronic migraine headaches like yours, with a normal neurologic exam, our specialists advise us that MRI scans simply don't add any new information.

Sometimes misguided requests represent an unrealistic quest for certainty.

PATIENT: Doctor, how can you be sure these are just migraines?

Rather than ordering more tests, consider addressing uncertainty together:

DOCTOR: Further testing won't really make us absolutely certain what you're feeling and may even be misleading. I'm confident that your headaches are following the pattern of what is called common migraine. I think that, with the opinions of specialists to guide us, we can follow you here in the office and be vigilant for signs of other diseases. You'll need to tell me about any changes in your symptoms, and I'll need to examine you periodically. In the meantime, we can help you cope with the headache symptoms.

A next step is to find ways to work with patients when their ideas or intentions conflict with your own. Acknowledge that a disagreement exists.

DOCTOR: This really puts us in a bind. We both have different ideas about what we should do to get you well.

Empathize with the patient's dilemma.

DOCTOR: I can see this hasn't worked out at all like you wanted. No wonder you're frustrated.

Consider using the following negotiation formula:

1. State the most specific goal on which you can both agree.
   DOCTOR: We seem to have solid agreement that the goal is to increase your comfort and control over this pain.

2. Respectfully acknowledge your different approaches to that goal.
   DOCTOR: Where we differ is on the role narcotics should play in achieving that goal.

3. Compromise where possible.
   DOCTOR: I'm willing to work with you on a plan that respects our different approaches and ultimately gives you the control you want without medications.

At times a mutually agreeable solution cannot be found, leaving both parties dissatisfied. It is important to acknowledge this dissatisfaction and to assert your belief that your relationship can withstand this impasse.

SEEING THE SPECIALIST

Case illustration 4:

PATIENT: I know how my insurance works. If you don't send me to the specialist, then you get to keep the money. But the gynecologist who did my conization said I should see him every 3 months. He really understood my care.

In this illustration, the patient's previous gynecologist is not a member of her new managed care plan. In the new plan, her primary doctor receives a fixed amount for her care, from which consultant expenses are deducted. The ongoing relationship she enjoyed with her gynecologist is gone, her new physician is cost-conscious, and she feels cheated and abandoned.

An early goal for the physician in this visit is to keep the focus on providing quality health care rather than the details of the new health plan. Address the patient's feelings of loss and frustration but explain her new plan in realistic, unbiased terms:

DOCTOR: I can understand how upsetting it must be to have your previous care interrupted. On the other hand, you've got a good plan. It allows you excellent medical care. It is restrictive on the use of specialists, however, and requires that I do things for you that we normally do in the office, such as pelvic exams and Pap smears. If something comes up that we both decide needs the input of a specialist, I'll help you get it.

The patient's ability to trust her new physician can also be dealt with explicitly:

> DOCTOR: It sounds as though you're not sure I'll have the knowledge or skills to take care of you properly, or worse, that I wouldn't act in your best interests. I want you to know that my goal, like yours, is to provide you the very best care we can. If at some point you feel we're not meeting that goal, I hope we can talk about it and reach a solution together.

Then do a thorough and careful examination as evidence of your competence and concern.

BENDING THE RULES

Case illustration 5:

> PATIENT: Doc, I haven't seen a dentist in years, and I can't afford to now. If you could make a referral saying that it aggravates my diabetes, then my plan will pay for it. Can you do that?

In some managed care plans, coverage for certain types of care (for example, dental, optometric, preventive, or mental health) is minimal or absent, depending on the level of care purchased. Physicians working in such plans should be familiar with what types of care are covered and denied, what specialists are available and their qualifications, and the physician's obligations to the plan and to the patient when specialty treatment is denied.

The physician in this case illustration has a number of options, reflecting her various roles. Administratively, she can refer the patient to a clerk or administrator, write in support of the patient's request, or become active in committees that determine eligibility rules. Clinically, she can request specialty consultation to evaluate the effect of the dental condition on diabetes (for example, "rule out dental infection"). At times this form of patient advocacy involves a degree of deception. For example, Novack found that physicians are willing to use deception in recording the reason for ordering a mammogram in a setting where tests ordered for "screening" are denied but those ordered to "rule out breast cancer" are approved. Ethically, the physician's duty to advocate for the individual patient conflicts with her duty to operate within the guidelines of the plan to provide cost-effective care to a population of patients. Professional society guidelines discourage physicians from engaging in "bedside rationing" and support the physician's role as an advocate for individual patients. Legally, if the plan denies care that the physician strongly feels

is indicated, she may have an obligation to contest the decision on the patient's behalf and to discuss all options with the patient including getting care outside the plan at the patient's expense. Although managed care plans may be held liable for a physician member's actions, courts may also hold physicians responsible for upholding community standards of care, even when this care is not covered by the plan.

In responding to requests to bend the rules, physician actions (and related communications to patients) can be impulsive, depending on their feelings about the individual patient, the ease of dealing with the managed care plan, and the time available to think about it. Such requests rarely require immediate action. The physician in this illustration should take time to consider the issues underlying the request, her various roles and goals in responding, and, if her roles conflict, which role takes priority. Then she should consider what she really wishes to communicate to the patient. An appropriate response might be:

> DOCTOR: I'm glad you mentioned this because hidden infections can cause problems with diabetes. You have some cavities, but I don't see any evidence of infection in your teeth or gums. At this point I can't really make the case that they are interfering with your diabetes. You should get them taken care of, however, before they cause a more serious condition.

Then document the episode and your response in the patient's chart.

MANAGED CARE CAN HELP DOCTOR-PATIENT RELATIONSHIPS

Managed care plans can help patients and physicians communicate more effectively. Plans can help patients by explicitly describing what to expect regarding time with the doctor, use of the telephone, use of the emergency room, the roles of other health care professionals (nurses and nurse practitioners, physician assistants, pharmacists, and others), referrals to specialists, and handling of grievances. Plans can help physicians by reviewing with them ways the plan's promises are marketed and limitations are disclosed to patients. Programs should be available to help patients self-manage common health problems and to educate providers in population-based as well as traditional dyadic medical care.

What is more, there should be a well-defined, physician-generated internal policy for dealing with difficult doctor-patient relationships, including a means for terminating a patient's relationship with an individual provider or with the entire plan. This can take the form of a standing interdisciplinary committee. There should also be a strong but sensitive central administrative physician to deal directly with patients who have insistent demands and contentious behaviors. This frees up primary providers to be advocates for good medical care and to negotiate about medical rather than administrative issues. Administrators and risk managers can unwittingly undermine physicians' efforts to provide safe, effective care for difficult patients by granting unreasonable requests for care or by using complaints about physicians as signs of inadequate care. Managed care plans may reasonably decide that for some patients who cannot cooperate with their physicians in obtaining safe, effective care, disenrollment is administratively preferable to provision of substandard care.

Finally, managed care plans should provide opportunities for communication skills training for providers. Administrators and providers should work together to identify mutual goals for such training and to ensure that the plan's overall policies support those goals. Goals for administrators and risk managers could include greater patient satisfaction and retention, and fewer complaints and lawsuits. Goals for providers could include fewer frustrating patient encounters, improved treatment compliance, and greater job satisfaction. All of these outcomes are demonstrably related to physician communication skills. Training is best conducted in a workshop format, with opportunities to review recent research findings in physician-patient communication, to practice new skills in realistic and relevant situations, and to work in small groups with liberal exchange of ideas and feedback. Such training is increasingly part of medical school, residency, and continuing education curricula.

SUGGESTED READINGS

Beckman HB et al: The doctor-patient relationship and malpractice. Arch Intern Med 1994;154:1365.

Cohen-Cole SA: *The Medical Interview: The Three-Function Approach.* Mosby-Year Book, 1991.

Emanuel EJ, Dubler NN: Preserving the physician-patient relationship in the era of managed care. JAMA 1995;273:323.

Epstein RM, Beckman HB: Health care reform and patient-physician communication. Am Fam Physician 1995; 49:1718.

Frankel RM et al: Can I really improve my listening skills with only 15 minutes to see my patients? HMO Practice 1991;5:114.

Hall RC: Legal precedents affecting managed care: The physician's responsibilities to patients. Psychosomatics 1993;34:166.

Lazare A: The interview as a clinical negotiation. In: Lipkin M Jr, Putnam SM, Lazare A (editors): *The Medical Interview: Clinical Care, Education, and Research.* Springer-Verlag, 1995.

Novack DH et al: Physicians' attitudes toward using deception to resolve difficult ethical problems. JAMA 1989;261:2980.

Quill TE: Partnerships in patient care: A contractual approach. Ann Intern Med 1983;98:228.

Schroeder JL, Clarke JT, Webster JR: Prepaid entitlements: A new challenge for physician-patient relationships. JAMA 1985;254:3080.

8

Physician Well-being

Anthony L. Suchman, MD, & Gita Ramamurthy, MD

INTRODUCTION

Case illustration: Don, a 38-year-old primary care physician, sighs as he sees Mrs. D.'s name as a last-minute addition to his patient list. It is midafternoon on Friday, and he had blacked out the last hour of the day to attend his son's final softball game. "Of all the days for one of her 'crying headaches,' " Don mutters to himself, "why today? "

Don's skill in handling patients with somatoform problems is respected throughout the health center. Since he assumed responsibility for Mrs. D.'s care, her emergency-department visits have fallen by 90%, and she has even taken a part-time job. Don has almost always been able to help her through these spells by sitting with her, holding her hands, and letting her talk.

When he was growing up, Don was always a leader; he was the pride of his home town, the young man people always thought would "make it out of this place." Now he is back home, as a founding partner in a successful regional health center—and with a waiting list of residents from the university hoping to rotate through his thriving primary care practice.

"Hey, Don!" The greeting comes from Grace, one of Don's partners. Briefcase in hand, she is moving toward the door. "What a great afternoon! My last patient just canceled—I'm going to go home, pour myself a glass of white wine, sit out on the deck, and catch up on some journals. Hope you have a great weekend."

The door opens, the door closes, and frustration, sadness, loneliness, and anger come together as Don watches Grace leave.

Primary care practice can be both an enriching source of personal growth and meaning and an unmerciful and depleting taskmaster. It provides us with access to a broad range of human experience—an intimate view of the characters and stories of a thousand novels—and an opportunity to have our very presence matter to others. At the same time, it makes constant demands and surrounds us with perpetual uncertainty; it relentlessly confronts us with our limitations of time, energy, knowledge, and compassion. It is a job that is never done; at best, problems are stabilized until something else goes wrong.

The balance each of us strikes between our own enrichment and depletion is critical to our own physical, emotional, and spiritual health and to our ability to care for others. All too often, however, we lose sight of this balance. We become so outwardly focused, attending to clinical problem-solving, that we do not tend to our own renewal. This lack of balance is not surprising; our education has taught us much more about how to care for others than how to care for ourselves. The socialization processes of medical school and residency have cultivated a variety of unrealistic self-expectations and attitudes while ignoring the basic communication and relationship skills essential to thriving in practice.

The result of this imbalance is a vague but increasing sense of demoralization. The joy of work is lost; patients seem increasingly annoying and adversarial. Work becomes the means to some other end—skiing trips or a vacation house—rather than meaningful in its own right. When the root causes of this dissatisfaction are invisible to us, we blame external sources such as the government, insurance companies, or lawyers. Although there are many legitimate complaints about restrictions and bureaucracy, the most fundamental determinants of satisfaction and well-being are not external but rather are found within.

This chapter discusses important values, attitudes, skills, and healthy work environments, but it must be remembered that simply reading a chapter is not enough to solve the personal problems that practitioners face. It can, however, help increase the practitioner's awareness of modifications that must be made and aid in addressing these essential changes.

BASIC NEEDS OF PRACTITIONERS

The foundation of our well-being is the acknowledgment that we are human, that we have needs and limits, and that to keep on giving we must know and have reliable access to those things that sustain and revitalize us. Unfortunately, the notion that we—clinicians—have needs has been virtually off-limits. An excessively narrow interpretation of the scientific model that guides our work has called on us to be detached and objective observers, leaving no room for our own subjective experience. Moreover, we are exposed early and repeatedly to the ideal of the clinician who is selfless, invulnerable, and omnipotent (the "iron man" model). This ideal is unrealistic at best and dangerous at worst, to both ourselves and our patients. Each of us has a variety of needs, both universal and neurotic, that will ultimately assert themselves. The more we can be aware of these needs and attend to them, consciously and purposefully, the healthier our lives will be.

Among our most fundamental needs are those for human connection, meaning, and self-transcendence—experiencing ourselves as part of something larger than we are. Clinical work is particularly rich with opportunity for human contact and appreciation. Many studies have shown the patient-clinician relationship to be the single most important factor contributing to physician satisfaction (mirroring its central importance to patients). When we are working under excessive pressure or in situations for which we are not adequately prepared, however, clinical work can interfere with the satisfaction of these needs, resulting in depersonalization and alienation from and hostility toward our patients.

Clinical work can also threaten the fulfillment of transpersonal needs through family and community life. Family and career often compete intensely for time and attention, too often to the detriment of the former. Moreover, we sometimes have difficulty shedding the white coat—leaving our professional caretaking role and expressing the spontaneity and vulnerability necessary for intimacy. As tensions build at home, putting more time into work can provide a short-term escape. In the long-term, however, avoidance of difficult relationship problems leads to alienation and potentially to the breakdown of a crucial support system.

In addition to our universal needs for connection and meaning, we also have very individual neurotic needs—born of pain and conflict—that are intimately related to our medical work. These needs influence both our motivation to go into medicine in the first place and the way we practice. Out of a need to feel loved or appreciated, we often find ourselves in the role of overfunctioning caretakers, and our difficulty saying no quickly leads to overcommitment. Feelings of impotence engendered by childhood experiences of illness—our own or that of a close friend or relative—

may be relieved through our work with patients, but the wishful fantasy of controlling disease is constantly challenged by reality. Voyeuristic desires, fear of death, and the fulfillment of parental expectations are other factors, conscious or unconscious, that can motivate our careers.

These darker, neurotic needs are no less legitimate than those less hidden; they, too, are a normal part of life. When these needs operate outside our awareness, however, they can drive us to work excessively, assume unrealistic degrees of responsibility, and otherwise distort our work lives, thereby causing us to suffer. If we invest ourselves in unrealistic solutions that must inevitably fail, we risk unsuccessful relationships, substance abuse, and even suicide. Through various processes of self-exploration (such as psychotherapy, peer support groups, or self-awareness workshops), we can become more aware of these needs that underlie our work and find healthier ways to satisfy them. We ignore them at our own peril.

PERSONAL PHILOSOPHY

Another important but underrecognized determinant of our well-being is personal philosophy—the deeply held beliefs and values that address the most fundamental questions of our lives: the meaning and purpose of life, death, joy, and suffering; why things happen the way they do; the nature of our relationship to other people and to the world; and the nature of our goals and responsibilities as human beings. Our personal philosophies define our expectations of ourselves and other people. They guide the way we perceive and respond to our world and help us identify our place in it. They define the framework by which we imbue things in our lives with meaning, joy, or pain and by which we determine what seems right and what seems wrong.

Developing a personal philosophy tends to be a subliminal process—a gradual internalization of attitudes and values from family, culture, education, and life experience. This process makes it possible for us to be entirely unaware of our core beliefs as an ideology; we may take them so completely for granted that they just seem to be part of the way things are. If we do not understand how these beliefs filter our perceptions and shape our behaviors, then we are unable to subject them to critical reflection and to decide which parts work well for us and which parts need to be changed.

The Control Model

An aspect of personal philosophy with special importance to clinical practice is our attitude towards control. Through the influence of Western culture in general and medical culture in particular, we often perceive being in control (of disease, of patients, of the health-care team) to be the ideal state (Table 8–1). We use specific intellectual tools for gathering and

Table 8–1. A comparison of control- and relationship-based personal philosophies.

Attribute	Control	Relational (I–Thou)*
Phenomenon of interest	Thing-in-itself	Thing-in-context
Epistemologic strategy	Reductionist; linear causality	Emergent; systems model
Clinician's stance	Detached observer	Participant observer
Information deemed relevant	Objective data only	Subjective and objective data
Model for patient-clinician relationship	Hierarchy	Partnership
Focus of attention	Outcome-oriented	Process-oriented

* Terms are from Martin Buber: *I and Thou.* Scribner, 1970.

applying knowledge—reductionism: "Sickle cell anemia is attributable to the substitution of a single nucleotide"; linear causality: "*A* causes *B*"; and moving away from the particular toward the general: "This is a case of asthma." All have a distinctly controlling, outcome-oriented focus, that is, to manipulate *A* so as to control *B*. Although this approach has led to important technologic advances, it also has important adverse consequences.

Expectations: The control model creates unrealistic expectations that limit our opportunities to feel successful. If we strive for complete control—or at least attempt to maintain that illusion—we are assuming responsibility for all outcomes. Consider, for instance, how our expectations of good control in caring for a diabetic patient allow us to feel successful only when the blood sugar is tightly regulated. The patient's blood sugar, however, is influenced by many factors over which we have no control, the patient's own behavior being foremost among them. We become angry at the patient whose noncompliance stands in the way of our success. If success for us is defined only in terms of controlling disease, we are precluded from feeling successful in many, if not most, situations. Accepting responsibility for outcomes over which we have little or no control is highly stressful and leads us to feel helpless, threatened, and angry.

Distance and Detachment: Our quest for control also creates distance and detachment in the patient-clinician relationship, which we have already seen to be an important factor in professional satisfaction. A strong orientation toward control leads to hierarchic relationships. This, coupled with the reductionism and labeling of medical thinking, turns patients into objects, and we find ourselves working more with *things*—organs, diseases, medications, tests—than with people. We, too, become depersonalized in this process, leaving no room for our subjective experience.

The Relational Model

An alternative philosophy that avoids many of these problems emphasizes relatedness rather than control. This model does not reject the insights of reductionism, but rather builds on them by adding an appreciation of context and relationship. Therefore, although *A* may seem to cause *B,* there are also other mediating factors and bidirectional interactions. For example, the tubercle bacillus causes tuberculosis, but not everyone who is exposed to this bacterium becomes ill; environmental and socioeconomic factors also contribute to the process. The illness, in turn, affects those contextual factors since no portion of the system exists in isolation.

In the relational model, we seek to be with and to understand the patient in a number of dimensions simultaneously—biological, experiential, functional, spiritual. As we come to understand patients' experiences, we may or may not identify opportunities to recommend strategies or undertake treatments to ameliorate their suffering. Patients retain responsibility for their lives; they may or may not accept our suggestions. In some cases, we may have no suggestions or treatment to offer, but we can still find success in offering empathic witnessing, honoring the patient's need for connection—a healing intervention in its own right.

This relational model helps us avoid unrealistic expectations of ourselves. It offers us the opportunity to feel successful in situations, such as untreatable illness or a patient's refusal to accept our good advice, that would seem like failures under the control model. The relational model also leads us to more effective action. In contrast to the control model, which attends exclusively to outcomes, this model calls for explicit attention to process, to the quality of communication and to the values embedded in the way we work together. Paradoxically, it is by letting go of outcomes and focusing more on making the process as good as possible that we achieve the best outcomes. The relational model also gives us more room to look outside ourselves for guidance and solutions—and to admit our own limitations or powerlessness.

Whereas the control model creates barriers between clinicians and patients, the relational model keeps us closer to the experience of both our patients and ourselves, thereby increasing the opportunities for our work to be meaningful and decreasing the potential for frustration, alienation, and burnout.

SKILLS

There are a number of skills that can spell the difference between depletion and thriving in practice.

Time-Management Skills: These skills are essential both within the office visit and in arranging work schedules (see the Suggested Readings at the end of the chapter). Negotiating an agenda at the start of each visit focuses attention on the issues that are most important to the patient and the clinician, minimizes time spent on unnecessary tasks, and vastly reduces the emergence of last-minute topics ("Oh, by the way, Doc, I've got this chest pain. . . .") that lay waste to office schedules. Informing patients at the outset how long their visits will last and reminding them a few minutes before ending allows them to share responsibility for using time effectively. On a more global level, time-management skills can help preserve the balance between work, family, community, and recreation that is so important to life satisfaction. Keeping time logs for several days can help us discover whether we are apportioning our time in accordance with our personal goals and priorities. Time logs can also point out time-wasters (eg, unnecessary interruptions) in daily work habits and help us devise more efficient office procedures.

Communication: Given the important contribution of the patient-clinician relationship as a source of meaning, communication and relationship skills become critical tools for well-being. Learning to *be with* the patient requires broadening the goal of the interview from making a diagnosis to understanding the story of the patient's illness as a lived experience. Rather than ending the interview after we can say, "This is a case of asthma," we need to understand the meaning of the illness to the patient—why this disease in this particular patient at this particular time, what its functional effect is, and what role it might be playing in the patient's life. Thus, we need skills for eliciting deeper levels of patients' stories and responding to their emotions. As we are more able to do this, it becomes apparent that there is no longer such a thing as a routine or uninteresting case—each patient is unique.

Negotiation & Coaching: Sharing responsibility more effectively and more realistically with patients requires both negotiation and coaching skills. Specifically, we must know how to facilitate patients in articulating their own values, goals, and opinions, including their feedback about their medical care. We must be willing to relinquish our traditional—and burdensome—role of unquestioned authority and adopt instead a more flexible stance, trying to combine synergistically our own knowledge of medicine with patients' knowledge of themselves and the patterns, problems, and balances of their daily lives. Knowing how and when to set firm boundaries without being judgmental and how to discuss communication and relationship problems openly can help to resolve impasses with many seemingly difficult patients, making their care less frustrating and more rewarding.

Self-Reflection: Finally, we need the ability to reflect on our own feelings and actions, to recognize when our own personal issues are influencing our perceptions of and behavior toward our patients. Rather than shutting out as "unprofessional" and "unobjective" feelings such as anger, attraction, arrogance, or insecurity that must inevitably arise in us, we can learn to use them to gain insights about ourselves and our patients. There are two basic catalysts for this kind of self-exploration. The first is protected time for quiet, solitary reflection or meditation, during which we can more thoroughly recognize and experience our inner states. Meditation can also be a valuable process in the transition from control toward relatedness as the core of one's personal philosophy. The other catalyst for self-awareness is talking with colleagues. This can take place in any setting that provides sufficient support, honesty, and confidentiality—from informal conversations to more organized formats such as Balint or other support groups, workshops, or psychotherapy. These opportunities to shed the mask of the iron man and disclose our vulnerabilities to each other are also key resources for working amid uncertainty and coping with mistakes; they offer many openings for connection.

The skills listed above have been introduced into medical education only recently. The vast majority of current practitioners were left to sink or swim on their own; most are somewhere in between. Fortunately, these skills are now well described in the medical literature and are the focus of a growing number of continuing medical education workshops, making it easier for physicians to assess their own strengths and weaknesses and to cultivate the critical skills they lack.

HEALTHY WORK ENVIRONMENTS

Our workplaces have an important effect on our well-being. The local culture of the institutions in which we work—be they hospitals, individual practices, or medical communities—subtly reinforces values through both formal educational processes and everyday policies and practices. The local culture can determine whether we feel able to disclose uncertainty and vulnerability to one another or feel constrained always to maintain the iron-man facade; whether we can discuss mistakes and ask for help—or be forced to work in perpetual isolation; whether we receive encouragement and respect for setting reasonable limits on our workload so we can be present in our families or feel shamed for being lazy.

The Person-Centered Environment

Creating person-centered environments that support person-centered care is a large topic; a few general principles must suffice for this discussion.

■ As clinicians, we tend to treat patients in the same way that we ourselves are treated within our institutions. Core values such as respect, partnership, honesty, and accountability must be explicitly articulated and embodied in institutional policies and procedures. Clinicians and administrators alike may need to learn new communication and relationship skills, and redesign processes for making decisions and maintaining accountability.

■ Respecting values and attending to the quality of process must be embraced as the most effective means to high-quality outcomes at the organizational level, just as at the clinical level. This requires that we abandon traditional, hierarchic approaches of top-down decision-making and control of the work process.

■ We can replace the current culture of rugged individualism with a culture of teamwork, accountability, and mutual support. Support groups for all staff, including physicians, may encourage self-awareness, increase sensitivity to patients' concerns, and diminish the isolation and depersonalization that both characterize and accelerate burnout. We can be vigilant to ways in which the local culture reinforces work addiction and inhibits collaboration and work to improve it.

Most clinicians have traditionally been reluctant to involve themselves in medical administration. Especially in this era of cost-control and managed care, we must become more active and work in partnership with all members of the health-care team to redesign our medical institutions, making them more respectful and humane, more oriented to partnership, more responsive to the needs of both the people they serve and the people who work within them. Risk management, clinical efficiency, patient satisfaction, and health outcomes may well be related to healthy work environments for health-care providers; institutions thus have a direct stake in maintaining the well-being of their clinicians and staff.

Whether the rigors of clinical work become sources of meaning or exhaustion depends on a number of factors. We must be able to know and address deliberately the personal needs that affect our work. The need for connection and meaning are particularly important and, when they are met, sustaining. A more mature perspective of balance, acceptance, and relation must replace the current preoccupation with control. The latter leads only to unrealistic (hence unachievable) expectations and the ongoing specter of inadequacy or failure. Skills must be acquired for working with uncertainty, sharing responsibility, and promoting relationship. We must become more attentive to the values expressed subliminally but powerfully in our work environments and begin to make necessary changes so that our environments call forth the best and healthiest of what we have to offer, as both professionals and as human beings. These approaches can help us to appreciate fully the privilege of caring for patients and to realize our best potential for personal fulfillment and growth.

SUGGESTED READINGS

Frankel RM et al: Can I really improve my listening skills with only 15 minutes to see my patients? HMO Practice 1991;5:114.

Gabbard GO, Menninger RW: The psychology of postponement in the medical marriage. JAMA 1989;261:2378.

Hobbs CR: *Time Power.* Harper, 1987.

Kleinman A: The healers: Varieties of experience in doctoring. In: Kleinman A, *The Illness Narratives: Suffering, Healing and the Human Condition.* Basic Books, 1988.

Matthews DA, Suchman AL, Branch WT: Making "connexions": Enhancing the therapeutic potential of patient-clinician relationships. Ann Intern Med 1993;118:973.

McKay B, Forbes JA, Bourner K: Empowerment in general practice: The trilogies of caring. Austral Fam Physcian 1990;19:513.

Quill TE: Partnerships in patient care: A contractual approach. Ann Intern Med 1983;98:228.

Quill TE, Williamson PR: Healthy approaches to physician stress. Arch Intern Med 1990;150:1857.

Reames HR, Dunstone DC: Professional satisfaction of physicians. Arch Int Med 1989;149:1951.

Suchman AL, Matthews DA: What makes the patient-doctor relationship therapeutic? Exploring the connexional dimension of medical care. Ann Intern Med 1988;108:125.

Vaillant, G: Some psychologic vulnerabilities of physicians. N Engl J Med 1972;287:372.

Williamson PR: Support groups: An important aspect of physician education (editorial). J Gen Intern Med 1991;6:179.

Zinn WM: Doctors have feelings too. JAMA 1988;259:3296.

Section II.
Working With Specific Populations

Families

9

Steven R. Hahn, MD

INTRODUCTION

Treating the patient in the context of the family has implications for every step of the clinical process, from basic assumptions about who the patient is, to the conceptual framework for the database, theories of causality, and the implementation of treatment. Although many physicians may feel they have an intuitive understanding about "the family" and how families work and develop, such intuition does not substitute for clinically useful understanding of family systems and of methods of assessment and intervention.

Caring for the patient in the context of the family goes beyond involving the families of some patients in the management of care. Two family case illustrations are presented in vignettes throughout the chapter. These cases lay the conceptual foundation and describe the basic skills and methods of family assessment and intervention in primary care.

THE FAMILY AS THE CONTEXT OF ILLNESS

The family is the primary social context of experience, including that of health and illness. The individual's very awareness and perception of symptoms are shaped by the family, as are decisions about whether, how, and from whom to seek help. Use of health care services and acceptance of and adherence to medical treatments are all influenced by the family.

Reciprocal Relationships: Family function has a reciprocal relationship with symptoms, illness, and health-care behavior. Ample research has demonstrated that physical symptoms and illness significantly influence the family's emotional state and behavior, often causing dysfunction in family relationships. At the same time, dysfunction in the family system can generate stress and lead to physical illness. A dysfunctional family system can incorporate a symptom and the complex of behaviors that evolve

around it into the family's behavioral patterns, thereby sustaining or exacerbating the symptom. In these "somatizing" families, the presence and persistence of the symptom or illness cannot be understood without examining its meaning in the family context.

Further reciprocal relationships—between individual and family, and between the health of the individual and the health of the family system—also make it necessary for the physician to care for the patient in the context of the family. This necessity is mandated by concerns ranging from the obvious, such as the need to discuss the diet of a diabetic patient with the family members who do the shopping and the food preparation; to the obscure, for example, understanding that the poor physiological control of a 10-year-old with diabetes is rooted in his family's adaptation to dysfunction in the marital relationship of his parents. In short, the doctor-patient relationship is more accurately described as a *doctor-patient-family relationship*.

What Is a Family?

Our own intuitive sense of what a family is, is based on an intimate personal experience of our own family and familiarity with the families of others. Despite this considerable personal knowledge, however, it is difficult to define the family because of the diversity of family structures. The variety of groups that are experienced as family is enormous: two-parent nuclear families; single-parent families; foster parents with children from different biological families; families of divorcees blended through remarriage; families with gay or lesbian couples as parents; married or cohabiting couples without any children at all. Isolated elderly individuals may think of their home health attendants as family, and for other solitary individuals the only family they may know is their pets.

All of these groups can be experienced as families. They share similarities in the structure of the relationships between their members and the role that the family group plays for the individuals and for the society in which the group exists. So, rather than define the family in terms of its members, we describe it as a *system having certain functional roles.*

The Role of the Family

Family relationships are better described by their roles than by the labels traditionally applied to individuals. For example, in one family an elderly woman may obtain companionship and emotional support from a home health attendant, a friend at the local senior citizen's center, and a daughter, whereas a woman in another family may find these needs met by her marital partner. In one society, the primary education of children may be accomplished in the household of the child's parent(s), and in schools to which the child travels each day. In another society, the children's group of a kibbutz or a boarding school far from the household of the parent may accomplish these educational tasks, thereby involving others in relationships with the child that approach the significance of the parent-child relationship. Hence, for physicians, the patient's family context must be understood as the individuals in the social system who are involved in the roles and tasks that are of central importance to the patient (Table 9–1).

The Family as a System

An understanding of the system properties of the family is the theoretic foundation for most schools of family therapy and "family systems medicine." Families as systems are characterized by:

- external and internal boundaries
- internal hierarchy
- self-regulation through feedback
- change with time, specifically family lifecycle changes.

The qualities of these four system characteristics in a particular family determine the family's internal milieu and functioning.

Boundaries: The family is imperfectly separated from that which is not-family by a set of behaviors and norms known as a "boundary." Family boundaries are created by norms that determine who interacts with whom, in what way, and around what activities. Different parts of the family system (ie, subsystems), such as "the parents" and "the children," or each "in-

Table 9–1. The role of the family: A partial list.

Reproduction
Supervision of children
Food, shelter, and clothing
Emotional support
Education: technical, social, and moral
Religious training
Health care—nursing
Financial support
Entertainment and recreation

dividual," are also separated from one another by boundaries. Teaching children "not to talk to strangers" creates a boundary around the family. Internal boundaries work in the same way: children who speak back to a parent may be told that they "don't know their place," that is, that they have crossed a boundary that defines their role. Healthy boundaries balance the individual identity of families' subsystems with the openness required for interaction and communication across boundaries. Boundaries may be excessively rigid, prohibiting communication between individuals and the world outside the family.

Internal Hierarchy: Subsystems of the family, including the individual, relate to one another hierarchically: parents have authority over the children, the older children over the younger children, and so on. A healthy hierarchy is clear, flexible enough to evolve with the needs of the family, and localizes power and control in those who are the most competent. Hierarchies may become dysfunctional when they are unable to adapt to change, when the allocation of power or authority is not consistent with the location of expertise or competence in the family, or when the lines of authority are blurred and effective decisions cannot be made.

Self-Regulation Through Feedback: Relationships within the boundaries of the family system and its subsystems are regulated by "feedback." Each individual act sets a series of actions in motion that in turn influence the original actor. It is through feedback that families shape the behavior of each member. All behaviors in the family have some effect on other members as feedback, and as such are a form of communication: often, actions speak louder than words. Families may be characterized as effectively communicating general information, thoughts, and feelings, or communication can be confused, contradictory, or simply absent.

Feedback maintains the integrity of the family system as a unit, establishes and maintains hierarchies, and regulates the function of boundaries in accordance with the individual family's norms and style. This tendency toward maintaining "homeostasis" is critical to the integrity of the family. The need for stability, however, inevitably conflicts with the need for change in family interactions.

Change & the Family Lifecycle: The family must continually adapt as its members evolve through the biological and social stages of individual development (Table 9–2). For example, the family with young children must keep them safely within the boundaries of the family's protective circle (or that of specific delegates, such as the schools). When the children become adolescents, they must be allowed to achieve a degree of independence and the ability to function without immediate adult or family supervision. To facilitate this, the family must develop new norms of behavior and relax the boundary between the child and the world (ie, allow more openness) and redraw the

Table 9–2. The family lifecycle.

Lifecycle Stage	Dominant Theme	Transitional Task
The single young adult	Separating from family of origin	Differentiation from family of origin. Developing intimate relationships with peers. Establishing career and financial independence.
Forming a committed relationship	Commitment to a new family	Formation of a committed relationship. Forming and changing relationships with both families of origin.
The family with young children	Adjusting to new family members	Adjusting the relationship to make time and space for children. Negotiating parenting responsibilities. Adjusting relationships with extended families to incorporate parenting and grandparenting.
The family with adolescents	Increasing flexibility of boundaries to allow for children's independence	Adjusting boundaries to allow children to move in and out of the family more freely. Attending to midlife relationship and career issues. Adjusting to aging parent's needs and role.
Launching children	Accepting exits and entries into the system	Adjusting committed relationship to absence of children in the household. Adjusting relationships with children to their independence and adult status. Including new in-laws and becoming grandparents. Adjusting to aging or dying parents' needs and role.
The family later in life	Adjusting to age and new roles	Maintaining functional status, developing new social and familial roles. Supporting central role of middle generation. Integrating the elderly into family life. Dealing with loss of parents, spouse, peers; life review and integration.

Source: Adapted, with permission, from Carter and McGoldrick; Doherty and Baird 1983; McDaniel, Campbell and Seaburn, 1990.

boundaries between parent and child (eg, provide more areas of autonomy and privacy and assert less parental authority). Each stage of the family lifecycle presents new challenges, and healthy families are able to change their hierarchic relationships and boundaries as they arise. Families whose boundaries, hierarchies, and self-regulatory feedback are dysfunctional have difficulties at each transition.

Family Cohesion: The ways in which families establish boundaries and internal hierarchies, regulate themselves through feedback, and adapt to change all contribute to the family's internal milieu. Different configurations of these characteristics result in varying degrees of family cohesion. A family's cohesiveness lies somewhere along a continuum ranging from "enmeshed" to "disengaged," with a functional level of cohesion lying between these two extremes.

1. Enmeshed Family: The enmeshed family has blurred or nonexistent boundaries: that is, everyone knows and is involved in everyone else's business. Moreover, internal hierarchies are unclear: individuals cannot determine who should be in control. Feedback in enmeshed families is overwhelming and controlling: everyone reacts to everyone else's emotional state and problems. These families have difficulty with the individuation of family members into the more mature roles that are part of every family lifecycle change, for example, allowing adolescents to develop autonomy and letting grown children leave home.

2. Disengaged Family: The disengaged family has impermeable and immutable boundaries: no one

knows how anyone else feels or thinks, rules about interaction tend to isolate members emotionally and interfere with healthy communication. Feedback in the disengaged family is sparse to nonexistent, that is, there is little guidance or supervision—family members are not "there for each other." It may or may not be clear who should be in control in the family, and the family hierarchy is likely to be dysfunctional because individuals may be too distant or isolated to exercise control. Furthermore, the inadequate feedback between members tends to make the hierarchy excessively rigid and unable to change with family lifecycle transitions. The disengaged family also has trouble with family lifecycle changes: younger members develop a premature autonomy, impoverished by the inability of the family to provide supervision and nurturance.

The Doctor-Patient-Family Relationship & the Compensatory Alliance

The doctor-patient relationship, typically thought and spoken of as dyadic, is part of the patient's larger social system and inevitably influences and is influenced by the other members of the family. The apparently dyadic doctor-patient relationship is actually part of the doctor-patient-family relationship, called a "therapeutic triangle" by Doherty and Baird. Developing a positive working relationship with an active and concerned family can be one of the physician's most powerful tools in caring for patients. On the other hand, when significant family problems exist, the doctor-patient relationship can become entangled in the family system's dysfunction.

The task of providing appropriate care for the patient's medical problems may even become subordinate to and subverted by the family dysfunction. Some families can only achieve internal stability and meet the needs of their members when one or more is perceived as being sick—Grandma only gets attention when she is not feeling well; a teenage daughter is only safe from parental abuse when her asthma is out of control; Mom and Dad only stop fighting when their 10-year-old son is in diabetic ketoacidosis; Mom and teenage daughter only stop fighting about her curfew when Dad gets a headache; and so on. The physician's role in determining that the patient is entitled to the special prerogatives and dispensations of the "sick role" makes the physician a central and powerful member of these family systems. The authority to prescribe changes in role function for the patient, and to offer support and validation as these changes take place, further involves the physician in the life of the entire family. In effect, the physician and patient develop an alliance that compensates for the dysfunction and deficit at home. Hahn, Feiner, and Bellin have termed this a *compensatory alliance.*

When the physician is unaware of underlying family dysfunction, the compensatory alliance can become dysfunctional and contribute to somatization, noncompliance, and functional regression. Although the therapeutic triangle may be more apparent when caring for pediatric patients than in adult medicine, where patients are often seen alone, a dysfunctional compensatory alliance may subvert the therapeutic triangle in either situation.

PATIENT CARE IN THE CONTEXT OF THE FAMILY: AN EIGHT-STEP APPROACH

General Considerations

Treating the patient in the context of the family requires a practical method that can be realistically acquired and employed by primary care providers within the context of their education and clinical practice. The large number of tasks that occupy the primary care provider places limits on the complexity and time requirements of the family assessment and intervention techniques that they can learn and employ. A primary care family assessment and intervention method must respect these limitations.

The first four steps of the method described here are designed to accomplish the "basic" family assessment and intervention goals that should be met with all patients in order to care for them in the context of the family (Table 9–3). A subset of more challenging patients with problems rooted in serious family dysfunction requires the more complex and advanced assessment and intervention techniques described in steps 5–8.

Treating the patient in the context of the family does not necessarily mean moving more people into the examining or consulting rooms with the patient and physician. In fact, in adult medicine a family-oriented approach is most often used with only the patient and physician in the room. In theory, each of the eight steps described in this approach can be accom-

Table 9–3. Goals of basic family assessment and intervention in primary care.

Understand the pattern of family involvement with the patient's medical problems.

Communicate with other family members about the management of patient's medical problems.

Recognize the presence of problem behaviors (eg, alcohol or drug abuse, somatization, domestic violence, physician experience of the patient as "difficult") and family dysfunction affecting the patient's medical problems or functional status, which require further assessment and intervention.

Assess the family's behavioral and emotional response to the patient's problems, and provide emotional support to the patient and family.

Provide counseling to enhance the family's emotional and functional adaptation to the patient's medical problems.

Perform a preliminary assessment of the doctor-patient-family relationship and recognize a "dysfunctional compensatory alliance" when present or developing.

Refer the patient or family for further assessment and intervention, or obtain a family systems consultation.

Understand the triangular relationships and repetitive patterns of interaction between members of the family system, including the development of a "dysfunctional compensatory alliance" in the doctor-patient-family triangle.

Understand the way that the patient's problems (ie, multiple or persistent symptoms, problem behaviors, noncompliance, or mental disorders) are embedded in the family's triangular relationships and repetitive patterns of interaction.

"Empathically witness" the family's pattern of interaction, experience of the problem and efforts to cope.

Reframe attention to underlying family system problems so that: (1) they can be addressed effectively, and (2) the doctor-patient-(family) relationship can be protected from the complications created by family systems dysfunction.

Use the experience of empathically witnessing and reframing the family problems as a foundation for counseling patients and family to make modest changes in the family system. Refer those who are unable to resolve their problems with modest intervention, and those with more profound family pathology for family therapy, other psychotherapy or consultation.

plished meeting exclusively with the patient. Meeting with other family members is very often desirable, however, and is sometimes necessary. Such meetings almost always enhance the physician's ability to provide care. A family systems orientation is also far easier to learn by watching a family in action.

Using a family systems orientation without meeting directly with other family members requires the ability to infer what is going on at home—to "see the family over the patient's shoulder"—and test those inferences with the patient despite the fact that patients may distort their presentation of family life; such distortion may be conscious, unknowing, or a combination thereof. It takes a great deal of experience working with and observing groups of family members to be able to make and test these inferences. With some patients and their families, it is impossible to test hypotheses about family functioning without direct contact, and impossible to correct the distortion of the patient-provided view of family life without the corrective power of a family meeting. When significant distortion is present, a direct relationship with other family members can help test the patient-provided view and maximize the patient's own efforts to present a less distorted picture.

BASIC FAMILY ASSESSMENT & INTERVENTION

Case illustration 1: The patient, Ariana, is a 40-year-old Italian-American woman with multiple somatic complaints. She has complained of chronic diarrhea but had normal stool collections and colonoscopy; dyspepsia, but with normal endoscopy; severe polyarthralgia without physical or serologic evidence of inflammation; and asthma, but without documented wheezing or abnormal spirometry. She has made multiple visits to her primary provider, to a walk-in urgent care clinic, and has been seen in several subspecialty clinics. She has made an average of 15 visits per year for the last several years and 40 visits in the last year.

Step 1: The Database—Constructing a Genogram

The first step to treating the patient in the context of the family is to gather a family database. Conducting a "genogram-based interview" is the ideal method for gathering these data. A genogram is a graphic representation of the members of a family. It uses the iconography of the genetic pedigree (Figures 9–1 and

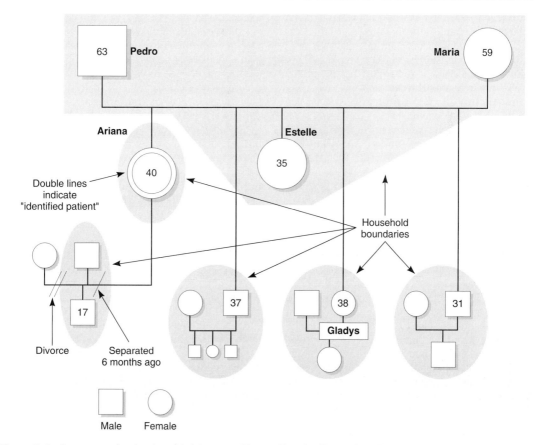

Figure 9–1. Genogram showing household composition and key family members in Ariana's family (case illustration 1).

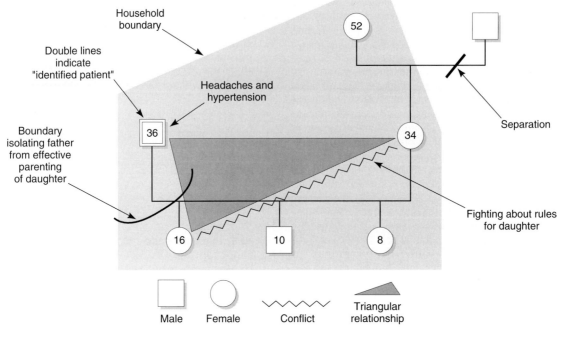

Household boundary

Double lines indicate "identified patient"

Headaches and hypertension

Boundary isolating father from effective parenting of daughter

52

36

34

Separation

Fighting about rules for daughter

16

10

8

Male   Female   Conflict   Triangular relationship

Figure 9–2. Genogram of the family of case illustration 2.

9–2) and can be used to record a wide variety of data ranging from the family's history of medical illnesses to life events, interpersonal conflicts and alliances, and important family stories. The overall objective of the genogram interview is to help the patient tell the family's story in relational terms.

Constructing a Genogram: The physician should begin with an empty sheet of paper (or a designated section of the patient's front flow-sheet), placed where the patient can look on. The family tree is created, and information about individuals and the family recorded as the interview progresses. Important dates such as marriages, divorces, and deaths can be noted, as can the addresses of individuals in other households. Family systems data can be recorded using lines to enclose household boundaries, double lines between individuals to indicate strong relationships or coalitions, jagged lines to indicate conflict, triple lines to indicate dysfunctional over-involvement, and lines perpendicular to the axis between two individuals to indicate boundaries. The genogram is a database and is therefore never "complete." Information is added to the genogram as the interview moves from the family tree per se to discussion of relevant family issues. By briefly looking at the genogram at the beginning of subsequent visits, the physician can be reminded of the family context of the patient, and the genogram may be expanded or altered at each visit as the family system changes and new issues arise.

Focused Versus Expanded Genograms: The type of information explored, even the number of

generations included in the genogram, depends on the objective of the interview and the physician's perception of the importance of family systems' issues. A comprehensive or "expanded" genogram interview is a powerful clinical tool but may be of limited utility in everyday primary care practice because of the amount of time required to perform an extended exploration of the family system. To use the genogram as an efficient tool in everyday practice, the physician must be able to perform a "focused" genogram, targeting the most clinically useful information while providing the foundation for planned family systems' interventions. As with most clinical databases, however, it is harder to know what can safely be excluded from the assessment than it is to include the entire possible range of family-oriented data. Therefore, performing a focused genogram interview takes practice and experience, and physicians will not be able to compose focused genograms without first learning how to do an expanded genogram interview.

The focused genogram limits inquiry initially to the core members of the family system, to the family's responses to the immediate or presenting problem, and to issues identified using the family lifecycle and screening questions described in steps 2 and 3 below. If no significant major problems or dysfunction are identified with these questions, the focused genogram interview stops when the physician understands the family well enough to talk to the patient and family about the patient's medical problems and their responses to them. When significant family problems are discovered, the physician should continue with steps 5–8 to assess and intervene whether performing a focused or expanded genogram.

Both the focused genogram and expanded genogram interviews begin with the same two tasks: (1) determine the nucleus of the patient's family system; and (2) identify the family lifecycle/stage of the family. This first stage of the genogram interview begins with the members of the patient's household and any of the patient's first-degree relatives not living in the household, especially parents, children, and past and present spouses. The physician can usually identify the family lifecycle/stage of the patient's family from the ages, relationships, and household composition of this nucleus of the patient's family. As described below, determining the lifecycle stage of the family enables the physician to predict the locus of stress, challenge, or conflict in the patient's family system, and this knowledge serves as an important guide to the rest of the interview.

Case 1 Discussion: Figure 9–1 shows the skeleton of the patient's genogram, indicating household composition and key members. After recording the nucleus of the patient's family and determining the family lifecycle stage, an expanded genogram interview extends the family tree centrifugally, going back to parental and grandparental generations of the patient (and the patient's spouse[s]), and forward to include all descendent generations. Brief descriptions of family members and characterizations of important relationships should be obtained. The patient and physician can explore repetitive intergenerational patterns of occupation, personality characteristics, religious affiliations, substance abuse, mental disorders, and so forth. The occurrence and effect of major life events, immigrations, or translocations should be explored as the patient is encouraged to tell the story of his or her family. Individual and family responses to the developmental tasks of the family lifecycle, both past and present, can be explored. The important relationships or data should be recorded on the genogram as the interview progresses, creating a picture of the family in view of the patient. The patient should actively participate in examining the family genogram and usually identifies patterns and relationships that are revelations to patient and physician alike.

Step 2: The Family Lifecycle/Predicting Stress & Conflict

Stage Assessment: Assessing the lifecycle stage of the family based on information obtained from a focused genogram is the first, orienting step that should be taken with every patient in the process of treatment in the context of the family. The stages of the lifecycle are a virtual road map for the clinician exploring the important issues in the life of a patient and family. The context provided by knowledge of the family's lifecycle stage is directly analogous to that provided by knowing a patient's age and gender before beginning to think about the causes or significance of a physical symptom.

The family lifecycle consists of six stages (Table 9–2). Each stage is grounded in biologically driven patterns of individual development. The cycle may be seen as beginning with the separation of the individual from the family of origin (stage 1), the formation of a new family of procreation (stage 2), the raising and "launching" of children into the world (stages 3, 4, and 5), and the family later in life (stage 6). Each of these stages is dominated by a theme or principle. Each task requires two to four major changes in family structure and function.

Refine Predictions: The general structure of the family system can be used to refine predictions about the locus of stress from the adaptational tasks of the family lifecycle. The structure of the parental subsystem is often the most powerful determinant of these major variations. For example, the adaptational strategies of families with one parent; one "working" and one "child-care" parent; two working parents; families with extended-family parenting; and blended families all have different developmental patterns that can be anticipated.

Case 1 Discussion (Contd.): Ariana's genogram (see Fig. 9–1) suggests that she is in the first stage of the family lifecycle, that is, between families, the unattached young adult. Her separation and divorce from her husband 6 months ago suggest difficulty forming a new family and moving on to the second stage of the family lifecycle. It is noteworthy that the patient's sister Estelle is having difficulty with the first phase of the lifecycle. The persistence of a dependent child-parental relationship raises concern about her parents' ability to make their transition into the grandparenting role and reorientation of marital relationships that characterize stages 5 and 6 of the family lifecycle.

Step 3: Screening for Family Function

After constructing the basic genogram and determining the lifecycle stage of the family, the physician's next step is to screen for family problems. The physician should be familiar with the patient's medical problems, particularly those that often have a significant influence on the family (Table 9–4). Once the physician has demonstrated genuine interest in the patient's family and the problems suggested by the screening, it is more likely that the patient will inform the physician about important family issues spontaneously and with less prompting.

Global Family Function: Screening for family problems should begin with open-ended questions about global family function (Table 9–5). The tone and content of the questions should be nonjudgmental, and even normalize the presence of family problems, for example, "I know that all families have their ups and downs, how is yours doing these days with all

Table 9–4. Presentations and problems associated with family dysfunction that should trigger screening for family dysfunction.

Noncompliance with self-care regimens
Alcohol or substance abuse
Mental disorders, especially psychotic, mood, and anxiety disorders
Unexplained medical symptoms and somatization
Physician experienced difficulty in the doctor-patient relationship, ie, the "difficult patient."
Health-related habitual behaviors—smoking, eating disorders
Newly diagnosed, rapidly deteriorating, or frightening illnesses, eg, HIV infection, cancer, end-stage renal disease, myocardial infarction
Disruptions and change in the family system—divorce, separation, death, immigration or emigration
Natural and social disaster or trauma—fires, floods, earthquakes, crimes
Sexually transmitted illness
Anniversary dates and important holidays
Domestic violence
Reproductive health: pregnancy, termination of pregnancy, family planning

that is going on in your life?" An effective initial inquiry directs the patient's attention to family issues in general but does not assume too much about what kind of problems may be present. Even though knowledge of the family lifecycle is highly predictive of the source of stress and conflict, the specifics in any particular family cannot be anticipated. If the patient is given permission to speak, and room to choose the focus, he or she may take the practitioner to the heart of the matter in response to this single, initial question.

Exploring Emotional Content: The remaining categories of screening questions are listed in Table 9–5, beginning with those that seem expected or routine by the patient and progressing to those that are increasingly likely to carry significant emotional content or distress and seem more removed from the narrow biomedical agenda that is usually the core of the patient's expectations. Although this sequence may seem the most obvious, it may not be the most efficient, especially when the physician is reasonably certain that a family systems problem is present. The physician may want to move directly to where prior knowledge of the patient's problems and intuition suggests the heart of the problem lies.

Screening for Family Problems With the Patient's Medical Conditions: The physician should screen for difficulty coping with the patient's medical problems, for example, "How is your family dealing with your diabetes?" Do not ask a question that can be answered with a yes or no, such as "Is your family having problems with your diabetes?" It is helpful to normalize problems, such as saying, "I know how hard it can be for family members to adjust to the needs of someone who has diabetes. There's the regular meal schedule, restricted diet, the expense of the home blood sugar monitoring, and everything else. Tell me a little about how your family is dealing with it."

Screening for Problems Likely to Be Associated With Family Dysfunction: Whenever a problem that is often associated with family dysfunction is revealed, the physician should screen for the family's reaction and adaptation (see Table 9–5). Many of these problems are emotionally charged and stigmatizing. Nonjudgmental, normalizing, and directive rather than closed-ended questions are therefore critical. Many of these issues have immediate clinical and legal implications and raise issues of confidentiality in the doctor-patient relationship. Appropriate assurances of confidentiality and the limits to confidentiality, if any, need to be discussed when asking the patient about these issues. Other "trigger problems" may seem quite mundane but are nevertheless important. For example, it is useful to routinely inquire about how the family is dealing with important holiday seasons.

Screening for Family Lifecycle Problems: After determining the family lifecycle stage, the physician should construct a few screening questions about

Table 9–5. Family assessment screening questions.

Category	Example
Open-ended assessment of family problems	"How are things going with your family? How is everyone getting along?" "Are you having any problems with (name the key individuals in the genogram)?"
Family problems with the patient's medical problems	"How is your family dealing with your medical problems?" "How is (name the key individuals in the genogram) dealing with it, what is their reaction?"
Problems associated with family dysfunction (see Table 9–4)	"I know you have been feeling quite depressed lately, how has your family reacted to that?" "What has (name the key individuals) said or done about your depression?"
Family lifecycle problems	"I see you have a houseful of adolescents. I know that can be quite difficult. How have you been bearing up?"
Problems in the doctor-patient-family relationship: the compensatory alliance	"What does your family think and feel about the suggestions I have made?" "What were you hoping I might say to or do about your family?"

the lifecycle tasks that confront the patient's family. For example, from the very limited information presented in Figure 9–2, we can discern that this family will be characterized by the tasks of stages 3 and 4 of the family lifecycle, that is, the family with young children and the family with adolescents (see Table 9–2). Thus, six questions can screen for problems with the lifecycle-related issues this family is facing (Table 9–6). In fact, it is likely that fewer than these six questions will be necessary to identify any sources of difficulty, especially if the unique features of any particular family are used to select the initial questions.

Screening for Problems in the Doctor-Patient-Family Relationship: Throughout the family assessment the physician should be considering what role he or she is playing in the family system, and be alert to the formation of a dysfunctional compensatory alliance. It may be useful to ask the patient or other family members what reactions the family has had to suggestions made by the physician or other health care providers. It is also useful to ask what the patient wishes the physician might say to other family members, or in what way the patient hopes the physician might intercede with the family. Often these hopes and expectations are implied by patient words or behavior rather than stated, because the patients are not fully aware of their implied request, they are embarrassed to make it, or they do not feel they have permission to make the request of the physician.

Case illustration 1 (Contd.): In response to an open-ended question about how things are going at home, Ariana immediately identifies the stress that Estelle's illness places on her mother and the pressure her mother puts on her (Ariana) to help out in caring for Estelle as the major problem. In response to a question about her family's reaction to her own medical problems, Ariana says her mom has difficulty understanding why she (Ariana) is always so sick. Ariana's sister Gladys has come right out and said that she doesn't think Ariana's problems should be taken

Table 9–6. Family lifecycle screening questions for families with young children and adolescents.

Stage 3—The family with young children.

How are you doing with making time and space in your lives for three children?
How are you and your wife managing with child care responsibilities?
How are you getting along with the children's grandparents, *particularly your mother*-in-law,* and your other in-laws?

Stage 4—The family with adolescents.

How are you doing with a teenager, *your daughter,* in the house, and setting rules and expectations?
How are you and your wife doing with your work or careers? *Your youngest is going to go to school all day now. Will that change you or your wife's responsibilities or activities?*
What concerns do you have about the health or functioning of your parents or in-laws, *particularly your mother-in-law?*

* Generic questions for this stage of the family lifecycle are shown in regular type, questions or elements in italic are modifications *specific for the family of the father,* see Figure 9–2.

seriously. Ariana admits to difficulty with the lifecycle task of forming a new family and to feeling lonely but suggests that the pressure of her mother's demands on her make it difficult to think about getting involved with anyone. She blames her divorce on her exstepson's wildness and her ex-husband's inability to control him. Ariana thinks her mother is definitely depressed about Estelle's illness, and suspects that her mother resents Estelle's continued dependence but would never admit it to herself or anyone else. Asked what she would like her physician to do in terms of her problems at home, Ariana says that she would like the physician to make her family understand that she really is sick. (Figure 9–3 shows the genogram at this stage of the family assessment.)

Step 4: Basic Family Intervention: Communicating About & Caring for the Patient's Medical Problem

After completing the basic genogram, assessing the family lifecycle stage, and screening for problems in family function, the physician should be able to provide basic primary care for the patient and the patient's medical problems in the context of the family (Table 9–7). With the majority of families, the interventions described in this step accomplish the basic goals of family assessment and intervention (see Table 9–3). For families in which serious family dysfunction, dysfunctional interactions between the family system and the patient's problems, or a compensatory alliance have been discovered, further family assessment and more complex interventions are required (as described in steps 5–8). Preparation for that assessment and intervention should be made by the physician as part of the basic family interventions of step 4.

Enhancing the Therapeutic Alliance: Perhaps the most important and fundamental family systems intervention is to enhance the therapeutic alliance between the patient, physician, and other family members, by demonstrating interest and concern about the patient's family and life situation. Patients' perception that their physician cares for them is probably the single most important variable in the formation of a successful doctor-patient relationship. Few things accomplish this better than talking to patients about the most important people in their lives.

Communicating With the Family: After performing the basic family assessment, the physician is much better able to communicate with the family about the patient's medical problems. (Issues of confidentiality and privacy must be discussed explicitly with the patient first, to determine what details the physician should share with which family member.) Communications with the family may involve answering questions and educating them about the patient's condition, discussing self-care regimens and monitoring family involvement with the medical regimen, facilitating the family's role in decision-making about medical management, and discussing and helping to adjust to changes in the patient's functional capacity and role.

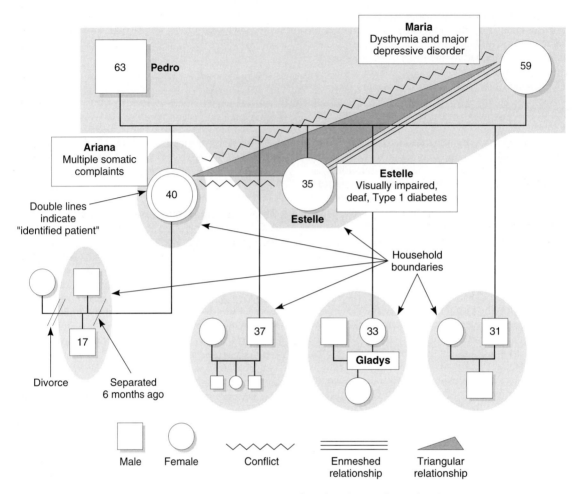

Figure 9–3. Annotated genogram for Ariana in case illustration 1.

Table 9–7. Basic family interventions in primary care.

Enhancing the therapeutic alliance by demonstrating interest and concern about the patient's family and life situation
Communicating with the family about the patient's medical condition
Providing information about the patient's problems: Discussing prognosis and answering family members' questions about medical problems
Discussing self-care and enlisting family assistance with medical management
Facilitating the family's participation in decision making about therapeutic options
Discussing and mediating the effect of the patient's loss of function on the roles of other family members
Providing emotional support to the patient and family
Counseling the family about simple family system problems
Identifying problems requiring attention from the family
Preparing for further family assessment, intervention, and referral for further family interventions
Working in collaboration with family therapists or other mental health specialists

Assessment & Support: Assessing the family's emotional response to the patient's problems and providing the needed support are among the most challenging and rewarding family-oriented tasks. It is often difficult for the physician to witness the emotional distress experienced by patient and family in the face of serious medical problems. The temptation to "stick to the facts" and restrict attention to biomedical issues is both strong and understandable. Perhaps one of the biggest barriers to providing emotional support to the family is the physician's perception that he or she "can do nothing" about the emotional pain. It is important to understand that empathically listening to the family and the patient is a powerful therapeutic intervention of itself—even if it appears to "fix" nothing (see Chapter 2). Furthermore, emotional distress is often a symptom of a treatable mood or anxiety disorder. Not acknowledging emotional distress is felt to be one of the reasons that even experienced clinicians may fail to recognize the presence of treatable mood and anxiety disorders in more than half of affected patients.

It is often possible to make simple family systems interventions by suggesting that families try new behaviors.

Case illustration 2: A 36-year-old man with hypertension presents to a walk-in clinic with 2 weeks of tension headaches. The focused genogram interview (see Figure 9–2 and Table 9–6) reveals that he is distressed by ongoing conflict between his wife and teenage daughter about rules governing her behavior with peers outside the home. At home the father remains silent until mother and daughter's fight becomes intolerable to him. Their fight only stops when he complains about the headache the fight has given him. He has never discussed his own perception of what the rules of his daughter's behavior—or of family arguments—should be, negotiated a common position with his wife, or tried to present a unified parental front to their daughter.

Case 2 Discussion: The suggestion that he and his wife discuss the situation before the fight begins and try to develop a plan that they both agree on would be an appropriate intervention. If the family has the flexibility to respond to this suggestion, it may help them with the developmental lifecycle challenge. If this intervention fails to help sufficiently, it may be a sign that further family assessment and intervention is required. It is important that suggestions be based on at least as thorough an evaluation as that produced by the preceding steps of this method; premature suggestions based on incomplete assessment are likely to fail.

Focusing on the Dysfunction: Many problems have an obvious and potentially devastating effect on the family. When basic family assessment has revealed such a problem, focusing the family's attention on the problems associated with family dysfunction is a crucial clinical task. For example, if a patient or a member of the patient's family has a problem with alcohol abuse or dependence, it is important to assess the family's response to that problem, help the family accept the reality of the problem, and support their need to address it. Sometimes the patient and family's denial is so strong that the basic family assessment described in the preceding steps is an insufficient foundation for helping the family organize appropriate action around the problem. In these cases it is necessary to proceed to the next level of intervention. On the other hand, many families are waiting for just the kind of professional, extrafamiliar attention that the physician can provide by validating their feelings, and providing information about resources such as Alcoholics Anonymous (AA), Al-Anon, and alcohol treatment facilities.

Preparing for Further Action: If significant family problems requiring more sophisticated intervention are identified, the physician must prepare patient and family for further assessment, intervention, or referral. If the primary care provider plans to take responsibility for the next steps, and does so with the patient alone, the task of preparing the patient, family, or both can be accomplished as a virtually imperceptible transition. On the other hand, if the primary care provider wishes to meet with other members of the family, involve a consultant, or refer to a mental health specialist, the patient and family must be prepared.

Resistance to a Family Meeting: It is not unusual for patients to express skepticism about the willingness of other family members to participate in family meetings or to fear confronting them with feelings that they may have been willing to show to the physician. Patients may also resist a family meeting if a compensatory alliance has been established and they fear that when other family members have the opportunity to "present their side" they may lose the physician's allegiance. Patients may also be afraid that the physician will become aware of the distortion they have introduced into their depiction of the other family members. This resistance to a family meeting must be negotiated, and the physician must decide how active a role to play in helping patients deal with whatever problems they anticipate.

Resistance to Counseling Referral: Similar resistance can be expressed to the idea of referral to a mental health specialist. Often a family meeting to discuss the problems helps patients and their families start therapy. If the physician encounters intractable difficulty at this stage of the process, an ideal solution is to invite a family systems consultant to participate in a visit with the patient or family in the clinic. It is often easier to involve a consultant on the physician's own turf than to refer the patient to another facility or provider.

Caregiver Collaboration: If a mental health specialist has been involved as a consultant or is treating the patient, the family, or both, the physician should actively collaborate with the mental health specialist. It is important to maintain boundaries between the roles of the mental health specialist and the primary care provider. Patients may attempt to play one health care provider against the other; for example, they may present somatic symptoms to the mental health specialist and attempt to engage the primary care provider in issues being examined in therapy. Patients or family members may complain about the therapist, especially when the family or patient is being challenged to change. The primary care physician and mental health specialist must maintain open and accessible lines of communication to prevent this kind of splitting and to use one another as resources when issues come up that are relevant to the other's expertise.

> *Case illustration 1 (Contd.):* Ariana greatly appreciated the opportunity to describe the situation at home, especially when the physician expressed sympathy for the burden that Estelle's illness placed on everyone and for the disappointment in Ariana's failed marriage. The physician felt that she now had a general feel for Ariana's family, a strong sense that Ariana needed to be labeled as "sick," and that a compensatory alliance had been established to that end that was enacted with every diagnostic test, referral to a specialist, and symptomatic treatment. Ariana, clearly feeling that the physician was on her side after the genogram interview, readily agreed to a family meeting.

ADVANCED FAMILY ASSESSMENT & INTERVENTION

If the physician has discovered that serious family dysfunction is interfering with patient self-care, with the doctor-patient relationship, or the patient's functional status and quality of life, a more intensive evaluation and intervention is required. The goals of advanced family assessment and intervention in primary care, as described here, do not focus on effecting the kinds of structural systems changes that are clearly the task of formal family therapy. Family systems experts have debated the wisdom of having primary care providers attempt family therapy at all. Some argue that with sufficient training, and in a delivery system in which adequate time is available (an increasing rarity that may make the whole debate moot), primary care providers can do family therapy with the families of their own patient (the identified patient). Others argue that the need that family therapists have to form shifting alliances with different family members threatens the trust that the identified patient must have in the physician in order to deal effectively with the existing medical problems.

There is one goal of family intervention, however, that most family therapists would agree is uniquely appropriate for the primary care provider. That goal is to refocus the patient and family's attention on family dysfunction so that the family can mobilize its resources and make the kind of commitment required to

work on changing dysfunctional patterns. Although this goal may be less than that of the family therapist, whose goals include facilitating the changes in the family system that are required, "reframing" the focus is nevertheless a critical goal and one that is not easily accomplished. The overall strategy of the advanced assessment and intervention is to make the nature of family dysfunction—as well as the pain and the impairment it causes—so palpable and real to the patient and family that they have little choice but to shift their attention to the family problems themselves; then the clinician must instill hope that something may be done to improve the situation.

Step 5: Assessing Family Structure & Patterns of Interaction

Assessing the family system as a foundation for further intervention requires a more complete understanding of the family dynamics. Three questions must be answered and one experience generated for the family and physician in the course of the assessment. The questions are:

1. What is the nature of the triangular relationships among members, including the triangles that involve the physician?
2. What is the circular pattern of interactions that constitute the family's "dance?"
3. How is the patient's problem symptom or behavior embedded in the family system, and what function does it serve?

In assessing the family system, the physician must work toward the objective of bringing the pain and dysfunction of the family system into the room so that it can be experienced by the patient and family and witnessed by the physician.

Triangular Relationships: Family interactions should be analyzed using triangular relationships in the family as the basic unit of structure, rather than in the dyadic terms that are most often used. For example, in their study of adolescents with brittle diabetes or poorly controlled asthma, Minuchin and colleagues often observed the following pattern: unresolved marital conflict erupts into an argument between the adolescent's parents; the adolescent, in response to the stress of the fight, becomes acutely ill; the parents stop arguing in order to take care of their child; the exacerbation of the child's illness resolves; the unresolved marital conflict erupts into another fight, and the process is repeated. From this point of view, it is clear that the outcome of the seemingly dyadic parental conflict cannot be understood without knowing that the child and the illness are "triangulated." It is impossible to understand the behavior of any member of this triangle without examining the interaction with both of the other two.

The triangular relationships among family members are caught up in circular patterns of interactions.

The sequence of events that take place in this family may be described in a linear fashion, that is, parents argue, the child is upset and gets sick, the parents stop arguing to help the child, the child gets better. The interruption of the fight, however, also prevents the parents from "finishing" their fight and resolving their problems, thu, the pattern inevitably repeats. Dysfunctional families are almost always stuck in such a repetitive, self-sustaining pattern. If they could modify the pattern, they would not be stuck, and they would not be dysfunctional.

It is important to understand how the patient's symptoms are embedded in the family system, and how the family dysfunction sustains the symptom. It is also important to see that there are no pure victims or villains in such a system. The child is not merely the "victim" of marital discord; the child and the acute exacerbations of illness have a powerful controlling influence on the inability of the spouses to resolve their conflicts. Looked at from a more positive vantage point, the child's illness is performing the important function of modulating a marital conflict that might otherwise threaten the integrity of the family system in a more fundamental way. The symptom is the product of and serves the needs of the entire family system. Though the price is high for all involved, and this "solution" is likely to fail in the long run, this dysfunctional family dance is the best that the family can do at the moment to cope with the totality of their problems.

Case illustration 1 (Contd.): During the family interview, the tremendous burden placed on the family by Estelle's visual impairment, deafness, and diabetes became painfully clear as the physician struggled to communicate with her; a process that required writing notes in letters six inches high, or having Ariana or her mother slowly and carefully speak so that Estelle could read their lips (Estelle was unable to read anyone else's lips, and the family had tried but failed to learn sign language). It became clear how much the family depended on Ariana and how she stepped ambivalently into the fray whenever Estelle needed attention.

When the subject turned to Ariana's failed marriage and current social life, the mother (Maria) expressed some hope, immediately labeled as ridiculous by Ariana, that she (Ariana) would get back together with her ex-husband. Ariana stated, as she had when interviewed alone, that "with all this," meaning the problems with Estelle, "how can I find time to get involved with anyone?"

Further discussion revealed that Maria was a worrier and constantly preoccupied with whichever of her children was having difficulties, especially medical problems. Next to Estelle, Ariana herself was labeled as being the most in need of attention by everyone except for Gladys. Gladys had been the most successful of the children in separating from her parents' household (she did not come to the family meeting despite being invited). In fact, Ariana made it clear that her own illnesses had no effect on Gladys' or anyone else's willingness to help out with Estelle. The family seemed to concur that Gladys' child and Ariana's brothers' jobs were legitimate reasons for them not being able to help out with Estelle.

On the other hand, Ariana's medical problems did elicit emotional support and sympathy from her mother, who suggested that, since Ariana was no longer married, she should move back into the family house. Ariana immediately rejected the offer and said that her medical problems were the biggest reason she couldn't move back into the house, the reason being that she didn't want her mother to see her when she was sick because the mother would worry too much. Ariana added that when she was feeling sick, she needed to stay home by herself, and at these times she didn't even answer the phone or know what was going on in her parents' house.

Case 1 Discussion (Contd.): The physician concluded that Ariana's somatization was embedded in the repetitive pattern of events dominated by her triangular relationship with Estelle and their mother. Ariana's physical symptoms served the purpose of allowing her to remain connected to her mother, enabling her to receive attention and emotional support, and at the same time was the only way she could control the family's expectations that she would always be there to help with Estelle. It seemed to be critical that Ariana's reason for remaining away from her mother and Estelle was an illness, that is, something beyond her control, as compelling as Gladys' childcare responsibilities or her brothers' jobs, and not merely the need to have more of her life to herself.

Step 6: Reframing Attention to the Underlying Family Problems

In exploring the triangular relationships and repetitive patterns in which the patient's problematic behavior is embedded, the physician must attempt to bring the patient and family's emotional experience into the interview. When the patient or family have displayed the pattern of behavior, and described—even reexperienced—the pain associated with it, the physician is able to reframe the patient and family's attention to the dysfunction. The physician is able to say, "It seems to me that the family situation you have just described is extremely painful, and that in addition to your [problematic symptom or behavior], this family problem is also worthy of attention." Note that the reframing does *not* state that the patient and family should attend to the underlying family problems *instead* of the presenting complaint, but rather *in addition to it*. If the patient and family are willing to accept the reframing so completely that the presenting symptom or problematic behavior is relinquished entirely, so much the better. This complete transformation, however, is not necessary for the subsequent steps of the method to have their beneficial effect. It is necessary, though, for the interview to succeed in recreating the family dance and capturing the emotional content of the experience with an intensity and reality that ensures that the patient and family cannot but agree that the family problems are worthy of attention.

To accomplish this effect it may be necessary to conduct an interview with the entire family and encourage them to actually enact their problem during the interview. With experience, this is not too difficult. It is usually sufficient to ask the family to begin talking about "the problem" and support individuals in stating how they truly feel. The result of such an enactment interview, which includes the steps described below, is usually both revealing and therapeutic. It can, however, be unnerving for the inexperienced physician to encourage a family to have their fight in the office. This technique therefore requires supervision from more experienced clinicians until the physician is reasonably confident that it will have a positive outcome.

Case 1 Discussion (Contd.): It was relatively easy to reframe the burden of caring for Estelle as a problem worthy of attention after the painful demonstration of just how difficult it was to have a conversation with her. It was also easy to reframe Ariana's desire to have some time for herself—a need she was unwilling to claim on her own—as something that would be important for "a woman her age" *even if she was not ill.* Ariana was willing to accept the suggestion that her failure to develop the kind of intimate relationship she desired was also a problem worthy of consideration.

Step 7: Empathic Witnessing

The most immediate way to ensure that family assessment and intervention have a positive and therapeutic effect—whether performed with a genogram-based interview of the individual patient or a full family enactment interview—is to use the assessment as the foundation for empathically witnessing the patient's and family's problems and their efforts to cope. If the interview has succeeded in exposing the distress and the family's best attempt to deal with their problems, the patient and family will know that the physician knows the family in a very intimate way. If the physician recognizes the special nature of this awareness, and responds empathically to the patient and family, the effect can be very therapeutic. The general format for empathic witnessing is to tell the patient and family that, having heard their story, and seen what they have to cope with, that you are very impressed with how well they have been doing despite the problems that afflict them. Empathic witnessing is a more intensive version of providing emotional support that was described in step 4 of basic family assessment and intervention.

Case illustration 1 (Contd.): The family was willing to admit that the current situation was indeed painful for everyone involved and that they themselves had not been able to solve the problem despite their best efforts to do so. The physician was able to tell Ariana and her mother how impressed she was with how well they were both doing, despite the tremendous problems they had to deal with. The physician remarked on the magnitude of the sacrifice Ariana had made, neglecting her own social life in order to be available to the family, and commented that developing the social aspect of her life was just as impor-

tant to her at her stage of life as caring for children was for Gladys. The physician also commented that it was easy to understand how this area of Ariana's life might be difficult for her to deal with because of her past difficulties.

Step 8: Referral for Family & Psychotherapy Overcoming Resistance:

Patient and family resistance to referral for psychotherapeutic intervention is common and is often one of the reasons why an advanced family assessment and intervention is required in the first place. Referral makes perfect sense to the provider because of the physician's understanding of the patient's problem. Resistance to referral shows that the patient does not share that understanding. The difference in perspective that leads to such resistance is not purely cognitive; patients may understand and even accept the physician's analysis intellectually but resist referral for psychotherapy out of fear of dealing directly with painful and powerful emotions. Acceding to a psychotherapy referral may also be perceived as an admission of personal or family failure. This is why the process of reframing must make the pain of the current situation so clearly unacceptable that the need to change, combined with the hope generated by their new understanding of the problem, outweighs the fear the patient and family have of further psychotherapeutic work.

Even when this approach is used skillfully, resistance to therapy can remain intractable. It may take years before the reframing and empathic witnessing bear fruit. It is not unusual for patients and families to finally go to a therapist only after there has been some further crisis or deterioration in family functioning such that they feel they have no choice but to seek help. Sometimes it is forced on them, for example, by the courts in criminal or custodial cases, or employer-mandated treatment for substance abuse. If the physician performs the family assessment and intervention described here when it first seems appropriate, the therapeutic alliance will be more effective in moving patient and family to the next step of treatment when the next crisis does arrive, as it inevitably will.

Not infrequently, patients and their families never get to therapy. Even in that case, the reframing and empathic witnessing of the patient's family story has a positive effect. Aside from the intrinsic therapeutic benefit mentioned earlier, repeated empathic witnessing offers a therapeutic response to the patient who continues to present with somatoform symptoms, neglect of self-care, or destructive health-related behaviors. *After* performing a family assessment and intervention, the physician may say to the patient who has not followed through with referral for therapy and who returns with persistent or recurrent symptoms (as did the father in case illustration 2):

Case illustration 2 (Conclusion): "I am sorry that your headache is still bothering you. Your wife and daughter are still fighting, aren't they? It's too bad that you haven't gotten to the therapist yet. I truly wish that there was more that I could do for you. Now, why don't we check your blood pressure."

Case 2 Discussion (Conclusion): The patient—aware that the physician has witnessed the family conflict—knows that the clinician understands the importance of the conflict at home and that this understanding is empathic. Hence, the physician does not have to repeat the assessment and intervention interview, merely recall it with the patient. The physician is in a position to respect the meaning of the patient's symptom without allowing it to divert the process of care into unnecessary testing, medication, or referrals for more evaluation. The physician is therefore able to maintain an emotionally supportive alliance with the patient, while avoiding a dysfunctional compensatory alliance. This is accomplished by responding to the patient's symptom in three ways: (1) making a therapeutic suggestion, (2) clarifying the limits of the provider's capacity to help, and (3) pointing out the patient's responsibility and opportunity to act on his own behalf.

Case illustration 1 (Conclusion): The physician referred the family for family therapy to explore better approaches to coping with the burden of Estelle's medical problems. The physician suggested that Ariana would

benefit from individual counseling to explore her difficulties in forming a satisfying intimate relationship. Maria's physician was asked to consider the diagnoses of dysthymia and major depression. The family agreed to try to obtain a home health aide for Estelle to give Maria *and* Estelle herself a break. The family agreed to all four of these suggestions at the time of the initial family interview. When Ariana returned for her next visit, she still had somatoform symptoms but spoke of them only briefly, allowing the physician to turn the discussion to what was going on at home. Ariana reported that the family had taken no steps toward family therapy and that she was still considering whether to go to individual therapy. She did report feeling more comfortable setting limits on her mother's expectations of assistance in dealing with Estelle and reported success in obtaining a home health aide for several hours three times per week. Maria had been placed on an antidepressant by her physician, made a few visits to a community mental health center, and was much less symptomatic.

Eight months later, Ariana entered individual therapy for about a year. Her somatization decreased dramatically and her limit-setting improved. Eventually she started dating and entered a steady relationship but has not married. The family subsequently weathered some major upheavals, including further deterioration in Estelle's physical and mental status and the death of a brother and sister-in-law from AIDS, leaving Ariana in custody of their son. The family never entered family therapy.

SUGGESTED READINGS

Carter CA, McGoldrick M (editors): *The Family Lifecycle: A Framework for Family Therapy.* Gardner Press, 1980.

Doherty WJ, Baird MA: *Family Therapy and Family Medicine.* Guilford Press, 1983.

Doherty WJ, Baird MA: *Family-Centered Medical Care: A Clinical Case Book.* Guilford Press, 1987.

Doherty WJ, Campbell TL: *Families and Health.* Sage Publications, 1988.

Hahn SR, Feiner JS, Bellin EH: The doctor-patient-family relationship: A compensatory alliance. Ann Intern Med, 1988;109:884.

Haley J: *Problem Solving Therapy.* Jossey-Bass, 1976.

McDaniel S, Campbell TL, Seaburn DB: *Family-Oriented Primary Care.* Springer-Verlag, 1990.

McGoldrick M, Gerson R: *Genograms in Family Assessment.* Norton, 1985.

Minuchin S: *Families and Family Therapy.* Harvard University Press, 1974.

Minuchin S, Bosman BL, Baker L: *Psychosomatic Families.* Harvard University Press, 1987.

10

Children

Howard L. Taras, MD

This chapter reviews common childhood behavioral problems and suggests some management guidelines. Pediatric behavioral medicine cannot be easily disassociated from child development because many problematic childhood behaviors have developmental roots.

UNDESIRABLE BEHAVIOR AS A NORMAL PART OF DEVELOPMENT

A child's ability to understand and interact with the environment is constantly evolving. To learn more about the world, a child experiments with ways of interacting with it. Most often, children test the reactions of the people they are closest to, their parents. Colloquial phrases such as *"the terrible twos," "She's going through a stage,"* and *"Boys will be boys,"* indicate that undesirable childhood behaviors are commonly accepted to be "normal." But when an undesirable behavior is manifesting in one's own child, the normalcy can be difficult to accept. And even when the cause is well understood, many parents still need the knowledge and skills to respond to the problem behavior.

EXTRAORDINARY STRESS

Behavioral problems associated with normal childhood development must be distinguished from problems with more complex causes. Aberrant childhood behaviors are often secondary to extraordinary life stresses. This applies to children who witness violence, those exposed to continuous marital discord, those with a chronic illness or a chronically ill sibling, and those who don't feel wanted. Children living under any condition that seriously threatens healthy and successful transition through a developmental stage are likely to pose serious behavioral problems.

Children, like adults, may appear to be the dysfunctional member of an otherwise healthy family unit even though the problem actually stems from family issues. This is particularly the case with childhood behaviors, however, because children are dependent on adults in almost every way. Take, for instance, the child who refuses to attend school. Classically, this behavior occurs when one or both parents send subliminal messages to the child to remain home. Although the primary problem is parental anxiety about separation, the child alone exhibits the apparent symptoms.

INHERENT DISORDERS

Besides problems stemming from normal development and extraordinary life stresses, a third general category of childhood behavioral problems are those caused by disorders inherent to the child. Attention deficit disorders are the most common and well known, but conduct disorders, depression, pervasive developmental disorders, and other psychiatric diagnoses may manifest during childhood. Complete histories, observation, and response to treatment help the primary care clinician distinguish these from other causes of behavior problems.

SCREENING FAMILIES FOR DIFFICULTIES WITH CHILDHOOD BEHAVIORS

Pediatric primary care providers must screen families for difficulties with undesirable childhood behaviors, sort out probable causes for the behaviors, recognize when a mental health referral is appropriate, and manage those problems that are likely to respond to simple environmental changes or to elementary behavioral management techniques.

Practitioner Concern Versus Time Constraints

Many parents do not know where to seek help for behavioral problems such as their baby's night awakenings, their toddler's tantrums, or their fourth grader's class-clown behavior. To overcome this barrier, health care providers should take every opportunity to initiate discussion on behavioral issues. This is done in the context of time limitations imposed on each office visit, especially given the recent expansion of managed health care. Time constraints curb a practitioner's ability to listen to histories that can be extensive. And should a parent begin to disclose matters that are difficult to speak about, practitioners do not want to appear insensitive by cutting the conversation short. What is more, many parents feel uncomfortable about being faced with questions for which they have no prior preparation. To meet such challenges clinicians need ways of screening for behavioral information that are expedient and that leave the clinician with time to reflect on issues that can be discussed more fully at another time.

Trigger Questions & Questionnaires

One such way to elicit information from parents is to ask a preset list of key questions, specific to each age group. An excellent source for such "trigger" questions is Green's *Bright Futures: Guidelines for Health Supervision of Infants, Children, and Adolescents.* Another option is to routinely use formal, standardized questionnaires that are designed for parents to respond to by mail in advance of an appointment or in the clinician's waiting room. The benefits of these are that they provide parents time to respond thoughtfully to physician inquiries and include the input of both parents—often exposing differences in parents' opinions. These questionnaires also minimize parents' discomfort with verbalizing certain family problems. They often yield information from a wide range of potential problem areas and do so effectively. Many of these tools are accompanied by a separate set of questions for teachers, which are useful when a problem has been identified.

Table 10–1 lists four behavioral screens that are popular and appropriate for use by primary care clinicians. Other available questionnaires were reviewed by Eisert and associates. This review is a useful guide for clinicians who wish to identify which tool is most suitable to their needs.

To effectively screen families for childhood behavioral problems, practitioners also need to develop their skills of observation and learn to apply their natural intuitions toward clinical use. Parent-child interaction in the office can be an excellent indicator of problems occurring at home. Incidents in the office that induce parents to discipline their child are opportunities for clinicians to better understand the parent-child relationship and to bring behavioral management issues into discussion. Experienced clinicians have learned to become aware of subtle signs in the office that are indicative of a family's dynamics. The way a mother is holding her baby is an example. If a mother seems uncomfortable feeding her baby, if there is a pattern of noncompliance, or if there is suspicion for the levels of interest mother or father show, this observation should register concern with the clinician for other issues. Involvement of grandparents and other extended family, references parents make about their own upbringing, and other family characteristics are also worth noting.

Although signs for concern do not always reveal problems, this information frequently becomes useful to the evaluation of a child behavioral issue, sometimes not until months or years later. Positive impressions that clinicians form about families also provide clinically useful information.

INTERVIEWING YOUNG CHILDREN

Primary care providers can find themselves in a quandary when they try to elicit information directly from the child. Most children by age 2 1/2–3 years are capable of communicating certain thoughts and feelings to an inquiring health provider. But children do not typically divulge such information to clinicians when questioned directly. Children freely offer their honest opinions on just about any topic, sensitive or banal, but they often do so when it is unsolicited. Parents themselves are often surprised when their

Table 10–1. Behavioral screening tools.

Name	Author/Reference	Characteristics
Achenbach Child Behavior Checklist	Achenbach, Edelbrock: *Manual for the Child Behavioral Checklist and Revised Child Behavior Profile.* Univ of Vermont, 1983.	112 items for ages 2–16 years.
Conners Parent Questionnaire	Goyette, Conners: J Abnorm Child Psychol 1978;6:221.	10 minutes/48 items for ages 5–15 years.
Eyberg Child Behavior Inventory	Eyberg, Ross: Am J Clin Psychol 1978; 7:12.	10 minutes/36 items for ages 2–17 years.
Pediatric Symptom Checklist	Jellinek, et al: J Pediatr 1988;112:201.	5 minutes/35 items for grades 1–12.

children first reveal their feelings about a delicate personal issue to an adult with whom they are not ostensibly very close (a preschool teacher, friend's mother in their car pool, etc).

To get around this problem, primary care providers should use tools that help children more freely and predictably disclose what's on their minds. One way is to ask children old enough to understand and comply, to draw a picture. Ask them to draw "anything they want," "something scary," "their family," or "the worst day at school," for example. This can yield important information about what they are thinking. The position of the characters in the drawings, facial expressions, and choice of colors may be indicative of how they are feeling and can be used as a starting point for discussion. Children often find it easier to speak about themselves when the conversation is in the third person, such as "Why would that little girl in the picture want to hit her mommy?"

To avoid alienating parents, you may go through a few such questions when both parent and child are in the room. But many children, and most of those older than age 4 years, respond differently when their parents are in the room. Explain to parents that you would like to interview the child in the same way without them. The general nature of children's responses can be discussed later with parents. Parents should be notified that this will occur. But the interviewer need not feel compelled to reveal children's specific responses to each interview item, particularly if information may be hurtful and not of therapeutic value at that time. Parents and children should know that too.

Other oblique ways of eliciting information from children are asking open-ended questions but using questions that children like to respond to: "Pretend a magical genie in a bottle wanted to grant you three wishes, what would they be?" And, "If you could magically turn into any animal you wanted, what would it be?" To their response to the last question, then ask, "Well that's wonderful! And why would you be happy as that animal?"

Sentence completion games are also useful. The clinician begins the first few words of a sentence and asks the child to complete the sentence by making something up. Examples of some are given in Table 10–2, and these (and others like them) can be typed onto colorful cards so that children can choose one at a time and

Table 10–2. Samples of "sentence completion" items for interviewing young children.

I really like it when . . .
I am ashamed . . .
I worry a lot about . . .
My mother . . .
I hate . . .
It makes me sad to . . .
It makes me happy to . . .
People think that I . . .
I really hope one day that I . . .

perceive it as a game, not a real interview. Allow the child to be imaginative with responses, and indicate that their responses can be the truth but don't have to be.

Toddlers and school age children often catch on to clinicians' actual intent when these interviewing techniques are used. Despite this, children seem to enjoy going along with this format of questioning and appreciate having an easy way to express themselves. Children respond best when they are comfortable with the clinician. Arranging a number of office visits can help to establish that relationship.

When using drawings, questions in the third person, or questions evoking the child's imagination; it is important not to read too deeply into children's responses. Children have active imaginations; they play around with frightening ideas and with wishful thinking. Sometimes they are merely obsessed with speaking about what they've recently seen on television. To be taken seriously, responses of young children should fit into a general pattern of what the clinician suspects from parent interview and symptoms. One or two worrisome responses should not stand on their own as proof for the etiology to a problem.

BEYOND THE PHYSICIAN-CHILD-PARENT TRIAD

A majority of toddlers have both parents who work outside of the home. These children are placed in the care of a day care provider, baby-sitter, or relative. Virtually all children older than age 5 spend a large portion of their waking hours in school. Yet despite this, clinicians traditionally rely almost exclusively on parents (and the children themselves) to gather a behavioral history. Some clinicians send questionnaires to school staff to elicit information, or they ask parents about their children's progress at school or daycare. It is rare, however, for clinicians to routinely engage in direct telephone contact with child care providers and teachers. Yet these people occupy many, and occasionally most, of children's waking hours. The value of attaining parent permission to speak directly with educational professionals in a child's life cannot be overstated. Teachers and child care providers can provide valuable insight. Many have numerous years of experience with all types of children, and their observations rarely include the emotional biases that sometimes confound a parent's interpretation and recollection of details. Once a behavior plan has been recommended, a relationship with daytime caretakers may extend the plan's implementation to that setting and render it more effective.

NORMAL CHILD DEVELOPMENT

To attribute an undesirable behavior to a developmental stage of childhood, health care providers need

Table 10–3. Highlights of child characteristics during stages of development.

Theory	Ages 0–2	Ages 2–6	Ages 6–12
Kohlberg (Development of moral judgment)	Pre-moral Stage Egocentric, no moral concepts Satisfaction of own needs	Moral Stage Desires to please others	Moral Stage Obligation to duty Respect for authority
Piaget (Cognitive development)	Sensorimotor/Preverbal Emergence of purposeful activities Learns that objects and people exist even when out of sight	Preoperational/Prelogical Can deal with one aspect of a problem at a time Learns to use symbols for language, etc	Concrete Operational/Logical Can deal with multiple aspects of a problem, if not abstract Ability to classify things
Erickson (Psychosocial development)	Oral Stage (early on) Initially gaining trust Once gained, seeks independence Uses words like "no" and "me" Anal Stage Initially learns self control Then, can develop self-esteem and good will Learns autonomy but struggles with shame and doubt	Phallic Stage Takes initiative, is curious Becomes more aggressive and competitive Starts to plan ahead Struggles with guilt	Latency Stage An industrious stage Focused on performance and producing results Struggles with inferiority/ inadequacy when meeting some meritable failures

to be knowledgeable about stages of normal childhood development, for which numerous theories have been proposed (Table 10–3) and for which there are some excellent summaries.

Maturational Theory

This theory teaches that behavioral sequences occur by a process of unfolding in all children, that these sequences are regulated by genes, and that detrimental environmental factors could impede this sequence.

Freudian Psychoanalytic Theories

Freud's theories emphasize unconscious and conscious mental processes that children go through. For example, in the anal stage at $1\frac{1}{2}$–3 years of age children are personally focused on elimination and interpersonally focused on "rebellion versus compliance" with parental demands. At this stage, they may fear loss of parental love.

Erikson's Stages of Child Development

Erickson's is an expanded version of psychoanalytic theory, and his teachings help clinicians understand children's psychosocial development.

Piagetian Theory

Paiget's staging of children's cognitive development describes, for example, that a child cannot be expected to see a situation from a perspective other than his or her own until school-age.

Kohlberg's Theory

Kohlberg's theory of children's moral development describes, for example, how young toddlers understand their actions to be good or bad based on the presence or absence of a resulting punishment or reward.

The five preceding theories do not necessarily contradict one other. None is complete on its own. Each theory can be viewed by the clinician as a different view of a single multidimensional entity we call "child development." Each describes child development from another perspective. If one theory throws more light than another on a given child's behavior, then try using it to explain an undesirable behavior and then to help guide parents toward a proper response.

MANAGEMENT & REFERRAL

The rise of managed health care has heightened the importance for primary care providers to evaluate and manage common child behavior problems in their own offices. In addition, mental health referrals are usually unnecessary since so many undesirable child behaviors are maladaptations or manifestations of normal child development. There are occasions when the need for psychiatric assessment, psychotherapy, or play therapy are apparent from the start. But for most problems that present to primary care practitioners, children respond well to brief, solution-focused strategies. As with the treatment of common medical problems, most clinicians find they need to use only a small number of management techniques. Clinicians should become comfortable with a number of these and ultimately in the variation of responses that occur among families. Although no single behavioral management technique works well for all children with similar problems and similar etiologies to their problems, clinicians can quickly learn to tailor their management plans to suit individual needs of each family. These plans should be based on families' cultural characteristics, size, work schedules, and other factors. A management failure should always first be considered a problem with the behavioral management technique prescribed, not with the child or family.

EXAMPLES OF COMMON BEHAVIORAL ISSUES

Infancy: Night-Waking

Case illustration 1: Parents of a 12-week-old girl complain that their daughter rarely sleeps more than a total of 4–5 hours between 8 PM and 6 AM. She may fall asleep at 8 PM, only to reawaken an hour later. She seems to fall asleep during or after short feeds and then remains awake for a period of hours later on. Each night is a struggle of long awakened periods between short spells of sleep. Parents note that she cries for long periods when left alone. She seems content at night when parents walk around with her.

Child development in early infancy is characterized by large fluctuations in temperament and schedules. In the first few weeks of life, infants often sleep as much during the day as at night. In the first 2 months of life, two night awakenings are common, and by 3 months of life most infants are sleeping for 5–6 hours uninterrupted. In this case, the child did not naturally "learn" the difference between night and day, and parents did not train her to do so. But if clinicians ask parents to let their young infants cry themselves to sleep, they set parents up for feelings of inadequacy or guilt. This, in turn, strains the relationship of attachment that parents are forming with their children.

Case illustration 1 (Contd.): On further questioning in this case, the parents reported that their baby falls asleep immediately after daytime feeds and sleeps for 3–5 consecutive hours thereafter. This baby did not adapt to an acceptable or optimal day/night schedule. In this case their doctor recommended waking the baby up after no more than 2–3 hours of daytime sleep. Parents were to try to occupy their infant's daytime hours by walking around, talking, playing music and offering other playful activities. It was recommended that nighttime feeds be made minimally stimulating. Soften the lights, produce minimal noise, and avoid "fun" interactions at night. Although sleeping and feeding "on demand" need not always be discouraged, in this case the infant's pattern needlessly disrupted parents' well-being and this justified modification. After 5–6 days of compliance with this schedule, it became easier for parents to keep their daughter awake during the day and the parents settled for a night-time feed at 11 PM before they retired and another feed at 4 AM.

It is important to note that likely causes for night awakenings change with developmental stages. This same sleep history told by parents of a 9-month-old would be more likely related to the child's cognitive ability to recognize that parents still "exist" after they leave the room. At that age, if there were no other likely cause, other recommendations are in order. A nightlight or a transitional object (favorite blanket or teddy bear) could prove to be helpful. The clinician, in the case of the 9-month-old, should devise a careful behavioral intervention schedule that includes parental reassurance for the child but may also include an allowance for the child to "cry it out" for a couple of nights.

Toddler: Aggression

Case illustration 2: The parents of a 3-year-old boy report that their son throws himself on the floor, throws objects, and screams . . . usually when he doesn't get his own way. This seems to happen daily. At his child care center, he has begun to bite other children when he is angry, and other parents have begun to complain about him.

Assessment of this behavior begins with elucidating, through history-gathering, the extent of the child's aggression and its likely etiology. Angry outbursts are common at 3 years of age, when children often begin to direct their anger at others. Parental response to a given level of aggression differs widely from family to family. Parents' expectations of children's behavior, not solely the magnitude of the child's behavior, help to define whether or not a behavior is a problem. Large discrepancies between childhood behaviors and parental thresholds may predict that a child will continue to be problematic in the future. A child who explores the environment very actively may be described as "curious" in one family but as "always climbing the walls" in another. A "difficult and stubborn" child to one family is "persistent—just like his successful grandpa" to another. Perhaps the more positive perspective creates a better self-image for a child and leads to fewer problems later on.

Certain questions may help clinicians assess the etiology of aggressive behavior: Is the child a cruel or unhappy child? Is the child exposed to frequent violent (physical or verbal) outbursts from others at home? Are the incidents that induce these behaviors unpredictable? Is the child cognitively not acting consistently with his or her age? Positive responses to these questions make a normal developmental etiology less likely.

When development is still the most likely cause, there are a number of possibilities to consider. First, children with well-developed cognitive abilities, but with comparatively delayed language abilities, often become frustrated with limited ways of expressing themselves. Second, children at this stage often strive for adult attention and have found aggressive behaviors to be a certain way of getting it. Third, children at this stage need to express their independence, yet some adults have not found enough acceptable ways to allow the child to do this. To ascertain the likely cause(s), clinicians should explore events surrounding these incidents of aggression. Detailed examples of what instigated the last one or two aggressive behaviors are more revealing than letting parents say, "Oh it happens for just about anything." Always ask parents how they feel when their child acts out. Feeling like "I just don't have time for this," may be a good indication that the child is trying to get attention. If their first reaction is to feel that this is a power struggle, then the child's strive for independence may be his or her primary incentive. Also ask what parents have done in response to a misbehavior and whether or not this reaction worked.

Case illustration 2 (Contd.): In this case, the child's degree of aggression was within reason for a child at his developmental stage. His tantrums began as a result of typical frustrations experienced by children his age. Over a period of months as his parents became busier with other family needs, however, he discovered that expressing anger was an excellent way to get adult attention, and the frequency of these behaviors increased. As part of the management plan, parents were instructed to ignore his anger and put him in his room for a few minutes when he became physically violent with others. Concomitantly, parents were to increase time spent doing happier things with him, like playing games, going on walks, and having him help them around the house. At day care, he was given increased individual attention during times he was behaving well. Child care providers were asked to ignore him when he attacked other children, and to shower a "noticeable" amount of attention on the attacked child. Within a couple of weeks their son stopped biting and seemed happier. Although he still had a terrible temper, these strategies gave his parents the feeling of some control with the situation.

Toddlers: Oppositional Behavior

Case illustration 3: A 3-year-old refuses to go to bed on time. He prolongs bedtime rituals by making numerous requests (eg, for water, use of bathroom, adjusting the door, etc). He repeatedly leaves his bed. On many nights he finally falls asleep in the living room or parents' bedroom while spending time with his parents.

Case illustration 4: A mother solicits your opinion on vitamin supplements to counterbalance her 28-month-old daughter's picky eating habits. She drinks apple juice, eats hot dogs, and Honey-Nut Cheerios, and little else. When these foods are not offered, she protests violently and eats nothing at all.

Behaviors described in these cases are typical for this age group. Toddlers commonly oppose parents for many sorts of issues, including the eating and bedtime cases illustrated here (eg, getting dressed, putting toys away, wearing seat belt, etc). A tendency to challenge parents' instructions subsides naturally as children grow older. But they need to be dealt with properly for those months or years they are present. When parents mistake a child's behavior as a personal offense, they react to the behavior in a way that creates

additional conflict and heightens oppositional behavior. Therefore, it is important for clinicians to emphasize the developmental component. Children in both illustrative cases have learned to exploit their parents' uncertainty with what exactly is in their child's best interest. In both cases, the clinician should rule out deeper problems by interviewing the parent and, to whatever extent possible, the child. Look for unusual fears, nightmares, and other symptoms that may indicate an unusual etiology to the oppositional behavior. None were found in these two cases.

Case illustration 3 (Contd.): In the first case, the pediatrician recommended to the parents that they explain to the child that from now on after his bedtime ritual he must remain in his bedroom whether he is able to sleep or not. They were to routinely ask their child before leaving his bedroom if he needed anything else. Thereafter, if the child cried, screamed, or tried to carry on a conversation with his parents, they were to ignore him. When he left his bed, they were to physically put him back without talking to him and with expressionless faces. They were to do this even in the middle of the night. They were warned that their child's behavior would likely worsen for one or two nights before improving. In less than a week, this boy resigned himself to making only one unenthusiastic, "face-saving" attempt to stay up before he fell asleep.

Parental persistence must be designed to outlast the child's. It is then almost always effective within 2 weeks, and often within 2 nights. If this child shared a room with a sibling, it would have been suggested that the sibling sleep in the parents' room until the index child's behavior became less disruptive.

Case illustration 4 (Contd.): In the second case, the same principles were applied to other behaviors. The child was offered three wholesome meals and one snack at preset times of the day. After telling their daughter once, parents were not to engage in any discussion with their child about the volume eaten. No other foods in the house were made available to her during this behavioral management period. Between meals this girl was allowed an unlimited quantity of water, but nothing else. After a difficult period of $1\frac{1}{2}$ days (thrown silverware, persistent crying, etc), she began to nibble at new foods and to enjoy the positive attention for doing so. Although the patient still enjoyed only a limited range of foods, parents were able to expand her repertoire to include broccoli, milk, and pasta.

Parents often worry about harming their child by restricting access to food after a missed meal, so they need to be reassured that this is not harmful and will ultimately improve nutrition. It is all too common for a well-meaning grandparent who resides in the home to "save" the child by sneaking her a cookie between meals (case 4) or lying down with the child after a designated bedtime (case 3). Such kindly motivated behaviors unwittingly prolong the child's maladaptive behavior, extending the period of inadequate nutrition and sleep. It is imperative that clinicians invite all adult household members to their offices when prescribing a management plan in order to be sure that all involved endorse both the intent and methods. It is useful to write behavioral management "rules" down on a prescription pad to be taped to the refrigerator door. This helps prevent conflict among adult household members that may arise later. Clinicians should also routinely recommend follow-up visits to their offices once the management plan has been implemented, in order to monitor progress.

Toddlers: Toilet Training

Children must be developmentally ready before toilet training is initiated by parents. First, physiologic sphincter control is necessary. This usually develops between ages 1 and 2 years, and parents often know when their child is beginning to sense a bowel movement because of a characteristic grimace or stance. The ability to follow sequential instructions, the motivation to imitate parents, and the patience to sit on a potty should also be present. It is reasonable to try toilet training at age 2 years if these milestones have been achieved. But disinterest or undue difficulty should alert parents to terminate their attempt and wait 2–3 months before trying again. Some children may not be ready until age 3. Others are ready at 18 months.

Although a number of effective toilet training methods exist, only one method is described here. Place the potty in the bathroom the child typically uses and explain what it is for by drawing parallels with the toilet parents uses. The child should be encouraged with praise to sit on the potty for a couple of minutes a day, initially with diaper and pants on and after a few days, without them. The child should accompany the parent to empty soiled diapers into the potty. Parents should avoid commenting on the foul odor of the stool, as some children identify what they've produced as extensions of themselves. Gradually, the child should be asked to sit on the potty more frequently during the day, particularly if there is a time when bowel movements are likely to occur. Encourage the child to let the potty "catch" the stool. Parents should never scold a child for inability to do this nor for any "accidents." Night training, standing at urination, and using a larger toilet are secondary skills that should be introduced only after the child has mastered the basics or if the child expresses interest.

School Age: Primary Nocturnal Enuresis

One workable definition for enuresis is at least one bed-wetting incident weekly for a boy older than age 6 or a girl older than age 5. It is considered secondary enuresis if a child had been dry previously for a period greater than 6 months. By this definition, 15% of children have this condition, making it one of the most commonly asked questions of pediatric health care providers. Absence of other urinary tract problems (in-fection, neurogenic bladder, etc) can be ruled out with a basic medical examination and history. It is important to recognize that the only problems with primary nocturnal enuresis are the reactions of the child and the parent. Otherwise, it is a self-limiting condition that resolves spontaneously. If a child and his or her parents are not bothered by it, then no treatment is necessary. This is worthwhile to point out to families whenever the option for intervention is offered.

To treat this condition, it is necessary that children themselves, not only their parents, are motivated. Verify that a child is truly motivated and determine the source of motivation by interviewing the child separately. When a child is not genuinely motivated to try something new in order to be dry, clinical efforts should be directed toward other family members. Gauge parental actions and anxieties and if necessary influence them so that their actions and anxieties are not causes of unnecessary stress for their child. Children should never be punished for their enuretic disorder. Even if parents insist that their child help to change wet bed sheets, this task should be carried out with the same attitude as other household responsibilities the child has been expected to take on.

Commercially available alarm devices assist clinicians and parents in instituting "conditioning therapy." This method is of clinically proven use. With this device, an alarm awakens the child with the first few drops of urine. Eventually this teaches the child to awaken with the sensation of a full bladder. The child is still responsible to get him or herself to the bathroom. The alarm is usually effective when used nightly for a couple of months. Setbacks occur after removing the alarm, but these are often corrected more permanently by one further trial period with the device.

Desmopressin (DDAVP), an analogue of antidiuretic hormone, is a pharmacologic therapy of choice. If children respond to this nasally administered medication they usually do so within 2 weeks. Relapses after withdrawal are not uncommon, however, and this therapy is best offered when the alarm device has failed. Imipramine has also been shown to be useful and may be indicated in certain circumstances. Sphincter control exercises, fluid restrictions in the evening hours, and urine retention training may be tried, but these methods have shown only limited success.

School Age: Attention Deficit Disorders

Unlike the behavioral problems described earlier, attention deficit/hyperactivity disorder (ADHD) is not a manifestation of normal child development but a disorder described in the *Diagnostic and Statistical Manual of Mental Disorders (DSM-IV)* of the American Psychiatric Association. It is characterized by inattention or hyperactivity/impulsivity for a period of at least 6 months. Symptoms begin prior to age 7 years. There must be clear evidence of clinically significant impairment in social or academic functioning with some impairment evident in more than one setting. Its diagnosis and management (and misdiagnosis and mismanagement) have become so popularized in the public press that clinicians are sometimes confronted with an unexpectedly emotionally charged situation when the diagnosis is being considered. Many school teachers and parents have strong opinions on both sides the spectrum, that is, that medications for this disorder are either grossly underprescribed or overprescribed. The first role of a clinician is to bring a level of pragmatism to the diagnostic process and to the management of the disorder. Clinicians need to carefully explain the rationale behind their investigative and management plans. Some useful strategies are described here.

Often it is classroom problems, not problems at home, that instigate a referral to a health care provider for suspected ADHD. Yet paradoxically little emphasis is placed on establishing direct communication between clinicians and appropriate school staff. Parents should be encouraged to provide consent to exchange such information and be reassured that they will participate at each stage of the process. Most elementary schools have multidisciplinary teams consisting of resource teachers, school psychologists, counselors, and so forth, whose function is to review students with learning or behavior problems. Clinicians are well advised to contact their patient's school to inquire about such teams and then suggest that their patient's case be presented there. This team's report can save the patient, the parent, and the clinician large amounts of time by avoiding unnecessary investigations. Multidisciplinary school teams provide excellent insight into children's behavior and help to assess the likelihood of an associated or an alternate diagnosis, like a learning disorder. This strategy is of particular importance economically because diagnoses and effective management occur after fewer office visits, and because third-party payers and managed health care plans do not frequently cover psychological tests to investigate learning disorders.

As with learning disorders, emotional and environmental problems can be mistaken for ADHD, or they may coexist with ADHD but exacerbate the symptoms. Primary care providers can usually fulfill their roles as diagnosticians by conducting thorough patient and family interviews (Table 10–4). Existing published questionnaires and rating scales simplify the elicitation of histories from educators and parents.

When medication is being contemplated, three factors should also be considered because they tend to enhance parent and child acceptance for medication. The first is to start the medication on a trial basis only, perhaps by alternating one week on medication with one week without for a period of a month. Keep the teacher blinded to this regimen, but ask the teacher for weekly feedback. It is reassuring to patients, families, and to prescribing physicians when the worth of a medication is demonstrated in this way. The second is to emphasize to patients that medication only serves

Table 10–4. A differential diagnosis of attention deficits.

Primary
Neurobiologically based
Inherited or secondary to factors affecting early brain development
Dysfunction of varying combinations of neural systems with varying clinical presentations (subtypes)

Secondary
Symptoms secondary to, associated with, or mimicked by:
Cognitive/processing disorder
    Language disorder
    Learning disorder
    Cognitive impairment/Mental retardation
Medical disorder

Neurologic	Metabolic
Seizures	Endocrine
Infections	Toxins
Choreiform disorder	Iron deficiency
Neurodegenerative conditions	Sensory impairment

Emotional/psychiatric disorders
    Anxiety
    Depression
    Autism
    Personality/behavioral factors
Environmental factors
    Disruptive/chaotic home situations
    Inappropriate school placement
    Mismatch of neurobehavioral styles and environmental expectations

Source: Reprinted, with permission, from Dr. Desmond Kelly: Attention deficits in school-aged children and adolescents. Pediatr Clin North Am 1992;39(3):487.

to help them perform as well as they want. It is important that improvements are attributed to the child's efforts, not only the tablet the child is swallowing. And third, medications should only be prescribed as one part of a larger management plan. Classroom strategies that assist students with attention deficits

Table 10–5. Examples of classroom strategies for students with ADHD.

Seat the child close to teacher, or ask the teacher to circulate around classroom near to student.
Teacher should frequently signal student to get on task.
Use signals classmates may not notice (eg, hand on shoulder).
Find enclosed spaces for student to work (cubicles, if possible).
Make frequent topic changes during the day for student (or class as a whole).
Reward progress and effort, not only achievement.
Avoid long written assignments (replace with oral examinations) and have tolerance for poor handwriting.
Break all tasks (tests, assignments, and worksheets) into smaller parts.
Regard inconsistency as part of ADHD, not student attitude.
Devise a behavioral modification plan for classroom behaviors (eg, impulsive behaviors like blurting out answers).
Be prepared to revise behavioral modification techniques frequently (eg, change reinforcements).
Specifically target organizational skills as a learning objective.
Minimize clutter on blackboard, desk, handouts, etc.

ADHD: attention deficit/hyperactivity disorder.

should be concomitantly implemented. Examples of these are listed in Table 10–5. These are best implemented through strong home-school-clinic communication lines. These techniques are most readily accepted in schools with programs that encourage teachers experienced with ADHD students to assist teachers who are new to these children.

CONCLUSION

With the elicitation of a good history and an understanding of child development, primary care clinicians can develop reasonable hypotheses about childhood behavioral problems. Clinicians who manage childhood behavioral problems become very comfortable with a set of behavioral management protocols that can be applied to many common misbehaviors. Most problems of a serious nature that require psychiatric or psychological intervention become apparent early on in the process. It is not only cost-effective to avoid unnecessary referrals; assisting families with behavioral issues that arise with their children in the primary care office improves the relationship that families develop with their primary care clinicians.

SUGGESTED READINGS

Christophersen E, Levine M (editors): Development and behavior: Older children and adolescents. Pediatr Clin North Am 1992;3:39.

Coleman W, Taylor E (editors): Family focused pediatrics. Pediatr Clin North Am 1995;42:[Entire issue].

Dixon S, Stein M. (editors): *Encounters with Children: Pediatric Behavior and Development,* 2nd ed. Mosby-Year Book, 1992.

Eisert D, Sturner R, Mabe PA: Questionnaires in behavioral pediatrics: Guidelines for selection and use. Dev Behav Pediatr 1991;12:42.

Glascoe F, Dworkin P: The role of parents in the detection of developmental and behavioral problems. Pediatrics 1995;95:829.

Green M (editor): *Bright Futures: Guidelines for Health Supervision of Infants, Children, and Adolescents.* National Center for Education in Maternal and Child Health, 1994.

Adolescents

11

Lawrence S. Friedman, MD

INTRODUCTION

This chapter offers a practical behavioral framework to assist those who provide health care to teenagers. Stages of adolescent development along with behavioral correlates are discussed, and suggestions for effective patient-doctor communication, interviewing, and provision of health services are presented.

DEFINITION

Adolescence is not a disease. From a physiologic perspective, adolescence is the interval between the onset of puberty and the cessation of body growth. Because *physical change* does not adequately describe cognitive, emotional, psychologic, or behavioral development, a purely physiologic definition is too confining. In psychosocial terms, adolescence is the period during which adult body image and sexual identity emerge; independent moral standards, intimate interpersonal relationships, vocational goals, and health behaviors develop; and the separation from parents takes place. Although some of these tasks may begin prior to puberty and continue evolving into adulthood, they provide the foundation for understanding adolescent behavior.

Health Status & Trends

Most teenagers are healthy. Compared with other age groups, mortality rates for teenagers are low. Even teenagers with serious chronic illness usually survive into early or middle adulthood. The majority of serious health problems in this population are behavior-related. The 1993 Youth Risk Behavior Survey sponsored by the Centers for Disease Control found epidemic proportions of unwanted pregnancy; sexually transmitted diseases; weapon carrying; interpersonal violence; suicidal ideation; and alcohol, cigarette, and illicit drug use. Nationally, accidents are the leading cause of death for teenagers, although gunshot wounds lead in some neighborhoods. Socioeconomic status rather than ethnic or racial grouping defines the neighborhoods most at risk for gunshot deaths. Despite these significant problems, however, the most common reasons for acute office visits for teenagers are routine or sports physicals, upper respiratory infections, and acne.

There is some argument that their relatively low rates of morbidity and mortality should make comprehensive health care for teenagers a rather low national health priority. Because most adolescent deaths are preventable and because adult sexual practices, dietary habits, and substance use usually begin in adolescence, however, ignoring this age group means missing a major public health opportunity.

In 1992, the American Medical Association produced the first set of developmentally and behaviorally appropriate comprehensive health-care guidelines for adolescents. These guidelines emphasize anticipatory, preventive, and patient-centered services. They suggest that adolescent health promotion and disease prevention be a partnership encompassing patients, parents, schools, communities, and health-care providers.

Although individual health care is vital, adolescent health outcomes—perhaps more than for any other population—are closely linked to cultural, educational, political, and economic policies. Handguns and tobacco are both relevant examples. For example, the availability of handguns is not a problem that the physician can resolve during an office visit, yet making them less available would substantially benefit the health of many teenagers. Many fewer teenagers would ever begin using tobacco if cigarette prices were significantly higher and advertising were not designed to attract teenagers.

STAGES OF DEVELOPMENT

Medical services for teenagers need to be developmentally appropriate. Each of the three recognized developmental stages is distinguished by physical, cognitive, and behavioral hallmarks. Not all adolescents fit perfectly into each phase, and they often progress at different rates from one phase to the next. In addition, rates of physical, cognitive, and behavioral development may not be congruent. For example, a 14-year-old girl who is physically mature may be emotionally unable to decide about sexual intimacy and the consequences of pregnancy—or even its possibility.

Early Adolescence (Ages 11–14)

Physical: Rapid growth causes physical and body-image changes. Many teenagers question whether their growth is "normal," and commonly there is a good deal of somatic preoccupation and worry. Gynecomastia, for example (a typical physical problem for boys), may cause anxiety and concern, and prevent participation in physical education class. Because the topic may be too embarrassing for an already self-conscious teenager to raise, physician-initiated reassurance is essential when the condition is identified during a physical examination. The early or later onset of puberty has widely variable effects. Early puberty may be associated with the increased likelihood of weight concern and excessive dieting and other eating disorders in girls, but it may result in greater self-esteem and athletic prowess in boys. Because self-esteem is linked closely with physical development and peer-group attractiveness, both boys and girls who develop later than their peers may have self-esteem problems. Among early adolescents, questions and concerns about menstruation, masturbation, wet dreams, and the size of their breasts (too large or too small) and genitals are common among young teenagers. These questions need to be anticipated and specifically and carefully addressed.

Social: Peer-group involvement increases, and family involvement decreases. Friendships are idealized and are mostly same gender. Close peer relationships coupled with curiosity about body development may result in homosexual and other sexual experimentation, anxiety, and fear. Although some heterosexual relationships are initiated, contact with the opposite sex frequently occurs in groups.

Cognitive: The transition from concrete to abstract thinking begins. Because experience and emotion play important roles in decision-making, improved cognition alone is not enough to prevent many teenagers from making impulsive decisions with little regard for consequences. Increased cognitive ability linked with the search for identity often leads teenagers to test limits both at home and at school. Daydreaming is common.

Middle Adolescence (Ages 15–17)

Physical: The issues of early adolescence may continue, although most physical development is complete by the end of this phase.

Social: The struggles around independence, identity, and autonomy intensify. Peer groups may become more important than family to some teenagers and result in increasing teen-parent conflict. Experimentation with alcohol, drugs, and sex is common. A sense of invincibility coupled with impulsiveness leads to high rates of automobile accidents, suicides, and interpersonal violence. Unfortunately, suicide, impulsively linked to failed love relationships, also occurs during this phase. Despite adhering to peer-group norms regarding music, dress, and appearance (including body piercing, hair color, and makeup) the expression of individuality is common. Many teenagers find identity and support in school, sports, community, or church activities. For teenagers whose support systems or community resources are inadequate, gangs may supplement personal strength and provide a sense of identity. Teenagers from alienated and disenfranchised ethnic groups are at particular risk for gang activity.

Cognitive: Improved reasoning and abstraction allow for closer interpersonal relationships and empathy in this group. Evaluation of future academic and vocational plans becomes important. Poor school performance may heighten anxiety and concern about vocational choices and lead to "escape" in drugs and alcohol. Practical guidance that identifies strengths and builds self-esteem can help avoid frustration and failure.

Late Adolescence (Ages 18–24)

Physical: Body growth is usually no longer a concern. The quest to become comfortable with one's physical appearance, however, usually continues throughout adulthood.

Social: If the adolescent's development has occurred within the context of a supportive family, community, school, and peer environment, individual identity formation and separation will be complete. In reality, however, at least some developmental issues usually remain unresolved into adulthood. Late adolescents typically spend more time developing monogamous interpersonal relationships and less in seeking peer-group support. Ideally, decision making, based on an individualized value system, is mediated by limit-setting and compromise.

Cognitive: Vocational goals are now set in practical terms, and there should be realistic expectations about education and work.

ADOLESCENTS & THE MEDICAL INTERVIEW

Flexibility and a sense of humor may be the most important interviewer qualities. A general health assessment should include a review of systems and an evaluation of health-related behavior, such as risk factors for accidents; sexually transmitted diseases (STDs) including HIV; pregnancy; interpersonal violence (including past physical or sexual abuse); diet; substance abuse; exercise; learning; and mental health problems. Guidance about promoting healthful behaviors and preventing disease should be integrated into the discussion. From the patient's perspective, the provider's inquiries and assessment of some behaviors may be viewed as embarrassing, intrusive, or trivial. It is therefore helpful to explain, prior to questioning, that: (1) the same questions are asked of all patients and that (2) the encounter goal is patient self-awareness and education. This preamble is especially reassuring to teenagers, who are usually preoccupied with their bodies.

Confidentiality

Certain ground rules are important. Assure the adolescent that, unless homicide or suicide is threatened or ongoing abuse is reported, all conversations are confidential, and the information will not be shared with parents, teachers, or other authorities without permission. Discussions about sex and drugs should always occur in private unless otherwise requested by the patient. If the patient is accompanied by a parent, solicit parental concerns, then ask the adult to leave the room and conduct the interview in private.

Although teenagers want to receive information and discuss sexual behavior, pregnancy prevention, AIDS prevention, and substance use, these discussions must generally be initiated by the physician. Most teenagers are not accustomed to interacting in such participatory conversations with adults. The willingness of a teenager to share personal or confidential information depends on the perceived receptiveness of the provider. Teenagers need to feel that they have permission to share personal and intimate information. For example, it is usually not difficult for patients and providers to discuss routine chronic medical conditions such as diabetes or asthma. Control of these conditions in some teenagers, however, may be more related to alcohol and marijuana consumption, respectively, than to insulin or inhaler use. Such health-compromising behaviors must be identified before they can be dealt with; disapproving comments, facial expression, or body language can undermine the patient's willingness to disclose confidential behavior (Table 11–1).

Legal Issues

Many practitioners worry about the legality of evaluating and treating teenagers without parental consent. Since laws vary by state, it is important to become familiar with the applicable local statutes. Almost all states allow for the diagnosis and treatment of teenagers with sex-, drug-, and alcohol-related problems without parental notification or consent. Likewise, most states also allow for providing med-

Table 11–1. Suggestions for dealing with adolescents.

1. Ensure doctor-patient confidentiality. Don't inquire about health-related behaviors in front of parents.
2. Use the HEADSS format to organize the interview.
3. Assess the patient's cognitive and developmental level through interactive dialogue.
4. Initiate discussions about behavior and offer anticipatory guidance that is culturally and developmentally appropriate.
5. Listen actively to patients' opinions and perspective.
6. Be familiar with and refer to local resources for cases of domestic violence, runaways, and substance abuse.
7. Include patients in discussing and making all diagnostic and therapeutic decisions.
8. Review the behavioral stages of development with parents. Emphasize the importance of instilling confidence and building self-esteem in their children.
9. Reinforce good behavior. Congratulate teenagers who do not use drugs and who are not sexually active.
10. Address all teenagers with respect, and be nonjudgmental about their behaviors and traits.

ical care to teenagers if the condition is potentially life-threatening. In reality, since it is often impossible to determine whether a condition is potentially life-threatening until after taking the history and performing a physical examination, there is usually some legal leeway in this area. For instance, it is easy to justify evaluating a 15-year-old girl with abdominal pain, because, until determined otherwise, the pain may be from an ectopic pregnancy.

The Interview Organization

A comprehensive health-risk assessment should cover issues concerning home, education, activities, drug use, sexual practices, and suicidal ideation (HEADSS). Using the HEADSS format helps with organization and standardization. Assessing cognitive ability, using interactive dialogue, needs to be done in the first few minutes of the interview. The following interview goals and questions facilitate communication.

Home

1. Goal–Determine the family's structure and function, its conflict-resolution skills, the possibility of domestic violence, and the presence of chronic illness in the family (see Chapter 9).

2. Questions–"Who lives where you live?" If one parent is at home, the interviewer should inquire about the other parent's whereabouts, visitation pattern, and reasons for leaving (especially domestic violence and substance abuse) and whether the teen has moved back and forth between parents. Teenagers caught between divorced parents or those who feel neglected may "act out" and get into trouble to gain parental attention, sometimes in the hope that their problems will reunite separated parents. For single-parent families, the patient can be asked, "Does your mom or dad date? How do you get along with the people he or she dates?" Questions about domestic violence should include

"What happens when people argue in your house?" and "Does anyone get hurt during arguments? How about you?" and "What if someone has been drinking or using drugs and they argue?" and "Have you ever seen your mother hit by anyone?" Ask about siblings, including their health and whereabouts. Somatization may be learned by observing a family member who receives attention for a chronic medical condition.

Education

1. Goal–Identify attention deficit hyperactivity disorder and other learning disabilities, and evaluate the patient's declining grades (if applicable), cognitive ability, and vocational potential.

2. Questions–"What grade are you in?" "What type of grades do you get?" "How do they compare with your grades last year?" Falling grades may indicate family, mental health, or substance-abuse problems. "Have you ever been told you had a learning problem?" "Can you see the blackboard?" Most teenagers respond that everything in school is okay. Specific questions about courses and content need to be asked, including the student's favorite and worst subjects and his or her career aspirations. Generally speaking, teenagers who perform well in school are less likely to participate in multiple risk behaviors. The physician should ask about attendance, and truancy or other school troubles. Teenagers with chemical dependency may enjoy going to school because, although they may never attend class, school is where they can visit friends and purchase drugs. Students who get all "A's " should be asked about school-related stress and what would happen if they didn't receive high grades. Some suicides are related to unrealistic grade expectations by teenagers and their parents.

Activities

1. Goal–Evaluate the patient's social interactions, interests, and self-esteem.

2. Questions–"What do you do for fun?" "Are you involved in school, community, or religious activities, such as youth groups, clubs, or sports?" Self-esteem is often related to successful participation in these activities. Teenagers actively involved in "productive" activities are less likely to participate in delinquent behavior. The clinician should ask about gang or fraternity or sorority membership, either of which can be a source of inappropriate peer pressure. For most members, belonging to a gang is a source of pride, so an honest answer can be expected. Gangs may provide the strongest sense of family or community that is available to some teenagers.

Questions should be asked about dietary habits, including the frequency and amount of fast food and "junk" food, who cooks at home, and dieting or self-induced vomiting (see Chapter 20). It is also important to inquire about patients' physical activities and to educate them and make recommendations about regular exercise.

Drugs

1. Goal–Evaluate the patient's current habits and

Table 11–2. Substance-abuse risk factors for adolescents.

1. Family history of use
2. Low self-esteem and body image
3. Depression or thought disorder
4. Antisocial personality traits
5. Peer and cultural pressures

patterns of use and the genetic or environmental risk factors (Table 11–2). Distinguish those who drink because of social, cultural, and peer pressure; from those who are genetically predisposed; and from those who drink or use illicit drugs because of comorbid mental health problems.

2. Questions–It is less threatening to begin by asking, "Are you aware of alcohol or drug use at your school?" and "Do any of your friends drink or use drugs?" followed by, "Have you ever tried alcohol or drugs?" The physician should inquire specifically about cigarettes, alcohol, marijuana, "pills," cocaine, LSD, crystal methamphetamine, anabolic steroids, and heroin. The quantity, frequency, circumstances, and family patterns of use are important. To learn about family drinking, ask specific questions about each parent and both maternal and paternal grandparents, including whether anyone in the family attends Alcoholics Anonymous (AA) or other self-help groups. When parents do not recognize or admit to a problem, a child may not identify them as "alcoholics." The teenager should be asked to describe the parent's pattern of alcohol use. "Have you ever seen your mother or father drunk?" If the answer is yes, "When and how frequently?"

Recognition of a parental problem is essential. Even the best treatment program will fail if a teenager is discharged back into the home of an actively using parent. It is unrealistic to expect a teenager to stop using drugs or alcohol when a parent uses either or both. The willingness of parents to change either their own drinking or family behavior patterns is one of the best predictors of adolescent treatment success.

Among many teenagers, the use of drugs and alcohol is not considered abnormal or dangerous. In fact, only 5–10% of teenage drinkers or drug users develop substance-abuse problems as adults. Because serious physical consequences, other than accidents, usually do not occur until later in life, there is little negative association with alcohol or drug use. Abused, neglected, disabled, or chronically ill teenagers, may consider drugs or alcohol one of the few things that, at least temporarily, make them feel good. If legal involvement, school problems, or family conflict are present, it is important to assess the role of alcohol and drugs. Even if use seems minimal, it should be pointed out that problems are best solved sober.

Referral to a substance-abuse expert is indicated when use significantly interferes with school, family, or social, or (legal) functioning. Frequently, all aspects of the teenager's life are negatively affected by significant abuse or dependency. Anticipatory guidance should address age-appropriate concerns. Advising teenagers to stop smoking cigarettes because of the possibility of future lung cancer and heart disease is meaningless to most of them. Talking about wrinkled skin, bad breath, and yellow teeth is much more relevant to body-image concerns and far more likely to prevent or stop cigarette use. Similarly, the association between alcohol and date rape is more important to teenage girls than are other far-off consequences.

Sex

1. Goal–Determine the level of the patient's sexual involvement and sexuality, use of birth control, protection against STDs, and any history of abuse.

2. Questions–An opening question such as "Have you ever been sexually involved with anyone?" is preferable to "Are you sexually active?" The word *active* is notoriously misinterpreted. Questions need to be open-ended and should not assume heterosexual orientation. Assumptions about boyfriends or girlfriends inhibits discussion or questions about homosexual partners or feelings. Since teenagers frequently practice serial monogamy, the sequential number of different partners and their ages should be determined. A 15-year-old with a peer-group partner is at less risk for STDs, especially HIV, than is one with a substantially older partner. Most HIV infection in teenage girls is through contact with older intravenous-drug–using partners. For the sexually involved, discuss birth control techniques and condoms. One of the most common reasons for not using a condom is the belief that birth control pills provide adequate STD protection. Most teenage boys report using condoms to prevent partner pregnancy rather than out of concern about STDs. The physician, however, should not expect every teenager to be sexually experienced and should reinforce sexual abstinence with congratulations and support.

Sexual abuse is unfortunately common, and a sexual abuse history should be sought by asking, "Have you ever been touched sexually when you did not want to be?" Obtaining this history may be pivotal in helping a teenager who has developed abuse-related behavioral problems, such as sexual promiscuity, depression, substance abuse, delinquency, or an eating or a somatization disorder.

Teenage pregnancy is at epidemic proportions. Risk factors are complex but include ignorance, lack of access to family-planning services, cultural acceptance, and poor self-esteem. Some girls fantasize that childbirth will heighten their self-esteem and ensure their getting attention. In addition, because gang entry and exit often involve violent hazing, pregnancy may also offer a safe and nonviolent exit from a gang.

Suicide

1. Goal–Identify serious mental health problems and distinguish them from normal adolescent affect and moodiness. Primary risk factors are listed in Table 11–3.

Table 11–3. Risk factors for major depression and suicide.

1. Prior episode of serious depression or suicide
2. Family history of suicide or mental health problems
3. History of victimization
4. Substance abuse or dependency
5. Gay or lesbian sexual identity
6. Availability of handguns (increases rate of success)
7. Recent loss of significant friends or family
8. Extreme family, school, or social stress

Distinguishing significant psychiatric disease from normal fluctuations in a teenager's affect is challenging. In spite of the general perception to the contrary, most teenagers are not maladjusted, and the rates of mental health problems are no higher than in adults. Few teenagers announce that they are feeling depressed or are in emotional turmoil. Depression is instead often reflected in sexual promiscuity, in drug and alcohol abuse, or in the commission of violent and delinquent acts. Chronic somatic complaints such as headache, abdominal pain, or chest pain without identifiable biological explanation may also indicate depression.

2. Questions–The physician should identify vegetative signs of depression, such as sleep disturbance, decreased appetite, hopelessness, lethargy, continuous thoughts about suicide, hallucinations, or illogical thoughts. It should also be noted that many of these symptoms may also be caused by substance abuse. Evaluation of lethargy should be done from the patient's perspective. Energy may be low relative to the parents' desires or expectations—but sufficient for the teenager. There may be insufficient energy to clean, help with household chores, or complete homework but plenty of energy available to play sports, go on a date, party with friends, or travel miles and wait for hours to obtain concert tickets.

Case illustration 1: Two days after being injured in a traffic accident, Jeff, a 16-year-old, comes to the physician's office complaining of left shoulder pain. He is accompanied by his mother, who is concerned because Jeff was recently arrested for driving under the influence of alcohol. There is no history of medical or behavioral problems, although, on questioning, his mother describes a 12-month history of moodiness and falling school grades. Using the HEADDS format assessment, the physician assesses Jeff's health risks:

Home: Jeff lives at home with his biological mother and father. The parents are first-generation immigrants who both work full-time. There are few arguments at home, and Jeff describes both parents as stoic, religious, and unemotional.

Education: Although he was an above-average student until last year, Jeff's education is now being adversely affected by his truancy and lack of interest.

Activity: Although Jeff previously played several sports at school, watching television is now his favorite activity.

Drugs: Jeff admits to using drugs frequently. He drinks alcohol at least twice a week and smokes marijuana on the other five days. Since this use is no more frequent than that of his friends, he does not consider it excessive.

Sex: Jeff has no steady sexual partners, but he has had several short-term relationships.

Suicide: Jeff denies being suicidal or depressed. When asked about significant losses, however, he becomes tearful and talks hesitantly about his older brother, a construction worker, who died accidentally 2 years ago. Since the religious burial, his brother was never talked about at home.

Comment: The connection between increased substance use, declining grades, and the brother's death seems obvious. Since the substance use began insidiously, and significant trouble did not occur until more than a year after his brother's death, neither Jeff nor his parents associated the events. Furthermore, this is a family that does not share emotions, and Jeff never learned how to discuss his feelings. In this case, simply learning about his drug use, home situation, school performance, and activities was not enough. The facts all confirmed his substance abuse but did not explain it. With a teenager who previously has been without significant behavioral problems, it is crucial to search for precipitating personal or family events, including losses, that underlie and precipitate the behavior change.

Both Jeff and his parents must be made aware of the connection between the substance use and the brother's death. It is imperative that Jeff acknowledge his drug problem and be referred to a practitioner experienced in treating adolescents with substance-abuse problems (see Chapter 21). Although Jeff should respond to psychotherapy that addresses his grief and loss, psychotherapy may not be effective if mind-altering substances are being used, and their use must be discontinued.

SPECIFIC AT-RISK POPULATIONS

Homeless & Runaway Teenagers

There is a heterogeneous group of between 500,000 and 2 million homeless teenagers in the United States. Some are homeless because their families are homeless, some live on the streets for brief periods of time, and others find shelter with friends or relatives. Runaways who leave home, do not return, and no longer depend on parents for financial support or shelter constitute a significant proportion and are more precisely called *throwaways*. Before they leave home, these teenagers have usually had repeated contacts with social service agencies and have histories of severe parental conflict and high rates of physical and sexual abuse. Family abandonment because of sexual orientation is not uncommon. The social network designed to protect them has failed, and their experience of neglect, abuse, and abandonment results in a distrust of adults and institutions.

Leaving home and living on the streets may initially be a liberating experience. Once on the street, multiple substance use is the rule, often becoming a short-term pleasant escape from an otherwise dismal existence. Survival often depends on trading sex for drugs, food, or shelter. Other survival techniques, such as selling drugs and stealing, create risks for interpersonal violence and victimization. Poor self-esteem, depression, and suicidal ideation are common in this group. Usually—within weeks or months—the liberating experience of independence becomes one of desperation and hopelessness.

The initial medical evaluation may seem overwhelming. Most of these patients qualify for emancipated-minor legal status and may be eligible for Medicaid. Distrust of adults, the inability to navigate a complicated health system, and reluctance to disclose personal information may, however, keep them from receiving Medicaid and proper health care. It is important for the provider to rank such a patient's health issues and be familiar with community referral sources. Shelter, food, safety, social support, substance-abuse and mental health counseling, and medical evaluation are all usually necessary. Developing a trusting working relationship is essential and may take several visits. Keeping medical appointments and complying with referrals may be complicated by a reversed sleep-wake cycle. As with other teenagers, questions about sex and drugs are best kept in a medical context; it should be made clear that they are raised solely because of their health implications. Rather than asking whether a teenager has been a "prostitute," asking, "Have you ever had sex in order to obtain drugs, food, or a place to sleep?" is nonjudgmental and will be readily understood. Questions about sexual orientation may be confusing to a teenager with a history of sexual abuse and survival sex and may provoke anxiety and shame. These issues are best raised after a stable living situation and support system have been established. Runaway youth exist in every community, and they seem to be increasing in both number and diversity. Health-care providers must support local and national efforts to reverse this disastrous national trend.

Chronic Disease & Disability

At least 2 million teenagers in the United States have chronic disabilities or diseases. Although this is a diverse group, its members share some similar behavioral issues. Unlike other teenagers whose identity and self-esteem are molded by the acceptance of their peer group, chronically ill or disabled teenagers have a limited ability to conform and often suffer poor self-esteem. Too frequently this leads to depression, family conflict, and social isolation.

Concerns—like those of other teenagers—usually revolve around physical, social, and sexual develop-

Table 11–4. Strategies for improving compliance.

1. Have patients participate in all therapeutic and diagnostic decisions.
2. Discuss developmentally appropriate consequences of noncompliance. For instance, the renal or neurologic complications of poor diabetes control will not seem very important to a 14-year-old. Emphasize the positive instead—such as how proper glucose control will allow continued participation in sports and other peer activities.
3. Parents need guidance on how to balance protectiveness with their teenager's need to make independent decisions. Role-playing in specific scenarios may be helpful.
4. When possible, communicate directly with the patient without using the parent as a conduit. Let patients know that their opinions and questions are important.
5. Refer patients and parents to local peer support groups such as diabetes, asthma, and epilepsy societies. Support groups exist for almost all chronic illnesses and can usually be found through local telephone directories or agencies such as United Way.

Table 11–5. Recommendations for addressing needs of gay or lesbian youth.

1. Assess the patient's level of comfort and self-acceptance.
2. Evaluate and discuss external stressors, such as parents, school, and the patient's social and religious environment. Refer the patient (and parents, if necessary) to mental health experts if the stressors are severe and interfere with daily activities.
3. Reassure the patient that, from a medical perspective, homosexuality is a normal variant like left-handedness.
4. Refer patients to local gay youth groups for peer support; most cities and colleges provide resources for lesbian and gay youth, and telephone directories usually list local resources. Refer parents to local parent support groups, especially the local chapter of Parents and Friends of Lesbian and Gay Youth (P-FLAG).

ment. Frank discussions, including realistic assessments of their hopes and expectations, need to be initiated by the physician. It is crucial to identify and encourage the interests and skills that may realistically be expected to strengthen these patients' self-esteem and lead to peer recognition and companionship. Predictors of successful coping include friendships with healthy as well as ill or disabled peers, parents who are not overly protective, involvement with family activities, and appropriate household responsibilities.

Chronically ill teenagers are often "noncompliant" with medical regimens. Adolescence is no less a time of experimentation, self-discovery, and limit testing for the chronically ill teen than for other teens, and chronically ill teenagers—like other teenagers—are often noncompliant. Issues about compliance are often issues about control and of limit testing. The struggle for independence runs head first into the limitations placed by disability, as well as those placed by parents and health-care providers. Table 11–4 lists some suggestions for ways of improving compliance.

Gay & Lesbian Youth

Gay and lesbian teenagers are at a greatly increased risk for social isolation, depression, STDs (including HIV), substance abuse, and interpersonal violence. The relationships they develop with their health-care providers may help avoid the severe negative stereotyping they will receive from many parts of society. A nonjudgmental and supportive attitude helps lessen the weight of such cultural negativity.

Although some teenagers may volunteer information about their homosexual concerns or ideation, many do not unless they are specifically asked or "given permission to do so." Some teens may have feelings of anxiety, shame, and guilt about same-sex experiences. Such experiences are common, especially among young adolescents who have not yet

recognized a sexual identity, and do not necessarily reflect sexual orientation. The risk of HIV infection increases when gay teenage boys have older partners, who themselves may often have had multiple partners and may provide easier access to alcohol and drugs. Table 11–5 lists some suggestions for working with gay and lesbian youth.

MANAGED CARE

There has not yet been any systematic evaluation of the effects of managed care on the health outcomes and welfare of teenagers. Theoretically, managed care's emphasis on primary care and preventive services benefits teenagers. Such benefits may become apparent as more organizations enter the managed Medicaid arena.

Since they are generally in good health, however, teenagers are easily ignored by managed care organizations and providers. Moreover, even when services are available, teenagers may not seek access because of their concerns over confidentiality and parental notification. In addition, since most teenagers will probably not be covered under the same managed care contract in adulthood, there is concern that managed care organizations have little financial incentive to provide anticipatory guidance and counseling for behaviors whose health consequences will not be evident for decades. A further frequent complaint about managed care is that mental health services are limited or difficult to access. There is, however, currently no information showing that teenagers enrolled in managed care plans have worse mental health outcomes than do those covered under traditional reimbursement models.

Managed care providers have the opportunity to rationalize controlling health expenditures while providing comprehensive health services. Whether the nation's health needs can be adequately met by a health-care delivery system driven by corporate profits is yet to be determined.

SUGGESTED READINGS

Blum WR, Geber G: Chronically ill youth. In: McAnarney ER et al (editors): *Textbook of Adolescent Medicine.* Saunders, 1992, p 222.

Carnegie Council on Adolescent Development: *Great Transitions: Preparing Adolescents for a New Century.* Carnegie Corporation, 1995.

Elster AB, Kuznets NJ (editors): *AMA Guidelines for Adolescent Preventive Services (GAPS).* Williams & Wilkins, 1994.

Emans SJ, Goldstein DP: *Pediatric and Adolescent Gynecology,* 3rd ed. Little, Brown, 1990.

Friedman LS et al: *Source Book of Substance Abuse and Addiction.* Williams & Wilkins, 1996.

Goldenring JM, Cohen E: Getting into adolescents' heads. Contemp Pediatr 1988;5:75.

Ingersoll GM: Psychological development. In: McAnarney ER et al (editors): *Textbook of Adolescent Medicine.* Saunders, 1992, p 91.

Kann L et al: Youth risk behavior surveillance: United States, 1993. MMWR CDC 1995;44(SS-1):1.

Weiner IB: Normality during adolescence. In: McAnarney ER et al (editors): *Textbook of Adolescent Medicine.* Saunders, 1992, p 86.

Older Patients

12

Clifford Singer, MD, Stephen Jones, MD, & Linda Ganzini, MD

INTRODUCTION

We are an aging society. By the year 2020, one in five Americans will be over the age of 65, compared with a little more than one in eight today. This percentage is considerably higher in some parts of the country, particularly in rural areas or the sunbelt region. The oldest old, those over 85, comprise the fastest growing age cohort of our population. These frail elderly persons make up large proportions of most primary care practices and require a special knowledge of their unique problems, physiology, and psychology.

Although temperament (eg, energy, intensity, reactivity) remains remarkably stable throughout adult life, personality (learned behavior patterns) undergoes refinement and change over time in most healthy adults. Mental illnesses and neurodegenerative diseases take their toll, but the majority of elderly persons actively continue to seek pleasure, to be curious, and to learn throughout their lives. Predictable changes in intellect occur in most people as they age. Although judgment, knowledge, and verbal skills increase through the lifespan, mental functions relying on new memory, the speed of information processing, and coping with distractions are slowed by aging.

Successful adaptation to old age is difficult to define and variably expressed. Signs of successful aging that clinicians might notice include acceptance of change, affectionate relationships with family and friends, and a positive view of one's life story. Another indicator might be the patient's ability to find new sources of self-esteem independent of raising children, career, physical strength, or beauty. Factors that promote successful adaptation include luck (good genes, avoiding injury), good health behaviors, enough money for basic needs, a culture that values old people, available confidants, strong kinship and extended family bonds, and for many people, spirituality. Opportunities to be productive and assist younger generations often provide a sense of connection to one's community and a feeling of complete-ness. Conditions that contribute to demoralization in old age include highly mobile and rapidly changing communities, youth-oriented aesthetics, the deaths of one's family (especially children or grandchildren) and peers, and forced retirement.

Declining hygiene, poor nutrition, falls, alcohol abuse, social withdrawal, chaotic finances, and denial of health problems are clues that an older person is failing because of diminishing physical, emotional, or intellectual function. Recognizing these problems can be difficult because elderly patients may avoid detection of problems by being reclusive, or they may show their best—most controlled—behavior when visiting the office, clinic, or hospital. Often it is neighbors, friends, or other nonprofessionals who have the best opportunity to recognize the patient's declining ability to function at home. Their observations should be sought and respected.

Elderly people both create and experience obstacles to seeking and obtaining treatment for mental and physical disorders in old age. They may deliberately avoid even asking for help, particularly for emotional and cognitive problems. People in the current older generation may view emotional distress as something not to be discussed with physicians. They may suffer silently or disguise their distress with physical symptoms or irritability and withdrawal from family, friends, or caregivers. Unfortunately, the prejudicial attitudes of some physicians and mental health providers about mental and emotional problems in old age play into this silence and contribute to their under-recognition and treatment. Providers may be reluctant to prescribe treatment for problems seen as inevitable parts of aging, or they may simply consider treatment to be futile.

Providing good medical care to the elderly requires an understanding of normal changes in mental and emotional functioning in old age and skill in detecting when help is needed. Addressing the concerns of family and caregiver, accessing community resources, and advising patients about appropriate living arrangements all require sensitivity and skill. Diagnosing mental disorders in the elderly can be challenging, as clinical syndromes—including medical illnesses—often overlap. Given a basic knowledge of clinical geriatrics, time to adequately assess symptoms adequately, strategic use of all sources of information, and a sense of hopefulness in treating problems associated with aging, clinicians can provide substantial help to their patients and ample gratification for themselves.

Case Examples

Case illustration 1: Martha is an 87-year-old woman, who never married and who lives alone in her own home, as she has for 48 years. Her doctor is a family practitioner in private practice who has been asked to see Martha by her niece, Joanne (a current patient). Martha's sister (Joanne's mother), the only person with whom she had much contact in recent years, died not long ago.

Joanne tells the physician that she recently went to see her aunt, as she had promised her mother, and was appalled by her living conditions. Martha had more than 20 cats, many of whom seemed sick. The house reeked of cat urine, and the entire first floor was full of undiscarded trash and newspapers. The food supplies consisted of cat food, soda, cookies, canned spaghetti, and candy bars. Although the house had gas, electricity, and running water, there was no phone. Paid and unpaid bills, bank statements, an uncashed social security check, and several dollar bills were stuffed into a coffee can in the kitchen sink.

The following week, Joanne brings her aunt to the doctor's office. Martha is a thin, disheveled, and foul-smelling woman with poor dentition. She shakes the doctor's hand and comments pleasantly on how nicely the staff has treated her. Although she has not seen a physician in 30 years, she has no physical complaints. She cooperates with a physical examination, which reveals that she weighs 82 pounds and is 5 feet 4 inches tall. Her blood pressure is 180/98. The remainder of the neurologic and physical examination is unremarkable. Her blood chemistries are unremarkable except for a hematocrit of 30 and an albumin of 3.0.

The doctor asks Martha how she is managing at home. This seems to irritate her, and as he is about to proceed with a mental status examination, she states politely but firmly that the interview is complete, and that she feels fine and has no need for his services. She dresses herself and says she will be sitting outside in the waiting room. When she is out of earshot, Joanne says, "See what I mean? Even when she worked she was odd, and now she's totally unreasonable. Can you help me get her into a nursing home?"

The physician must now consider what other information would help determine whether Martha has a mental or neurologic illness, which kind of illness would be most likely, and how different diagnoses would affect his approach to this situation. Some important questions need to be asked: Should Martha stay in her home? What else should the physician know about her physical and cognitive functioning? How does Joanne fit into the evaluation?

Case illustration 2: Mr. and Mrs. J. have been patients in this internal medicine practice for several years. Mr. J., a retired engineer, is 89 years old. Mrs. J. also 89, is a retired teacher who until recently had volunteered as a church secretary. In their retirement they have been very active, particularly in church-related activities. The couple has two daughters living in the area, but one is in ill health, and the other—a single mother—has a demanding job and children to care for. Neither of the daughters is in a position to help care for their father.

Mr. J. has had a progressive decline in memory, reasoning, and ability to function independently. He has been diagnosed with a degenerative dementia, probably Alzheimer's disease. Now, 3 years later, he has almost caused a fire by leaving a glue gun burning in the garage and has had to give up his favorite activity, woodworking. Mrs. J. is greatly concerned because her husband has wandered away from the house several times—on at least one occasion he had to be brought home by the police. His behavioral changes in recent months have been particularly difficult. At church several months ago, Mr. J. began swearing audibly during the service, and they were forced to leave abruptly. Mrs. J. has been too embarrassed to return. Nighttime has also become especially difficult in that Mr. J. has stopped sleeping through the night and gets up and wanders around the house. Sometimes at night he does not recognize Mrs. J. and calls her a "hag," demanding that she leave his home.

Today Mrs. J. brings her husband in for an evaluation. During the appointment she begins to cry, saying that she feels she cannot go on much longer. She believes that God is punishing her for being a bad wife, and she feels guilty because she has been losing her temper with her husband. She believes that the pastor of their church and the congregation would like her to leave the church because of Mr. J.'s behavior. Through more questioning, the physician discovers that she has been getting very little sleep and has lost 15 pounds.

In this case, what kinds of interventions could make Mr. J. more manageable at home? What kinds of services might help give Mrs. J. some respite from the burden of providing constant supervision and care for her husband? Does Mrs. J. need further medical or psychiatric evaluation?

Case illustration 3: Mr. L. is a 79-year-old man whose wife of 45 years died unexpectedly 2 months ago. Theirs was a difficult marriage for much of that time; Mr. L. drank heavily, had numerous affairs, and was verbally abusive to his wife. Since his retirement at age 65, however, their relationship had been much more stable and Mr. L. seemed much more appreciative of his wife. This physician has attended to them for several years.

Mr. L.'s daughter, Eleanor, calls the physician to say that she believes her father is becoming senile. He seems to be at a complete loss since his wife died: He has not paid any bills, and the only food in his refrigerator is what neighbors and his daughter bring. Eleanor believes that her father has not changed his clothes or bathed for a week. One of the neighbors called her last week to saying that Mr. L. was wandering around the yard at night. Even more alarming to Eleanor, she has found him talking to his deceased wife as if she were there.

Eleanor makes an appointment for her father. When he comes to his appointment, the doctor is taken aback by Mr. L.'s haggard appearance. Although he seems distracted, on mental status examination, Mr. L. proves to be oriented. It seems that everything he is asked reminds him of his wife and makes him tearful. Mr. L. requests some sleep medication.

What is happening to Mr. L.? Is he mentally ill, or are his symptoms consistent with normal grieving? Is his daughter being overprotective? What kinds of interventions should the physician consider?

DIAGNOSTIC TECHNIQUES

The Clinical Interview

The Clinical Setting: Environmental conditions in the office can impair communication and rapport between elderly patients and health-care providers. Providers should be sensitive to noise, glare, and physical layout. Rooms must be wheelchair-accessible and large enough to accommodate family and caregivers when necessary.

The Patient Interview: Extra time should be allowed for elderly persons to tell their stories. Current generations of elderly people grew up in more formal times and many prefer to be called by their last names. Clinicians should inquire early in the interview whether they are being heard and understood. Some patients need clinicians to speak loudly and slowly. Active listening methods, such as maintaining eye contact, nodding, and paraphrasing the patient's questions and statements, should be used (see Chapter 1). When the patient is confused, special efforts may be necessary to make the person feel included in medical decision-making.

Family and Caregiver Interview: Optimally, frail elderly patients should be accompanied by a family member or caregiver so that the clinician can obtain a complete view of the problem. Elderly patients may be unaware of their cognitive and memory problems, or they may actively deny that any problems exist. They may have limited insight into the severity of depressive symptoms. Delusional thoughts may seem perfectly legitimate concerns until the caregiver is consulted (sometimes, of course, the patient is correct). The health-care provider risks alienating the patient while interviewing caregivers or family members if the patient is new to the physician or does not trust the physician or the family member or caregiver (see later discussion). One approach is to see everybody together in the first few minutes to establish the nature of the problem. Then the clinician can spend time alone with the patient for physical, neurologic, and mental status examinations, taking the opportunity to inquire about special concerns that the patient might have been unwilling to mention in the presence of others. Meanwhile, a second staff member, after obtaining the patient's permission, can interview the caregiver to obtain a more detailed history or a description of symptoms he or she did not feel free to describe in the presence of the patient.

Assessment

History: The health-care provider should inquire about past episodes of similar symptoms, recent changes in functional capacities, the time and course of symptom development, and all medication and substance use. The review of systems should emphasize changes in interest, motivation, sleep, and appetite as well as anxiety symptoms, weight loss, and pain.

Medical Assessment: The most important elements of assessment in older patients include the following:

- Vital sign changes may reflect cardiovascular problems that are contributing to confusion, lethargy, dizziness, panic symptoms, infection, or withdrawal states. Note that fever and tachycardia are less reliable as diagnostic markers in the very old. Checking for extreme orthostatic blood pressure changes is especially important to detect volume depletion from dehydration or bleeding; this should be done before prescribing psychotropic medications, which affect postural vascular control.
- General appearance, hygiene, and nutritional status in demented patients and in those who fail to thrive should be noted in order to detect either the patient's inability to live alone or the caregiver's inability to deliver necessary care.
- A general physical examination can detect endocrinopathy, neoplasia, cardiopulmonary disease, and bowel or bladder dysfunction.
- A neurologic screening examination should assess cranial nerve function; muscle tone, bulk, and strength; gait, balance, and postural control; muscle tenderness; and cortical integration (language, praxis, visuospatial abilities, perceptions, cortical sensory function). Special note should be taken of vision and hearing deficits.
- The mental status examination should include assessment of reasoning, insight, abstraction, motivation, hopefulness, the presence of paranoid interpretations, suicidal intentions, and the quality of affect and mood. Mood symptoms can be quantified and systematically evaluated with a clinical rating scale validated for use in elderly patients. Instruments such as the Mini-Mental State Examination or the more comprehensive Neurobehavioral Cognitive Status Examination are useful in evaluating cognitive impairment. Referral to a psychologist who is skilled in neuropsychologic assessment may be helpful in detecting subtle brain dysfunction or quantifying and characterizing more severe dementia as an aid to diagnosis and treatment planning.

Personality Assessment: Clinicians should note the patient's personality traits, such as the nature of their relationships with family and care providers, their health beliefs, and attitudes toward physicians and health-care providers.

Functional Assessment: Changes in activities of daily living (ADLs), such as bathing, dressing, grooming, eating, transferring from beds or chairs, and using the toilet; and instrumental activities of daily living (IADLs), such as telephone use, shopping, food preparation, tool use, laundry, driving, household chores, traveling, and money management, should be noted. Such changes tell the clinician how illness has actually changed a patient's ability to function. This information is critical in making treatment decisions. For example, if the illness causes no functional impairment, does the benefit of treatment still outweigh the risk? This information is also important for planning care that relies on other resources, from senior day care centers or other community-based services to private retirement or nursing homes.

Social System Assessment: Several questions need to be addressed when considering the care needs of frail elderly patients. Who are the primary caregivers and how are they coping? Have there been recent changes in caregivers? Are the caregivers competent in meeting the patient's needs? The clinician should probe carefully for indicators of stress, burden, and the capacity to function as a caregiver. A caregiver's potential for patient abuse should also be assessed. The healthcare provider must remember that neglect and hostile remarks can be as abusive as direct physical aggression (Chapter 32). Some states require physicians to report suspected abuse to local senior service agencies. Clinicians should be familiar with the laws in their state that protect vulnerable elderly persons.

Environmental Assessment: Organizations such as the Visiting Nurse Association or the local council or agency on aging may be able to assist healthcare providers by assessing frail elderly patients in their own homes. Evaluations should focus on safety issues (fall risk, fire safety, ability to access emergency services) and the patient's ability to provide for basic needs and comply with complex treatment protocols. When possible, home visits by the physician can have great benefits, by providing first-hand assessment and by increasing patient trust and rapport.

DIAGNOSIS

Diagnosing the Major Mental Disorders of Old Age

Mood Disorders: Major depression is the most common mood disorder of old age, occurring in 2–4% of elderly persons residing in the community. It is even more common in frailer populations, being found in more than 10% of those who are medically ill or living in long-term care facilities. Major depression in elderly people manifests in all the usual ways it does in younger adults (see Chapter 22), but symptoms that may be atypical in young adults, however,

are relatively common in the elderly and may dominate the clinical picture. Anxiety, fearfulness, irritability, and vague somatic concerns should arouse suspicion for depression, even when the patient denies being depressed. This diagnosis should always be considered in patients who are failing at home, losing weight, or coming to the physician frequently. Use of standardized instruments such as the Geriatric Depression Scale is an excellent screen for detecting buried depressive symptoms in primary care settings. The prognosis for depression in old age is fairly good, although relapses are common. Negative predictors include health problems that severely compromise the patient's level of function or comfort or many previous episodes of depression. Treatment usually requires both medication and psychosocial support.

Many old people look and act depressed but do not have a depressed mood or meet the criteria for major depression. This problem often occurs in the context of chronic medical conditions and functional decline, creating a syndrome known as "failure to thrive." Some of these patients experience a slow recovery from an acute physical illness, with poor oral intake and little motivation to become more active. Standard treatments for depression can often help improve motivation, appetite, energy, and pain tolerance in failing patients when there are many—or unclear—underlying reasons. Psychostimulants such as methylphenidate may have a special role in these cases as alternative or adjunctive treatments.

Although bipolar affective disorder rarely develops de novo in old age, it is not uncommon to make the diagnosis for the first time in an elderly person. Medical illness and medications can be the cause of late-onset manic symptoms unrelated to bipolar disorder. The diagnostic criteria are the same as for younger patients, although—as is the case for depression—elderly people may manifest mania without overt change in mood. Irritability, paranoia, and hyperactivity, for example, may be the primary symptoms. Previous episodes of depression, hypomanic surges in energy, or periodic psychotic symptoms are strongly suggestive of the diagnosis.

Anxiety Disorders: Elderly patients have the highest per capita use of antianxiety medications (11% of men and 25% of women); these figures are probably higher than necessary, considering that many of these anxious elderly patients are actually suffering from depression. Antidepressant medications tend to be underused in this cohort. Apart from depression, the differential diagnosis of anxiety in the elderly includes transient apprehension and fear about changes in environment, adjustments to major life changes, phobic disorders with avoidant behavior, obsessive compulsive disorder, generalized anxiety, and panic disorder. Secondary anxiety disorders are also very common; medications, chronic obstructive pulmonary disease, and endocrinopathies are often implicated in producing the symptoms.

Delusional Disorders: Delusional thinking arises from a number of disturbances in old age. A primary delusional disorder of unknown etiology, previously known as paranoia, is typically seen in elderly women who live alone. While these patients describe persecutory delusions of an intense nature, highly suggestive of schizophrenia, they do not have the other manifestations of this disease, such as hallucinations, loose associations, disorganized behavior, and functional decline. Elderly persons who do exhibit these cardinal symptoms of schizophrenia have usually had the disease for many years, although it can develop in late life on rare occasion. Paranoia and delusions can also be the presenting symptom of dementia, depression, mania, and alcohol abuse.

Dementing Disorders: The presence of dementia increases with age, approaching 20% of the 80-year-old group and 50% of those aged 90. Patients are diagnosed with dementia if they have memory and intellectual impairment that is sufficiently severe to affect independent functioning (Chapter 26). Alzheimer's disease is the most common cause of dementia in the elderly, and can be diagnosed with fairly good accuracy by using formal diagnostic criteria (Table 12–1). The presence of slowly progressive severe memory impairment, a normal motor examination (without weakness, ataxia, or parkinsonism) and multiple higher cortical deficits (impaired word-finding and aphasia, impaired ability to copy geometric figures or draw a clock face, an inability to perform simple calculations, poor abstract reasoning) are highly supportive of the diagnosis.

There are atypical variations of Alzheimer's disease that produce rigidity, bradykinesia, and tremor, and these findings should lessen confidence in the diagnosis of Alzheimer's disease. Distinguishing these cases from Parkinson's disease is difficult. In addition, there are other neurodegenerative diseases that cause parkinsonian changes in movement, gait, and postural control. A neurologic consultation may aid in making an accurate diagnosis.

Table 12–1. Diagnostic criteria for Alzheimer's dementia.*

- The patient develops multiple cognitive deficits, including both of the following:
  - Memory impairment
  - Impairment in at least one of the following: language (aphasia), complex motor tasks (apraxia), object recognition (agnosia), or complex reasoning and task execution
- The cognitive deficits cause significant functional impairment and a decline from a previous level of functioning.
- The cognitive impairments are not due to another known neurodegenerative disease; to acute illness, medications, intoxication, or delirium; or to a major mental illness.
- The course of the illness is characterized by gradual onset and progressive decline in function.

* Adapted, with permission, from American Psychiatric Association: *Diagnostic and Statistical Manual of Mental Disorders,* 4th ed. American Psychiatric Association Press, 1994.

Vascular dementias are the second most common dementias of old age. Also known as "multi-infarct dementias," they may develop from large cortical or small subcortical infarctions, and they have highly varied presentations. Accurate diagnosis based on stroke risk factors, focal neurologic signs, or evidence of stroke or advanced ischemic changes on CT or MRI will help with prognosis and treatment planning. Vascular dementias have different implications for patients and families than does Alzheimer's disease (Chapter 26).

Delirium: This syndrome is characterized by acute (within hours) or subacute (within days) development of disorientation and confusion. Apart from acute confusion, an inability to focus and sustain attention are key to the diagnosis. Hallucinations, fearful or paranoid perceptions, fluctuating awareness, and alterations in the sleep-wake cycle are other frequent symptoms. In patients with mild delirium, the decreased level of alertness may not be obvious, but the patient will have psychomotor slowing and be withdrawn, listless, and apathetic. These patients are frequently misdiagnosed as depressed. Delirium is often the first symptom of medical illness in frail elderly persons. The most common causes of delirium in the elderly include infection (usually urinary or pulmonary), medications, metabolic abnormalities, intoxication or withdrawal from alcohol, stroke, and cardiopulmonary disorders. In the frail old patient who cannot verbalize symptoms, even problems such as pain, bowel impaction, or urinary retention can cause rapid changes in mental status and behavior.

Substance Abuse & Polypharmacy: Often overlooked, substance abuse is very common in the elderly—and alcohol abuse is the third most common mental disorder in old men. Unexplained falls, ataxia, confusion, malnutrition, burns, head trauma, and depression may be signs of surreptitious alcohol abuse. Sedative-hypnotic medications and over-the-counter remedies for constipation, sleeplessness, and pain are also overused. An archetypal condition is chronic salicylism, which may result when an elderly person regularly takes otherwise acceptable doses of aspirin that are not cleared because of diminished renal function. Using multiple physicians and patronizing several pharmacies are clues to the clinician that prescription medication abuse is highly likely. Polypharmacy greatly increases the risk of adverse drug reactions, a leading cause of confusion, depression, falls, and functional decline in the elderly (see Chapter 21).

Somatization Syndromes: The elderly are not immune to somatic perceptions for which there are no physical bases. The physician must avoid unnecessary interventions while continuously supporting the needs of the elderly patient to be heard and understood, just as would be the case with younger patients. While regularly scheduled appointments with brief, focused examinations that allow the "laying-on of hands" continue to be the most effective interventions, major depression and anxiety disorders commonly underlie hypochondriasis. Antidepressant medication and psychotherapy may improve function and sense of well-being in somatically focused patients (see Chapter 24).

TREATMENT

Helping Old People Stay at Home: The focus of treatment planning with the frail elderly patient is always the provision of comfort and the maintenance of independent functioning. Although there are clearly times when safety becomes the paramount issue, as in the case of the elderly driver who is becoming a hazard behind the wheel, independence is usually the shared goal of patient and clinician. Consequently, achieving a cure becomes less of a goal than is keeping patients in their most desired living setting for as long as possible. To achieve this, treatment planning must include utilization of community care resources, skillful medical treatment, and functional rehabilitation therapies.

Community Care Options for the Frail Elderly: Clinicians should become familiar with the services available in the community that provide direct assistance and emotional support and advice to elderly patients and caregivers. Local or county agencies on aging, private case-management firms, local chapters of the Alzheimer's Association, and various home-health-care agencies are excellent resources when arranging the services necessary to keep patients at home longer than would otherwise be safe or desirable. In areas without such resources, family, neighbors, and networks of lay helpers can sometimes fill in the gaps to care for frail elders at home.

Persons with complex, round-the-clock care needs will eventually exhaust most family caregivers. Some patients with dementia-induced agitation and misperceptions can be combative at time and injure the caregivers who are trying to calm, clean, or feed them. In either case, nursing home placement may be necessary for the safety and well-being of both the patient and family. Clinicians can be tremendously important in helping families recognize when this step becomes necessary, aiding them in anticipating and minimizing the guilt that is often felt in such situations. Finding appropriate long-term care for a family member is typically frustrating and bewildering. Physicians and nurses who are knowledgeable about local care facilities can provide guidance by recommending specific homes or senior case-management services that can ease this difficult process.

Medical Treatment Planning: The motto of the British Geriatrics Society, "Adding Life to Years," is useful to keep in mind when treating elderly patients. Comfort and increased activity become the goals of treatment. Reducing polypharmacy, providing adequate pain relief, physical therapy, and treatment of depression are all integrated into comprehensive treatment plans.

Preventive care—immunizations, stress reduction, smoking cessation, exercise, and proper nutrition—must not be ignored in the elderly. It is also important to explore the expectations of both the patient and the caregiver and to discuss end-of-life treatment decisions. If possible, this discussion should take place before an acute medical condition forces interventions that may be invasive, futile, and unwanted. The plans should extend beyond cardiopulmonary resuscitation and include the patient's desires concerning fluids and nutrition, the use of antibiotics, and hospitalization. If the decision is to forego these interventions, the clinician should provide assurances that the comfort of the patient will be maintained.

Functional Rehabilitation: Effective rehabilitation of elderly patients with mental disorders uses a team approach to treat the primary disability, while preventing secondary disabilities such as immobility, or incontinence, and complications like skin ulcerations and infections. The composition of the team varies widely and may include rehabilitation professionals such as physical and occupational therapists as well as other professionals including the physician's office staff. The rehabilitation plan, like the medical care plan, must have realistic goals that are individualized to the patient.

MANAGED CARE

The philosophy of modern geriatric medicine can be compatible with managed health care at its best. Preventive medicine, reducing disability, reducing unnecessary medication use, and keeping patients as independent as possible in their environments are goals physicians and health insurance corporations can share. There are also potential conflicts of interest, however, about which clinicians should not become complacent. Caring for frail elderly patients will always require more resources of time and personnel than are necessary for the care of other adults. These patients need more hospital time to recover from acute illness, they need more time in the physician's office at each visit, and they need more attention from staff in the office or on the telephone. Elderly patients require a great deal from clinicians, and health-care providers should not be financially penalized for their willingness to take on the challenge. Despite limited Medicare reimbursement, health maintenance organizations and other managed-care plans that offer coordinated home-care services and reimburse physicians for the increased time spent with elderly patients provide better care per dollar for their clients. Ironically, such care often proves to be cost-effective in preventing falls and other injuries, adverse drug reactions, and unnecessary hospital admissions.

Case Discussions

Case Illustration 1 (Contd.): Despite her niece's concerns, Martha may be only eccentric and highly individualistic—or an impoverished person who does not ask for help easily. One does, however, need to be concerned about dementia or other conditions such as alcoholism or schizophrenia. A mental status examination and functional assessment would be helpful. Knowing she is paranoid or has memory and self-care deficits may alter the physician's approach to eliciting her cooperation with care and treatment planning. Awareness of ADL and IADL abilities, safety issues (fire, emergency services access, and fall risk) will help determine whether more intervention is necessary to ensure her safety. Her paid electricity and water bills suggest that she has some cognitive abilities. With in-home evaluations by one of the social service agencies; medical evaluation in the home or office; and help with housekeeping, shopping, and nutrition, she may be able to stay at home safely. A phone would also be helpful, assuming she can afford one and is able—or willing—to use it.

Several things will determine the success of the physician's efforts to help. First, because Martha seems to be sensitive and defensive, the doctor needs to approach her in a delicate manner, emphasizing the shared goal of her staying healthy and independent. Second, Martha's financial situation may limit her options. She needs a good social worker to help her manage her money and deal with the various agencies, organizations, and bureaucracies.

Martha needs to give away most of her cats; those remaining will need to receive veterinary care and be neutered. Because the cats seem to be important to her well-being, if other living arrangements must be made, placement should be in a facility that will allow her to have a pet or two.

Joanne may be Martha's only living relative, and she needs information about her aunt's diagnosis and prognosis, as well as support and education regarding serving as her aunt's advocate. If Martha is found to have impaired decision-making capacity based on dementia or a mental illness, Joanne may have to assume some formal role as guardian or conservator. Her ability to serve as Martha's advocate and surrogate decision maker will need ongoing evaluation by both the clinician and the court.

Case illustration 2 (Contd.): Like many caregivers, Mrs. J. is overwhelmed by the problems she faces and needs to use more support services. Options available in most areas include caregiver support groups, respite care, day programs, and housekeeping services. Learning how to manage the behavioral symptoms of her husband's dementia will decrease her feeling of helplessness. Sleep medication for Mr. J. may give both the patient and caregiver both some much-needed rest.

Mrs. J. may have a major depression, as evidenced by her sense of being punished by God, her poor self-esteem, her feelings of guilt, and her sleeplessness and weight loss. She should be evaluated for this and treated if necessary. She is also at risk for other stress-related problems. Education about how common anger is in these cases and finding ways to express her feelings so that she does not act on her anger with her husband might be helpful. In the event that Mr. J.'s symptoms cannot be improved by medication, or Mrs. J. cannot cope with his severe behavioral symptoms or his declining level of function, recommending a move to an appropriate care facility can preserve the level of care for the patient and improve the quality of life for his overwhelmed wife.

Case illustration 3 (Contd.): The major diagnostic considerations in Mr. L's case are bereavement, major depression, dementia, and alcoholism—which can all co-exist. His symptoms are consistent with bereavement: disorganization, dishevelment, talking to the deceased, and poor sleep. Benzodiazepines are a risky choice for him, given his past alcoholism, advanced age, and potential cognitive impairment. Antidepressant medication might be indicated if severe symptoms persist. Grief counseling and in-home support services could both be helpful. Although making major life decisions should be avoided during a period of acute grief, a move to an assisted-living retirement center might provide the perfect balance of privacy, socialization, independence, and support for his daily activities.

CONTINUING EDUCATION RESOURCES

The American Geriatric Society (770 Lexington Avenue, Suite 300, New York, NY 10021), The Gerontological Society of America (1275 K Street NW, Suite 350, Washington DC 20005-4006), and the American Association of Geriatric Psychiatry (Post Office Box 376 A, Greenbelt, MD 20768) publish outstanding journals and sponsor educational conferences for physicians and other health-care providers and gerontologists. Local academic medical centers may have divisions of geriatric medicine or psychiatry that provide journal clubs or grand round presentations. They may also include geriatric education and research centers that can be sources of information and referral.

SUGGESTED READINGS

Alexopoulos GS (editor): Psychiatric disorders in late life. Clin Geriatr Med 1992;8(2).

Butler RN et al: *Aging and Mental Health: Positive Psychosocial and Biomedical Approaches,* 4th ed. Macmillan, 1991.

Coffey CE, Cummings JL (editors): *Textbook of Geriatric Neuropsychiatry.* American Psychiatric Press, 1994.

Folstein MF, Folstein SE, McHugh PR: Mini-mental state: A practical method for grading the cognitive state of patients for the clinician. J Psychiatr Res 1975;12:189.

Kiernan RJ et al: The neurobehavioral cognitive status examination: A brief but differentiated approach to cognitive assessment. Ann Intern Med 1987;107:481.

Salzman C (editor): *Clinical Geriatric Psychopharmacology,* 2nd ed. Williams & Wilkins, 1992.

Spar JE, LaRue A: *Concise Guide to Geriatric Psychiatry.* American Psychiatric Press, 1990.

Yeasavage JA, Brink TL: Development and validation of a geriatric depression screening scale: A preliminary report. J Psychiatr Res 1983;17:37

Cross-cultural Communication   13

Melissa Welch, MD, MPH, & Mitchell D. Feldman, MD, MPhil

INTRODUCTION

By the year 2000, 40% of the United States population will be immigrants or first-generation Americans, and by the year 2050 half of the US population will be people of color. In addition, the composition of the major ethnic groups in the United States has changed significantly between 1980 and 1990 (Table 13–1). As a result, primary care providers will increasingly have to communicate with and treat patients of varying backgrounds and cultures. This requires not only a solid understanding of and respect for patients' differing health beliefs and practices, but also an appreciation of the physicians' own cultural beliefs and how they influence their behavior.

This chapter reviews important issues in cross-cultural communication. Cases are used to illustrate major concepts and to demonstrate effective and ineffective cross-cultural communication strategies. The knowledge, skills, and attitudes necessary for successful cross-cultural interactions are emphasized. Specific examples of provider and patient cultural experiences are included to highlight the importance of considering both viewpoints for an effective therapeutic alliance. Challenges posed by immigrant and refugee populations are discussed as well as traditional health belief systems and practices. Finally, a summary of strategies for effective cross-cultural communication is presented.

WHAT DEFINES A PATIENT FROM ANOTHER CULTURE?

Concepts of Race, Culture & Ethnicity

Culture is a system of learned and shared knowledge, beliefs, and rules that people use to direct patterns of social interactions and interpret experiences. Ethnicity is a group identity based on commonalties, such as religion, nationality, place of birth, or shared cultural patterns; over time these commonalties form a common history. The concept of race, originally referring to biological origin and physical appearance, has acquired a social meaning. Race may take on an ethnic meaning when members with similar biological and phenotypic characteristics evolve specific patterns of living. An extreme, negative example of race as a social construct occurs when, through stereotyping, social status is assigned based on skin color. Racism occurs when one group believes themselves to be inherently superior to another based on a genetically transmitted characteristic such as skin color and then attempts to assert power and control over the supposedly inferior group. Differences between groups become exaggerated, and some groups are afforded different opportunities or may experience differences in quality of life.

Defining a Patient's Cultural & Ethnic Identity

How does one define a patient from another culture? The black, Cuban physician who speaks only Spanish may not be viewed by others as being of a different cultural or ethnic background than any other black person in the United States. Alternatively, the young Asian college student, raised in the United States by first-generation Asian immigrant parents, may define his culture by traditional American standards. Cultural identity is based on personal preference; it is not determined by phenotypic racial characteristics. It is often in part determined by language preferences, religion, lifestyle, or birthplace and may be modified by individual life experiences and exposures. A patient's cultural identity must be validated and understood in order for physicians to appreciate the ways in which culture influences patients' beliefs, behaviors, and values. Similarly, providers must be comfortable with and understand their own cultural identities, values, and biases to be the most effective with patients.

Although cultural identification may provide understanding and a sense of belonging for patients, it

Table 13–1. Composition of US population in 1990 and percent change, 1980–1990.

| | US Population, 1990 | | |
	Number	Percent (%)	Change Since 1980 (%)
Total Race	248,709,873	100	10
White	199,686,060	83	6
African-American	29,986,060	12	13
American Native	1,959,234	1	38
American Asian and Pacific Islander	7,273,662	3	108
Hispanic*	22,354,059	9	53
All Other	9,804,847	4	45

* Hispanic denotes origination of Spanish-speaking people from the Caribbean, Central or South America, Spain, or elsewhere. It is distinct from race; thus persons of Spanish or Hispanic origin may be of any race.
Source: Bureau of the Census, Economics and Statistics Administration, US Department of Commerce: 1990 Census, "US population estimates by age, sex, race, and Hispanic origin: 1980 to 1991," Current Population Reports, p 25.

may also pose challenges, conflicts, and feelings of isolation when acculturation and assimilation into the traditional American mainstream occurs. This is often seen with second-generation Americans.

> *Case illustration 1:* Catherine, a 26-year-old Korean-American college student presented to her primary physician for a new patient evaluation. The provider had minimal prior contact with Korean cultural traditions but had some awareness of the value placed on high achievement and respect. Catherine expressed long-standing anxiety related to the family's desire for her to be a high achiever; Catherine's siblings were all high achievers. She also described a strained parental relationship; she believed her parents never should have had children and were "emotionally abusive." She identified with mainstream North American societal values, which favor an individual-centered orientation, self-reliance, and independence; she resented the pressure placed on her by her family. Catherine had been in prior psychotherapy and flippantly remarked on how the whole "damn" family was crazy.

Catherine's chosen cultural identification with an American value system conflicted with the traditional Asian values with which she was raised. In many Asian cultures, Confucianism, a deeply ingrained way of life, teaches respect for elders, emphasizes educational achievement, and lends great importance to family ties. The patient's primary health care provider, like the patient's family, expected her to ascribe to more traditional cultural values and was unprepared and surprised at her identified beliefs. Her physician was not accustomed to assertive Asian women and felt ill-prepared to address Catherine's needs. During the course of the encounter, the provider realized how she had stereotyped Catherine and had failed to recognize the generational and acculturation factors that influenced Catherine's values. The provider needed to abandon prior stereotypes and myths about Asian women to begin to understand and address her patient's concerns.

Heterogeneity Within Ethnic Groups

Assumptions that ethnic groups are monolithic in their beliefs and behaviors may lead to unfounded ideas about ethnicity and to stereotyping. In this latter circumstance, intracultural heterogeneity complicates the provider-patient encounter. For example, the intragroup heterogeneity of Asian and Latino groups has been well documented. Among Asians, some 15 distinct nationalities and cultures can be defined. In addition, although African-Americans are usually thought of as homogenous, in fact there is vast ethnic diversity among African-Americans. African-American heterogeneity is most prevalent in New York and Florida where blacks from Central America, the Caribbean, and Africa maintain diverse cultural practices, beliefs, and languages. In these geographic areas, in particular, stereotypes of blacks from different ethnic backgrounds to American blacks has caused friction among groups that would likely appear homogeneous to an outsider. Health behaviors and birth outcomes have also been shown to be different among these groups of black women, suggesting that traditionally identified health beliefs and practices are heavily influenced by cultural and ethnic factors. Intragroup diversity is one of the most compelling reasons for providers to encourage and validate a patient's chosen cultural identification. Lack of homogeneity within groups (both cultural and genetic) also suggests that race should not be used as a sole predictor of health outcomes.

Factors Influencing Cultural & Ethnic Identification

Validation of the patient's cultural identification also entails recognizing the social and environmental factors that influence individual and family functioning. For many people who do not belong to the white middle class, these factors are often related to inequalities stemming from racial discrimination, socioeconomic inequality, class status, family responsibilities, or environmental factors such as violence in the community.

> *Case illustration 2:* Ann, a young African-American woman with AIDS cannot attend to her HIV care needs due to multiple family challenges, lack of consistent insurance, and a severely strained marital relationship. She was relied on to be the family caretaker, despite her own chronic disease. Lack of health insurance, violence in her neighborhood, a drug-addicted daughter, an unem-

ployed and nonsupportive spouse, and inconsistent income often delayed needed medical evaluations and constantly threatened her living situation. She became withdrawn, angry, and depressed as she struggled to give priority to her health needs while attending to family and other demands.

Ann embodies the African-American matriarch. The matriarchal nature of African-American culture has functioned to enhance survival and longevity: African-American women historically have had to care for, not only their own families, but the families of others. Therefore, they are often unable to give priority to their own health care needs. This caretaking role is often in the context of other competing life priorities. When treating African-American women it is important to simultaneously recognize the importance of caring for family, but also encourage and permit the patient to care for her own well-being. Ann's health care provider included extensive social and psychiatric support services, a culturally specific community AIDS support group, and frequent follow-up visits in Ann's care plan. Ann was encouraged to develop specific goals to achieve each visit to maintain her health and give her a sense of empowerment. Failure to attend to this patient's competing life needs and family circumstances risks unheard health messages and an ineffective therapeutic alliance. Recognition of the context of Ann's chronic illness validates the cultural and ethnic context of her life, facilitating and directing the support necessary to attend to her chronic illness. Many less-advantaged and minority groups suffer from similar competing demands; this is part of their cultural identity and must be considered in the context of addressing their health care needs.

For health services to be effective in a multicultural society, providers must become culturally sensitive, learn and understand their own cultural biases, and avoid stereotyping. Allowing patients to define their cultural identities, putting this identity into a social context, demonstrating flexibility, avoiding generaliz-

izations, and demonstrating an appreciation for differences is the starting point for healthy cross-cultural communication.

IMMIGRATION

Immigrant Trends

Immigrants are coming to the United States in increasing numbers and from increasingly diverse backgrounds (Table 13–2). The reasons for immigration to the United States include education, economic benefit, family reunification, and escape from political oppression or war (as with refugees). Between 1985 and 1990 immigration to the United States was highest to California, representing one third of total immigration. Many of these immigrants are from refugee groups, including Southeast Asians (Cambodians and Hmong), Middle Easterners (Iranian), and Eastern Europeans (predominantly Russians). The ethnic diversity of these groups and the continuing increasing trends in the US ethnic immigrant and refugee populations are telling of the cross-cultural challenges we face in medicine.

Challenges Presented by Immigrants & Refugees in Primary Care

Barriers to health care for immigrant populations include structural, educational, sociocultural, linguistic, and economic. For many immigrants, anti-immigrant sentiments may also pose a barrier. Many immigrant and refugee groups experience difficult resettlement issues compounded by the fact that they often have left their countries under traumatic circumstances or are trying to adapt to a change from a rural to an urban lifestyle. Often individual members within cultural groups may differ from one another to such an extent that socioeconomic and educational differences may be more influential than cultural or ethnic ones. Many immigrants are unfamiliar with Western biomedical principles and are more oriented

Table 13–2. Selected US minority and refugee population (x10^6) by region and percent change (Δ) in population, 1980-1990.

Population Group	Population by Region							
	Northeast		Midwest		South		West	
	No.	Δ	No.	Δ	No.	Δ	No.	Δ
African-Americans	5.6	16	5.7	7	15.8	13	2.8	25
American Indian	0.12	59	0.33	36	0.56	51	0.87	29
Chinese	0.45	105	0.13	83	0.20	124	0.86	103
East (Asian) Indian	0.29	136	0.15	72	0.15	116	0.19	162
Cambodian	0.03	1222	0.01	472	0.02	650	0.08	853
Hmong	0.001	390	0.037	1237	0.002	1218	0.050	2446
Hispanic Origin	3.75	44	1.73	35	6.77	51	10.1	52
Afghan	0.005	475	0.001	425	0.005	627	0.009	722
Ethiopian	0.003	759	0.003	694	0.008	741	0.007	632
Iranian	0.006	3360	0.001	2180	0.004	1996	0.022	4680
Russian	0.075	10.366	0.018	13.395	0.013	11.908	0.048	11.319

toward family or traditional healers as the source of medical decision making. Some immigrant groups may pose particular challenges for health care providers when, for example, American values conflict with the group's culturally specific values, beliefs, and traditions, or when language barriers or differing communication styles hinder successful clinical assessment and management.

Case illustration 3: Olga was indifferent to her demanding communication style with her primary health care provider. She did not care to find the appropriately sized colostomy bag (her Russian bag "fit perfectly"); she felt dirty and unhealed by the leakage. Her tears and anger were directed not only at her poorly fitting colostomy bag, but also at her recurrent cancer, the tedious American system of health care, her perceived inability to clearly communicate her needs (knowing little English), and her lack of health insurance. She believed the United States to be cold and insensitive and wished only to return to Russia.

Olga was experiencing a cultural disequilibrium in the United States that was affecting her health care. As with many older Russian immigrants, she expected health care in the United States to be technologically advanced, readily accessible, and immediately available and accommodating. These high standards and expectations fell short in reality. In Russia she had to fight to get care, given the scarcity of resources. The only way Olga knew to get what she wanted was to be demanding and "pushy" or go without; she did not understand that the cultural norm of aggressively pursuing ones needs was counterproductive in the American health care system; she risked alienating health care providers. Despite the greater resources available to her in the United States, Olga was still unhappy because she did not leave Russia by choice but because her family left and the Russian government did not allow elderly relatives to stay behind. She felt frustrated and displaced.

Disequilibrium in cultural values and beliefs among immigrants such as the patient just described are not uncommon. It suggests that providers must learn about the social and political conditions, cultural influences, behaviors, and values that influence immigrant and refugee populations. Behaviors learned by patients under vastly different social and political systems may be difficult to understand and appreciate without this prior knowledge. Establishing links with community resources specific to the immigrant groups in your area is important, as is using professional translators with an appreciation for the cultures as well as the languages of the populations you serve. Many immigrant groups are unlikely to relinquish their previously held cultural norms, beliefs, and values and adopt those of this country, but both the immigrant and provider can, through educational efforts and increased awareness of each other's values, reduce the conflict posed by cultural disequilibrium in clinical interactions.

LANGUAGE FLUENCY

Language Competency

Providers need to be fluent in a language to conduct a truly effective interview. The interaction of language and culture in medical encounters greatly affects communication between provider and patient. Nuances are important, and much information may be lost if only a crude meaning of the interchange between health care provider and patient is being understood. The extent to which a patient fully understands English (or a provider fully understands the patient's language) is often underestimated by both patient and provider. For example, although a majority (75%) of Latinos speak English well, Spanish is the predominant language spoken at home for about 60% of this population nationally and may be the language of choice for patients to fully express their health concerns or beliefs. Furthermore, research has demonstrated that Spanish monolingual patients report a higher level of functioning and well-being when cared for by physicians who speak Spanish, suggesting that optimal care of Spanish monolingual patients may be provided by Spanish-speaking physicians.

Misuse or mispronunciation of words or expressions by physicians may also lead to confusion during interviews. For example, *ma* can mean mother or horse in Mandarin Chinese, depending on the inflection. Even when both patients and providers speak English, they may not always "speak the same language." Misuse of terms of address may be perceived as offensive to the patient. Providers should be aware, for example, that permission is often needed before addressing an African-American patient (especially men) by their first name. Among young and working class African-Americans there are differences in communication styles. For example, public health messages have notoriously failed to reach the so-called "Hip-Hop Generation" because they usually neglect to incorporate a communication style that includes the use of slang, rap, and street terms to convey their messages. Youth and young adults in this subculture are less apt to respond to health messages that tell them what to do, but respond well to instructions that allow for peer approval. Physicians may need to learn about local slang to improve their effectiveness in counseling patients on a variety of behavioral issues (eg, substance use or safe sex). Asking for clarification from the patient when slang is used in the clinical encounter is important to avoid the loss of important clinical symptoms or signs or to clarify the patient's understanding.

Use & Misuse of Translators

Trained translators can greatly facilitate patient-provider communication and improve the quality of care provided. Unfortunately, translators are vastly underused in the primary care setting. This may be due to economic constraints in some settings or because providers attempt to "get by" with a limited grasp of the patient's language and culture. This approach can compromise the quality of the care provided. For example, although a physician with adequate conversational Spanish language abilities may assume that he understands what a patient means when she describes an "ataque de nervios" (literally a "nervous attack"), the patient is actually referring to a culturally specific syndrome with identifiable precipitants and clear symptoms that has little to do with nerves or nervousness. A good translator would understand and explain to the physician not only the patient's words but also the health beliefs that give the words their true meaning. Thus, an effective translator should also function as a cultural interpreter, giving the physician insight into the patient's culture—insight that is necessary to truly understand and provide care for the patient.

To enhance the translator's effectiveness as a cultural interpreter, the translator should be explicitly incorporated as a full member of the health care team. The provider should meet with the translator briefly just prior to interviewing the patient to review together the goals for a particular visit. The provider may ask the translator to focus on a certain aspect of the interaction (for example, the patient's understanding of the need for compliance with a particular medication regimen) that has previously been problematic. In addition, the provider may want to stop the interview to seek clarification from the translator: "The patient has mentioned 'nerves' a few times, I was assuming that she simply meant that she felt nervous, but now I'm not so sure; could you explain to me what she means?"

When using a translator, some thought should go into how the chairs are arranged for physician, patient, and translator. Traditionally it was recommended that the chairs be placed in a "triadic," or triangular, arrangement that was thought to facilitate communication. Many physicians have found it difficult to maintain eye contact with the patient with this set-up, however. An alternative configuration that may help to enhance communication is having the translator sit next to the physician. The doctor can then look directly at the patient while speaking, and the patient can look in the direction of the doctor while speaking to the translator. Note that for some patients it may be threatening to have the translator and physician together on one side of the room, so the same objectives can be met by having the patient and translator sit side-by-side.

Family members may be called on to act as translators. Although convenient, family members introduce unknown variables and barriers into the interaction. For example, an adult son or daughter may heighten the language barrier by being overprotective of their

Table 13–3. Tips for effective interactions with a translator.

- Use professional translators, ideally skilled in the language and familiar with the patient's culture.
- Arrange the physical space in such a way that the provider can maintain direct eye contact with the patient; this may be best facilitated by having the physician (or patient) and interpreter seated next to each other; in this way, the patient can more easily maintain eye contact with the provider.
- Whenever asking questions or requesting clarification, address the patient.
- Request translation of all questions you ask—do not allow the translator to respond to a question before the patient has spoken.
- Request some translation of all patient-translator interactions.
- Nonverbal communication in the presence of significant language barriers is particularly important. By maintaining eye contact with the patient (rather than with the translator) you will be able to enhance communication with nonverbal cues such as facial expressions and gestures.

mother or father. They "already know" what is wrong with their parent and may not want to bother the doctor with their parent's complaints, thus neglecting what may be the most important symptom. Similarly, adolescents are inappropriate translators for an adult patient given the many intimate issues that may arise during a medical interview (sex, depression, stress, abuse, death). Children are also inappropriate translators, often having only limited mastery of their own language, much less of complicated medical situations or terminology. One translator described the unfortunate circumstance of a young child, frightened and distressed at being used as an interpreter during an ultrasound examination performed on her pregnant mother who may have been experiencing a stillbirth. The child explained to the translator (who had been called to the scene) how she was unable to explain to her mother all that the doctors were telling her.

In sum, disregard for the appropriate type and use of translators threatens effective cross-cultural communication. The increased time that may be required to communicate when using translators is outweighed by the value of a skilled translator for reliable and effective communication. The general guidelines for the effective use of translators shown in Table 13–3 may help primary care providers achieve optimal use of translation during patient interviews.

TRADITIONAL MEDICINE PRACTICES

The different health beliefs that exist throughout the world can be generally grouped into three major systems. All health beliefs may not be characterized by the systems described, but an understanding of the three most common health traditions gives providers a framework for beginning to understand patient health beliefs and choices. Within these health belief systems are curers or healers whose expertise may often be sought to treat folk illnesses and disease even before clinicians are consulted. The roles of folk illness and traditional healers are considered more closely after a review of traditional health belief systems.

Traditional Health Belief Systems

Western System: The Western health belief system, also referred to as **biomedicine,** was developed and is dominant in the Western world. According to this belief system, disease is a result of abnormalities in the structure and function of body organs and systems. Basic cause-and-effect mechanisms as seen in physics and chemistry are invoked. Pathogens (bacteria and viruses), toxins, biochemical alterations, stress, injury, or aging may be causes of disease. Diagnosis involves taking a health history and conducting examinations, which may entail a physical examination of the patient and laboratory and technologically advanced radiographic procedures. Treatment is effected by removing the pathogen or by repairing, modifying, or eliminating the affected body system. Healers or curers in Western medicine are highly trained clinicians. Prevention of disease is stressed by avoiding exposure to pathogens or other agents or conditions that alter the body's function.

Naturalistic: Naturalistic health beliefs remove the sources of disease from the personal, individual focus. Health and disease occurs when an imbalance occurs in insensate elements, especially heat and cold. Health exists when these elements are in balance and appropriate to the age and natural and social environment of the individual. An example of a naturalistic system is the *ayurvedic* (*ayur* = longevity, *veda* = science) tradition in India. In the Indian tradition *ayurveda* translates to a positive attitude toward health and is achieved by maintaining a balance among the five major elements (water, fire, earth, wind, and ether). Consuming certain foods can upset the humoral balance of these elements and cause disease (eg, consumption of garlic, a hot food, introduces heat into the body). Most Asian countries (Japan, Vietnam, Korea, Taiwan, Singapore, Hong Kong, China) also maintain natural health belief traditions. As a result of east-west migrations, some components of naturalistic systems are also seen in rural areas in Latin America and among some groups in the United States.

Most contemporary naturalistic health systems, irrespective of traditional origins, maintain the teaching of a balance between "heat" and "cold" in the body. Diagnosis and treatment of disease are concerned with discerning whether the cause of disease is excess heat or cold. The treatment for cold conditions in the naturalistic belief system is heat, and, conversely, cold remedies are used to treat hot conditions. Curers in naturalistic systems are often physicians, herbalists, or others who are familiar with medicine and treatments that can restore the body's equilibrium. Prevention is equated with maintaining a balance between hot and cold forces in the body.

Personalistic: The personalistic health belief tradition also posits that health and disease occur through sensate agents; however, these agents may be a supernatural being (eg, a god or deity), a nonhuman being (eg, ghost, evil spirits), or human beings (eg, a witch or sorcerer). Illness occurs when the individual becomes a victim of the agent as a result of techniques such as witchcraft, possession of the soul, or poison. Treatment involves identifying the agent causing disease and making it harmless through lifting of spells or reversing the techniques used by the agent. Healers or curers must then have supernatural or magical powers to elucidate who caused the disease, by what means, and how it should be reversed. Prevention is achieved when individuals ensure that their social systems and networks with fellow human beings and ancestors are in order. Personalistic systems are found in parts of Africa, the Caribbean and West Indies, among lower income blacks in the United States (most likely through West Indian and Caribbean descent), and the Navajo and other Indian tribes.

Examples of health and disease under the three traditional health belief systems are summarized in Table 13–4. These traditional systems may often coexist within individuals and within groups and society. Thus, features of each system may be accepted within cultural and ethnic groups. Concepts of health, disease, and treatment in Jamaica, for example, contain features of all three health belief systems.

Folk Illnesses, Beliefs, & Behaviors

There is a growing literature on the diverse health beliefs and practices of various ethnic groups. These explanatory models are passed down within cultures or groups and serve to validate their health beliefs and behaviors. Several explanatory models are more frequently encountered in the primary care setting and should be explored in the appropriate clinical encounter. Selected beliefs are summarized in the following sections.

Fear of Blood Loss: The loss of blood may have spiritual meaning for some cultures or religions (eg, Jehovah's Witnesses). Many Southeast Asian refugees are fearful of the loss of blood through blood draws and thus may need more thorough explanations about their importance. For others, venipuncture may be viewed as upsetting the hot and cold balance, and some refugees may associate blood draws with the military's need to give blood to American troops. Some patients may not understand that the body is usually able to replenish its supply of blood. Exploration of these various beliefs about blood should help to ensure enhanced compliance with needed laboratory tests as well as patients' satisfaction with their care.

Notions of High & Low Blood: The notion of "high" and "low" blood is often seen among low-income African Americans and white southerners in the United States. The terms *high* and *low* refer to the

Table 13–4. Diagnosis and treatment of disease under three health belief systems.

Western or Biomedical Tradition
The assessment and treatment of a patient with meningococcal meningitis is an example of using a biomedical health system. The patient may present with a change in mentation, fever, and rash; the patient is examined and a lumbar puncture is performed. The fluid from the central nervous system is tested to determine the offending pathogen. Treatment with antibiotics is initiated to avoid a rapid decline in body functioning. Others exposed to the patient try to prevent catching the disease pathogen by taking prophylactic antibiotics.

Naturalistic Health Tradition
A common example of a naturalistic health system is Chinese traditional medicine in which anger is viewed as a hot (yang) emotion. Cold (yin) may occur if a person eats too much of a cold food such as ice cream or melon. Among lower income African Americans *natural illness* occurs as a result of cold or impurities in the blood, as a punishment for sins, or during periods when the body's balance is altered or fragile. Pregnancy for example is considered to be a cold condition among low-income blacks, in poor southern whites, and in many Latin American naturalistic systems. Protection after the delivery of the child is afforded by keeping warm; this is also a preventive measure.

Personalistic Health Tradition
A West Indian woman has multiple stresses in her life including spousal difficulty, family stress due to alcoholism in her mother, and a recent job injury. She is experiencing headaches. While in church one day she experienced a headache and was given aspirin by a woman. The aspirin removed the headache, but made the woman sick to her stomach. The woman then had visions of the lady giving her pills and telling her if she did not take the pills, she would die. After discussing the visions with her sister-in-law, the woman suspected that the woman who gave her the aspirin wanted to take her husband from her and was poisoning her with the pills. On the advice of her sister-in-law, the woman went to a special healer who cast a spell to remove the lady's "power" over her.

amount of blood in the body or the shifts in its location. For example, high blood can signify either too much blood or a relocation of blood suddenly to the head. These changes are believed to result from changes in the diet or emotional shock. Similarly, low blood may signify anemia or may be confused with low blood pressure. The clinical importance of these beliefs are obvious. The magnitude of their significance is further seen in the treatment remedies sought. Often, treatment for low blood, experienced as fatigue, weakness, or "falling out" may be to eat *hot* foods as building blocks, or foods thought to build strength and stamina. High blood treatments include herbal remedies meant to "loosen," or weaken, the blood or to "cut it down." This latter remedy may cause a low-income African-American patient to discontinue taking his medication for hypertension. Notions of high and low are also ascribed to the presence of excessive or low levels of blood sugar.

Fatalism: Many African Americans are pessimistic about the ability of their physicians to cure cancer, and many view it as a "death sentence." This fatalistic view of cancer is also seen among Latinos

and is referred to as *fatalismo*. Fatalismo is the acceptance of things that one cannot control and supports the perception that there is no protection against adversity. These views are also often accompanied by cancer myths: a belief that one can get cancer from the air, that a bump or bruise can cause cancer, or that cancer is a punishment from God. These beliefs are a challenge to health education efforts in these communities. Health education for African-American and Latino patients must be framed in positive messages that both reduce cancer fears and increase the use of cancer-screening tests.

Among Asians, a loss of hope in the future is believed to occur if a patient is advised that she has a terminal illness; often family members may challenge providers not to divulge a diagnosis of terminal disease to patients so that the ill family member does not lose hope (see case illustration 5). "Truth telling" is equated with withdrawal of hope for these patients and their families, but withholding medical information may come into direct conflict with Western bioethical precepts of patient autonomy and informed consent. The anxiety that can evolve from such bioethical dilemmas between providers and patients and families may be lessened by understanding the cultural context of the patient's belief system.

Conservatism in Sexual Matters: Modesty and conservatism in sexual matters is common among women from many different cultures. Sexuality may be viewed only as a means of procreation. Women from these cultures may only come to medical attention for issues of sexuality during childbirth or at the time of marriage to prevent conception. Understanding the roots of modesty among these women is important for effective prevention strategies. Same sex providers for pelvic and breast examinations may be helpful for some patients.

Reluctance to Accept Mental Illnesses: Presentation of mental and behavioral illnesses varies among different cultural groups. For many cultures, including Middle Eastern, Latino, and Asian, mental illness is severely stigmatized, and many patients present with somatic manifestations of mental illness. Chinese families, for example, may be embarrassed to have family members with a mental illness; these family members may not be brought into care until very late in their illness.

Traditional Healers
The Western trained physician may not be initially sought for medical treatment by many persons in the United States. Traditional healers and informal networks are often used first or solely. For example, among African Americans, ideas about illness and treatments are discussed among informal networks of peers before professional medical advice or treatment is sought. This reliance on informal oral networks is a legacy of slavery; slaves could not keep written records, so information was passed on from person to

person. Today, this oral tradition may serve as a means of spreading prevention messages (eg, AIDS prevention). Jamaican bush doctors are another example of traditional healers who may be sought for herbal teas to treat conditions such as diabetes before the patient considers evaluation and treatment by a Western-trained physician. Among some Latinos, a minor illness may first be treated at home at the suggestion of a *señora* (usually an older woman), then the sick person may go to a folk curer. The folk curer, or *curandero,* is sought out because the illness may be considered to be "unnatural" and caused by saints as punishment. In this *curanderismo,* or folk-healing system, *curanderos* may be sought to assist with physiological, psychological, and social maladjustments.

Many of the healing traditions, beliefs, and behaviors reviewed in this chapter demonstrate a mixture of traditional health philosophies. Western-trained physicians may recognize some behaviors and practices but not others. Similarly, patients from other cultures may encounter Western medical traditions and practices for the first time in our offices. Providers must be flexible enough to appreciate the existence of differing health traditions, value the virtues of each, and integrate non-Western traditions into patient education and treatment plans.

CULTURAL FACTORS IN INTERVIEWING PATIENTS

The Role of Family

Families may play a central role in medical decision making and treatment plans among many cultural groups. For example, for many Middle Eastern patients, the extended family is seen as one of the most central and durable social institutions. Accordingly, the family plays a central role during crises brought on by disease, and especially around issues of death and dying. In these cases, the dying patient defers to the family for decision making. The family, by cultural tradition, never gives up hope and is not permitted to show grief. They expect that physicians will do everything possible to postpone death.

Case illustration 4: Omer, a 75-year-old Iranian man, was suffering from chronic renal insufficiency requiring dialysis, chronic obstructive pulmonary disease, and cardiovascular disease. He had been in and out of the intensive care unit throughout his hospitalization and required intubation on three occasions with successful extubation. The medical teams managing his case had long discussions with the family about Omer's worsening prognosis and raised questions of whether further reintubation was in his best interest. Discussions with Omer, who was fully competent to make decisions, always resulted in his deferring decisions to his eldest son. Several of Omer's sons were involved in his care and all stated they wanted to have "everything" done, "the best

care possible." The sons would on several occasions inquire about whether Omer could be transported back to Iran to be with his wife.

Unlike North American cultural values that emphasize the rights of the individual in health care decision making, other cultures elevate the role of family members or extended family networks as primary decision makers. Omer's case is exemplary. Latinos also tend to have a collective loyalty to the extended family that ranks higher than the individual, referred to as *familismo.* African-American extended families are an important resource for effective prevention strategies and behavioral change. They are often broadly defined to include extended relationships rooted in the father's or mother's lineage. Persons identified as being valuable to the family are often given titles, such as "Aunt" or "Uncle," "Brother" or "Sister." These individuals may be very helpful allies in the medical context. They may be called on to lend support during times of terminal illness or death, or may be influential in bringing about behavioral change needed to prevent disease or stop its worsening.

Cultural perspectives on illness affect how families act toward a patient's illness. In cultures where illness is viewed as a sin or punishment or represents weakening of the soul, families may demonstrate less caring, nurturing, and support. Without this cultural perspective, physicians may misinterpret family dynamics as being negligent or overbearing. Meeting with the family along with the patient may offer valuable insights for primary care providers.

Gender & Cross-Cultural Communication

Traditional roles can heavily influence the cross-cultural interview. In many African-American and Filipino elderly couples, for example, when wives accompany their husbands to the office visit, the roles are defined such that the wives are the primary decision makers for the husband's health concerns. Physicians often observe that they can proceed more efficiently with the care plan if the wife acts as the historian and is integrated into the care plan. In many traditional Chinese families, however, the husband is often the center of the interaction, and may not allow the wife to be the primary spokesperson even when she is the patient.

Case illustration 5: Mrs. Woo, a Chinese patient diagnosed with a recurrence of nasopharyngeal cancer, had a poor prognosis. At her first primary care visit, her husband approached the physician and advised her that his wife was unaware of her recurrent cancer and to inform her of this diagnosis would cause her to give up hope. Mr. Woo also advised the physician that he knew what was best for his wife and would be in charge of her care plan. "Everything will be through me," he said.

Gender roles may be challenged as couples assimilate American values that see women more as equals in the family. This difference again may create conflict and change for immigrant couples in the United States, as is shown by the next case illustration.

Case illustration 6: Mrs. Singh, an Indian woman, was always accompanied to medical visits by her husband. He spoke English and insisted on being in the room to interpret. Over time, it became apparent through facial expressions and recurrent stress-related symptoms, that there was some underlying conflict between the couple. The primary provider was able to gain Mr. Singh's trust overtime so that he agreed not to accompany his wife into the office, and another translator was obtained. Mrs. Singh confided to her physician that she was not in love with her husband, that their marriage had been arranged, and that they had slept in separate rooms for the last 10 years, but that she would never leave her husband because, "this is the culture." The physician asked what she could do to help. Mrs. Singh said that she wanted to work as a baby sitter but did not know English. The doctor encouraged Mrs. Singh to take a course in English. Mr. Singh truly loved his wife and did not want to see her unhappy, so he assisted in enrolling her in English classes. Mrs. Singh eventually learned enough English to apply for baby-sitting jobs. This opportunity may have never been afforded to her in India and suggests some influence of North American values in this couple's relationship (ie, women viewed more as equals, with their talents both in the home and work being valued).

Sex roles may not always be clear in the medical encounter. Because many gay and lesbian couples defy stereotypes, providers must be cognizant of maintaining an impartial stance, particularly in the depth and types of questions that are asked. Assuming a heterosexual orientation and asking multiple questions about birth control is clearly inappropriate for lesbian or gay patients. Instead, nonjudgmental questions should be used (Table 13–5). Similarly, failing to ask specific questions may not reveal that a Latino male is homosexual, since many Latino males do not consider themselves homosexual unless they are the receptive partner during intercourse. Attention to proper address of gay and lesbian couples is also important; most couples prefer the use of the term *partner* to denote their significant other (See Chapter 14).

Culturally Diverse Communication Styles

Although language skill and competency is important to successful communication with patients, an understanding of cultural styles of communication is equally important. Communication styles may in-

Table 13–5. Nonjudgmental questions about sexual orientation.

- Are you single, partnered, or married?
- Is your partner a man or a woman?
- Who is in your immediate family?
- What is the relationship with your roommate?
- Have you been sexually active with men, women, or both?

clude nonverbal and verbal cues, as well as interpretation of symptoms in culturally specific ways (eg, differences in perceptions of pain). Although care must be taken to avoid generalizations, some patterns and styles of communication characterize specific ethnic groups. Caution must be taken to remember that each individual in an ethnic group has unique experiences that shape their communication style. A comprehensive discussion of every ethnic group is not possible; the following descriptions give some general aspects of communication styles for selected ethnic groups in the United States.

African-Americans: African-American communication styles include direct eye contact, conveying a sense of concern for the person and the problem, and a nonjudgmental approach. African-Americans often use eye contact differently than whites: they tend to look at a person when speaking to him or her but may look away when listening to that person. Giving personal space without appearing cold, insensitive, or discriminatory is critical.

Case illustration 6: Vera suffered from severe osteoarthritis, advanced cardiomyopathy, and hypertension. She had been used to being very independent and achievement-oriented. She was in tears, pleading with her new, requested, African-American provider not to have her see a specific orthopedic specialist she had recently visited. Vera described the specialist as "insensitive to her needs;" he never looked at her during the visit and seemed not to care. "He made me feel so small and worthless, as if I wasn't even there."

When the orthopedist failed to acknowledge Vera's presence by not looking at her, she interpreted this to mean her problems were either irrelevant or not worthy of medical attention. Providers must avoid "talking down" to African-American patients; this conveys a message that they are in some way inferior and undeserving of care simply by virtue of their race, background, or class.

Latinos: Latino patients expect a friend in their physician; he or she must be both authoritative and demonstrate formal friendliness, referred to as *personalismo.* Latino patients often evaluate providers on the basis of their verbal communication skills rather than their medical knowledge. Therapeutic relations are enhanced if a tone of respect, *respeto,* is maintained. For example, many Latino patients expect a handshake in greeting and not offering this may be interpreted as rude. As the patient-provider relationship is more established, touching, other than during the examination, is culturally accepted behavior.

Case illustration 7: Julia advised her provider that she spoke highly of her all the time. Julia made a special request of her provider to give her son advice about what he could do to get into medical school. At the end of the encounter, Julia again spoke admiringly of her provider and hugged and kissed her.

Manner and style of communication is thus as important as language skills when addressing Latino patients. They expect freedom of communication in their description of symptoms and complaints and demonstrated respect by the provider through listening to and repeating or paraphrasing the concerns they raise. Latinos are more likely to expect positive social interactions, referred to as the cultural script of *simpatico*. Accordingly, they are less likely to engage in adversarial or confrontational encounters and more likely to agree with recommendations, even if they do not understand or may have reservations about them. Out of respect for the provider, they may not often admit when they are ambivalent about a treatment or medication.

Asian and Pacific Islanders: Although tremendously diverse in their cultural beliefs and traditions, Asian and Pacific Islanders share some similar communicative patterns. Humility is valued in most Asian and Pacific island cultures. Filipino patients, for example, demonstrate a subtle, indirect style of communication and may be less responsive to direct or abrupt ways of talking or giving instructions. Many Asians may not directly show emotions but instead may somatize emotional problems or concerns.

Middle Class White Americans: This group is rarely thought of and rarely thinks of themselves as a cultural group with distinct styles of communication, mostly because traditional Western medical training takes this style for granted. These patients often expect a lot of information during medical encounters. They may use more sophisticated technical language or seek additional information from other health care sources when communicating with their provider, including copying articles from major medical journals brought to the medical encounter, use of fax machines, or increasingly, electronic mail. These patients do not view this as an infringement on the provider's time and expect timely responses and complete explanations of questions posed. They may not always admit their ignorance about health problems to avoid the appearance of being less informed. It is therefore very important for providers to be aware that these patients may not fully understand their medical situation or fail to report relevant symptoms to avoid appearing less knowledgeable. Concerns or problems, and disagreements with recommended assessments or treatments, may often be intellectualized to avoid confrontation.

Russians: Some Russian patients may appear aggressive and demanding in their request for medical assessment and treatment. Many Russian immigrants had to be assertive to get medical attention and other essential resources in the former Soviet Union, which may be the basis for this behavior. (See case illustration 3.)

Again, these are general patterns of communication styles, and variations undoubtedly exist within and across cultural groups.

Models of Cross-Cultural Communication

Effective cross-cultural communication requires elicitation of patient health beliefs, cultural perspectives, and negotiation of treatment plans to avoid stereotypes and improve clinical outcomes. Missed opportunities for effective prevention and education can occur when providers fail in this capacity. Assumptions and stereotypes are rarely maliciously intended and in fact often go unrecognized, but may have major consequences.

> *Case illustration 8:* Bertice, a well-educated, young African-American woman, felt insulted and "dirty" after her primary care encounter. When she admitted to no longer using an oral contraceptive, Bertice felt that her physician assumed her to be sexually promiscuous and inattentive to birth control methods (a stereotype often ascribed to low-income African-American women of childbearing age). Despite telling the provider of her monogamous relationship with her husband, she was lectured on the importance of birth control usage. Bertice had a significant side effect with the contraceptive pill and was seeking birth control education and information. Her provider was never able to elicit this information from Bertice, because she became immediately defensive after the initial moments of the encounter. Bertice immediately requested to transfer her care to a physician who was more culturally sensitive.

Two models of cross-cultural communication may serve as guidelines for physicians in eliciting, understanding, and negotiating treatment plans with patients (Table 13–6). These models can be integrated into a strategy for effective cross-cultural communication in primary care (Table 13–7).

CULTURAL EXPECTATIONS OF PHYSICIANS

Respect for Physician and Patient

Respect and formal friendliness toward authority figures such as physicians are often central to many cultural groups. Many cultural groups in the United States value and respect the formal, authoritative role that physicians have traditionally played. Rarely however, disrespect of physicians by patients may hinder effective cross-cultural communication. For example, many international medical graduates practicing in the United States may be unfairly treated by patients who do not understand some of the cultural and job-specific challenges faced by physicians of another culture. Disrespect for a physician may stem from the patient's concentration on differences in the physician's language, socioeconomic status, or upbringing, which may give rise to inherent stereotypes and biases on the patient's part. Throughout the United States, minority physicians and residents in training may face discriminatory treatment that often influences their effectiveness as providers.

Table 13–6. Models of cross-cultural communication.

L.E.A.R.N. Model

- Listen with empathy and understanding to the patient's perceptions of the problem.
- Explain your perceptions of the problem.
- Acknowledge and discuss the differences and similarities.
- Recommend treatment.
- Negotiate treatment.

R.E.S.P.E.C.T. Model

- Rapport
  Connect on a social level.
  Seek the patient's point of view.
  Consciously attempt to suspend judgment.
  Recognize and avoid making assumptions.
- Empathy
  Remember that the patient has to come to you for help.
  Seek out and understand the patient's rationale for his or her behaviors or illness.
  Verbally acknowledge and legitimize the patient's feelings.
- Support
  Ask questions about and try to understand barriers to care and compliance.
  Help the patient overcome barriers.
  Involve family members if appropriate.
  Reassure the patient you will be able to help.
- Partnership
  Be flexible with regard to issues of control.
  Negotiate roles when necessary.
  Stress that you will be working *together* to address medical problems.
- Explanations
  Check often for understanding.
  Use verbal clarification techniques.
- Cultural Competence
  Respect the patient and his or her culture and beliefs.
  Be aware of your own biases and preconceptions.
  Know your limitation in addressing medical issues across cultures.
  Understand your personal style and recognize when it may not be working with a given patient.
- Trust
  Self-disclosure may be an issue for some patients who are not accustomed to Western medical approaches.
  Take the necessary time and consciously work to establish trust.

Case illustration 9: Misa, a first-year intern at a major academic medical center, had grown accustomed to patients questioning her ability because of her gender and apparent youth. She continued to be resentful of patients who refused her care because of her black skin color, however. Twice in her medical training she was confronted by a patient who said: "I don't want a black doctor." She tired of always having to prove herself. Such discrimination was a part of Misa's everyday life, and despite her achievements, it haunted her even in the context of health care delivery. Both patients were advised by the intern and the health care team that discriminatory treatment toward a physician was unacceptable. The intern was able to continue caring for one of the two patients.

Table 13–7. Strategies for effective cross-cultural communication in primary care.

1. Demonstrate genuine interest and caring and a motivation to serve.
2. Elicit health beliefs and negotiate treatment plans using models for cross-cultural communication (eg, R.E.S.P.E.C.T., L.E.A.R.N.).
3. Engage the family in the care plan, especially in family-centered cultures.
4. Learn about the diverse cultures in your area of practice, their traditional health beliefs and practices.
5. Know when and how to effectively use professional translators.

Like race, differences due to gender, gender preferences, or body habits may also be sources of physician disrespect and discriminatory treatment. As primary care providers, we must be aware of our own as well as our patient's biases and remain objective toward patients who demonstrate discriminatory attitudes. Our role is not to try to change our patients' social consciousness, but we can take the opportunity to educate them. By maintaining a professional demeanor under all circumstances, we are more likely to establish the trust that will allow our patients to appreciate us as skilled practitioners, irrespective of our cultural backgrounds or differences. Patients who demonstrate persistent disrespect should be advised that such behavior is not acceptable. Although obliged to care for patients under any emergency circumstances, physicians are not obligated to maintain a therapeutic alliance that is nonproductive for the patient or provider.

Physicians' Cultural & Ethnic Identity & Biases

Though programs in cross-cultural health care are increasing, there is presently a lack of comprehensive, formal training in cultural competency in medical school and residency. Accordingly, few providers have thought about the biases they bring to patient encounters or about their own cultural and ethnic background, health beliefs, and practices. Pinderhughes has defined the perspectives, capacities, competencies, and abilities that enable practitioners to focus successfully on culture in their work. These include: (1) becoming comfortable with differences; (2) acquiring the ability to control and change false beliefs and assumptions; (3) respecting and appreciating the values and beliefs of those who are different; (4) thinking flexibly; and (5) behaving flexibly.

To begin to unravel the challenges inherent in cross-cultural encounters with patients and colleagues, physicians need to take steps toward becoming more culturally competent. **Cultural competency** has been defined as a set of congruent behaviors, attitudes, and policies that come together in a system, agency, or among professionals that enable that system, agency, or those professionals to work effectively in cross-cultural situations. Providers (and institutions) can take steps toward improving cultural competency in health care encounters. Several phases of cultural responsiveness must be addressed before full integration of other world views and values occurs in the health care encounter. These phases include:

- Resolving fear and frustration of unfamiliar cultural beliefs and values.
- Overcoming denial that cultural and class differences do not exist.

- Overcoming negative stereotypes and belief in the superiority of your own ethnic group.
- Avoiding minimization of psycho-socio-cultural variables.
- Demonstrating relativism, in which cultural differences are acknowledged and respected, but having no real appreciation of what this implies for health care or how to address differences.
- Progression to empathy, in which a true understanding of patients' world views and values occur, but without full ethical decision making and counseling ability.
- Cultural integration, the final phase in which one acquires an ability to understand numerous world views and value systems with a critical assessment of each, and a clear understanding of one's own values. This phase is marked by the ability to recognize cultural and individual norms and distinguish between "normal" and "abnormal" behaviors within the context of patients' belief systems.

An increased awareness of where one is on the continuum of acquiring cultural competency is important. The progression from one phase to another may not be linear. It is only through the demonstration of flexibility of approach in communication and assessment of patients from culturally diverse backgrounds or lifestyles that we can effectively treat patients from the tremendously diverse cultures we are now and will continue to encounter in our examination rooms.

SUGGESTED READINGS

Barker J: Cross-cultural medicine: A decade later. West J Med 1992;157[special edition(3)]:(entire issue).

Erzinger S: Communication between Spanish speaking patients and their doctors. Cult Med Psychiatry 1991;15:91.

Helman C: *Culture, Health, and Illness,* 2nd ed. Butterworth-Heinemann, 1992.

Kleinman A: *Patients and Healers in the Context of Culture.* University of California Press, 1980.

Mull JD: Cross-cultural communication in the physician's office. West J Med 1993;159(5):609.

Pinderhughes E: *Understanding Race, Ethnicity, and Power: The Key to Efficacy in Clinical Practice.* The Free Press, 1989.

Lesbian & Gay Patients

14

Jocelyn C. White, MD

INTRODUCTION

Since the mid-1980s, acquired immunodeficiency syndrome (AIDS) has caused health-care providers to become more aware of the specific health needs of gay men. Similarly, the recent interest in women's health issues has led to a greater awareness of the unique health needs of lesbians. Before this time, the medical literature rarely discussed the health needs of either lesbians or gay men. Consequently, few primary care providers felt competent or comfortable caring for this population. Knowledge and skill are essential for the primary care provider to be able to identify the sexual orientation of patients; communicate acceptance and understanding of lesbian, gay, and bisexual health issues; screen for conditions amenable to behavioral medicine; and provide information and resources specific to the needs of lesbian, gay, and bisexual patients. By acquiring and using these skills, primary care providers can give lesbians and gay men access to competent medical care.

Lesbians and gay men make up anywhere from 1 to 10% of the general population—depending on the source quoted and the sampling method used in the study. In most studies, self-identified bisexuals are a small fraction of the lesbian or gay population. Whatever the exact percentage, however, in absolute terms, lesbians and gay men are a large group of patients with unique medical, psychologic, and social needs. Many primary care providers currently care for lesbian and gay patients without recognizing or acknowledging the patients' sexual orientation or unique needs.

Defining Sexual Orientation

Sexual orientation refers to sexual attraction to another person, including fantasies and the desire for sex, affection, and love. Sexual orientation is not necessarily predictive of sexual behavior, which refers only to sexual activities. Being a lesbian or a gay man involves awareness of a sexual attraction to a person of the same gender and, often, formation of a personal identity influenced by this awareness. This identity is formed by emotions, psychologic responses, societal expectations, and the individual's own choices in identity formation. Most self-identified lesbians and gay men are sexually active with a partner of their own gender. In addition, some women and men identify themselves as lesbian or gay, although they are currently celibate or sexually active with a partner of the opposite gender. On the other hand, some men and women, particularly in the African-American and Latino cultures, for example, are sexually active with a partner of their own gender but do not identify themselves as lesbian or gay. Most lesbians and gay men prefer the terms *lesbian* and *gay* to *homosexual,* because such terms refer to emotions, behavior, and a cultural system, as well as sexual orientation, and are nonjudgmental. Patients often see the term *homosexual* as a clinical term and may perceive it as pejorative.

Recent research suggests that a combination of both biological and environmental factors probably determines sexual orientation—heterosexual, homosexual, and bisexual. Studies of neuroanatomy, twins, and genetic markers in the families of gay brothers support a biological basis for homosexuality. The care and treatment of lesbian and gay patients remains the same, however, whether homosexuality is primarily a biological or an environmental phenomenon.

Homophobia

Homophobia: Homophobia has been defined as an irrational fear of or prejudice against homosexuals. In daily life, lesbians and gay men experience homophobia as interpersonal, workplace, societal, or political bias. In other words, homophobia is prejudice or hatred based solely on perceived homosexual orientation, and lesbians and gay men often find it difficult to act in accordance with their identity for fear of homophobic responses. They may experience stress and confusion in response to societal attitudes, identity-disclosure conflict, and internalized homophobia from years of living in an intolerant society. Despite the myths to the contrary, however, the potential for positive self-esteem in lesbians and gay men is generally similar to that of heterosexuals.

Provider Homophobia: Gay men and lesbians report frequent and often-detrimental experiences of homophobia from health-care providers. The manifestations of discomfort with homosexuality in health-care providers cover a wide range. Some providers assume the patient is heterosexual and fail to allow opportunities for sexual orientation disclosure. Others make frankly homophobic comments or jokes about the fact that the patient is lesbian or gay. Patients and physicians have reported observing substandard patient care because a provider failed to recognize a lesbian or gay sexual orientation or became overtly hostile to a lesbian or gay patient. A man with a perirectal abscess, for example, was lectured about being gay and was denied treatment. He sought care elsewhere and was hospitalized. In another instance, a woman visiting her partner in the recovery room after surgery for breast cancer called her "lover" and "honey." A nursing assistant walked by, shoving her a bit, and said "queer."

Health-care providers must recognize that patients of all sexual orientations are likely to be encountered in the daily practice of medicine (see the discussion of doctor-patient interactions, below). Providers can do several things to project a nonjudgmental attitude to all patients. Most important, they can communicate with a patient in a way that does not assume heterosexuality. They can also ensure that office forms, support staff, and environment all convey an accepting attitude to patients—whatever their sexual orientation. Any health-care provider who feels uncomfortable in treating gay or lesbian patients should explain this to the patient and refer him or her to another competent provider.

DOCTOR-PATIENT INTERACTIONS

The doctor-patient relationship is the key to providing primary care to gay and lesbian patients. Without a good provider-patient relationship, patients may avoid medical care, especially primary care screening. Providers who are uncomfortable working with lesbian and gay patients, or who fail to recognize the sexual orientation of a patient, will manage patients incorrectly. They will fail to obtain pertinent information or to recognize important elements of the evaluation and treatment of these patients. Patients who do not obtain competent primary care services, including screening and health-risk and psychosocial counseling, are likely to have a lower health status than do their heterosexual counterparts. Providers can develop a good relationship with gay, lesbian, and bisexual patients by showing an understanding of their health needs and communicating a nonjudgmental attitude.

Case illustration 1: Robert, a middle-aged high school teacher, comes to the doctor's office. This is his first visit, and he hasn't completed the intake history form. After the introductions, the physician looks at the form and prepares to take a social history.

Overcoming Barriers to Communication

Many lesbians and gay men are reluctant to share their sexual orientation with health-care providers for fear of negative judgments and homophobic responses. Some fail to share this information even when asked directly. Unpleasant experiences with health-care providers have made lesbians and gay men more likely to avoid health-care and routine screening. Even sympathetic health-care providers are often uncomfortable with the interaction. They may lack experience with lesbian, gay, and bisexual health issues or feel unsure as to what language to use to elicit information respectfully from these patients. When both patient and provider are uncomfortable, important information is not shared.

The Sexual History: Gathering information about a patient's gay or lesbian sexual orientation, or sexual practices, is often the first stumbling block encountered by health-care providers. Asking about orientation while taking a sexual history can limit the opportunity to learn whether the patient is gay or lesbian to only those visits in which a sexual history is taken. In addition, the most commonly used questions set up barriers between the provider and patient, and can lead to inaccurate or incomplete information: "What form of birth control do you use?" "Are you married, single, widowed, or divorced?" "When was the last time you had intercourse?" When lesbians or gay men hear these questions, they may not know how to answer because these questions are based on the assumption that the patient is heterosexual. Because the options given don't necessarily pertain to a lesbian or gay patient, the patient must either provide false information or awkwardly stop and explain. Needing to give such explanations can make the already challenging sexual history even more difficult for both parties. To avoid this awkwardness, patients may opt to play along with the assumption of heterosexuality, which can significantly affect the diagnosis of any illnesses and treatment of the patient.

The Social History: This is a more comfortable part of the interview in which to raise issues of sexual orientation. By using questions with no heterosexual assumptions in taking the social history, the provider can increase the opportunities for, and comfort level in, discussing these issues. In asking about spouses, partners, children, and support systems, providers and patients explore how patients are most likely to cope with difficult situations. Providers learn what the patient's family structure is, what stressors the patient might have, and what personal and community resources patients would be likely to draw on (see Chapter 9). Thus, the social history can be a more appropriate and comfortable place for exploring the sexual orientation of all patients and how it affects their health.

Sensitive Communication: Sensitive questions make no assumptions about sexual orientation and are easily phrased: "Are you single, partnered, married, widowed, or divorced?" "Who is in your immediate family?" "Over your lifetime, have your sexual partners been men, women, or both?" "If you become ill, is there someone important whom I should involve in your care?" "How do you feel about my documenting your sexual orientation on the chart?" "What percentage of the time do you use safer sex?"

Because lesbians and gay men come in all shapes, sizes, ages, and colors, providers need to use questions such as these with all men and women, not just those they suspect of being lesbian or gay. In taking a sensitive sexual history, it is often helpful for providers to explain that they need information on sexual practices to make an accurate diagnosis or provide appropriate education.

In the initial visit with the patient, it is important to discuss explicitly the documentation of sexual orientation in the chart. Many lesbians and gay men are forced to keep their sexual orientation hidden for legal, employment, or child-custody reasons. When a lesbian or gay patient does not want sexual orientation documented, providers may use a coded entry and inform the patient that this is being done. The code serves to remind providers of the patient's sexual orientation for medical purposes but will prevent inadvertent breaches of confidentiality.

> *Case illustration 1 (Contd.):* The doctor starts the social history:
>
> DOCTOR: Are you single, partnered, married, widowed, or divorced?
>
> ROBERT: I'm divorced, with a 20-year-old son, and I'm partnered now. His name is Tim.
>
> DOCTOR: How long have you been together? How's the relationship?
>
> ROBERT: Six years, and there's some tension now.
>
> Further questioning reveals that Tim is younger than Robert—and openly gay. Robert is uncomfortable being that open; he is afraid of a scandal at school and the loss of his job. As the history-taking continues, the physician asks how Robert feels about having the fact that he is gay documented in the chart. After some discussion, the two decide on a coded entry of the information. At the end of the visit, Robert thanks the doctor for being so understanding; the doctor is also happy with the visit because he has been able to screen the patient appropriately and provide him with his first physical examination in 6 years.

Enhancing the Relationship

Providers who show a nonjudgmental attitude are much more likely to develop trusting relationships with gay and lesbian patients. Providers can improve the relationship in several simple ways: offering to include a partner in the discussions, ensuring that a gay or lesbian patient's partner is treated as a spouse in the office and the hospital, including partners in discussions of next-of-kin policies and advance directives, and using office and hospital forms with words that do not assume a heterosexual family structure.

Gay & Lesbian Providers: Gay and lesbian patients often prefer working with gay and lesbian health-care providers because of the presumed absence of homophobia in the relationship. Unfortunately, however, like their heterosexual colleagues, many gay and lesbian providers have learned communication skills without recognizing heterosexual bias. Medical schools and the literature are just beginning to provide information about lesbian and gay health issues. In learning to take care of these patients, providers—current and future—need to learn new language habits for bias-free communication.

Lesbian and gay providers may find themselves in a situation in which the question of whether to disclose their own sexual orientation to their patients arises. As in any other situation, the question is whether disclosure of sexual orientation is in the best interest of the patient. In many cases, such disclosure may be beneficial. When a patient clearly needs to understand that there will be no overt homophobia in the interaction before agreeing to remain in care, it may be reassuring to know that the provider is lesbian or gay. As patient-provider relationships develop, patients often want more personal information about the provider. Gay and lesbian providers must weigh for themselves the therapeutic benefit to the patient, the patient's need for information, and their own level of comfort in self-disclosure. Although many gay and lesbian physicians have reported ostracism, harassment, and professional discrimination from colleagues, teachers, administrators, and health plans, others report being open about their sexual orientation without experiencing any negative consequences.

Managed Care: As more providers and patients take part in managed care plans, access to sensitive, competent care for lesbian and gay patients has become even more important. Patients may have difficulty learning which doctors on the provider panel are sensitive to lesbian and gay issues and knowledgeable about lesbian and gay health. Lesbian and gay physicians and others with expertise in the area rarely disclose this information to the managed care plan. Some plans have therefore erroneously told patients that they have no lesbian and gay providers or lesbian- and gay-sensitive providers. To afford access to sensitive and competent care for lesbian and gay patients, providers need to mention to the health-care plan that they have expertise in this area. Managed care plans can then make referrals for patients by matching expertise with needs.

PROBLEMS

Coming Out

The process of discovering one's sexual orientation and revealing it to others is known as *coming out* and can occur at any age. Stage theories for coming out have been well described and have been summarized as a four-step process:

1. Awareness of homosexual feelings
2. Testing and exploration
3. Identity acceptance
4. Identity integration and self-disclosure

The process of coming out involves a shift in core identity that can be associated with significant emotional distress, especially if family and peers respond negatively. Prevailing social attitudes also influence the experience. Societal and internalized homophobia often causes lesbians and gay men to perform a fatiguing cost-benefit analysis for each situation in which they consider coming out. If the costs of self-disclosure are repeatedly high, an individual may ultimately become socially isolated or revert to denying gay or lesbian identity.

Adolescents: Lesbian and gay adolescents are particularly vulnerable to the emotional distress of coming out, and this distress can make adolescent development even more difficult (see Chapter 11). Parental acceptance of the adolescent during the coming-out process may be the primary determinant of healthy self-esteem. Primary care providers need to screen for signs of sexual-orientation confusion in their adolescent patients. These signs may include depression, diminished school performance, alcohol and substance abuse, acting out, and suicidal ideation. Providers noting these signs need to consider sexual-orientation confusion in the differential diagnosis, along with depression and substance abuse.

Older Adults: Coming out, as noted previously, can occur at any age, even among older patients. Because there are varying degrees of disclosure, older individuals may be "out" to themselves and a partner or close friends but no one else beyond that trusted circle. Older lesbians and gay men are vulnerable to social isolation, and primary care providers are often among the primary support resources for older individuals. In exploring the social support network for their older patients, primary care providers need to be alert to the possibility of a lesbian or gay identity and the needs this engenders.

Relationships

Community: A gay or lesbian individual's support network may not include the family, as many families have difficulties accepting a lesbian or gay relative's sexual orientation. Lesbian and gay individuals have reported receiving support mostly from partners, friends, and lesbian and gay community or-

ganizations. Primary care providers should be aware of a few useful resources in the lesbian and gay community to which they can direct patients (some resources are listed at the end of this chapter). For many gay men and lesbians, the gay and lesbian community serves as an extended family. Discussion groups, activity clubs, gay and lesbian religious organizations, and book stores often serve as a focal point for activities and the means of constructing and maintaining a support network. Lesbian and gay community organizations, newspapers, and book stores are usually the most useful and most commonly available.

Partners: Like most heterosexuals, the majority of lesbians and gay men express a desire to find a partner and develop a relationship. And just like heterosexuals, lesbians and gay men can form and maintain long-lasting primary relationships. Lesbians and gay men may have commitment ceremonies, own homes together, share finances, and raise children.

Because of potential isolation from family, coworkers and religious organizations, the relationship with a partner can be particularly important to a lesbian's or gay man's psychological well-being. As a result, discord in the relationship may be even more stressful than it might be for a heterosexual couple. In times of relationship stress, an individual may have limited resources for help in coping with the situation. Primary care providers should screen for relationship stress and be able to provide referrals for lesbian- and gay-sensitive couple therapy when appropriate.

Parenthood: Parenthood plays a role in the lives of many lesbians and gay men, and the decision to become parents is usually deliberate and carefully made. Gay men and lesbians may have children from previous heterosexual relationships or through adoption, artificial insemination, heterosexual intercourse, or serving as foster parents. Occasionally, a lesbian couple and a gay couple will agree to have and bring up a child together.

Some members of society oppose parenthood for lesbian and gay men because of concerns about the psychological development and sexual orientation of the children. Studies have shown that there are no demonstrated differences between children raised by lesbians and gay men and those raised by heterosexuals. Open communication with children about their parents' sexual orientation appears to benefit family function, and the children themselves appreciate such openness.

A pregnant lesbian may find it difficult to get support for her pregnancy. The development of her identity as a mother may also be more complex. A primary care provider can support a pregnant lesbian by showing nonjudgmental attitudes and encouraging acceptance of lesbian motherhood among members of the delivery team and childbearing classes. Providers should encourage patients' partners and donor fathers, when appropriate, to participate in all phases of the fertility assessment, preconception and prenatal care, and delivery. It should be noted that partners and donor fathers may also need emotional support after delivery.

Loss

1. Grief–Grieving the loss of a partner may be more difficult for a lesbian or gay man if a support system is not available. Lesbians grieve the loss of partners and friends to breast cancer and other illnesses. Gay men and lesbians are particularly affected by deaths of partners and many friends from AIDS. Some gay men and lesbians report losing 10 or more friends or family members in a single year. In cases such as this, grief becomes a life constant. When a partner dies, the survivor, in effect, loses a spouse. This fact often goes unrecognized in the survivor's own social network. Frequently, the family of the deceased partner excludes the survivor or will not allow him or her to take part as a spouse in the funeral. A close-knit network of surviving friends is often neglected when a grieving family takes over funeral plans.

Occasionally, parents and family of the deceased are shocked and embarrassed to learn of the individual's sexual orientation or AIDS diagnosis. In such cases, the family may feel intense guilt or the need to hide their grief, unable to share it with their support network because of embarrassment. Family members of gay or lesbian individuals can find information and support for this and other issues by contacting Parents and Friends of Lesbians and Gays, a national organization with local chapters (see the list of resources at the end of this chapter).

Primary care providers can assist surviving partners and friends in the grieving process in several ways. Providers can assist the survivor in talking about the loss and expressing his or her feelings, identify and interpret normal grieving behavior and timelines, provide on-going support throughout the grief process, encourage the survivor to develop new relationships and support structures, and help the survivor adapt to new roles and patterns of living. In some cases, the health-care provider may be the only individual in whom the survivor can completely confide (see Chapters 3 and 35).

2. Advance directives–In recent years, discussions of advance directives, such as a health-care proxy or durable power of attorney for health care, have become more common between patients and their providers. The durable power of attorney for health care is particularly important for lesbians and gay men. Because they are unable to marry legally, lesbians and gay men need to execute these documents to appoint their partners as surrogate health decision makers. Without such a document, the next of kin is considered the surrogate decision maker. Completing this document is the best way to avoid tragic decision-making conflicts between a partner and the estranged family members of seriously ill patients in time of crisis. As with all patients, a discussion of advance directives should be included in the preventive medicine check-up (see Chapter 35).

CLINICAL ISSUES

The American Psychiatric Association removed homosexuality from its list of mental illnesses in 1973. Psychiatric and behavioral interventions used in the past to "cure" patients of homosexuality have proven neither effective nor necessary. Overall, mental illness is no more common in lesbians or gay men than in the heterosexual population. Nonetheless, primary care providers must be aware of the unique psychosocial issues that some lesbians and gay men face.

Depression & Suicide: Some reports have suggested that lesbians and gay men are at higher risk for depression and suicide than the general population. This higher risk may be particularly true for HIV-infected gay men (see Chapter 31). As noted earlier, lesbians and gay men have unique psychosocial stressors, including societal bias, which can put them at risk for depression. African-American lesbians and gay men are particularly vulnerable to depressive distress in the United States, presumably from the pressures of being members of two minority populations that face pervasive discrimination.

Adolescents are particularly vulnerable to depression and suicide. One report suggests that approximately one third of adolescent suicides are gay adolescents. This number is an alarmingly high proportion of youth suicides in a population that has few resources for counseling on sexual orientation issues. Further studies on depression and suicide in adolescent and adult gay men and lesbians are needed to confirm and update information on risk and prevalence. As part of a comprehensive clinical evaluation, primary care providers should screen all patients, including their lesbian and gay patients, for depression and suicidal ideation. Treatment of these conditions should be nonjudgmental with regard to sexual orientation and sensitive to the needs of specific individuals.

Substance Abuse: As part of the social history with any patient, including gay and lesbian patients, it is important to ask about drug and alcohol use (see Chapter 21). A provider should specifically explore the types of substances, the frequency and quantity, and whether patients use them during or preceding sexual activity. Many substances have a disinhibiting effect on the user and may make individuals more likely to engage in unsafe sex practices than they would be otherwise.

There is controversy about the extent of drug and alcohol use in the gay and lesbian community. Older studies are flawed, but methodologically sound studies now exist. Based on some of these latter studies, alcohol and drug use among gay men is probably the same as or slightly more prevalent than among heterosexual men, and gay male drug users may use drugs more heavily than do their heterosexual counterparts. According to a comparision of a population-based sample of lesbians in the San Francisco Bay area with a control group, alcohol use appears to be no more prevalent among lesbians than among heterosexual women. There are no population-based studies of drug use among lesbians compared with heterosexual women, but such use does occur.

Treatment for alcohol and other substance addiction can be challenging for both provider and patient. Homophobia, both societal and internalized, compounds the challenges. In many communities, there may be no treatment programs or counselors who are gay-sensitive or gay-affirmative. Although there are gay and lesbian 12-step meetings in many communities, many people have not come out publicly or do not feel comfortable in such meetings.

Domestic Violence: Contrary to some popular beliefs, battery of lesbians and gay men by their partners exists. The prevalence of battery in gay and lesbian relationships is not known; it often appears to be related to alcohol or drug use. Lesbians perceive that interpersonal power imbalances contribute to battery. They also report that many women's shelters are not responsive to their specific needs. Gay men may find it even more difficult to obtain services related to battery. Primary care providers should screen their gay and lesbian patients—and all patients—for the possibility of domestic violence and be able to give referrals to lesbian- and gay-sensitive resources, including shelters and counselors (see Chapter 33).

Hate Crimes: Also known as bias crimes, these are words or actions directed at an individual because of membership in a minority group. The US Department of Justice reports that gay men and lesbians may be the most victimized group in the nation. Many studies report crimes ranging from verbal abuse and threats of violence to property damage, physical violence, and murder. The number of hate crimes reported by gay men and lesbians is increasing every year. Lesbians at universities, for example, report being victims of sexual assault twice as often as do heterosexual women.

Perpetrators of hate crimes often include family members and community authorities. Many gay and lesbian adolescents leave home because of an abusive family member, and homeless gay and lesbian youths are of increasing social concern. When patients present with symptoms of depression or anxiety, providers should consider violence, including hate crimes, as a possible correlate.

EDUCATION, REFERRALS, & RESOURCES

Patient Education: This is a cornerstone of primary care. Providers who care for lesbian and gay patients must know how to advise patients in health issues, refer them to appropriate educational and community resources, and provide appropriate reference materials to hand out at visits.

Instruction: Instruction in preventing the spread of HIV and other sexually transmitted diseases should be clear and specific to lesbian and gay sexual practices. Physicians should be able to educate lesbians and gay men about risks and screening for sexually transmitted diseases and cancers. They also should be able to counsel patients, or refer them for counseling, about such issues as safer sex, parenting, coming out, battery, drug and alcohol use, depression, and hate crimes.

Referrals: Referrals should include other providers and community-based resources sensitive to the needs of lesbians and gay men. Hot lines, book stores, and bibliographies can help educate. Youth groups, senior groups, community centers, lesbian and gay religious organizations, retirement centers, and counselors who deal with lesbian and gay issues can all provide support. Gay and lesbian 12-step programs and substance-abuse support groups are also available. In areas where such local resources are not available, a central hot line, book store, or gay and lesbian newspaper elsewhere in the state usually can provide referrals or information.

Provider Education: Health-care providers can obtain additional information dealing with health issues and communicating with lesbian and gay patients through textbooks, review articles, teaching videos, and workshops at both national and regional medical conferences. Further information and educational materials are available from the Gay and Lesbian Medical Association at (415) 255-4547 (Internet address: GayLesMed@aol.com). Other resources include the following:

- National AIDS Hotline
  (800) 342-AIDS
- National Center for Lesbian Rights
  Lesbian Health Project
  (415) 392-6257
- National Federation of Parents and Friends of Lesbians and Gays, Inc.
  (202) 638-4200
- National Gay and Lesbian Task Force
  (202) 332-6483
- National Women's Health Network
  Resource packet on lesbian health issues
  (202) 347-1140

Caring for lesbian and gay patients can be an educational and rewarding experience. For those providers who, for whatever reason, feel unable to care for lesbian or gay patients, making a referral to another provider is appropriate. Hospital physician referral services may have listings for lesbian- and gay-sensitive providers. Local community organizations may keep lists of providers willing to work with lesbian and gay patients. Polling colleagues to find those educated about lesbian and gay health issues can be fruitful. When referring a lesbian or gay patient to another provider for this reason, a brief but open discussion about the reason for the referral is both appropriate and respectful of the patient.

SUGGESTED READINGS

Alcohol, Drug Abuse, and Mental Health Administration: Report of the secretary's task force on youth suicide. In: Vol 3. *Prevention and Interventions in Youth Suicide.* DHHS Pub. No. (ADM)89-1623. Superintendent of Documents, US Government Printing Office, 1989.

Bloomfield K: A comparison of alcohol consumption between lesbians and heterosexual women in an urban population. Drug Alcohol Depend 1993;33:257.

Byne W, Parsons B: Human sexual orientation: The biologic theories reappraised. Arch Gen Psychiatry 1993;50:228.

Cabaj RP: AIDS and chemical dependency: Special issues and treatment barriers for gay and bisexual men. J Psychoactive Drugs 1989;21(4):387.

Diamond M: Homosexuality and bisexuality in different populations. Arch Sex Behav 1993;22(4):291.

Fawzy FI, Fawzy NW, Pasnau RO: Bereavement in AIDS. Psychiatr Med 1991;9(3):469.

Lamendola F, Wells M: Letting grief out of the closet. RN 1992;May:23.

National Gay and Lesbian Task Force: Anti-gay violence: Causes, consequences, responses. National Gay and Lesbian Task Force, 1986.

O'Neill JF, Shalit P: Healthcare of the gay male patient. Prim Care 1992;19(1):191.

Patterson CJ: Children of lesbian and gay parents. Child Dev 1992;63:1025.

Quam JK, Whitford G: Adaptation and age-related expectations of older gay and lesbian adults. Gerontologist 1992;32(3):367.

Savin-Williams RC: Coming out to parents and self-esteem among gay and lesbian youths. J Homosex 1989;18 (1-2):1.

Schatz B, O'Hanlan K: Anti-gay discrimination in medicine: Results of a national survey of lesbian, gay and bisexual physicians. American Association of Physicians for Human Rights (AAPHR), May 1994.

Stevens PE: Lesbian health care research: A review of the literature from 1970 to 1990. Health Care Women Int 1992;13:91.

White J, Levinson W: Primary care of lesbian patients. J Gen Intern Med 1993;8:41.

Wismount JM, Reame NE: The lesbian childbearing experience: Assessing development tasks. Image: J Nurs Schol 1989;21(3):137.

15

Women

E. Montez Mutzig, MD

INTRODUCTION

The past decade has seen an increased concern for the overall health of women and the health care they receive. The interest in and information about women's health has become one of the fastest growing areas of medicine. Current research shows that diseases occurring in both men and women may have different prevalence rates, presentations, and treatments. The medical community is beginning to realize that women have unique medical needs. Providing good health care for women not only involves addressing the patient's medical problems but also requires attending to the emotional and psychosocial needs of women.

For too many years, women's health was considered only related to reproduction, and other health issues were thought to be gender-neutral. This thinking has led to gaps and fragmented knowledge in the medical literature. As a result, physicians may be uncertain how to diagnose and manage such chronic diseases as coronary artery disease in women.

Since the identification of gender bias and gender-related differences, great strides have been made in the federal government and the scientific community in emphasizing research on women. Efforts are now underway to understand many of those chronic diseases that are unique to women or for which the diagnosis and treatment may vary from that provided to men.

USE OF & ACCESS TO HEALTH CARE

Health Care Providers of Women

Data from the National Ambulatory Medical Care Survey reveal that the specialties differ in their delivery of care to women. For example, gynecologists are twice as likely to perform a clinical breast examination, Pap smear, and pelvic examination as are general internists and family practitioners. Mammograms are more likely to be ordered by internists. Because women seek care from a variety of health care specialties, some primary care clinicians may experience difficulty and feel uncomfortable in treating certain aspects of women's care such as gynecology and mental health. These providers may feel inadequately trained or prefer not to deal with certain diseases, psychosocial issues, or lifestyle concerns. Some providers may feel that taking the time to understand the psychological well-being of the patient will require too much time or open up a Pandora's box—attitudes that may contribute to inadequate or fragmented care for women.

A current and popular health care trend has been the formation of women's health centers. These centers apply a multidisciplinary approach to women's health by offering many services at a single site. Many of these sites offer mental health and educational services as well as primary care and gynecological services. The stimulus for these health centers has predominately been market-driven, and it is unknown whether the centers either represent or provide a better model of health care delivery.

Clinicians who care for female patients need to be able to provide comprehensive and continuous care. The care needs to focus not only on acute and chronic diseases but also on gynecologic disorders, diseases of mental health, psychosocial concerns, and lifestyle issues. It is only by incorporating the entire needs of women into their practice that health care providers can successfully treat their female patients.

Health Insurance

In the United States, women are more likely than men to have some form of health insurance but are also more apt to be underinsured or at higher risk of losing their insurance than men. Women are twice as likely as men to have limited coverage that requires them to bear a higher financial burden of their health care costs. Medicaid benefits provide help for many patients, but 14 million women of childbearing age are without insurance.

As women age, they continue to experience problems in either purchasing or obtaining health insurance. Middle-aged women pay higher premiums, are less likely to have insurance through employers, and are twice as likely to have no insurance as compared with men. Insurance discrepancies are compounded in elderly women. Seventy-one percent of those over age 85 are women, and this demographic trend appears to be continuing. It is vital that health care policy makers provide women greater access to health insurance.

Managed Care

Managed care and health maintenance organizations (HMOs) are rapidly growing in our current health care system. Historically, they have provided more preventive and screening services than private indemnity plans. Many HMOs also provide benefits that allow patients the choice of either a primary care physician or an obstetrician/gynecologist to perform yearly Papanicolaou (Pap) smears and pelvic examinations.

Women enrolled in HMOs tend to be younger and of childbearing age. They are more likely to receive regular preventive services, such as Pap smears, pelvic examinations, clinical breast examinations, and mammograms than are patients not enrolled in an HMO.

The challenge for managed care is to balance the cost, access, and quality of care for all patients. Health care providers must balance time management and patient satisfaction. Through the use of patient-centered interview techniques, providers can successfully meet both agendas while maintaining quality care and their own personal satisfaction. Quality health care for women will also require further refinement in standards of care that target women's specific health care needs. Quality care also demands that women have a choice in services, treatment options, and health care providers.

GENDER & THE MEDICAL ENCOUNTER

Gender is a complex issue that has a profound effect on the medical encounter. Differences in gender may lead to miscommunication, unmet expectations, and, ultimately, frustration for both physician and patient.

Gender & the Doctor-Patient Relationship

The doctor-patient relationship is vital to the success of the medical encounter (see Chapter 1). Multiple factors can influence this relationship, including gender, attitudes, and behaviors of both the patient and the physician.

If given a choice, women are more likely to seek out a female physician, especially if they are requesting a breast or pelvic examination. They also report much greater satisfaction when seeing a female physician. Female patients are also more likely to ask and

to receive information from their physicians than are male patients.

Both male and female physicians perceive that female patients are more emotionally labile and more likely to have somatic complaints. In general, women tend to be viewed as more demanding and more difficult to care for than men.

Recent studies on physician-patient communication indicate that female physicians spend more time with their patients, and the majority of this time is spent talking. The extra time spent with patients is largely due to a longer and more interactive history taking by female physicians. Regardless of the patient's gender, female physicians engage in more positive interaction, more counseling, more guidance, and more discussion of psychosocial issues with their patients than do male physicians.

Effect of Physician's Gender on Preventive Care

Recent studies found that the physician's gender may affect the delivery of preventive health care for medical problems unique to women. There does not, however, appear to be a gender difference in the delivery of preventive care in the areas of blood pressure and cholesterol screening.

In one study, female physicians were more likely to perform Pap smears and mammograms on their patients than were male physicians. There was a similar but not statistically significant trend for breast examination. The gender differences were most pronounced in young male physicians who performed the fewest preventive care services for their female patients.

Multiple reasons may contribute to the differences noted in providing preventive health care for women. Young male physicians may feel embarrassed or have inadequate training in performing pelvic examinations. Patients of young male doctors may also contribute to the problem by delaying their pelvic examinations or by minimizing the importance of the screening examination.

SPECIFIC TOPICS IN WOMEN'S HEALTH

Health care professionals who treat female patients must understand the diseases and psychosocial issues that are unique to them. The following topics highlight important behavioral aspects of women's reproductive health care in greater detail. Strategies to help clinicians integrate the psychosocial aspects of their patients' care are also included.

Preventive Health Care

Preventive health care is an important part of providing total care to patients. Immunizations and screening tests have been the mainstays of prevention; however, counseling is equally important in the following areas: injury prevention, substance abuse, sexual behavior, diet and exercise, and dental health. Each patient should be screened annually for individual risk factors based on age. Areas relevant for women include cancer screening, preconception planning, prevention of sexually transmitted diseases, screening for domestic violence (see Chapter 33), and osteoporosis prevention.

The current recommendations for screening for breast and cervical cancer are listed in Table 15–1. Although professional opinion differs regarding the time intervals for screening, the consensus is for routine Pap smears and mammograms. Patients undergoing these procedures may encounter emotional, social, and cultural barriers, which physicians should anticipate and address.

Gynecologic Examinations: Gynecologic examinations are an essential component of preventive health care for women. Unlike many other medical examinations that are viewed as routine for good health maintenance, the pelvic examination can be associated with negative feelings and attitudes. The most important predictor of a patient's current acceptance of a routine gynecologic examination is her past gynecologic care.

Most patients, but especially adolescents, are reluctant to and anxious about having a pelvic examination. The most common concerns of adolescent females are fear of pain, discovering that something is physically wrong, and embarrassment about their sexual activity, their personal hygiene, or being unclothed.

Adult women have many of the same feelings, attitudes, and experiences. Some women report negative feelings about their last pelvic examination and describe the experience as feeling vulnerable, humiliating, dehumanizing, and anxiety provoking.

Cervical Cancer Screening: Age, race, and socioeconomic factors play a role in the likelihood of women receiving Pap smears. Women who are most likely to have never received a Pap smear are those who have never been married, Hispanic women, and Caucasian women below the poverty level. In one study, nearly 80% of the women who had never received a Pap smear reported having seen a physician in the past 2 years, and 90% reported contact in the past 5 years. Women age 65 and older and all minority women, especially older African-American women, are at the greatest risk of not having a current Pap smear. The most frequently reported reason was procrastination or not believing that a Pap smear was necessary.

Over the past two decades, the incidence of abnormal Pap smears has risen dramatically. Receiving the news of cervical dysplasia can be one of the most stressful situations that women encounter. They may experience anxiety, depression, guilt, and concerns about their sexual function. When faced with the possibility of cancer, women tend either to reexperience the event of being notified of the diagnosis or avoid reminders, thoughts, and triggers of the experience. Adolescents diagnosed with cervical dysplasia are concerned about their current and future health, especially the ability to become pregnant. They report a lower sexual interest and negative feelings about intercourse, and many of them change their sexual behavior by using condoms or practicing abstinence.

Breast Cancer Screening: Breast cancer is currently the leading type of cancer in women. Unfortunately, not all women receive mammograms to screen for breast cancer. Studies have shown that older women, minority women, and those of lower socioeconomic class are less likely to have had a mammogram. Many barriers have been cited as reasons why some women do not follow breast cancer screening guide-

Table 15–1. Cancer screening recommendations for women.

Test	USPTF	ACP	ACOG
Pap smear	Onset sexual activity or age 18; every 3 years or earlier based on risk factors and physician recommendation; consider discontinuing at age 65 if previous Pap smears are normal.	Onset sexual activity; every 3 years age 20–65; every 2 years if high risk; age 66–75 screen every 3 years if not screened in the 10 years prior to age 66.	Onset sexual activity or age 18 annually for 3 years then may be 1–3 year intervals at physician discretion.
Mammography	Every 1–2 years from age 50–69; insufficient evidence for recommendation age 40–49 or >70 years of age.	Every 2 years age 50–74; recommendation against screening women <50 or >75 years of age and baseline mammograms.	Every 1–2 years beginning at age 40; annually at age 50 and greater.
Clinical breast examination (CBE)	Recommendation only in combination with mammography; insufficient evidence to recommend for CBE alone.	No recommendation.	Annually beginning at age 40.

USPTF = US Preventive Task Force; ACP = American College of Physicians; ACOG = American College of Obstetrics and Gynecology.

lines, the two most important of which are (1) the patient's belief that mammograms are only appropriate when symptoms are present and (2) their physicians never recommending the screening test. Other barriers include the patient's misunderstanding of recommended frequency of testing and concerns with radiation exposure, cost, and access-related factors. Anxiety and fear of finding a cancer have also been associated with women not obtaining screening mammograms.

Strategies to Help: Health care providers should exhibit sensitivity and compassion during exams in which a woman feels vulnerable. Communication is key (see Chapter 1). Rapport building and patient education prior to the pelvic examination is critical. The patient should be encouraged to ask questions. Providing information about the procedure and its necessity as well as explaining each part of the examination before performing it helps place the patient at ease and demonstrates respect and sensitivity. A sense of caring and concern can be conveyed during the pelvic examination by ensuring that the patient is comfortable. Respect for the patient's privacy is also important. Lowering the drape and not placing it on the patient's knees may remove a barrier and can allow the clinician to observe the patient's facial expressions. Most women prefer that the physician talk about the examination while they are performing it. Lastly, clinician expertise in performing breast and pelvis examinations can ensure gentle and relatively painless experiences for all women.

As previously noted, gender plays a role in whether women receive necessary preventive care. Male physicians may therefore need to place an increased emphasis on communication skills, specifically rapport building, eliciting patient concerns about the examination, and patient education. Empathy can be an important tool in these circumstances, allowing the doctor to acknowledge that undergoing a pelvic examination can be embarrassing. Physicians can improve cervical cancer screening rates for their patients by being more aware of the influence of gender on cancer screening, obtaining the necessary expertise in performing pelvic examinations, and understanding the importance of routine cancer surveillance.

Ensuring that women experience a comfortable and sensitive pelvic examination may be crucial in obtaining routine Pap smears. Prior to having a Pap smear taken, women need to be informed why screening is necessary and what an abnormal Pap smear would mean. Women who receive complete, accurate, and specifically written information about cervical dysplasia are less likely to experience psychological distress.

When an abnormal Pap smear is identified, the clinician should make every effort to inform the patient in a timely manner (see Chapter 3). Ideally, a follow-up office visit can allow the patient to ask questions and clarify information. An educational brochure needs to be enclosed if a written message is sent.

It is important to explore with patients their beliefs and attitudes about screening for preventable diseases. By understanding the patients' views, clinicians can appropriately educate them and facilitate the necessary screening test, whether it be a Pap smear or a mammogram. In addition, clinicians should recommend testing to all women who meet current screening recommendations.

Premenstrual Syndrome

Premenstrual syndrome (PMS) is common in menstruating women and is characterized by cyclic occurrences of a variety of somatic, affective, and behavioral symptoms. As many as 150 symptoms have been attributed to PMS. The most common signs and symptoms are shown in Table 15–2. Manifestation of symptoms typically occurs 7–10 days prior to menstruation and usually resolves within a few days after the onset of menses.

Approximately 80% of women experience either emotional or physical changes prior to menstruation. PMS occurs in only about one third of women, however. These women tend to experience symptoms that are problematic but not severe enough to interfere with daily activities. Four percent of women experience significant impairment in their life or work and may be diagnosed with premenstrual dysphoric disorder (PDD) as classified by the *Diagnostic and Statistical Manual* of the American Psychiatric Association (DSM-IV). As many as 50–60% of women with PDD have a coexisting psychiatric disorder. Therefore, it is important to evaluate and treat any underlying psychiatric disorder if it is present in this group of patients.

The most important tool that a clinician can use in making the diagnosis of PMS is a prospective daily

Table 15–2. Common symptoms of PMS.

Symptom	Women With PMS Showing Symptom (%)
Behavioral	
Fatigue	92
Irritability	91
Labile mood with alternating sadness and anger	81
Depression	80
Oversensitivity	69
Crying spells	65
Social withdrawal	65
Forgetfulness	56
Difficulty concentrating	47
Physical	
Abdominal bloating	90
Breast tenderness	85
Acne	71
Appetite changes and food cravings	70
Swelling of the extremities	67
Headache	60
Gastrointestinal upset	48

Source: Reprinted, with permission, from American College of Obstetricians and Gynecologists: Premenstrual Syndrome. Committee Opinion #155. Washington, DC, ACOG, © 1995.

Date	Menstru-ating?	Headaches	Back, joint, or muscle pain	Abdominal pain	Breast pain
6/25	N	1 2 3 4 5 (6)	(1)2 3 4 5 6	1 2 3 4(5)6	1 2 3 4 5(6)
6/26	N	1 2 3 4 5(6)	(1)2 3 4 5 6	(1)2 3 4 5 6	1(2)3 4 5 6
6/27	N	1 2 3(4)5 6	1 2(3)4 5 6	1 2 3(4)5 6	1 2 3(4)5 6
6/28	N	1 2(3)4 5 6	1 2 3(4)5 6	1(2)3 4 5 6	1 2 3 4(5)6
6/29	N	1 2 3 4 5 6	1 2 3 4 5 6	1 2 3 4 5 6	1 2 3 4 5 6
6/30	N	1 2 3 4 5 6	1 2 3 4 5 6	1 2 3 4 5 6	1 2 3 4 5 6
7/01	N	1 2 3(4)5 6	1 2 3 4(5)6	1 2 3(4)5 6	1 2 3 4(5)6
7/02	N	1 2 3 4(5)6	1 2 3(4)5 6	1 2 3 4(5)6	1 2 3 4 5(6)
7/03	N	1 2 3 4 5(6)	1 2 3 4 5(6)	1 2 3 4 5(6)	1 2 3 4 5(6)
7/04	Y	1 2 3(4)5 6	1 2 3 4(5)6	1 2 3 4 5(6)	1 2 3 4 5(6)
7/05	Y	1(2)3 4 5 6	1 2(3)4 5 6	1 2 3(4)5 6	1 2 3 4(5)6
7/06	Y	1 2(3)4 5 6	1 2 3 4(5)6	1 2 3 4(5)6	1 2 3 4 5(6)
7/07	Y	1(2)3 4 5 6	1 2 3 4(5)6	1 2 3 4(5)6	1 2 3 4 5(6)
7/08	Y	(1)2 3 4 5 6	1 2 3 4(5)6	1 2 3 4(5)6	1 2 3 4 5(6)

Figure 15–1. Daily rating form: No association between symptoms and cycle. Four items from the patient's full 21-item form are shown. Severity ratings: 1 = not at all; 2 = minimal; 3 = mild; 4 = moderate; 5 = severe; 6 = extreme. (Reproduced, with permission, from Gise LH: Premenstrual syndrome: Which treatments help? Med Aspects Hum Sex 1991:67. Daily rating forms are reproduced with permission from Jean Endicott, PhD.)

symptom scale (Figures 15–1 and 15–2). The patient is instructed to chart and rate her symptoms daily for 2 months. The timing of the symptoms around the time of ovulation and a symptom-free period are crucial to the diagnosis. The chart is helpful not only as a diagnostic aid but can also be therapeutic to the patient.

Psychosocial Issues: The underlying etiology of PMS is unknown. Numerous studies have attempted to identify various stressors in the exacerbation or maintenance of premenstrual symptoms. Lifestyles, stressful life events, general stress levels, family dynamics, and work environment have all been found to increase the symptoms of PMS.

Many women with PMS often feel misunderstood by their friends, family, and health care provider. They are frequently told that their symptoms are "all in their head" or "it is just something that you have to live with." Therefore, it is critical that primary care providers educate patients that this is a legitimate chronic medical disorder and that treatment can either alleviate or improve symptoms.

Strategies to Help: Treatment for PMS is an ongoing process for both the patient and the clinician. As mentioned earlier, the prospective daily symptom scale can be therapeutic. It helps patients identify their symptoms and how they relate to the menstrual

Date	Menstru-ating?	Active, restless	Mood swings	Depressed, sad, low, blue, lonely	Anxious, jittery, nervous
2/29	N	1(2)3 4 5 6	(1)2 3 4 5 6	(1)2 3 4 5 6	(1)2 3 4 5 6
3/01	N	1(2)3 4 5 6	1 2(3)4 5 6	1(2)3 4 5 6	1(2)3 4 5 6
3/02	N	1 2 3(4)5 6	1 2 3(4)5 6	1 2 3(4)5 6	1 2 3(4)5 6
3/03	N	1 2 3(4)5 6	1 2 3 4 5(6)	1 2 3 4 5(6)	1 2 3 4 5(6)
3/04	N	1 2 3(4)5 6	1 2 3 4 5(6)	1 2 3 4 5(6)	1 2 3 4 5(6)
3/05	N	1 2 3(4)5 6	1 2 3 4 5(6)	1 2 3 4 5(6)	1 2 3 4 5(6)
3/06	N	1 2 3(4)5 6	1 2 3 4 5(6)	1 2 3 4 5(6)	1 2 3 4 5(6)
3/07	N	1 2 3 4(5)6	1 2 3 4 5(6)	1 2 3 4 5(6)	1 2 3 4 5(6)
3/08	Y	1 2(3)4 5 6	1(2)3 4 5 6	(1)2 3 4 5 6	(1)2 3 4 5 6
3/09	Y	(1)2 3 4 5 6	(1)2 3 4 5 6	(1)2 3 4 5 6	(1)2 3 4 5 6
3/10	Y	(1)2 3 4 5 6	(1)2 3 4 5 6	(1)2 3 4 5 6	(1)2 3 4 5 6
3/11	Y	(1)2 3 4 5 6	(1)2 3 4 5 6	(1)2 3 4 5 6	(1)2 3 4 5 6
3/12	Y	(1)2 3 4 5 6	(1)2 3 4 5 6	(1)2 3 4 5 6	(1)2 3 4 5 6
3/13	Y	(1)2 3 4 5 6	(1)2 3 4 5 6	(1)2 3 4 5 6	(1)2 3 4 5 6

Figure 15–2 Daily rating form: Clear menstrual pattern. (Reproduced, with permission, from Gise LH: Premenstrual syndrome: Which treatments help? Med Aspects Hum Sex 1991:66.)

cycle and allows them to be proactive in anticipating, managing, and avoiding symptoms. By planning ahead the patient can be in control of her illness and not feel as though she is a victim.

Various treatment strategies have been studied in attempting to treat PMS. Although numerous drugs have been used, only antianxiety and antidepressant medications have been found to be effective. Benzodiazepines and the nonaddictive anxiolytic, buspirone, used only during the symptomatic phase of the cycle can help decrease symptoms. The selective serotonin reuptake inhibitors (SSRIs) used daily have led to dramatic improvements in the symptoms of PMS. A recent study of fluoxetine used in the treatment of PMS showed a significant reduction in symptoms of tension, irritability, and dysphoria compared with a placebo. Lifestyle modification appears to be a critical component of the treatment for PMS. Regular aerobic exercise, sleep, hygiene techniques, and modification of diet (decrease in caffeine and salt) have all been shown to reduce the symptoms of PMS. Stress reduction through relaxation exercise, counseling, developing appropriate coping strategies, and psychotherapy have also proved to be effective.

It is important that clinicians who interact with women that have PMS be empathetic and actively listen to their patients. Reassurance, legitimization, and education can help women begin to understand and to cope with the symptoms of PMS. These approaches can contribute to a sense of empowerment in which women are more likely to take charge of their disease and their life.

Chronic Pelvic Pain

Chronic pelvic pain (CPP) is defined as persistent pain in the pelvis for greater than 6 months duration. In addition, there is a high incidence of other somatic symptoms, such as headache, low back pain, dizziness, shortness of breath, fatigue, and weakness. CPP is one of the most common and perplexing diseases that female patients present to a provider. CPP can be frustrating and difficult to manage. In the majority of cases no organic pathology can be found; however, a rare exception may be ovarian cancer. Because of the possible life-threatening ramifications of leaving this cancer untreated, such a diagnosis should be ruled out. Many women have had extensive evaluations, including surgical procedures, for their complaints.

Psychosocial Issues: Women diagnosed with CPP tend to experience depression, anxiety, somatization disorders, sexual dysfunction, substance abuse, or other chronic pain syndromes. It appears that a substantial number of women with CPP have been the victims of sexual abuse, particularly during childhood.

Women with CPP are also at risk of having other somatic diseases. Irritable bowel syndrome is highly associated with CPP. Other less common findings include urethral syndrome and abdominal wall trigger points.

Although there are several organic causes of CPP

(Table 15–3), in 50% of cases psychopathology is the only identifiable diagnosis and can be a cofactor 30% of the time when an organic cause is determined. Therefore, all patients that present with CPP need to be evaluated for a psychiatric component.

Strategies to Help: CPP is a complicated disease that can be exacerbated by multiple confounding stressors. It is important that both women patients and health care providers understand the role of stress in this disease. Clinicians need to inquire and understand the patient's, spouse's, and family's perceptions and beliefs about CPP. Knowing the patient's work, personal relationships, sexual functioning, family responsibilities, and daily living activities is crucial to understanding how the disease affects the patient's life. By using patient-centered interviewing techniques (see Chapter 1), clinicians can explore the patient's stressors and elicit the triggers of the pain.

Empathic and active listening can be a valuable tool in treating patients with CPP. Reassurance, legitimization, and education are equally important. Lastly, a referral for professional counseling may be required. A psychiatrist, social worker, or psychologist may be useful in dealing with many of the underlying psychological issues associated with CPP.

Case illustration 1: The patient is a 24-year-old female who presents for relief of her CPP. The pain is constant and has been present for 4–5 years. Extensive medical evaluations and surgical procedures have failed to elicit a cause.

DOCTOR: Tell me how the pain has affected your life.

PATIENT: What part has it not affected! My marriage, my job!

DOCTOR: Tell me more about that.

PATIENT: My husband and I fight all of the time. He has threatened to leave because I'm sick a lot. In fact, I don't care if he does. All he wants to do is have sex all of the time even when he knows how painful it is for me.

Table 15–3. Organic factors related to chronic pelvic pain.

Gynecologic
  Adhesions
  Chronic pelvic infection
  Endometriosis
  Adenomyosis
  Fibroids
  Retained ovary syndrome
  Pelvic floor myalgia or congestion
  Ovarian cancer
Gastrointestinal
  Irritable bowel syndrome
  Inflammatory bowel disease
  Constipation
Urologic
  Interstitial cystitis
  Urethral syndrome
Musculoskeletal
  Myofascial pain syndrome
  Abdominal wall trigger points

DOCTOR: When did your sexual difficulties begin?

PATIENT: I guess it all began on our honeymoon. Every time we have sex it hurts and then the fighting begins.

DOCTOR: Have you ever been sexually abused or forced to do something against your wishes?

PATIENT: (Long pause) I was molested by my older step-brother.

The provider, through exploring the psychosocial aspects of the patient's life, has identified sexual abuse as a potential etiology of her CPP. After a thorough history and physical examination, a referral was made for professional counseling.

Infertility

Infertility is experienced by approximately 5 million couples in the United States. Since the first successful in vitro fertilization in 1978, great technological advances have been made in the area of infertility. As more couples began taking advantage of these reproductive technologies, the psychological effect of infertility on men and women has become more apparent.

Psychosocial Issues: For most couples, treating infertility is a chronic and exhausting process. Extensive evaluations, side effects from medications, recovery from surgery, frequent doctor's appointments, and enormous financial burdens are all stressful events. Most infertile couples experience monthly cycles of hope and optimism, followed by tremendous sadness and despair when menstruation occurs. This cycle leads to chronic sorrow for what is perceived as lost and the acute distress of another failure.

Common responses to infertility include feelings of anger, denial, guilt, anxiety, depression, isolation, grief, and decreased self-esteem. Feelings of inadequacy may occur when patients experience both a loss of control and low self-esteem. The psychological effect of infertility has been found to affect men and women differently (Table 15–4). Women initially seem more vulnerable to the infertility crisis than their male partners. They tend to experience more distress and report disruption in their personal lives. They worry over role failure, decreased self-esteem, and a significant sense of loss. Because of their distress,

they are more likely to increase their use of medical and mental health services.

Women tend to use a variety of coping mechanisms in dealing with their infertility. Social coping is frequently used. Women talk about their problems, seek support from others, and gather information on infertility from reading and attending lectures or seminars. Wishing and hoping is a form of emotional coping that is commonly used by infertile women.

Strategies to Help: Primary care providers can play a valuable role in helping patients deal with the issues of infertility. Many times primary care physicians are the first contact for an infertile couple. In addition to making an appropriate referral to an infertility specialist, clinicians need to remain accessible to their patients. Accessibility includes not only dealing with other health care issues, but providing emotional and psychological support.

The use of empathy and active listening may be extremely therapeutic for a woman involved in the chronic daily stress of dealing with infertility. Counseling, validation, and information-giving may also be helpful tools. Explaining to infertile couples that the emotions and coping responses they may be experiencing are normal reactions may relieve a tremendous psychological burden. Educational materials and referrals to support groups may also be beneficial.

Hysterectomy

Hysterectomy is the second most frequent major surgical operation performed in the United States. Numerous studies have tried to determine the psychological effect of hysterectomy on women. The results have been variable, from hysterectomy having no effect to having positive or negative effects on women's lives.

Psychosocial Issues: Prior to surgery, the majority of women have mixed feelings about having a hysterectomy. Women who have negative feelings about hysterectomy list the conflicting information they received prior to surgery as the main reason for their misgivings about the procedure. These women tended to get their information from friends or family members who have previously undergone a

Table 15–4. Common responses to infertility by gender.

Area	Male Response	Female Response
Communication	Less need or desire to discuss infertility. Use of conversation primarily to problem-solve or compete.	Needs and desires to discuss repeatedly. Use of conversation primarily to connect, relax, and discuss feelings.
Coping	Private coping. Primarily problem-focused.	Social coping. Primarily emotion-focused, variety of strategies.
Isolation	Some; generally able to compartmentalize infertility.	Often significant; infertility pervades all areas of life; feels separate from other women.
Options for parenting	Often able to consider child-free life earlier.	Usually strong drive for motherhood.

Source: Reprinted, with permission, from Draye, Mary Ann: Emotional aspects of infertility. In: *Primary Care of Women.* Lemcke DP et al (editors), Appleton & Lange, 1995.

hysterectomy. The other woman's previous experience has a tremendous effect on the patient's attitudes before and after surgery. For example, if a family member has reported sexual difficulty after her hysterectomy, then the patient is likely to experience the same problem. Most women, however, view surgery as positive, and they are glad they no longer have to worry about birth control or having menstrual periods.

Most women do not report negative psychological experiences due to their hysterectomy. Occasionally, they may experience feelings of loss, emptiness, diminished femininity, and concerns about sexual activity. Most women do experience a minimal amount of anxiety about reengaging in sexual activity after surgery, but this resolves quickly without any sequelae.

Strategies to Help: Once the decision has been made that a hysterectomy is the best treatment option, clinicians need to take the time to explore the patient's knowledge and beliefs about the upcoming surgery. Often the psychological significance of the surgical event will have a bearing on the patient's outcome. Stressing positive outcomes prior to surgery can have a significant effect on the patient's quality of life (see Chapter 6).

> *Case illustration 2:* The patient is a 43-year-old female needing preoperative medical clearance for a hysterectomy.
>
> DOCTOR: What is your understanding of the need for your surgery?
>
> PATIENT: I need it because my uterus has fibroids and they cause me to bleed all of the time. Taking it out will solve my bleeding problems.
>
> DOCTOR: Do you have any concerns or questions about the hysterectomy?
>
> PATIENT: Well, I have been worried that after the surgery my husband will find me undesirable.
>
> DOCTOR: What do you mean?
>
> PATIENT: My aunt had a hysterectomy and all she does is complain how it ruined her sex life. My husband and I are worried that the same thing may happen to us.
>
> DOCTOR: I can understand your concerns, however most women who have a hysterectomy experience no sexual problems. A few women may have some anxiety about having sex after surgery, but this usually resolves quickly.
>
> PATIENT: Oh, what a relief! I have been worried that I would have sexual problems like my aunt.

Physician inquiry about the patient's concerns or questions has uncovered an opportunity for patient education and reassurance.

Menopause

Currently, 40 million US women are now perimenopausal or postmenopausal, and another 20 million will reach this stage in life over the next decade.

As the life expectancy of women increases, they will likely live one-third or more of their lives after menopause. Because menopause affects a significant portion of our female population, it is important that health care providers understand the physiological, cultural, and psychosocial factors that influence a woman's perception of menopause.

Psychosocial Issues: Each woman's experience of menopause appears to depend on a number of factors. Cultural background, age, health, surgical versus natural menopause, the desire for more children, and interaction with a health care provider all may play a role in a woman's response to menopause.

Various cultures respond to menopause differently. For example, in the Asian and Arab cultures, women report little or no menopausal symptoms and are unlikely to seek medical help. East Indian women view menopause as a positive event and eagerly await the end of menses. Western cultures tend to value fertility and youth; therefore, menopause may have a more negative effect on women.

Even though menopause is a normal physiological event, women's attitudes and beliefs regarding menopause are often mixed. The majority of women welcome the cessation of menses and menstrual-related problems. They may be relieved with not having to deal with issues of pregnancy or migraine headaches. Others tend to harbor negative views and dread menopause. They believe that they will experience more physical and psychological problems because of menopause or that "the change of life" is a sign of old age. Some women may become saddened by their loss of reproductive capabilities.

Women's attitudes toward and expectations about menopause may be a result of inaccurate information. In fact, recent evidence reveals that most women do not receive their information from physicians, and one-third of patients have never discussed their concerns about menopause with their physician. Women are more likely to gain knowledge of menopause from magazines, books, television, newspaper, and friends or family members. Many patients may be misinformed or not informed at all about the long-term health concerns associated with menopause.

Women who do receive information on menopause from their physicians appear to be dissatisfied in what they receive. Physicians are more likely to discuss short-term physical effects, such as hot flashes, and not address patient concerns. Female patients, however, appear to be most concerned with issues of osteoporosis, emotional well-being, and coronary artery disease.

Strategies to Help: Clinicians should inquire about their patients' knowledge and perceptions of menopause. Knowing the patients' beliefs about menopause, their reactions to hot flashes and long-term risk factors, their feelings about fertility, and their partner's response to menopause can aid the provider in understanding how best to help them with appropriate support, education, and counseling.

Explanation and reassurance have been shown to be effective strategies in 40% of women who seek medical care for menopausal symptoms. Clinicians, however, should inquire about their patients' perceptions and their knowledge of menopause and long-term health risks before providing information. It is only after knowing patients' level of information or misinformation that physicians can give appropriate and balanced information.

Multiple studies have shown that women are more likely to be compliant with hormone replacement therapy when informed and involved in the decision-making process. Clinicians should not make treatment decisions for patients; the role of the clinician is to act as a facilitator in aiding women in their decision-making process (see Chapter 17).

SUMMARY

The knowledge and treatment of diseases in women is rapidly growing. It is important that clinicians understand that gender differences exist in many chronic diseases and that gender plays a vital role in the doctor-patient relationship. In addition, clinicians should inquire about and understand the emotional, cultural, and psychosocial factors that may play an integral part in their patient's illness. It is only by understanding the illness in the context of the patient's life that health care providers can begin to provide complete and comprehensive care to all of their female patients.

SUGGESTED READINGS

Bernhard LA: Consequences of hysterectomy in the lives of women. Health Care Women Int 1992;13:281.

Biro FM, Rosenthal SL, Wildey LS: Self-reported health concerns and sexual behaviors in adolescents with cervical dysplasia. J Adolesc Health 1993;12:391.

Calle EE et al: Demographic predictors of mammography and Pap smear screening in US women. Am J Public Health 1993;83(1):53.

Collins KS, Simon LJ: Women's health and managed care: Promises and challenges. Women's Health Iss 1996;6(1):39.

Committee on Gynecologic Practice: Premenstrual syndrome. ACOG Comm Opin 1995;155:1.

Davis DC, Dearman CN: Coping strategies of infertile women. J Obstet Gynecol Neonatal Nurs 1991; 20(3):221.

Draye MA: Emotional aspects of infertility. In: Lemcke DP et al (editors): *Primary Care of Women.* Appleton & Lange, 1995.

Franks P, Clancy CM: Physician gender bias in clinical decision making: Screening for cancer in primary care. Med Care 1993;31(3):213.

Frye CA, Weisberg RB: Increasing the incidence of routine pelvic examinations: Behavioral medicine's contribution. Women Health 1994;21(1):33.

Gise LH: Premenstrual syndromes. In: Lemcke DP et al (editors): *Primary Care of Women.* Appleton & Lange, 1995.

Harlan LC, Bernstein AB, Kessler LG: Cervical cancer screening: Who is not screened and why? Am J Pub Health 1991;81(7):885.

Hunter MS: Predictors of menopausal symptoms: Psychosocial aspects. Bailliere's Clin Endocrin Metabol 1993;7(1):33.

Kreuter MW et al: Are patients of women physicians screened more aggressively? J Gen Inter Med 1995;10(3):119.

Longstreth GF: Irritable bowel syndrome and chronic pelvic pain. Obstet Gynecol Surv. 1994;49(7):505.

Lurie N et al: Preventive care for women: Does the sex of the physician matter? N Engl J Med 1993;329(7):478.

Massion CT, Clancy MC, Maxwell ME: Women's access to health care. In: Lemcke DP et al (editors): *Primary Care of Women.* Appleton & Lange, 1995.

Roter D, Lipkin M, Korsgarrd A: Sex differences in patients' and physicians' communication during primary care medical visits. Med Care 1991;29(11):1083.

Severino SK, Moling ML: Premenstrual syndrome identification and management. Drugs 1995;49(1):71.

Stein M et al: Fluoxetine in the treatment of premenstrual dysphoria, N Engl J Med 1995;332(23):1529.

US Preventive Services Task Force: *Guide to Clinical Preventive Services,* 2nd ed. International Medical Publishing, 1996.

Utian WH, Schiff I: NAMS-Gallup survey on women's knowledge, information sources, and attitudes to menopause and hormone replacement therapy. Menopause 1994;1(1):39.

Walling MK et al: Abuse history and chronic pain in women: A multivariate analysis of abuse and psychological morbidity. Obstet Gynecol 1994;84(2):200.

Section III.
Health-Related Behavior

Behavior Change

16

Daniel O'Connell, PhD

INTRODUCTION

Despite the advances in medical technology that help physicians identify and treat problems from broken bones to rare bacterial infections, one aspect of treating patients defies neat categorization and clinical-manual roadmaps; that is, the behavior of patients—how patients react to illness, how they interact with their physicians, and how their attitudes and actions affect their health. Health-related problem behaviors can range from simply denying the fact of an illness to refusing either to discuss or to end smoking, drinking, or unhealthful eating. In dealing with such behaviors, physicians must be able to gauge the patient's readiness to change.

Development of the stages-of-change model discussed in this chapter was developed by Prochaska and DiClemente in the 1970s and can be applied to most of the health-related behaviors of concern found in primary care practice. The model posits that most people move through predictable stages in their efforts to change their health-related behaviors (Table 16–1). It provides a powerful framework for recognizing where patients are on a continuum of behavior change and how to influence their ultimate success.

ASSESSING STAGES OF CHANGE

In trying to modify patient behavior, it is essential to recognize the patient's readiness for and stage of change (see Chapter 21). For example, a 60-year-old widow whose drinking appears to be problematic might be asked whether she has noticed any problems arising from the consequences of her drinking. What has she tried to do so far about her alcohol use? To address a 25-year-old gay patient's risky sexual behavior, the clinician should ask specific questions to determine his present stage in thinking about and acting safely in sexual relationships: Does he recognize problems in his behavior? How could he reduce risks?

Is he already taking some action to reduce risks? Has he relapsed into riskier behavior after ending a long-term relationship in which safe sex was routine? The most valuable question for assessing the stage of change is "What thoughts have you had about [the problem behavior] and its effect on your health and life satisfaction?"

A key point to keep in mind is that stages of change are specific to each problem behavior: they are not global aspects of an individual's personality. For example, while a patient may be in the precontemplation stage for modifying his high-fat diet, he may already have moved through to maintenance on smoking cessation. Clinicians should also guard against the tendency to conclude prematurely that patients are completely ignoring or denying obvious problems.

For example, it is a common—but erroneous—belief that most problem drinkers and drug users are precontemplators, and that alcohol and drug addiction are diseases of denial. This concept assumes that the individual involved neither thinks about nor tries to modify the drinking or drug-use behavior. This situation is actually quite rare. It is common for problem drinkers to stop drinking hard liquor and switch to beer or wine in an effort to manage their drinking and its consequences. Although this approach is not likely to solve the drinking problem, such patients have clearly thought about (contemplated) the effects of various strengths of liquor. They have committed themselves to a different behavior (drinking wine or beer rather than hard liquor) and perhaps even achieved maintenance at this level.

Although many people do try to address their problems, they typically do not think their strategies through carefully enough, or they apply them inconsistently and without the skill to succeed. Astute clinicians will take note of such efforts at self-change and inquire about their effectiveness in ending the behavior—and its undesirable consequences—that prompted the effort to change in the first place.

Understanding the stages-of-change model gives

Table 16–1. Stages of change and patient characteristics.

Stage	Patient Characteristics
Precontemplation	The problem exists, but the patient minimizes or denies it.
Contemplation	The patient is thinking about the problem and the costs and benefits of continuing with the problem or trying to change.
Preparation	The patient commits to a time and plan for resolving the problem.
Action	The patient makes daily efforts to overcome the problem.
Maintenance	The patient has overcome the problem and remains vigilant to prevent backsliding.
Relapse	The patient has gone back to the problem behavior on a regular basis after a period of successful resolution.

clinicians a valuable tool for promoting behavior change. This is not an approach that encourages impassioned pleas, long exhortations, or ugly confrontations. Instead, clinicians are urged to focus on brief interventions that target specific obstacles to the patient's movement to the next stage (Table 16–2). The goal is to induct and maintain the patient in the change process until long-term success is achieved and, when possible, to shorten the amount of time required to accomplish a sustained behavior change.

Precontemplation

In this stage patients minimize or deny the existence of a problem behavior. Typically, the problem has been identified by others; patients try not to think about the problem and avoid listening to pertinent information and want others to do the same.

Patients are likely to deny the extent of the problem and its influence on themselves or others; they resist discussion of the problem, often with irritation, impatience, and defensive body language. Children and teens may claim to be bored by the topic. Adults may indicate that they are in a hurry, or that far more pressing concerns need their attention. In some form, "Get off my back!" is a common message from these patients.

It is important for clinicians to differentiate between true precontemplation and the reluctance to discuss uncomfortable issues that stems from other dynamics. The patient's reluctance to discuss the problem may reflect shame, demoralization, or a lack of trust in the clinician. Some patients are only too well aware of the problem and its costs to them and others (contemplation); they may feel overwhelmed by it and powerless to succeed in its resolution. They are often afraid of being embarrassed or shamed in front of the physician. In addition, whereas their resistance to discussion may appear to be precontemplation-stage behavior, some patients are actually demoralized long-term contemplators or relapsers. Although the clinician's interview style can influence the patient's willingness to discuss the problem, arguments, frustration, and antagonism on the part of both patient and clinician are highly likely.

Case illustration 1: Jack is 50 years old and is being seen by his internist. The appointment was made by Jack's wife Clara, ostensibly for follow-up of treatment for persistent high blood pressure. The actual reason, as explained to the nurse-receptionist, is Clara's concern about her husband's drinking and his failure to follow the clinician's latest recommendations for blood pressure control. During the appointment, Jack does not mention any problems with alcohol or any difficulty following the recommended regimen. When the doctor presses Jack for more details about the amount of alcohol he is consuming, Jack becomes evasive and irritated. The physician backs off and ends the visit with only a change in medication—and a feeling of frustration.

To avoid this impasse, the physician should express curiosity about Jack's own thoughts and feelings about his use of alcohol and its possible effect on his health. Pressing for details about problem behaviors often provokes defensiveness in precontemplators who quickly suspect that they are being trapped through interrogation. The physician's goal is to promote the patient's own willingness to contemplate potential health problems related to his behavior.

Clinicians often believe that their practices are overrun with patients in the precontemplation stage. As they listen more carefully to their patients' thoughts about such behavior, however, they often find that many of the patients are already wondering about the problem and how to resolve it. The psychologic theory of **reactance** posits that individuals are strongly motivated to maintain a sense of autonomy and to resist coercion by others. Because people resolutely protest and resist the perception that another's will is being imposed on them, the best way to influence patients' behavior is to create the perception that the change was their idea in the first place. Reactance creates its own logic, and patients who might otherwise have admitted their concern over a problem may instead feel compelled to defend their behavior.

At some point the precontemplator may begin to think about the problem and how it might be solved. This movement could be prompted by threats from others, developmental pressures (eg, "Now that I'm a father, I don't feel as much like partying"), a compelling example in real life or fiction, or a skillful interaction that makes the person aware of the negative consequences of the behavior without increasing defensiveness. The patient can then move into the contemplation stage of change.

Table 16–2. Stages of change and clinician strategies.

Stage of Change	Patient Characteristics	Clinician Strategies
Precontemplation	Denies problem and its importance. Is reluctant to discuss problem. Problem is identified by others. Shows reactance when pressured. High risk of argument.	Ask permission to discuss problem. Inquire about patient's thoughts. Gently point out discrepancies. Express concern. Ask patient to think, talk, or read about situation between visits.
Contemplation	Shows openness to talk, read, and think about problem. Weighs pros and cons. Dabbles in action. Can be obsessive about problem and can prolong stage.	Elicit patient's perspective first. Help identify pros and cons of change. Ask what would promote commitment. Suggest trials.
Preparation/ Determination	Understands that change is needed. Begins to form commitment to specific goals, methods, and timetables. Can picture overcoming obstacles. May procrastinate about setting start date for change.	Summarize patient's reasons for change. Negotiate a start date to begin some or all change activities. Encourage to announce publicly. Arrange a follow-up contact at or shortly after start date.
Action	Follows a plan of regular activity to change problem. Can describe plan in detail (unlike dabbling in action of contemplator). Shows commitment in facing obstacles. Resists slips. Is particularly vulnerable to abandoning effort impulsively.	Show interest in specifics of plan. Discuss difference between slip and relapse. Help anticipate how to handle a slip. Support and reemphasize pros of changing. Help to modify action plan if aspects are not working well. Arrange follow-up contact for support.
Maintenance	Has accomplished change or improvement through focused action. Has varying levels of awareness regarding importance of long-term vigilance. May already be losing ground through slips or wavering commitment. Has feelings about how much the change has actually improved life. May be developing lifestyle that precludes relapse into former problem.	Show support and admiration. Inquire about feelings and expectations and how well they were met. Ask about slips, any signs of wavering commitment. Help create plan for intensifying activity should slips occur. Support lifestyle and personal redefinition that reduce risk of relapse. Reflect on the long-term—and possibly permanent—nature of this stage as opposed to the more immediate gratification of initial success.
Relapse	Consistent return to problem behavior after period of resolution. Begins as slips that are not effectively resisted. May have cycled back to precontemplation, contemplation, or determination stages. Lessening time spent in this stage is a key to making greater progress toward fully integrated, successful, long-term change.	Frame relapse as a learning opportunity in preparation for next action stage. Ask about specifics of change and relapse. Remind patient that contemplation work is still valid (reasons for changing). Use "when," rather than "if," in describing next change attempt. Normalize relapse as the common experience on the path to successful long-term change.

Contemplation

In this stage the patient is thinking about the problem and potential solutions, weighing the pros and cons of each scenario, and showing behaviors characteristic of contemplation.

- The patient is open to thinking about and discussing the problem.
- The patient appears interested, may ask for additional information, or try to explain why the problem has persisted.
- The patient weighs the pros and cons of changing or not changing the problem behavior.
- Unless the patient is pushed to make a specific commitment to take appropriate action, there is less risk of irritation and argument.
- The contemplation stage can be prolonged or obsessive. Patients who have been in contemplation for a long time often request more convincing data and look for the ideal time and situation in which to initiate change.
- Patients may seem to be dabbling in action without a commitment to overcome obstacles that arise. They may, for example, decline an occasional dessert, not drink on weekdays, or make early-morning promises to change—and break them by midafternoon.

■ Contemplators may view obstacles from too limited a framework, for example, doubting that they
have sufficient "will-power" to follow through.

Some contemplation behavior appears to be necessary for later successful resolution of the problem.
Patients must anticipate costs and obstacles, identify
their motivations, understand how easy or difficult
the behavior change might be, and feel that they are
making informed and independent decisions, rather
than being coerced by others. Although some people
claim that they impulsively threw away their cigarettes, or that they quit drinking and never once
looked back, research suggests that even these people
may have been quietly doing contemplation work in
the years and months leading up to the presumably
impulsive action.

Case illustration 2: Joanna is 44 years old and has been
smoking a pack of cigarettes a day since she was 17.
When prompted by her family practice clinician she is
very willing to discuss the pros and cons of smoking.
Joanna tells her doctor that she is being pressured by her
children about secondary smoke and that she agrees with
their position. She thinks that the habit is both expensive
and stupid. On the other hand, she believes that smoking
is one of the few things that relax her throughout the day
at work and at home. One of her friends quit smoking and
gained 25 pounds; this possibility is frightening to
Joanna, who is already concerned about her weight. She
wonders whether medication or a nicotine patch or gum
would make quitting easier and perhaps keep her from
gaining weight. She has often promised herself in the
morning that she would cut down drastically on cigarettes
but has lost her resolve with her coffee break. She wonders aloud whether there is any better or worse time to try
to quit. By the end of the discussion, Joanna has promised
her doctor to think even more seriously about quitting.

Often the physician can help the contemplator
move toward being more determined to change simply by eliciting the pros and cons the patient has been
weighing as he or she thinks about trying to change.
In this case, the doctor's empathic summary brings
the contemplator's dilemma into clearer focus:

DOCTOR: It sounds as though you realize that changing
your behavior—not smoking—will be best for you in
the long term, but you're still trying to anticipate your
short-term sacrifices and need to decide how you'll cope
with them.

Following a period of contemplation—which can
be a few days or several years—many people move
toward a greater resolve and sense of urgency about
changing the problem behavior. There may be a convergence of information and threat or pressure (eg, the
alcoholic husband whose wife threatens divorce, the
smoker who learns she is pregnant), an inspiring
model, the chance for increased social support with
others undergoing similar changes, or opportunity for

a fresh start, such as a job transfer or move. Such
changes leads to the preparation/determination stage.

Preparation/Determination

In this stage the patient experiences a mounting
sense of urgency and commitment to change.

■ The patient talks about having made the decision to
change, in contrast with the contemplator's desire
or hope to change.
■ The patient has committed to a specific goal: "I am
going to stop smoking completely." "I will exercise
three times a week."
■ The patient mentions a specific time to begin the
activity: "On my next birthday. . . ." "After my
surgery. . . ." "When the kids start school in
September. . . ."
■ The patient has chosen a specific course of action,
such as joining a commercial weight-loss program
or Alcoholics or Narcotics Anonymous (AA, NA),
or is asking for a referral so the health plan will
cover the treatment.
■ The patient is willing to pay the costs of change, including out-of-pocket expenses, the time required
for the change, physical discomfort, embarrassment, and public exposure.
■ The patient considers the potential reactions of important people who may resist or be threatened by
the change. A spouse or partner who smokes or
drinks or is overweight, for example, may react
negatively to the patient's plans to overcome the
problem. Sometimes this occurs because such individuals anticipate pressure to face their own problems. In other cases, spouses, partners, and friends
may resist the patient's decision to change because
of some anticipated personal inconvenience (eg, the
husband who must watch the children while his
wife goes to an aerobics class) or embarrassment
over the possibility of exposing a weakness to
friends or neighbors.
■ The patient can envision overcoming obstacles that
lie ahead and how to overcome them.

Case illustration 3: Mike is a 15-year-old boy who has
been doing poorly in school for several years. Although
he has been diagnosed with attention deficit hyperactivity disorder, his parents, teachers, and pediatrician has
been unable to convince him to take his medication regularly. Now he has asked for an appointment with his pediatrician to discuss the situation. During the visit, Mike
confesses that he is tired of his problem behavior and
poor school performance. Further questioning by the
physician reveals that one of Mike's friends admitted being treated for attention deficit hyperactivity disorder.
Mike noticed and envied his friend's success; he asks the
physician to prescribe "whatever it will take to get me
out of this."

The pediatrician probes a bit to establish that Mike
has thought through the pros and cons of taking stimulant medicine and that his parents are still committed to

such a plan. The parents are invited into the examining room, and all agree on a plan that will begin with a trial of stimulant medicine. The effects of the medication will be reassessed in a month, based on questionnaires filled out by Mike and his parents and teachers.

By allowing Mike to work through the contemplation stage at his own pace, the pediatrician has helped establish an informal commitment to a treatment plan. He is treating Mike as a young person who can understand and assimilate information and who is capable of weighing the costs and benefits of treatment and then committing himself to the plan.

The day finally arrives when the individual begins to put the chosen plan into action. Some people may move back and forth between determination and contemplation a few times without going on to take action against the problem. They may feel—and claim to others—that a major effort at change is imminent, only to back off to the contemplator's lower level of urgency. The clinician can help patients at the determination stage intensify their commitment to a specific course of action (see discussion under "Promoting Behavior Change"). Patients at this point may talk about "gearing up" for action—the next stage.

Action

In the action stage, patients follow specific activities intended to achieve the goals they have set. While the patient's goal—cutting down on drug use, for example, rather than quitting completely—may not be exactly what the clinician prefers, the patient believes it is worthwhile and achievable on the basis of the previous period of contemplation.

- The patient has begun a set of actions intended to solve the problem. He or she has joined and is attending a weight-reduction group; has started going to AA and cut down or stopped drinking in the last few weeks; has recently quit or cut down on smoking and may be wearing a nicotine patch; or is exercising regularly.
- The patient may be focusing on one day at a time or trying to look past the initial discomfort by focusing on the long term.
- The patient recognizes and deals with the obstacles that arise before they can derail the program. The work done previously in the contemplation and preparation/determination stages is evident in the patient's comments during discussions with the clinician.
- Unlike the contemplator, the action patient does not allow exceptions to the course of action. This is not experimental dabbling in change to see what it might be like. At this stage, the patient has already decided that the discomfort of changing will be worthwhile. It remains to be seen whether the actual experience will be more difficult than was ex-

pected and whether the action plan can be maintained.
- By keeping the motivation for change in mind, the patient reinforces his or her commitment.

This is a time of maximum focus and effort. The greatest risk is that second thoughts may plague the patient, who is now particularly vulnerable to abandoning the change effort in a moment of weakness. Unexpected discomfort, resistance from others, or temptations that were neither anticipated nor planned for may overwhelm the patient's commitment to change. The action plan may then be abandoned precipitously.

Case illustration 4: Martha is a 45-year-old diabetic patient of a family practice. Over the last few years, her doctor has encouraged her to lose weight and exercise regularly, without much success. Martha comes in today and proudly reports that she has joined a weight-loss group that is held at her work site. Two colleagues have also joined, and they all have been attending faithfully and following the dietary recommendations for the last 3 weeks. The doctor encourages Martha to talk about her efforts. She is eager to talk; she reports feeling a great sense of pride and satisfaction. She admits that although she had been disgusted with herself for getting so heavy, she never before felt ready and able to tackle the problem. When her friends suggested that they join the group together, she was surprised at her enthusiastic response. She understands that this is the situation she had been hoping for, one that could provide support in making a difficult change.

Martha also admits to anxiety, since many people now know that she is trying to lose weight, and she does not want to fail publicly. Although she has been tempted to cheat on the diet, she has resisted the urge. She tells the doctor that she had felt somewhat discouraged when she did not lose as much weight as she had hoped the previous week. She asks the doctor to look over the program's dietary recommendations to be sure that they are safe in light of her diabetes.

After checking the weight-loss program's recommendations, Martha's doctor encourages her to discuss both the action steps she is taking and the reasoning (the contemplation work) that led to the effort. By asking open-ended questions about what Martha is doing and how the effort is going, the clinician reinforces the effort at change. Given enough time during the visit, he can make additional helpful suggestions to reduce the risk of early relapse and orient Martha more firmly toward long-term maintenance. The clinician's warm, curious, and engaged demeanor has reverberations beyond the visit. Martha can use the pleasant memory of the encounter to further internalize the value of the effort toward change.

The action stage is a time of concerted effort to resolve the problem. Once change has begun, however, many individuals are surprised to find that their resolution has faded, and all the ground gained during the action stage can be lost in relapse. Long-term vigilance and occasional (or even frequent and prolonged) supportive activity are necessary to prevent backsliding into a full relapse. This period of sustained vigilance and activity is known as the maintenance stage of change. For people who must control their weight, this stage may last a lifetime. In one study, former smokers reported some temptation to smoke 18 months after quitting. Problem drinkers may continue in AA for many years before they feel comfortable that their risk of relapse is low. Clinicians should be concerned about patients who have made good progress on resolving health-behavior problems but cannot describe their long-term plans to prevent relapse. Helping patients anticipate and find answers to the questions addressed in the next section is an important way in which clinicians can promote success at this stage.

Maintenance

The maintenance stage is the period of sustained vigilance and activity needed to preserve the improvements achieved during the action stage.

- The patient has achieved a period of success—as he or she has defined it—in overcoming the problem. The patient may have cut down or stopped drinking, reduced to the desired weight, or gone without cigarettes for several months. He or she is managing time and commitments better so that stress is no longer overwhelming, has gained consistent control over a short temper, or has accomplished any other desired outcome.
- Some patients assume a positive identity, seeing themselves as people who have overcome a problem and who are able to continue the action for a protracted period to prevent relapse. Patients who begin an exercise and diet program in order to lose weight, for example, may become avid hikers whose leisure time is devoted to rigorous outdoor adventures. These people have made a life-style and identity change in which the former problem behavior has no place.

To continue this period successfully, the patient must be able to handle both predictable and unpredictable obstacles and accept the constraints of abstinence. This requires dealing appropriately with the temptations and frustrations that inevitably arise in the months and years following successful action.

- Some patients may be frustrated that success in dealing with one problem has not brought about hoped-for changes in other areas. For example, while the weight loss may produce a slimmer, healthier body, it does not necessarily lead to an idealized slenderness and attractiveness. Abstinence from crack cocaine may not be enough to end all marital, job, and financial problems.

Patients who reduce their workaholic schedules so as to spend more time with their families may find they've traded more admiration at home for less at work. They must first take satisfaction in accomplishing their stated goals and then be ready to go to work on other dissatisfactions.

- The initial intensity of effort may be tapering off. Attendance at support-group meetings, for example, may have become erratic. The patient may be wondering whether it is now safe to quit the group or treatment program or to end a diet. It is hard to know when one is "out of the woods" and the problem resolved; successful maintenance requires both accurate self-appraisal and ongoing vigilance.
- Slips into the problem behavior may begin to be tolerated or justified: "I'll have just one glass of wine when I'm out with friends." "I'll only have a cigarette if I'm feeling really tense." These seductive thoughts must be resisted if successful maintenance is to continue; it may be necessary to renew the intense efforts of the action stage to do so.

Case illustration 5: At 55 years of age, Bill is—overall—doing very well, seeing his internist, periodically for health maintenance. Bill had been a very heavy drinker for 20 years; 5 years ago, a citation for driving under the influence of alcohol and the threat of divorce by his second wife pushed him into an alcohol treatment program. He achieved abstinence while attending the formal, court-mandated, 2-year outpatient treatment program. Since that time he has continued in AA, attending at least two meetings a week and occasional weekend conferences and workshops. Bill also sponsors a younger man in the group. In his conversations with his doctor, Bill describes himself as a recovering alcoholic. He schedules an appointment to discuss his distress over problems his son is experiencing—for which he holds himself partly responsible. The doctor thinks antidepressant medicine might be helpful, particularly in light of Bill's disturbed sleep and preoccupied demeanor. Bill questions the internist closely about the risk of addiction and explains his reluctance to use "another crutch" to control his moods.

Bill's doctor can be helpful here by recognizing that because Bill is consciously in maintenance he is extremely vigilant about anything he sees as a threat to his sobriety. The doctor asks directly and respectfully why Bill believes antidepressant medication might undermine his sobriety or stimulate a new addiction. Bill says that he is basically afraid of becoming dependent on the medication. The physician advises him to think about the recommendation and to speak with other AA members or friends. He also suggests that Bill read some related articles before his follow-up appointment so that he can make an informed commitment to addressing the depression through psychotherapy or a self-help group or by taking the prescribed medication.

Unfortunately, the odds favor relapse over any other outcome for a single attempt at health-behavior change. Clinicians know from both research and experience that too often patients' attempts to lose weight, stop alcohol or drug abuse, change their lifestyles to reduce stress, alter their diets in a more healthful direction, and even to floss their teeth daily are most likely to end in relapse. The false starts, failed promises, and pounds lost and promptly regained tend to obscure the reality that persistent effort often does result in successful resolution of the problem. Although any single effort to change is likely to get derailed before the patient achieves successful long-term maintenance, repeated efforts tend to yield the desired result eventually (this is borne out by Schacter's classic 1982 study). It is worth noting that more than 40 million Americans have quit smoking, many on their third or fourth serious try.

Many patients who appear to have reached the maintenance stage—for however brief a time—relapse, reverting to the undesirable behavior. Using the stages-of-change model, clinicians can encourage patients to keep working at the process of change, learning from each stage and experience, until the patient finally manages to reach—and maintain—the desired outcome.

Relapse

All relapse begins with a "slip," a deviation from the action plan. In a slip, the patient has an episode of problem behavior after a period of self-defined success in having overcome the problem. A slip might constitute engaging in an undesirable behavior such as smoking, or not engaging in a desirable behavior such as exercising. In the actual relapse stage, patients return to consistent problem behavior. With prompting by the clinician, patients may be able to describe the circumstances that led to the slips and eventually to relapse. They can learn how to anticipate and correct these vulnerabilities when they take action again.

- The typical patient in relapse has regained the weight lost, has begun drinking heavily again, has started smoking cigarettes after a period of nonsmoking during pregnancy, or has stopped using condoms during sexual intercourse with new partners.
- The patient may now talk or act like a person in an earlier stage of change. He or she may have entered a period of resistance and avoidance that is characteristic of the precontemplation stage. Alternatively, the patient may be contemplating change again, possibly even considering action in the near future.
- Relapsing patients' stories are more complex than those of patients who have never relapsed or are in earlier stages, and the reasons offered for the relapse provide many clues to the steps that must be taken to reinvigorate the patient's willingness to tackle the problem again. One patient may think: "I did it once, I can do it again!" Another patient may instead think: "I guess I don't have the willpower to do this."

The time the patient spends in relapse before initiating the next action stage of change accounts for much of the observed slowness in achieving final success for many health-behavior problems. Relapse is the norm for any single attempt at change. Even in professional treatment, as many as two thirds of the participants are likely to have relapsed within a year after achieving initial alcohol or drug sobriety. Success in smoking cessation, weight control, or alcohol and drug sobriety is usually achieved after a number of separate, unsuccessful attempts at change. In one study of smoking cessation, it took an average of 7 years to move from precontemplation to maintenance of smoking cessation. The typical participant had three relapses during that period, in which he or she had resumed regular smoking.

If handled empathically, patients in this stage are usually not too entrenched in denial or resistance. They had already concluded at least once that change was needed and can often recount the costs of continuing the problem behavior. It is the uneasiness they feel in anticipation of trying again to change that often has them stuck. Knowing this, the clinician can save much time that might otherwise be wasted on lecturing patients about things they already know and with which they agree.

Case illustration 6: Barbara is a 28-year-old woman who is being seen 2 months after the birth of her second child for renewal of her birth control prescription. Her physician is delighted to see Barbara again. As the interview evolves, Barbara sheepishly reveals that she is back to smoking a pack of cigarettes a day. The clinician is both disappointed and surprised, since Barbara had been quite proud of the fact that she stopped smoking during the pregnancy. The doctor takes a deep breath and calmly asks Barbara how that could have happened so quickly. Barbara talks about how frazzled she has felt taking care of both her baby and her 3-year-old son. She explains how, at first, she found it relaxing to smoke a cigarette or two after dinner with her husband (who is also a smoker); she had not pictured herself smoking a pack a day again. Soon, however, she was smoking with a friend who stopped in to visit. Now she has begun looking forward to a cigarette whenever she has a break from the immediate demands of her family. She tells her doctor that although she tries never to smoke when the baby is up, even this control is starting to erode.

The doctor's first challenge is to manage her own frustration and not leave Barbara feeling judged and ashamed. She points out Barbara's success in caring for her (then) 2-year-old child and dealing with the mood swings and physical discomforts of pregnancy without smoking. She also expresses her support and encouragement for the Barbara's recommitment to abstinence. Reaffirming the health benefits of not smoking—for both the patient and her children—helps reinforce the commitment. As a further step, the clinician suggests making and enforcing a no-smoking rule in the house.

PROMOTING BEHAVIOR CHANGE

The clinician's first task is to identify the patient's stage of change for each behavior of concern. The more accurately the clinician can differentiate the stages, the easier it will be to make a brief—but effective—intervention during a regular medical visit.

The clinician's main task is to promote movement from one stage to the next. Clinicians who are aware of the theory of reactance avoid forcing change on patients out of their own sense of urgency. Forgetting that most people strive to be self-directed and resist coercion only frustrates the clinician and impairs the doctor-patient relationship, which over time is a key to exerting influence. Shame or embarrassment might lead the patient to avoid facing the clinician again. Clinicians must also remember that they are neither powerless nor all-powerful. Addressing only the aspects of the present situation that hinder movement to the next stage makes the best use of primary care clinicians' time and energy to help change behavior.

Because behavior change is an area of practice that many clinicians find frustrating, it is important to guard against feeling either irritation or apathy. By reflecting on their own attempts at change, clinicians can better appreciate the time, false starts, and circular nature of the change process. This makes it easier to feel and express empathy to patients for their difficulties along the path to changing patterned behavior. Research has consistently demonstrated the power of an empathic and involved supporter in promoting growth and change.

It also helps to adopt an attitude of curiosity whenever patients behave in ways that seem illogical or counterproductive. Dismissing such behavior as stupidity, dependency, irresponsibility, or the manifestation of a personality disorder can block a more helpful line of inquiry. The clinician can instead ponder why this patient waited weeks for an appointment, sat in the reception area for an additional half hour because the doctor was running late, paid for some or all of the cost of the visit, felt physically and emotionally uncomfortable enough about a problem to discuss it, and then didn't follow through on the recommendations that were made to resolve or ameliorate it. The clinician can express that curiosity to the patient, saying, for example, "I'm curious as to why you think you couldn't start the exercise program we discussed at your last visit. What do you think is the most important thing you must do to get that exercise program into your regular schedule?" The most productive questions are those that convey a respectful curiosity and that focus the patient on identifying and overcoming specific obstacles to change.

Success entails helping patients view themselves as engaged in an ongoing process of changing the specific behavior, and the clinician can help make that the most efficient process possible. If the average patient (as reported in one study) takes 7 years to move from precontemplation to maintenance, cutting that time to 4 years through skillful intervention is a significant improvement. Understanding the length of time required to make such changes can relieve clinicians of the urgency and pressure that come with unrealistic goals.

Strategies for the Precontemplation Stage

The clinician should ask pertinent questions before attempting to persuade patients to change their behavior, for example, "What effect do you think your smoking has on your asthma?" Questions of this kind, asking patients to *contemplate* the possible connections between the physical symptoms that bother them and the behaviors that may be provoking those symptoms, are among the most helpful to precontemplators.

Patient defensiveness can often be defused if practitioners ask the precontemplator's permission before talking about the problem, for instance, "Would it be all right if we talk a little more about how your drinking might be contributing to some of the problems you mentioned today?" The physician's agenda should be linked with concerns the patient has already expressed. If a female patient asks for birth control, the clinician can use her concern about pregnancy as a basis for asking how else she had previously been protecting herself when having sex. Patients who complain about headaches can be asked what is going on in their lives that could affect the headaches. This is a way of examining patients' life stresses by placing them in a natural context and so avoiding the patients' suspicion that the physician is dismissing the problem as "all in your head."

Discrepancies between the patient's present behavior and the expressed goal of feeling better and worrying less should be pointed out gently. Physicians should also express their concern that the patient may not achieve the desired improvement without addressing the specific problem:

> DOCTOR: I'm concerned that you'll always worry about another heart attack unless you know you've changed your life-style and lowered the risk.
> I'm concerned that none of these medicines will be able to relieve your stomach discomfort as long as you drink alcohol and caffeine.

The goal with precontemplators is to increase their willingness to understand (contemplate) the connections between behavioral health and physical health as the first step toward change. Much of the actual contemplation work is done between visits, and clinicians can ask whether the patient is willing to think about, keep track of, and read about the problem and potential solutions—or talk to someone else about them—before the next appointment. The clinician should be sure to note the patient's response and mention it at the next visit.

Strategies for the Contemplation Stage

In this stage also, the clinician should elicit the patient's perspective before offering advice, with questions that acknowledge movement toward change:

> DOCTOR: What have you been thinking about your cigarette smoking and what you might be able to do about it?

Patients can be helped to identify the pros and cons of change and to examine the current pleasures and ultimate consequences of the problem behavior, as well as the anticipated consequences of trying to change it. It seems axiomatic that people do unhealthful things because they desire the pleasures such acts bring. Many patients already believe that they would be better off if they ate differently, exercised more, drank less, stopped or cut down on drug use, lost weight, reduced stress, and so on. Contemplators frequently become stuck in ambivalence over the possibility that the change process itself will be psychologically or physically unpleasant, costly, and likely to fail; they may need help identifying and working their way through these anticipated obstacles. Clinicians can ask the patient what the greatest obstacle has been in taking action to resolve or ameliorate the problem and focus their curiosity on this obstacle.

Patients who claim that—because of insufficient will power—they are powerless to stop smoking, quit drug or alcohol abuse, or change any other behavior should be asked such questions as, "If you were convinced that your wife's life depended on your not smoking for 3 months, do you think you could resist temptation that long? Where would the ability to do it come from?"

Similarly, patients should be asked what they think would bring about a commitment to change the behavior:

> DOCTOR: If I were to meet you years from now and find that you had completely stopped using crack cocaine, what do you think you would tell me was the reason you finally decided to stop?

Depending on the answer, the next questions might be,

> DOCTOR: Knowing that such an event (eg, arrest) is likely to come about, what do think about trying to resolve the problem before that happens?
> What approach do you think you would use to overcome the problems if you believed you really had to?
> What obstacles would you encounter if you were to start using that approach now?

Clinicians can encourage patients to think about an upcoming time in which taking action to resolve or improve the problem situation would be least taxing.

Suggestions for limited trials of possible solutions might include the following questions:

> DOCTOR: Would you be willing to cut down from 20 to 15 cigarettes a day and make a note of how hard or easy this is for you?
> I know you want to resolve the argument you and your wife are having about how much you actually drink. Would you be willing to write down in a notebook every alcoholic drink you have for the next 2 weeks?

Even when the patient objects to this strategy as being unrealistic, the suggestion raises the possibility that such data can help answer previously unresolvable questions and arguments.

> DOCTOR: Would you be willing to always carry a condom with you so that it's available the next time you have intercourse?
> Before our next appointment, would you be willing to check with your health plan about your options for getting alcohol treatment in the evening? That way, if you should decide to start treatment, you wouldn't miss work and no one there would have to know about the problem.

Strategies for the Preparation/ Determination Stage

Patients should be encouraged to set a date to start action on the problem. They should be helped to understand more clearly the program they are planning to follow, including structured activities or referrals. Summaries can be used for clarification:

> DOCTOR: So you're planning to start Weight Watchers at work next month with the goal of losing 35 pounds?
> You've committed yourself to getting 30 minutes of aerobic exercise four times a week.

These comments should be noted in the chart in the patient's presence, and the patient should be told that the clinician is looking forward to hearing about what happens next.

Patients should be supported with reassurance that initiating action to change problem behavior is always the right thing to try. Even when the attempt is not fully successful, the experience will yield helpful information about how to succeed eventually. It is important not to appear so enthusiastic, confident, and hopeful that patients who are unsuccessful in taking the agreed-on step feel too ashamed to see their physicians that they avoid them. Because public commitments are more likely to be kept than private ones, patients should be encouraged to tell others about their commitment to change.

Follow-up is also important, whether it involves scheduling an appointment, sending a postcard, or requesting a note or phone message soon after the proposed start date. Clinicians should highlight the patient's commitment as being an important step beyond prior contemplation and thus deserving of special attention.

Strategies for the Action Stage

A warm inquiry about the specifics of the patient's activities to promote change adds the support and encouragement of a professional person to the patient's other social supports. Clinicians should also ask about any obstacles the patients encounter (obstacles and second thoughts are to be expected) and how they are handling the problems. The clinician can suggest that patients write out the pros of making the change and post them prominently as an aid to maintaining their motivation. An accepting attitude encourages patients to try problem solving rather than yield to the urge to give up.

Patients should be asked for permission to consult with any other professionals involved in the program. A brief contact with a chemical-dependency counselor, smoking-cessation group leader, psychotherapist, and so on demonstrates that the physician values and supports the patient's efforts during the most vulnerable period of active change.

It is important to help patients prepare for recovery from slips—smoking a cigarette, having a drink, missing an exercise session or AA meeting, or having seconds at a meal. A slip need not become a fall if patients have anticipated the possibility and prepared how they will think about the slip and react once it is recognized: throw out the rest of the cigarette pack; pour out the remainder of the bottle; add another exercise session or AA meeting; eat a smaller-than-usual portion at the next meal; and reaffirm the commitment to conquer this problem.

Some type of follow-up (eg, a note, a call, an appointment) should be scheduled both to get a progress update and to show support for the patient. Physicians can give patients preaddressed postcards and ask them to write brief notes on their progress 2 or 4 weeks into a new change effort. A telephone call from the office nurse can reassure the patient and provide a progress report. Making a note on the chart will remind the physician and office staff to inquire about the change effort at the next patient contact.

Strategies for the Maintenance Stage

Inquiring about how well the patient is maintaining the improvements achieved in the action stage is an important first step:

DOCTOR: What have you been doing to keep your weight down?
Have you been going to your support-group meetings regularly?
How well have you been doing with your exercise program?

Successful maintenance often involves making lifestyle changes that turn out to have significant positive effects beyond control of the original problem. The sedentary patient who starts a program of physical activity for cardiovascular conditioning may find, as a bonus, both long-term weight control and unexpected skill on the tennis court. In addition, clinicians who have successfully stopped smoking, lost weight, or become more physically active can sometimes use themselves as examples of the real possibility of maintaining change. The key here is to emphasize that the new behavior can become an integral part of a more healthful and satisfying life-style.

Patients should be asked about slips that have already occurred and how they responded. Even when patients say that they have stopped drinking or smoking, it makes a great deal of sense to ask neutrally, "Have you had even one drink (or cigarette) since you quit?" Many quitters have at least one slip to report, and discussing how a full relapse was prevented can reinforce their commitment and identify risky situations.

It is important to emphasize the difference between a slip and a full relapse. Because many patients do not even want to consider making a slip, they may be unprepared to react appropriately if it occurs. Patients should be prepared for the likelihood of a slip and have a plan for how to deal with it at once. They may protest that the clinician is being too pessimistic; explaining to patients that such preparation is a way of protecting their newly achieved change can provide a more positive tone.

Patients should also be asked what they have learned so far about the change process as well as how confident they are that they will maintain the improvement over the next time period. They should further be asked to describe their highest-risk situations for a slip or relapse—an event such as a party, or an emotion such as anger, sadness, or exuberance—and how prepared they feel to handle these high-risk situations without a slip.

Each of these recommendations involves showing interest, support, and curiosity and suggesting that anticipation and vigilance are the keys to successful maintenance.

Clinicians must be alert for any signs of waning enthusiasm and express their curiosity about the cause. As noted earlier, patients often become discouraged when improvement in one area does not resolve other life dissatisfactions. They may feel that others do not recognize and appreciate the effort that they have made to change. A sincere compliment from a clinician accompanied by a message that "I am rooting for you" creates a memory that can be recalled during moments of discouragement.

Strategies for the Relapse Stage

The key to dealing with relapse is to reframe it as a valuable learning experience that will shed light on how best to go about the next attempt at change. It is therefore essential that clinicians express their interest in the last attempt at change and ask the patient to describe exactly how initial success was achieved and how slips led to a full-blown relapse.

Some patients promptly—and erroneously—conclude, "I tried it and it didn't work; therefore, it never will work." This is too global a statement; it obscures the successful components that could be used in the next change effort. The physician's response might be:

> DOCTOR: It sounds as though you were very successful in quitting smoking using the action strategies you described, and they might work well again. Where you fell down was in thinking that you could have one cigarette and not recognizing how dangerous this could be for you.

The next attempt at change should be discussed as inevitable—*when* rather than *if.* Patients should be reminded that all the analysis and conclusions that led to deciding to change last time remain valid. If chang-

ing was the right decision then, it is still the right decision now. The question the relapser must answer is "What is the next step for you to get moving again toward change?"

Clinicians should remember that many patients think of themselves as relapsers, even if the care and commitment they put into previous attempts at change seem inadequate. The relapser may feel more demoralized than makes sense since from our point of view a good deal of constructive work must have been done leading up to the failed effort to maintain the desired change. One of the most helpful aspects of using the stages-of-change model is the optimism it generates for both clinician and patient. The concept that pursuing the process knowledgeably and persistently over time almost inevitably brings about the desired change is a welcome counter to the frustration and pessimism so often reported by clinicians and patients alike.

SUGGESTED READINGS

DiClemente CC: Motivational interviewing and the stages of change. In: Miller WR, Rollnick S (editors): *Motivational Interviewing: Preparing People to Change Addictive Behavior.* Guilford, 1991.

Marlatt GA, Gordon JR: *Relapse Prevention.* Guilford, 1985.

Prochaska JO, DiClemente CC, Norcross JC: In search of how people change: Applications to addictive behaviors. Am Psychol 1992;47:1102.

Prochaska JO, Norcross JC, DiClemente CC: *Changing for Good.* Guilford, 1994.

Schacter S: Recidivism and self-cure of smoking and obesity. Am Psychol 1982;37:436.

17

Adherence

M. Robin DiMatteo, PhD

INTRODUCTION

The failure of patients to comply with treatment regimens that their physicians have recommended is a significant problem in clinical practice. This problem, known as **nonadherence,** typically consists of patient actions such as taking antibiotics incorrectly (eg, only until the symptoms abate), forgetting or refusing to take longer-term medications (such as those for hypertension), and persisting in dangerous and unhealthy activities (such as smoking and high-risk sexual activity). As a result of their failure to adhere to the recommended treatment, patients can become more seriously ill, or treatment-resistant pathogens may develop. Physicians may then inappropriately alter the treatment (by increasing medication dosages, for example) or become misled about the correct diagnosis. Practitioners and patients become frustrated, and the time and money spent on the medical visit are wasted.

On average, 40% of patients in the United States are nonadherent; rates vary with the type of regimen that is prescribed. Approximately 20% of patients fail to follow short-term treatments for acute conditions (such as taking an antibiotic correctly). About 40–50% of patients are nonadherent to longer-term regimens (such as taking regular medication for a chronic disease), and more than 75% of patients fail to adhere to such recommended life-style changes as limiting the consumption of alcohol and dietary fat, exercising, or ceasing the use of tobacco products.

Research on patient adherence shows that patients do only what they believe in and only what they feel they are able to do. Primary care providers should remember that the medical provider is but one influence in what is often experienced by the patient as a cacophony of health messages, ranging from the ridiculous to helpful information that may be better geared to the patient's quality of life and personal concerns than what the provider has to offer. The most important ingredients in achieving patient adherence are effective communication and patients' informed collaboration with the physician.

RECOGNIZING NONADHERENCE

Nonadherence can be difficult to recognize (Table 17–1). Few patients readily admit to having difficulties following their treatment regimens—and they rarely indicate to their providers that they have no intention of following the recommendations that they disagree with or feel incapable of following. Patients weigh the physician's recommendations against both their own beliefs and what has been told to them by others (including sources of information outside the health-care field).

Patients who are passive and uninvolved and appear to be unquestioningly obedient are often nonadherent. This kind of patient is more likely to disregard the directions than is a patient who questions recommendations, offers opinions, and even attempts to negotiate a more acceptable regimen. Nonadherence should always be considered whenever a patient is inconsistently responsive—or remains unresponsive—to treatment and when the clinical picture is confusing or does not appear to make sense.

Case illustration: Clark is a 46-year-old civil engineering professor who has moderate essential hypertension, is overweight, and lives a sedentary life-style. Despite recommendations to follow a low-fat diet and an exercise program, Clark remains more than 20% over his ideal weight and appears to be physically out of condition. Antihypertensive medication has been prescribed for 4 months, with little or no reduction in blood pres-

Table 17–1. Typical clues to nonadherence.

- Patient passivity and lack of involvement
- Appearance of unquestioning obedience
- Lack of response or inconsistent response to treatment
- Confusing or indistinct clinical picture

sure. After returning several times for scheduled office visits, Clark starts to cancel appointments.

Eventually Clark returns for a follow-up visit, but his clinical parameters remain unchanged. The physician's task now is twofold: to impress on the patient the very real dangers of excessive weight and hypertension and to develop a treatment regimen that he can believe in and integrate into his life, while maintaining Clark's trust and his commitment to improving his health. Once Clark understands that his noncompliance can lead to a stroke or heart attack, the physician can discuss treatment with him. At the very least, this will involve establishing and monitoring a graduated regimen of physical activity that Clark enjoys, a gradual modification of his diet—most likely with support from nutritional counseling or a self-help group—and considerable education about and negotiation of drug-treatment choices, with regular assessment of the medications' effects on his quality of life. These goals will be achieved over the course of regular office visits.

UNDERSTANDING ADHERENCE PROBLEMS

The first step in understanding adherence problems is to talk openly with the patient about his condition and its treatment while maintaining respect for his beliefs. When Clark's physician does this, it becomes clear that although the patient is a highly educated person, he does not fully understand the meaning of hypertension, the risks of leaving it untreated, or the role of medication and life-style changes in lowering his blood pressure. The physician is surprised to learn, for example, that Clark takes his medication only when he feels what he describes as "hyper," or "tense." He does not understand or believe in the efficacy of taking medication regularly; in fact, he thinks it might be dangerous. He also feels somewhat embarrassed by being "the kind of person who has to take medicine." Furthermore, he experiences unpleasant side effects (primarily impotence) that he attributes to the medication. Clark does not follow the recommended fat-reduction diet and does not exercise because he finds too many barriers in his daily life to doing so. He works extremely hard at his profession and claims that he has little time to devote to such pursuits as exercise and regular, nutritious meals.

Psychological Mechanisms

Adherence problems have not been linked to any particular personality type, gender, ethnicity, class, or educational attainment. Very affluent and highly educated patients may be as nonadherent as those who are poor and uneducated. The primary causes of nonadherence (Table 17–2) are poor provider-patient communication, resulting in the patient's lack of understanding of the treatment regimen and the reasons for its importance; poor provider-patient relationships in which there exists a lack of trust and mutual caring, in which patients do not feel listened to, and in which

Table 17–2. Causes of nonadherence.

- Poor provider-patient communication about the regimen
- Lack of trust and mutual caring in provider-patient relationship
- Controlling, paternalistic provider behavior
- Patient's failure to understand costs, benefits, and efficacy of regimen
- Patient's lack of commitment to regimen
- Provider's failure to anticipate and overcome practical barriers to adherence

the provider behaves in a controlling, paternalistic manner; the patient's failure to understand fully the costs, benefits, and efficacy of the recommended regimen and to believe in the regimen as a valuable undertaking, worthy of commitment; and the physician's failure to anticipate and overcome barriers to adherence or to work within the patient's constraints (eg, the inability to afford costly medication, a hectic or irregular daily schedule).

Nonadherence may sometimes be the patient's way of equalizing the balance of power in the physician-patient relationship. When patients feel they cannot assert their preferences, they often make private plans for their own medical well-being, even to the point of not adhering to medical regimens. Nonadherence may thus be thought of as a strategy for restoring a lost sense of control. Patients who offer little resistance to a recommendation or prescription during a medical encounter may be adapting to a social situation they feel unable to resist. Their apparently passive acceptance is likely to be interpreted by the physician as a sign of commitment instead of as a warning of nonadherence. Although the patient may be agreeing verbally, body language—crossed arms, stiff posture, lack of eye contact—may indicate the opposite. Without further persuasion, the patient may fail to follow the prescribed regimen.

Assessing Adherence

Studies show that physicians are not very accurate in their determination of which patients are adherent and which are not. Adherence problems can be particularly difficult to detect if they are viewed as aberrant behavior rather than patients' rational choices. It should be assumed that every patient is potentially nonadherent—often for good reason—and physicians might think back to their own personal instances of nonadherence to gain perspective on how reasonable such a choice might sometimes seem to be. Patients may attempt to hide adherence difficulties to avoid disappointing the physician and because of the social and normative pressures to be a "good patient." They are especially circumspect if they anticipate any criticism from their providers or negation of their right to make choices. Conversely, providers may be reluctant to inquire about nonadherence for fear that such revelation might be awkward and frustrating. The goal in questioning patients about their adherence is to help them improve their health, not to catch and reprimand them or to assert physician authority. Patients must be helped to understand the value of making collaborative choices with their physicians instead of unilateral choices that may jeopardize their health.

The most effective approach to adherence assessment involves recognition and acceptance that patients are autonomous and appropriately make personal choices to maximize their quality of life *as they see it*. Patients are experts about their own values, preferences, and capabilities, just as physicians and other primary care providers are experts in medical diagnosis and treatment. The provider's task is to be a sensitive, supportive advocate, not an authoritarian adversary. In addition, the patient is a complex person with unique values, life-style, and beliefs about quality of life that must be incorporated into medical treatment decisions.

Adherence depends greatly on patient involvement in making medical choices and treatment decisions. Patient responsibility for self-management and adherence requires effective practitioner-patient communication and collaboration. The cost of not establishing this collaboration is high for both patients and health professionals. Without discussion and its inevitable but manageable conflicts, providers and patients create relationships in which their expectations for their interaction and for the course and outcome of treatment are never discussed. Furthermore, when patients are not informed of and involved in their care, they give less adequate histories and they tend to delay in reporting important symptoms to their physicians.

MANAGING NONADHERENCE

Behavioral Techniques

The relationship between medical interventions and patient outcomes is mediated by patient adherence to treatment, a phenomenon that is highly dependent on the physician's mastery of the behavioral elements listed in Table 17–3.

The provider must build the two essential elements of provider-patient communication: accurate transmittal of information from patient to practitioner and from practitioner to patient, and emotional support and understanding of the patient as a unique person and of his or her emotional needs and personal experience in medical care.

Effective, Accurate Communication of Information: Unfortunately, this is not the norm in medical practice. Research has demonstrated that close to one half of all patients leave their doctors' offices not knowing what they have been told and what they are supposed to do to take care of themselves. Physicians regularly use medical terms that patients do not understand, and patients are unwilling or lack sufficient skill to articulate their questions. Although the vast majority of patients greatly value obtaining as

Table 17–3. Essential elements of achieving patient adherence.

- Accurate transmission of information between patient and provider
- Emotional support and understanding of patient
- Help in choosing an acceptable course of action to which a commitment can be made
- Help in overcoming barriers to adherence
- Focus on the overall quality of life of the patient
- Acceptance of the value of provider-patient negotiation
- Development of a specific plan to implement the regimen

much information about their conditions as possible and want to know about potential outcomes of and the range of possible treatments, such information is rarely provided to them. Usually less than 5% of the medical visit is spent giving patients any information at all. Physicians often unwittingly discourage patients from voicing their concerns and requests for information by exhibiting rushed behaviors, such as looking at their wristwatches and interrupting patients' questions.

In response to these cues, patients tend to ask few questions and provide little information beyond what is directly requested. Despite their confusion over the technical terms and medical jargon used by their physicians, patients typically do not ask for clarification. It should be noted that although educating patients and answering their questions may initially take a few extra minutes, those few minutes are very well spent in the long run.

Emotional Support and Understanding: The second element of provider-patient communication involves empathy, the understanding of patients' feelings, and the building of interpersonal trust in the physician-patient relationship (see Chapter 2). This aspect of care has traditionally been a source of discomfort for physicians and other primary care providers. If, however, the physician attends only to disease and ignores the patient's suffering, both physical and emotional, he or she may fail to support the patient's healing.

Physicians' behavior and communication style during office visits are directly linked to patients' satisfaction with medical care, their recall of medical information, and their subsequent adherence to prescribed regimens. Patient satisfaction with medical treatment is greater if patients trust their providers. Emotional support of patients appears to enhance positive expectations for healing and patients' fulfillment of those expectations. Providers who are more sensitive to and emotionally expressive with nonverbal communication have more satisfied patients and patients who are more likely to adhere to the recommended treatments. Providers who make patients feel rushed or ignored, devalue patients' views, fail to respect and listen to them, and fail to understand their perspectives are more likely to be sued for medical malpractice. It is important to note that there is empiric evidence that technical skill is not sacrificed in developing the capacity to respond to patients' feelings.

Acceptable Course of Action: The physician should help the patient choose an acceptable course of action to which a commitment can be made. Patient adherence depends on commitment to what may be a disruptive, difficult course of action. Commitment depends on the patient's clear understanding of the regimen and belief that it is worth following; that it is likely to be effective; and that the benefits outweigh the costs in time, money, discomfort, possible embarrassment, and life-style adjustment. Such a commitment by the patient requires detailed discussion about the recommendation, including its value compared with other courses of action and any potential risks or problems that may be encountered. The time for discussion of any disadvantage to an alternative is before the choice is made, not after, when the patient's sudden awareness of the adverse effects results in abandonment of the regimen.

Quality of Life: It is essential to focus on the patient's overall quality of life. Paradoxically, striving for patient adherence to precisely what the provider has chosen will likely result in nonadherence and poor health outcomes. The goal of treatment should not be to achieve the provider's unilaterally conceived agenda. In all approaches to medical decision making, there needs to be an emphasis on the patient's personal quality of life and a recognition that the patient always knows more about himself or herself than the clinician ever will. The patient is the one who has to live with the results of medical treatment decisions. The physician and patient must explore together and discuss the chances of achieving the goals that they have jointly chosen. They must consider the chances of achieving the entire goal picture, which is life as the patient would like to live it. Together, they must work to consider various alternative futures for the patient that may result from various courses of action, such as different treatment regimens—or even no treatment at all.

Provider-Patient Negotiation: The physician must accept the inevitability—and the value—of disagreements with the patient. Choosing the best course of action to enhance a patient's quality of life and solve a medical problem is something that should be expected to take some time and effort. The mutual exploration of alternatives toward the goal of agreement can help physician and patient form realistic expectations of outcomes and learn to work together despite their likely differing perspectives on the clinical situation. Patients tend to be more risk-averse than their physicians, and they usually favor more conservative interventions. Since patient involvement in the decision process is likely to lead to more satisfactory outcomes, physicians should actively pursue with patients any possible conflict and work to unearth patients' objections in the process of negotiation and collaborative decision making. Negotiation and con-

structive challenge lead physician and patient to examine their points of disagreement; they may also forestall such expressions of patient dissatisfaction as nonadherence and malpractice litigation. The purpose of the negotiation is not just to have the patient accept the clinician's definition of the problem and preferred solution, rather, it is to have the clinician accept the possibility that the patient has a different definition of the problem, different goals, and a different idea of what methods are acceptable for achieving those goals. There must be a recognition that the most effective interaction occurs if each party fully understands the goals and preferences of the other.

The process of resolving conflict brings the primary care provider and patient closer to mutually acceptable solutions. If provider and patient have such disparate views that conflict cannot be resolved, it is better to know sooner rather than later in their relationship. When the patient's perspective is not known to the clinician, continuity of conflict rather than resolution is inevitable. Thus, physicians should invite conflict by exploring patients' assessments and feelings about all proposed actions. Clinicians should actually lead therapeutic conversations to legitimate expressions of differences and conflicts, making it clear that the encounter is one in which differences can be resolved through negotiation. Steps to effective negotiation include stating principles and goals on which doctor and patient agree, eliciting the patient's feelings and concerns about alternative methods, respectfully acknowledging physician-patient differences, and compromising where possible.

Patient Education

After a commitment has been made by the patient—that is, after the patient has truly come to understand and believe in the value of the regimen—the clinician should work with the patient to develop a plan for how the recommended treatment is to be incorporated into the patient's life. Physician and patient must identify ways to overcome practical problems that may serve as barriers to adherence. For example, many patients are likely to have difficulty taking medication four times a day (and will typically settle on two or three times as their best compromise). A more appropriate clinical regimen that the patient can follow correctly might be a medication that can be taken only three times or—even better—twice a day and that is associated with such regular activities as eating meals or brushing teeth. The clinician might recommend other ways for the patient to be reminded of medication, such as setting a wristwatch alarm or posting a medication schedule on the refrigerator. The most important educational tool at this stage of adherence advancement is to work with the patient to determine precisely how the regimen can be implemented for maximum clinical effectiveness.

It is important to develop—with the patient—methods for follow-up and continued maintenance, such as regular telephone calls and office visits to check on progress and solve inevitable problems or to modify the regimen when necessary. Some physicians write out brief contracts with their patients, specifying what the patient is to do (the details of the treatment regimen) and what the physician is to do in return (eg, regular telephone contact for encouragement or even a free office visit after 3 months of acceptable blood pressure readings).

Patients who are involved in both choosing and planning the implementation of their treatment regimens are much more involved in their own care, ask more questions, and express greater satisfaction with their care than are those who are not. Involved patients also have greater alleviation of their symptoms and better control of their chronic conditions, less distress and concern about their illnesses, and better responses to surgery and invasive diagnostic procedures. Patients who are involved in their care also feel a greater sense of control over their health and their lives. They demonstrate better adherence to the treatment they have helped to decide on, and they have more positive expectations for their health. Patients who participate in and share responsibility for their health decisions are less likely to blame their physicians if something goes wrong.

Effective therapeutic communication also involves the recognition that both physician and patient bring unique areas of expertise to the medical encounter. The physician's expertise involves medical knowledge and clinical experience; the patient's involves knowing the effect of the problem on his or her quality of life and goals and the effects of many variables on character and control of symptoms. The patient also knows his or her degree of commitment to any proposed treatment plan and the barriers that may be encountered in attempting to follow it. Education, therefore, cannot be one-sided; the physician needs to be educated about the patient's needs, wants, and expectations for care—elements that cannot be assumed without asking.

Indications for Referral

In many cases, primary care providers may find it difficult or impossible to devote extended time to patient education, follow-up, and maintenance. Written materials can be helpful, but only if those materials are used to supplement what has been discussed with the patient. Although office nurses or health educators can provide valuable adjunctive care to patients, their role in education should never fully take the place of the physician's. Patients often need additional referrals, such as to a nutritionist for dietary modification or an exercise counselor/personal trainer for fitness education and training. The primary provider should always remain involved, consulting with these ancillary providers and monitoring the patient's own views of progress. The primary provider should be familiar with and believe in the methods used by referral providers; his or her enthusiasm for these referrals affects patient adherence to their recommendations as well.

Some patients, particularly those with a chronic disease, may do well with a support group in which ideas for coping as well as practical help may be provided by others with the same illness experience.

Finally, patients with truly bizarre behavior may be referred for a mental health evaluation. The clinician must, however, avoid overinterpreting nonadherence as a behavioral or mental disorder.

SUGGESTED READINGS

Brody H: *The Healer's Power.* Yale University Press, 1992.

Cassell EJ: *Talking with Patients,* Vol. 1: *The Theory of Doctor-Patient Communication.* MIT, 1985.

DiMatteo MR: Enhancing patient adherence to medical recommendations. JAMA 1994;271:79.

DiMatteo MR, DiNicola DD: *Achieving Patient Compliance.* Pergamon, 1982.

DiMatteo MR, Reiter RC, Gambone JC: Enhancing medication adherence through communication and informed collaborative choice. Health Commun 1994;6:253.

Eddy D: Anatomy of a decision. JAMA 1990;263:441.

Kaplan RM: Health-related quality of life in patient decision making. J Soc Iss 1991;47:69.

Katz J: *The Silent World of Doctor and Patient.* Free Press, 1984.

Levinson W: Physician-patient communication: A key to malpractice prevention. JAMA 1994;272:1619.

Roter DL, Hall JA: *Doctors Talking with Patients/Patients Talking with Doctors.* Auburn House, 1992.

Smoking

18

Nancy A. Rigotti, M.D.

INTRODUCTION

Cigarette smoking is the leading preventable cause of death in the United States, responsible for an estimated 419,000 deaths per year, or one in every five deaths. Physicians must take care of the health consequences of their patients' tobacco use. It is equally important for them to prevent smoking-related disease by treating their patients' smoking habits.

PATTERNS OF TOBACCO USE

Cigarette smoking in the United States and its health consequences are largely 20th-century phenomena. Smoking was uncommon before 1900, rose rapidly in the first half of the century, and peaked in 1965, when 40% of adult Americans smoked cigarettes. Since then, smoking rates have declined, reflecting growing public awareness of the health risks of tobacco use. By 1994, adult smoking prevalence had fallen to 25.5%. This decline is primarily attributable to smoking cessation. Smoking initiation rates have not decreased since 1980, despite a concurrent fall in smoking prevalence. In both sexes, smoking starts during childhood and adolescence; 90% of smokers begin to smoke before the age of 20.

These aggregate data conceal dramatic differences in the smoking patterns of men and women that have led to substantial gender differences in smoking-related disease mortality. American women did not take up smoking in large numbers until World War II, three decades later than men. When smoking prevalence peaked in 1965, only 32% of adult women smoked, compared with 50% of men. After 1965, smoking rates fell four times faster in men than in women. The result has been a convergence in the smoking rates of men and women. By 1994, 23.1% of adult women and 28.2% of men smoked cigarettes.

In the United States, smoking is more closely linked to education than it is to age, race, occupation, or any other sociodemographic factor. Educational attainment is a marker for socioeconomic status, and these data indicate that smoking is a problem that is becoming concentrated in lower socioeconomic groups.

HEALTH CONSEQUENCES OF TOBACCO USE

Cigarette smoking increases the overall mortality and morbidity rates of both men women. In both sexes, smoking is a cause of cardiovascular disease (including myocardial infarction and sudden death); cerebrovascular disease; peripheral vascular disease; chronic obstructive pulmonary disease; and cancers of the lung, larynx, oral cavity, and esophagus.

Lung cancer, once a rare disease, has increased dramatically. Since 1955, it has been the leading cause of cancer death in men, and by 1986, lung cancer surpassed breast cancer to become the leading cause of cancer death in women. Cigarette smokers also have higher rates of cancers of the bladder, pancreas, kidney, stomach, and uterine cervix. Smoking interacts with alcohol to increase the risk of laryngeal, oral cavity, and esophageal cancers. Tobacco also interacts with occupational exposures such as from asbestos to greatly increase cancer risk.

Smoking is associated with many pregnancy complications. It is a cause of low birth weight (<2500 g) in infants. Babies born to smokers weigh, on average, 200 g (7 oz) less than the babies of nonsmoking moth-

Selected portions of this chapter are based on material written by the author and Lela Polivogianis, MD, for a chapter entitled, "Smoking Cessation" in: *Primary Care of Women.* Carlson et al (editors). Mosby-Year Book, Inc, 1995.

ers. This is primarily attributable to intrauterine growth retardation (IUGR), although smoking in pregnancy also increases the risk of preterm delivery. Smoking is the major known cause of IUGR in the developed world, responsible for an estimated 30% of cases. Other adverse pregnancy outcomes linked to smoking are miscarriage (spontaneous abortion), stillbirth, and neonatal death. Placenta previa, abruptio placenta, and bleeding occur more often in smokers than nonsmokers, suggesting that smoking impairs placental function.

Smoking during pregnancy affects children even after birth. Sudden infant death syndrome is two to four times more common in infants born to mothers who smoked during pregnancy. Cognitive deficits and developmental problems in childhood have also been linked to maternal smoking during pregnancy, although the relationships are not clearly causal. The adverse health effects of smoking extend to reproductive function before pregnancy. Smoking has been associated with reduced fertility in both men and women, though a causal link remains to be established. Smoking also increases the risk of serious cardiovascular disease among women using oral contraceptives. Compared with nonsmokers, women smokers who also use oral contraceptives have a substantially increased risk of myocardial infarction, subarachnoid hemorrhage, and stroke.

There is debate about whether smoking increases a woman's risk of developing postmenopausal osteoporosis. Some, but not all, studies link smoking with reduced bone mass and osteoporosis. There is also conflicting evidence about whether smokers have a higher risk of osteoporotic fracture than nonsmokers. Women who smoke are thinner and have menopause 1–2 years earlier than nonsmokers, both of which are risk factors for osteoporosis. Smoking may also have an antiestrogen effect.

Smokers have higher rates of peptic ulcer disease, poorer ulcer healing, and higher recurrence rates than nonsmokers. They are more susceptible to upper respiratory infections and have more cataracts than nonsmokers. Smokers have more prominent skin wrinkling than nonsmokers, an association independent of sun exposure. The majority of residential fire deaths are caused by smoking.

There is no safe level of tobacco use. Smoking as few as one to four cigarettes per day increases the risk of myocardial infarction and cardiovascular mortality. Smoking cigarettes with reduced tar and nicotine content does not protect against the health hazards of smoking.

The health hazards of smoking are not limited to those suffered by smokers. Nonsmokers are harmed by chronic exposure to environmental tobacco smoke (ETS). The children of parents who smoke have more serious respiratory infections during infancy and childhood, more respiratory symptoms, and a higher rate of chronic otitis media and asthma than the children of nonsmokers. Nonsmoking women whose hus-

bands smoke have a higher lung cancer risk than nonsmoking women whose husbands do not smoke. A 1993 Environmental Protection Agency report identified ETS as a source of carcinogens, responsible for approximately 3000 lung cancer deaths per year in US nonsmokers. Passive smoke exposure also appears to increase nonsmokers' risk of coronary heart disease.

HEALTH BENEFITS OF SMOKING CESSATION

Epidemiologic data demonstrate that smoking cessation has health benefits for men and women of all ages. Even those who stop smoking after the age of 65 or who quit after the development of a smoking-related disease derive benefit. Smoking cessation decreases the risk of lung cancer and other cancers, heart attack, stroke, chronic lung disease, and peptic ulcer disease. After 10–15 years of abstinence, overall mortality rates for smokers approaches that of those who never smoked. The cardiovascular risk reduction occurs more rapidly than the risk reduction for lung cancer or overall mortality. Half of the excess risk of cardiovascular mortality is eliminated in the first year of quitting, whereas for lung cancer, 30–50% of the excess risk is still evident 10 years after quitting and some excess risk remains after 15 years.

The benefits of stopping smoking translate into a longer life expectancy for former smokers, compared with continuing smokers. The degree to which former smokers benefit from cessation depends on their previous lifetime dose of tobacco, their health status at the time of quitting, and the elapsed time since quitting. Smokers who benefit the most are those who quit when they are younger, have fewer pack-years of tobacco exposure, and are free of smoking-related disease. The health benefits of smoking cessation far exceed any risks from the small weight gain that occurs with cessation. The benefits of smoking cessation were summarized in the *1990 Surgeon General's Report on Smoking.*

Smoking cessation reverses the hazards of smoking to the fetus. Women who stop smoking before pregnancy or during the first 3–4 months of gestation have infants who weigh the same as those born to women who never smoked. Pregnant smokers who stop smoking at any time up to the 30th week of gestation have infants with higher birth weights than women who smoke throughout pregnancy. Reducing daily cigarette consumption without quitting smoking is of less benefit in preventing low birth weight.

SMOKING CESSATION

Approximately half of living Americans who ever smoked have quit smoking. According to surveys, a majority of the remaining smokers would like to stop smoking and have made at least one serious attempt to do so.

Surveys of former smokers reveal how and why smokers stop smoking. The reason most often cited by former smokers for stopping smoking is fear of illness. Awareness of health risks is not sufficient to motivate smoking cessation, however. Over 90% of current smokers know that smoking is harmful to health, yet they continue to smoke. Many smokers rationalize that they are immune to the health risks of smoking until these risks become personally salient. Current symptoms (eg, cough, breathlessness, chest pain), even if they represent minor illness rather than the onset of a smoking-related disease, stimulate change in smoking behavior more powerfully than does fear of future disease. Illness in a family member may also motivate smoking cessation. Another frequently cited reason for quitting is growing social pressure from work, family, and friends not to smoke.

In surveys, 90% of former smokers say that they quit on their own. Most quit abruptly ("cold turkey"), although smokers can progressively reduce daily cigarette intake in preparation for quitting. A variety of programs are available to smokers who seek help. The best evidence for efficacy supports behavior modification programs; hypnosis is poorly evaluated, and acupuncture is not effective for smoking cessation.

The majority of former smokers did not succeed in stopping on their first try. About 30% of smokers who attend formal programs are not smoking 1 year later; most resume smoking within 3 months. Behavioral scientists liken smoking cessation to a learning process rather than to a discrete episode of will power. Smokers learn from mistakes made during a prior attempt at quitting, thereby increasing the likelihood that the next attempt will succeed. Psychologists have identified a series of cognitive stages through which smokers pass as they move toward nonsmoking: (1) initial disinterest in quitting; (2) thinking about health risks and contemplating quitting; (3) actively preparing to quit within the next month; (4) currently taking action to stop smoking; and (5) maintained nonsmoking (see Chapter 16.)

MANAGEMENT OF BARRIERS TO SMOKING CESSATION

Nicotine Withdrawal Syndrome

Cigarettes and other tobacco products are addicting. Evidence summarized in the *1988 Surgeon General's Report on Smoking* identified nicotine as the addictive drug in tobacco that is capable of creating tolerance, physical dependence, and a withdrawal syndrome in habitual users. Nicotine withdrawal symptoms include (1) cravings for a cigarette; (2) irritability, anxiety, impatience, and anger; (3) difficulty concentrating; (4) excessive hunger; and (5) sleep disturbance. These symptoms begin within a few hours of the last cigarette, are strongest during the first 2–3 days after quitting, and gradually diminish over 2–3 weeks. The severity of nicotine withdrawal is variable and related to the level of prior nicotine intake. Other than craving for a cigarette, the symptoms are nonspecific, and many smokers fail to recognize them as nicotine withdrawal.

The discomfort of nicotine withdrawal is one reason why smokers fail in their efforts to stop. Nicotine replacement therapy relieves the symptoms, but pharmacological treatment is not mandatory, because mild symptoms can be managed with behavioral methods.

Behavioral Factors

The attractiveness of smoking is attributable to more than nicotine dependence. Smoking is also a habit, a behavior that has become an integral part of a daily routine. Smokers come to associate cigarettes with enjoyable activities, such as finishing a meal or having a cup of coffee. These actions trigger the desire for a cigarette in smokers who are trying to quit. Smokers also use cigarettes to cope with stress and negative emotions such as anger, anxiety, loneliness, or frustration. Quitting smoking represents the loss of a valuable coping tool.

Behavior modification strategies address these barriers to quitting smoking and are effective in aiding smoking cessation. Smokers monitor their cigarette intake to identify cues to smoking, change their habits to break the link between the trigger and smoking, and learn to anticipate and handle the urges to smoke that do occur. The skills can be taught in formal group programs or packaged into booklets or videotapes for at-home use.

Weight & Smoking Cessation

Smokers weigh 5–10 lb. less than nonsmokers of comparable age and height. When smokers quit, 80/% of them gain weight. The average weight gain of 5 lb. (2.3 kg) poses a minimal health risk, especially when compared with the benefits of smoking cessation. Women gain more weight than men; their average weight gain in one national sample was 8 lb. (3.8 kg). Though many smokers fear large weight gains, only about 10% gain more than 25 lb. after cessation. Heavier smokers (>25 cigarettes/day) gain more than lighter smokers. The mechanism is incompletely understood, but a nicotine-related decrease in metabolic rate and possibly increases in food intake appear to be largely responsible. The weight gain occurs in both sexes, but survey data reveal that it concerns female smokers more than male smokers, presumably because women experience greater cultural pressure to be slender. Although weight gain has been considered a trigger to relapse, some studies show that successful abstainers gain more weight than relapsers. Smokers who use nicotine gum gain less weight than those who quit with a placebo, though weight gain may just be delayed until after gum use stops. Use of the nicotine patch does not reduce weight gain. Behavior modification approaches to avoiding weight gain have not been successful.

The best approach to the problem may be a change in attitude. Smokers can learn that although some weight gain is likely, the amount is less than they fear. Accepting a small increase in weight until smoking cessation is secure is a better strategy than attempting to stop smoking and lose weight simultaneously. The chance of a large weight gain may be reduced by avoiding high-calorie snacks and increasing physical activity during smoking cessation. Nicotine gum may provide a way to delay and possibly avoid weight gain.

Social Support

Smokers with nonsmoking spouses are more likely to quit than smokers whose partners smoke. Smokers whose efforts to stop are supported by partners, family, and friends are more likely to succeed than smokers without this support. This is especially true for women smokers. Those who live with smokers can ask them to restrict smoking to outdoor areas or to limited areas of the home in order to provide a smoke-free area in the home. Formal cessation programs provide an additional source of social support.

Mood Disorders

Stopping smoking represents a loss for many smokers. Cigarettes have been reliable "companions" as well as coping tools. Transient sadness is common and requires no special treatment. Acknowledgment that this is normal can be helpful. There is, however, growing evidence of an association between smoking and mood disorders. Smokers have more depressive symptoms than nonsmokers and are more likely to have a history of major depression. Depressed smokers are less likely to stop smoking than nondepressed smokers. There are case reports that smoking cessation precipitated depression in smokers with a history of major depression and that resuming smoking restored mood. These observations suggest that some smokers use nicotine to regulate mood. Clinicians should be alert to the possibility of depression in smokers. If present, it should be treated before cessation is attempted. Smokers with a history of depression should be watched for the reemergence of symptoms during smoking cessation.

Substance Abuse

Smokers use more drugs—including coffee and alcohol—than nonsmokers. Because alcohol is frequently an ingredient in relapse situations, smokers attempting to quit are commonly advised to avoid alcohol temporarily after quitting. Smoking increases caffeine excretion. Smokers who stop should be advised to reduce caffeine intake to avoid increased blood levels and jitteriness. There is a high rate of smoking among abusers of alcohol, cocaine, and heroin. Depression and substance abuse should be considered as potential comorbid disorders in smokers who repeatedly try and fail to quit.

THE PHYSICIAN'S ROLE

The optimal way to avoid the health hazards of tobacco is never to smoke. Because smoking behavior begins so early, preventing smoking is particularly the task of physicians who care for children and adolescents. The challenge for physicians taking care of adults is smoking cessation. Physicians have the opportunity to intervene with smokers, because each year, they see an estimated 70% of the smokers in the United States. Primary care physicians have the advantage of repeated contact with smokers. Physicians have the additional opportunity of seeing smokers at times when symptoms have made them concerned about their health and therefore more likely to change their smoking behavior. For example, the diagnosis of coronary artery disease motivates behavior change. Approximately one third of smokers stop smoking after a myocardial infarction, and this proportion can be increased with brief counseling delivered by a physician or nurse. For women, pregnancy encourages smoking cessation. Approximately 30% of female smokers stop smoking while pregnant, though many resume smoking after delivery. Other smoking-related conditions may also provide "teachable moments" when smokers are more receptive to advice to stop smoking.

Although physicians report advising most patients to stop smoking, fewer than half of smokers recall having ever received this advice. Providing brief advice to stop smoking to all patients seen in the office increases patients' smoking cessation rates, as was demonstrated in a randomized controlled trial of British general practitioners. Although advice alone is effective, randomized controlled trials in general medicine and family practices have demonstrated that supplementing advice with brief counseling is more effective. Programs shown to be effective consist of brief structured counseling during which the physician asks the patient to set a quit date, provides written materials, offers nicotine replacement, and schedules a follow-up visit. Cost-effectiveness analyses demonstrate that counseling smokers in office practice is as cost-effective as, or more so, than other accepted medical practices and that counseling smokers as part of prenatal care is cost-saving.

SMOKING CESSATION COUNSELING STRATEGY FOR OFFICE PRACTICE

Detailed evidence-based clinical guidelines for smoking cessation treatment by primary care providers have been developed by the Agency for Health Care Policy and Research. These guidelines recommend that the primary care of adults should include a routine assessment of smoking status in all patients, strong advice to all smokers to quit, and assistance for those smokers who are ready to stop. The National Cancer Institute has organized the common elements of effective smoking cessation counseling programs into a four-step protocol intended to require only a few minutes of an office visit (Box 18–1).

1. **ASK:** Physicians should routinely ask all patients at every visit whether they smoke cigarettes. Those who smoke should be asked whether they are interested in quitting smoking. This permits the physician to determine the smokers' readiness to change. Categorizing smokers in this way is a clinically useful approach that helps the physician to determine what counseling strategy is appropriate and to set achievable goals for that encounter. Although the clinician's overall goal is to assist the smoker to stop permanently, a realistic goal for a single office visit is to move the smoker to the next stage of readiness to stop smoking.

2. **ADVISE:** Regardless of a smoker's degree of interest in quitting, it is the physician's responsibility to deliver clear advice to each smoker about the importance of stopping smoking. The message should be strong and unequivocal; for example, "Quitting smoking now is the most important health advice I can give you." If appropriate, advice should be tailored to the clinical situation, either current symptoms or family history. For example, smokers can be informed that they will have fewer colds, less asthma, or healthier babies if they stop smoking. Advice is more effective when phrased in a positive way; for instance, emphasizing the benefits to be gained from quitting rather than the harms of continuing to smoke.

3. **ASSIST:** The third step is to assist the smoker in quitting smoking. The physician's approach should vary according to the smoker's readiness to stop smoking.

   If the smokers are interested in quitting smoking, the physician should ask whether they are ready to set a "quit date," a date within the next 4 weeks when they will stop smoking. If so, the date should be recorded in the chart and on material given to them to take home. The physician should discuss with the patients what approach is most likely to be successful. A stepped-care model of smoking treatment can guide the physician in making this recommendation. For smokers making a first attempt to quit, the

Box 18–1. Smoking cessation counseling protocol for physicians.

1. **ASK**—about smoking at every visit.
   a. "Do you smoke?"
   b. "Are you interested in stopping smoking?"
2. **ADVISE**—every smoker to stop.
   a. Make advice clear: "Stopping smoking now is the most important action you can take to stay healthy."
   b. Tailor advice to the patient's clinical situation (symptoms or family history).
3. **ASSIST**—the smoker in stopping smoking.
   a. For smokers ready to quit
      (1) Ask smoker to set a "quit date."
      (2) Provide self-help material to take home.
      (3) Consider nicotine replacement therapy.
      (4) Consider referral to a formal cessation program.
   b. For smokers not ready to quit
      (1) Discuss advantages and barriers to cessation, from smokers' viewpoint.
      (2) Provide motivational booklet to take home.
      (3) Advise smoker to avoid exposing family members to passive smoke.
      (4) Indicate willingness to help when the smoker is ready.
      (5) Ask again about smoking at the next visit.
4. **ARRANGE**—follow-up visits.
   a. Make follow-up appointment 1 week after quit date.
   b. At follow-up, ask about smoking status.
   c. For smokers who have quit:
      (1) Congratulate!
      (2) Ask smoker to identify future high-risk situations.
      (3) Rehearse coping strategies for future high-risk situations.
   d. For smokers who have not quit:
      (1) Ask: "What were you doing when you had that first cigarette?"
      (2) Ask: "What did you learn from the experience?"
      (3) Ask smoker to set a new "quit date."

Source: Adapted, with permission, from Glynn TJ, Manley MW: *How to Help Your Patients Stop Smoking: A National Cancer Institute Manual for Physicians.* US Department of Health and Human Services, Public Health Service, National Institutes of Health, National Cancer Institute, Division of Cancer Prevention and Control. NIH Publication No. 89-3064, 1989. [Available free by calling 1-800-4-CANCER.]

physician should assist them in quitting on their own; this can be done most simply by providing a take-home booklet containing standard behavioral modification strategies (Box 18–2). Alternatively, this information can be provided by office staff or on a videotape. The physician should be prepared to discuss management of barriers to cessation if the smokers ask.

Nicotine replacement therapy should also be considered. Although it is especially appropriate for smokers likely to have severe nicotine withdrawal symptoms, it has been demonstrated to benefit smokers of all types. Smokers who suffered nicotine withdrawal symptoms on previous attempts to quit or who smoke more than 25 cigarettes daily, have their first cigarette within 30 minutes of awakening, or are uncomfortable when forced to refrain from smoking for more than a few hours are likely to suffer nicotine withdrawal.

More intensive treatment is indicated for smokers who have been unsuccessful in previous attempts to quit. The option at this second level is referral to a formal smoking cessation program, with or without prescription of nicotine replacement therapy. Smoking cessation programs provide intensive training in behavioral smoking cessation skills combined with social support from the counselor and other group members. Combinations of nicotine replacement and a behavioral counseling program are more effective than either one alone.

For smokers not interested in quitting or not ready to set a quit date, the physician should ask them what they consider to be the benefits and harms of smoking. From an understanding of the patients' perspective, the physician can provide missing information about health risks and correct misconceptions about the process of smoking cessation. The discussion should focus on short-term benefits rather than distant risks, and the physician should be prepared to discuss common barriers to smoking cessation. The clinician should advise the smokers not to expose family members to passive smoke (eg, not to smoke inside the home if nonsmokers are present), provide a take-home booklet about smoking cessation, and indicate future availability to help them when they are ready to quit.

4. **ARRANGE:** Randomized trials have demonstrated that arranging follow-up visits to discuss smoking increases the success of physician counseling. Smokers should be asked to return shortly after the quit date to monitor progress; this is especially important for smokers using nicotine replacement.

If smokers are not smoking at the follow-up visit, they should be congratulated but warned that continued vigilance is necessary to maintain abstinence. The level of nicotine withdrawal symptoms should be assessed, and if indicated, treated. To prevent relapse to smoking, patients should be asked to identify future situations in which they anticipate difficulty remaining abstinent. The physician can help to plan and rehearse coping strategies for these times. Further follow-up visits or telephone calls should be offered.

If smokers have not been able to remain abstinent, the physician's role is to redefine an experience that the smokers feel has been a failure into a partial success. They can be told that even one day without cigarettes is the first step toward quitting and reminded that it takes time to learn to quit, just as it took time to learn to smoke. To help smokers learn from the experience, the physician should ask in detail about the circumstances surrounding the first cigarette smoked after the quit date. They should be asked what they learned from the experience that can be used for the next attempt to quit. Finally, these smokers should be asked whether they are ready to set a new quit date.

Office Organization

Smoking counseling in an office need not and should not be limited to the physician's actions. A system-wide approach is at least as effective as a

Box 18–2. Selected smoking cessation guidelines for physicians and patients.

For Physicians
1. *How to Help Your Patients Stop Smoking.* A National Cancer Institute Manual for Physicians.
2. *Smoking Cessation.* Clinical Practice Guideline No. 18. Agency for Health Care Policy and Research. AHCPR Publication No. 96-0692, April 1996.
3. *Clinical Opportunities for Smoking Intervention—A Guide for the Busy Physician.* National Heart Lung and Blood Institute.
4. *Family Physician's Guide to Smoking Cessation.* American Academy of Family Physicians.
5. *A Healthy Beginning Counseling Kit.* American Lung Association.

For Patients
1. *Clearing the Air.* National Cancer Institute. (Order from 1-800-4-CANCER).
2. *Smart Move.* American Cancer Society.
3. *Freedom from Smoking for You and Your Family.* American Lung Association.
4. *Freedom from Smoking for You and Your Baby.* American Lung Association.

physician-focused model, and it reduces the burden on a busy physician. In this model, the patients' smoking status is assessed before the physician sees them. The staff member who checks weight or blood pressure asks about smoking and labels the chart to remind the physician to discuss smoking. Simple reminder systems like this increase the amount of time physicians spend counseling smokers. The physician's prime role is to provide advice to stop smoking and ask the patient to set a quit date. Office personnel build on physician advice to provide counseling, medication instruction, or referrals to outside programs.

PHARMACOLOGICAL TREATMENT

Nicotine Replacement Therapy

The rationale of nicotine replacement is to supply nicotine in a form other than tobacco in order to block the symptoms of nicotine withdrawal. Nicotine replacement permits the smoker to break the smoking habit first and taper off nicotine later. Three forms of nicotine replacement are currently approved for use in the United States: nicotine polacrilex (a gum), a transdermal skin patch, and a nicotine nasal spray (Table 18–1). The first two produce relatively constant blood levels of nicotine, a substantially different pattern from the fluctuating nicotine levels produced by cigarette smoking. The nasal spray produces nicotine levels that more closely resemble those produced by smoking. The nicotine supplied by the gum, patch, or nasal spray is sufficient to block nicotine withdrawal symptoms but not to reproduce the pleasures of smoking.

Randomized placebo-controlled trials demonstrate that nicotine gum, patch, and nasal spray all reduce nicotine withdrawal symptoms and increase smoking cessation rates. A meta-analysis of nicotine patch trials found that the patch more than doubled smoking cessa-

tion rates, compared with a placebo, though the cessation rates in individual trials varied widely. A meta analysis of nicotine gum demonstrated its effectiveness in special clinics treating smokers but not when used in medical settings. The effectiveness of all products depends on what instruction and counseling accompany it. This is particularly true for the gum and nasal spray, which require careful instruction for proper use. Compliance is less of a problem with the nicotine patch. The most effective use of any product, however, requires that the physician provide the smoker with concurrent behavioral counseling of some type that teaches how to break the cigarette habit.

Nicotine replacement has been used safely, even in smokers with stable coronary artery disease. Contraindications to nicotine replacement include acute or recent cardiovascular events (myocardial infarction, unstable angina, or serious arrhythmias). Anecdotal reports of myocardial infarction in patients who were smoking while using the patch were not borne out by more careful study, but smoking is contraindicated in patch users; it increases blood nicotine levels and, more importantly, is not a pattern of behavior that leads to smoking cessation. The gum is contraindicated in patients with temporomandibular disease; the patch is contraindicated in patients with widespread skin eruptions. The safety of any product in pregnancy is not established. Nicotine replacement is almost certainly safer than smoking cigarettes, but medicolegal concerns have limited its use. Clinicians who have used it reserve it for use in patients who have failed a behavioral smoking cessation program and prescribed it only after documenting a risk-benefit discussion with the patient.

Transdermal Nicotine Patch: The nicotine patch contains a reservoir of nicotine that is released at fixed doses that are absorbed through the skin. Each of the four products available is more effective than placebo in relieving withdrawal symptoms and pro-

Table 18–1. Nicotine replacement products.

Brand Name	Dosage per Day	Recommended Duration of Use
Transdermal Nicotine Patch		
Habitrol	21 mg/24 h	4 weeks
	14 mg/24 h	2 weeks
	7 mg/24 h	2 weeks
Nicoderm CQ	21 mg/24 h	4 weeks
	14 mg/24 h	2 weeks
	7 mg/24 h	2 weeks
Nicotrol	15 mg/16 h	8 weeks
Prostep	22 mg/24 h	4 weeks
Nicotine Gum		
Nicorette CQ 2 mg	9–12 pieces/day* (maximum 30)	2–3 months (maximum 6)
Nicorette CQ 4 mg	9–12 pieces/day (maximum 20)	2–3 months (maximum 6)
Nicotine Nasal Spray		
Nicotrol NS	1–2 doses/h (maximum 8/day)	3 months

* Chew as needed or 1 piece every 1–2 h while awake.

moting smoking cessation. No studies have directly compared different patches; therefore, there are insufficient data to recommend any one patch as most effective or safest. The most common side effect is local skin irritation, which rarely requires discontinuation of treatment and can be treated with topical steroids. Vivid dreams, insomnia, and nervousness have also been reported; they can be managed by removing the patch at bedtime or using a lower-dose patch.

The smoker applies the first patch on the morning of the quit day and applies a new patch to rotating skin sites each morning afterward. Three products are intended for 24-hour use; the fourth is removed after 16 hours (eg, at bedtime). Smokers started on the patch should be monitored after 1 week to assess level of withdrawal symptoms and to screen for smoking during patch use. Some patches are available in three sizes to permit tapering, and data suggest that patch use continue for 2 months. Lower starting doses are recommended for patients weighing under 100 lb. or smoking fewer than 10 cigarettes/day. Long-term dependence on the nicotine patch appears to be uncommon. Four nicotine patches (Habitrol, Nicoderm, Nicotrol, and Prostep) have been available by prescription since 1972; in 1996 two of them (Nicoderm and Nicotrol) were granted permission to be sold as over-the-counter products.

Nicotine Gum: Nicotine gum is available without prescription in 2-mg and 4-mg strengths. Careful instruction in proper chewing technique is essential for it to be effective and to avoid side effects; for this reason, compliance is more problematic than with the nicotine patch. The gum should not be chewed like regular gum. A piece is chewed only long enough to release the nicotine, producing a peppery taste, then placed between the gums and buccal mucosa to allow for nicotine absorption. After 30 minutes, it is discarded. No liquid should be drunk while the gum is in the mouth, and acidic beverages (eg, coffee) should be avoided for 1–2 h before gum use. Side effects are common but minor; they include those related to nicotine (nausea, dyspepsia, hiccups, dizziness) and to chewing (sore jaw, mouth ulcers). The product is approved for use as needed to handle urges to smoke; however, its effect is slower than smoking. Most patients chew fewer than the recommended 9–12 pieces daily. Consequently, some clinicians use fixed-dose schedules (eg, chewing one piece every hour) to achieve adequate blood nicotine levels to prevent withdrawal. Approximately 5–10% of gum users develop long-term dependence on the gum.

Nicotine Nasal Spray: A nicotine nasal spray became available in 1996. Nicotine is rapidly absorbed from the nasal mucosa, reaching a peak within 15 minutes, then declining over 1–2 hours. The variable pattern of nicotine exposure produced from repeated use of the nasal spray resembles that produced by smoking cigarettes, raising concerns that the nasal spray will have a greater potential for producing dependence than has been observed with other nicotine replacement products. It is superior to placebo in randomized controlled trials, but its high incidence of side effects (nose and throat irritation, watery eyes, sneezing and cough) and concerns about its potential for producing dependence are likely to limit its appeal, except in smokers who have failed with other nicotine replacement products. Nicotine nasal spray is not recommended for smokers with asthma or chronic rhinitis or sinusitis, and careful instruction is required for its proper use.

Other Pharmacological Agents

Clonidine, a centrally acting alpha-adrenergic agonist, is used to treat craving for psychoactive drugs other than nicotine. In randomized, placebo-controlled trials, both oral and transdermal clonidine reduced withdrawal symptoms, but there is inconsistent evidence that either product increases smoking cessation rates in the long term. Clonidine is not approved for use as an aid for smoking cessation.

There is no evidence to support the use of tranquilizers or benzodiazepines for smoking cessation. The growing awareness of the link between smoking and mood disorders has stimulated interest in the use of antidepressants to treat smoking in individuals with a history of depression. Until more is known, it is appropriate to use these agents to treat depression in a smoker and to continue their use when the patient attempts to stop smoking. Whether they have any role in smokers who are not currently depressed is not known.

SUGGESTED READINGS

Agency for Health Care Policy and Research: Smoking cessation clinical practice guideline. JAMA 1996;275:1270.

Bartecchi CE, MacKenzie TK, Schrier RW: The human cost of tobacco use. N Engl J Med 1994; 330:907-912, 975-980.

Benowitz NL: Nicotine replacement therapy during pregnancy. JAMA 1991; 266:3174-3177.

Cohen SJ, Stookey GK, Katz BP et al: Encouraging primary care physicians to help smokers quit: a randomized controlled trial. Ann Intern Med 1989; 110:648-52.

Cummings SR, Coates TJ, Richard RJ et al: Training physicians in counseling about smoking cessation: a randomized trial of the "Quit for Life" program. Ann Intern Med 1989; 110:641-647.

Fiore MC, Smith SS, Jorenby DE, et al:. The effectiveness of the nicotine patch for smoking cessation: a meta-analysis. JAMA 1994; 271:1940-1947.

Glassman A: Cigarette smoking: implications for psychiatric illness. Am J Psychiatry 1993; 150:546-553.

Glynn TJ, Manley MW: *How to Help Your Patients Stop Smoking. A National Cancer Institute Manual for Physicians.* U.S. Department of Health and Human Services, Public Health Service, National Institutes of Health, National Cancer Institute, Division of Cancer Prevention and Control. NIH Publication No. 89-3064, 1989. [Available free by calling 1-800-4-CANCER.]

Hollis JF, Lichtenstein E, Vogt TM, et al: Nurse-assisted counseling for smokers in primary care. Ann Intern Med. 1993; 118:521-525.

Lam W, Sacks HS, Sze P, et al: Meta-analysis of randomized controlled trials of nicotine chewing gum. Lancet 1987; 2:27-29.

Manley MW, Epps RP, Glynn TJ: The clinician's role in promoting smoking cessation among clinic patients. Med Clin North Amer 1992; 76:477-494. (Part of an entire volume on smoking cessation.)

Russell MAH, Wilson C, Taylor C, et al: Effect of a general practitioner's advice against smoking. Br Med J. 1979; 2:231-235.

Williamson DF, Madans J, Anda RF, et al: Smoking cessation and severity of weight gain in a national cohort. N Engl J Med 1991; 324:739-745.

Wilson DM, Taylor DW, Gilbert JR, et al: A randomized trial of a family physician intervention for smoking cessation. JAMA 1988; 260:1570-1574.

Cummings SR, Rubin SM, Oster G: The cost-effectiveness of counseling smokers to quit. JAMA 1989; 261:75-79.

Working group for the study of transdermal nicotine in patients with coronary artery disease. Nicotine replacement therapy for patients with coronary artery disease. Arch Intern Med 1994; 154:989-995.

19

Obesity

Robert B. Baron MD, MS

INTRODUCTION

Obesity is one of the most common problems in clinical practice. Defined as a body weight 20% or more above "desirable" weight, over one third of adult Americans are overweight. Perched at the center of chronic disease risk and psychosocial disability for millions of Americans, the prevention and treatment of obesity offers unique patient care and public health opportunities. If all Americans were to achieve a normal body weight, it has been estimated that life expectancy would increase by 3 years, coronary heart disease would decrease by 25%, and congestive heart failure and stroke would decrease by 35%.

Unfortunately, obesity is often one of the most difficult and frustrating problems in primary care for both patients and physicians. Considerable effort is expended by primary care providers and patients with little benefit. Using standard treatments in university settings, only 20% of patients lose 20 pounds at 2-year follow-up, and only 5% of patients lose 40 pounds. This lack of clinical success has created a never-ending demand for new weight-loss treatments. Approximately 45% of women and 25% of men are "dieting" at any one time, spending over 0 billion each year on diet books, diet meals, weight-loss classes, diet drugs, exercise tapes, "fat farms," and other weight-loss aids. The challenge for health care providers is to identify those patients with obesity who are most likely to benefit medically from treatment and most likely to maintain weight loss, and to provide them with sound advice, skills for long-term lifestyle change, and support. For patients not motivated to attempt a weight-loss program, health providers must continue to be respectful and empathic and focus on other health concerns (see Chapter 16). Whenever possible, health providers should emphasize prevention of obesity and further weight gain.

DEFINITIONS

Obesity represents an excess of body fat; being overweight means having an excess of body weight, including all components of body composition (muscle, bone, water, and fat). In clinical practice, the two are used interchangeably to refer to excess body fat. The two most commonly used terms to quantify obesity are relative weight (RW) and body mass index (BMI). The RW is the actual weight divided by the "desirable weight" (derived from "acceptable weight" tables). The BMI, or Quetelet index, is the actual body weight divided by the height squared (kilograms per square meter). This index more closely corresponds to measurements of body fat and better differentiates being "overweight" due to an increase in muscle mass from that caused by true obesity.

The National Institute of Health defines obesity (somewhat arbitrarily) as a RW of greater than 120% (BMI > 27 kg/m^2). "Morbid" obesity is commonly defined as a RW greater than 200% (BMI > 40 kg/m^2).

HEALTH CONSEQUENCES OF OBESITY

The relationship between body weight and mortality is curvilinear, similar to other cardiovascular risk factors. Most studies have demonstrated a {J}-shaped or {U}-shaped relationship, suggesting that the thinnest portion of the population also have an excess mortality. This is primarily due to the higher rate of cigarette smoking in the thinnest group, except in the elderly, in whom malnutrition is predictive of excess mortality independent of cigarette use.

The increase in total mortality related to obesity results predominantly from coronary heart disease (CHD). Although it is not fully established that obesity is an "independent" risk factor for CHD, obesity is clearly an important risk factor for the development of many other CHD risk factors. Obese individuals age 20–44, for example, have a three- to fourfold greater risk of type II diabetes, five- to sixfold greater risk of hypertension, and twice the risk of hypercholesterolemia. The obese also have an increased risk of some cancers, including those of the colon, rectum, and prostate in men; and those of the uterus, biliary tract, breast, and ovary in women.

As a result of these conditions, relative weights of 130% are associated with an excess mortality of 35%. Relative weights of 150% have a greater than twofold excess death rate. Patients with "morbid" obesity (relative weights greater than 200%) have a greater than 10-fold increase in death rates.

Obesity is also associated with a variety of other medical disorders, including degenerative joint disease of both weight-bearing and non-weight-bearing joints, diseases of the digestive tract (gallstones, reflux esophagitis), thromboembolic disorders, heart failure (both systolic and diastolic), respiratory impairment, and skin disorders. Obese patients also have a greater incidence of surgical and obstetric complications, are more prone to accidents and are at increased risk of social discrimination. Obesity is not, however, associated with an increased risk of major psychiatric or psychological disorders.

In addition to the total amount of excess body fat, the location of the excess body fat (regional fat distribution) is a major determinant of the degree of excess morbidity and mortality due to obesity. Increased upper body fat (abdomen and flank) is independently associated with increased cardiovascular and total mortality. Body fat distribution can be assessed by a number of measurement techniques. Measurements of skin folds (subscapular and triceps) reflect subcutaneous fat. Measurement of circumferences (waist and hip) reflect both abdominal and visceral fat. Computed tomography (CT) and magnetic resonance image (MRI) scans measure subcutaneous and visceral fat. Clinically, measurement of the waist and hip circumference is most useful. The waist is measured at the umbilicus and the hips at the greater trochanter. A waist-to-hip ratio of 1.0 and 0.8 are considered normal in men and women, respectively. Ratios above these values reflect abdominal or visceral obesity (or both) and a greater risk of obesity-related disorders.

ETIOLOGY OF OBESITY

Numerous lines of evidence, including both epidemiologic studies of adoptees and twins and animal studies, suggest strong genetic influences on the development of obesity. In a study of 800 Danish adoptees, for example, there was no relationship between the body weight of adoptees and their adopting parents but a close correlation with the body weights of their biological parents. In a study of approximately 4000 twins, a much closer correlation between body weights was found in monozygotic than in dizygotic twins. In this study, genetic factors accounted for approximately two thirds of the variation in weights. More recent studies of twins reared apart and the response of twins to overfeeding showed similar results. Studies of regional fat distribution in twins has also shown a significant (but not complete) genetic influence.

Recent molecular genetic studies have confirmed important genetic determinants of some types of obesity. Studies in animals have identified a gene that, when made useless by mutation, causes obesity. The normal gene produces the protein leptin, which controls appetite. When leptin is defective, mice grow profoundly fat; when leptin is supplemented, the mice lose weight. Human studies have recently confirmed the existence of an almost identical human gene. Although mutations in this gene are rare, it is hypothesized that extra doses of leptin may be effective in reducing human obesity. Recently, a high-affinity receptor for leptin has been identified in the mouse hypothalamus and a possible leptin-induced satiety factor, glucagon-like peptide-1 has been identified. Human studies have also identified a mutation in the gene for the beta-3 receptor in adipose tissue, involved in lipolysis and thermogenesis, that markedly increases the risk of obesity. These studies suggest that genetic factors may result in changes in both energy intake and energy expenditure. Genetic influences on control of appetite and eating behavior have long been considered. Animal studies have demonstrated the influence of dozens of factors on eating behavior, and it is likely that similar factors are at work in humans.

Differences in energy expenditure are also likely to be at least partially determined by genetic influences. Differences in the resting metabolic expenditure (RME), for example, could easily result in considerable differences in body weight since RME accounts for approximately 60–75% of total energy expenditure. The RME can vary by as much as 20% between individuals of the same age, sex, and body build; such differences could account for approximately 400 kcal of energy expenditure per day. Recent evidence suggests that the metabolic rate is similar in family members, and as expected, individuals with lower metabolic rates are more likely to gain weight. Differences in the thermic effect of food, the amount of energy expended following a meal, may also contribute to obesity. Although some investigators have shown a decreased thermic effect of food in the obese, others have not.

Environmental factors are also clearly important in the development of obesity. Decreased physical activity and food choices that result in increased energy intake also clearly contribute to the development of obesity. Medical illness and some medications can also result in obesity, but such instances account for less than 1% of cases. Hypothyroidism and

Cushing's syndrome are the most common. Diseases of the hypothalamus can also result in obesity, but these are quite rare. Major depression, which more typically results in weight loss, can sometimes present with weight gain. Consideration of these causes is particularly important when evaluating unexplained, recent weight gain.

PATIENT SELECTION FOR WEIGHT LOSS

Weight loss is indicated to assist in the management of obesity-related conditions, particularly hypertension, diabetes mellitus (type II), and hyperlipidemia, in any patient who is obese (RW > 120%, BMI > 27 kg/m²). Many patients with relative weights of 100–120% (BMI 25–27 kg/m²) who have one of these conditions (particularly hypertension, diabetes, lipid disorders, or significant psychosocial disability) also often dramatically benefit from weight reduction.

Weight loss to prevent complications of obesity in patients without current medical, metabolic, or behavioral consequences of obesity is more controversial. In young and middle-aged individuals, particularly those with a family history of obesity-related disorders, treatment should be based on the degree of obesity (RW > 120%) and body fat distribution. Such individuals with upper body obesity (waist-hip ratios > 1.0 in men and > 0.8 in women) should be considered for treatment; those individuals with lower body obesity and no significant consequences of obesity, can be reassured and followed for development of additional upper body obesity and its metabolic consequences. Many such patients, however, desire weight loss for psychological, social, and cosmetic reasons. A careful discussion of the risks and benefits of weight loss in such instances helps patients make informed decisions about various weight-loss strategies.

A medical or psychosocial indication for weight loss is necessary but not sufficient, however, to begin treatment. Only motivated patients should be treated. Considerable effort should be made to assess the patient's motivation for significant diet and exercise changes. Questions should focus on how the current attempt compares with previous attempts, a realistic assessment of the patient's goals for the amount and rate of weight loss; the extent to which outside stresses, mood disorders, or substance abuse might impair the attempt; and the degree to which others can provide support. Patient motivation can be further assessed by requiring the patient to complete specific pretreatment assignments. For example, patients can be asked to complete a 3-day diet record and to submit an exercise plan that includes both the type of aerobic exercise the patient plans to begin and how the patient plans to fit it into his or her schedule. When obesity coexists with other significant psychiatric disorders, particularly depression and substance abuse,

treatment should initially be directed at the concurrent disorder. (See Chapter 16 for further discussion of assessment of patients' readiness to change.)

DIET THERAPY

Standard dietary treatment of obesity should use the same nutritional principles as diet recommendations for healthy people. Total fat intake should be limited to 30% or less of total calories, protein to 15%, and carbohydrate (primarily complex carbohydrates) to 55% or greater. A total energy intake should be recommended to result in a daily energy deficit of 500–1000 kcal. Since 1 pound of fat equals approximately 3500 kcal, these deficits should result in a 1–2 pound weight loss per week. No dietary manipulation of macronutrients or other nutritional components can change these basic thermodynamic concepts, yet, virtually all popular diets are based on attempts to circumvent thermodynamics. Diets can easily be designed in medical settings with the assistance of clinical dietitians or other health professionals, or patients can be referred to well-established community resources that follow these principles.

A major development in the dietary treatment of obesity is the use of safe and effective very-low-calorie diets (VLCDs). Also known as protein-sparing modified fasts and protein-formula liquid diets, these diets restrict calorie intake to 400–800 kcal/day. Patients ingest only preformulated, usually liquid, food that provides adequate protein, vitamins, and minerals. Additional intake is limited to 2–3 quarts of calorie-free beverages per day. The major advantage of these diets is the "complete removal of patients from the food environment" to facilitate compliance. In addition, the significant energy deficit results in rapid weight loss, usually 2–4 pounds per week, encouraging the patient to continue. Ongoing concerns about these diets include their cost, side effects and complications, and long-term results. Recent studies suggest that the use of 800-kcal VLCDs can lower cost and prevent most of the significant side effects associated with the lower-calorie (400–600) VLCDs, including gallstones and fluid and electrolyte disorders, with equal long-term efficacy.

As with standard diet therapy of obesity, VLCDs require compliance during the diet, and long-term nutritional and behavioral changes to maintain weight loss. Well-planned programs that combine VLCDs with behavior modification, exercise, and social support report improved long-term results. For example, Nunn and colleagues report an average weight loss of 55 pounds with 75% and 52% of the loss maintained at 1- and 2¹/₂-year follow-up, respectively, and Hartman and associates reported maintenance of an average of 24 pounds after 2- to 3-year follow-up. Although these results are significantly better than results from published reviews of standard weight-loss programs (in which approximately only 5% of patients lose and maintain 40 pounds at 1-year follow-up), the even-longer-term efficacy and cost-effectiveness of VLCDs programs remains controversial.

HEALTH CONSEQUENCES
OF DIETING & WEIGHT LOSS

Surprisingly few studies have examined the effects of weight loss on morbidity and mortality. Studies examining the effect of weight loss on cardiovascular risk factors generally show beneficial changes with weight loss as predicted. Descriptive studies on mortality, however, show inconsistent results. Such descriptive studies are unable to clarify if changes in mortality are caused by the weight change, if disease or other factors that contribute to disease, such as cigarette smoking, cause weight loss, or if both are related to a third factor. No randomized trials of long-term effects of voluntary weight loss on mortality have been published.

Since so many Americans are dieting at any one time, and having so little long-term success, considerable interest has been focused on the potential adverse effects of weight cycling ("yo-yo" dieting). Numerous adverse effects of weight cycling have been hypothesized, primarily from animal studies. These include making further weight loss more difficult, increasing total body fat and central obesity, increasing subsequent calorie intake, increasing food efficiency, decreasing energy expenditure, increasing levels of adipose-tissue lipolytic enzymes and liver lipogenic enzymes, increasing insulin resistance, increasing blood pressure, and increasing blood cholesterol and triglyceride levels. Most experts currently feel that these phenomena occur inconsistently, if at all. Descriptive studies that have addressed this question by looking at the impact of weight fluctuations on CHD incidence, CHD mortality, and total mortality have shown mixed results.

There is also debate over whether weight loss diets cause eating disorders or binge eating. Although a history of dieting often precedes the development of eating disorders, there is no evidence proving a causal link. In addition, approximately half of individuals with binge eating disorder report that binging preceded dieting. There is also some evidence to suggest that successful weight loss may reduce binge eating in the obese (see Chapter 20).

Thus, there is only indirect evidence suggesting that dieting has negative health effects. This remains an important question, however, and reinforces the idea that casual attempts at quick weight loss should be avoided. At the present time, however, committed attempts at long-term weight loss should not be discouraged because of adverse health effects or the potential of regaining weight.

Dieting also has a significant effect on energy balance both during and after weight loss. As every successful dieter has observed, the rate of weight loss slows during the course of dieting. Because this can be quite discouraging to the unwary patient (or uninformed health care provider), it is important to inform the patient prior to initiating a weight-loss diet that this is likely to occur. Weight loss is most rapid during the initial days of hypocaloric feeding due to changes in sodium and water balance. This is due to early loss of glycogen and protein (both contain water) and, depending on the degree of calorie deficit and type of diet, to sodium losses associated with ketonuria. Following this initial phase, weight loss depends on the extent of energy deficit. With time, however, the rate of weight loss slows again as the body's metabolic rate decreases and the energy deficit becomes smaller. This change in metabolic rate can be two to three times greater than that predicted from changes in body weight. The lower the energy content of the diet, the lower the metabolic rate. Although it was initially suggested that exercise occurring during a period of hypocaloric feeding could prevent this decrease in metabolic rate, recent studies have suggested that it has no direct effect during hypocaloric feeding (but exercise does increase the postdiet metabolic rate by preserving lean body mass).

Following the period of hypocaloric feeding (resumption of normal energy intakes), the resting metabolic rate increases, but to a level below that observed before beginning the diet. This reduction is in part a reflection of the loss of lean body mass and in part due to additional, poorly understood effects on energy metabolism. Overall energy expenditure is further reduced due to a decrease in the thermic effect of food (the individual eats less) and in differences in physical activity (it takes less energy to perform the same amount of activity for a smaller person). Thus, in order to maintain weight loss, individuals need to consume less energy than before dieting (and increase energy expenditure by increasing the amount of physical activity).

EXERCISE

Exercise offers a number of significant advantages to patients attempting to achieve long-term weight loss. First and foremost, exercise increases energy expenditure, helping to create the energy deficit necessary for weight loss. Unfortunately, the amount of energy expended during most aerobic exercises (walking, jogging, swimming, etc) for the typical periods performed (20–30 minutes four to five times per week) is modest, approximately 500–1000 kcal per week. Thus, exercise can be predicted to have little effect on short-term weight loss. Clinical trials reflect this modest effect: some studies demonstrate weight loss with exercise alone or extra weight loss when exercise plus diet is compared with diet alone, but other studies do not show such an effect.

The importance of exercise for successful maintenance of weight loss is more clearly established. In addition to the cumulative effect of increased energy expenditure (500–1000 kcal/week × 52 weeks = 7–15 pounds per year), exercise affects the composition of the body substance lost during weight loss. When exercise is directly compared with diet, or when exercise plus diet is compared with diet alone, exercise results in greater preservation of lean body mass. That is, for each pound of weight lost, less fat and more muscle is lost during weight-loss programs without exercise. This is particularly important since the body's resting metabolic expenditure (a major portion of the total daily energy expenditure) is closely correlated with lean body mass.

The observation that much of the long-term effect of exercise is through preservation of lean body mass has resulted in an increased interest in the potential role of resistance training (weight lifting, circuit training, etc). Preliminary results suggest that resistance training during dieting does result in maintenance of lean body mass compared with the result from dieting alone. Thus, highly motivated patients can be instructed to add resistance training to their aerobic exercise program.

Regular aerobic exercise results in a number of other benefits to the obese patient, including improved cardiovascular training effect (increased exercise tolerance), decreased appetite (per calorie expended), a general sense of well-being, decreased blood pressure (in hypertensives), improved glucose metabolism and insulin action (in diabetics), improved blood lipids (in lipid disorders), and, in the long-term, decreased mortality from cardiovascular disease and all other causes.

Young patients with mild-to-moderate obesity can be started directly on a regular aerobic exercise program. Patients are commonly instructed to select two exercises and to perform either one of them four to five times per week for 30 minutes per day. Patients are taught to take their pulse and to generate a sustained tachycardia at 70–80% of their maximum predicted heart rate. Sedentary patients, older patients, and patients with severe obesity are instructed to begin walking programs without initial concern about meeting target heart rates. As weight loss proceeds, and patients become used to exercising regularly, they can be advanced to formal aerobic programs.

BEHAVIOR MODIFICATION & SOCIAL SUPPORT

Sustained weight loss requires long-term changes in eating behavior. Patients must learn specific skills to facilitate decreased calorie intake and increased energy expenditure. Although formal behavior modification programs are available, most patients can be taught basic behavioral strategies in the office.

The single most useful behavioral skill is planning and record keeping. Patients can be taught to plan both menus and exercise programs in advance. Patients are instructed to record actual food intake and exercise behaviors. The act of record keeping itself aids in behavioral change, and the availability of records also helps the health care provider assess progress and make specific suggestions for additional problem solving. Specific reward systems are also useful for many patients. Refundable financial contracts have been shown to be effective in a number of small studies. Additional behavioral strategies include breaking behaviors into identifiable parts (antecedents, consequences, etc) and specific techniques for stimulus control. Methods for slowing eating may also be effective. Efforts to identify and understand lapses and to prevent relapses are particularly important for long-term weight maintenance.

Social support is an additional essential component for any successful weight-loss program. Most successful programs use peer group support. Diet partnerships are effective for some patients. Involvement of family members is also important. A comprehensive review of published results of weight-loss programs strongly suggests that close provider-patient contact is a better predictor of success than the particular weight-loss intervention.

MEDICATIONS FOR TREATMENT OF OBESITY

Medications for the treatment of obesity are widely available, both over the counter and with prescription. Amphetamines (DEA schedule II) have extremely high abuse potential and are almost never recommended for weight loss. The most commonly prescribed appetite suppressants are fenfluramine (Pondimin), phentermine (Adipex-P, Fastin, Ionamin), diethylpropion (Tenuate, Tepanil), mazindol (Sanorex, Mazanor), and the antidepressants fluoxetine (Prozac) and sertraline (Zoloft). Dexfenfluramine (Redux), an isomer of fenfluramine, was approved by the FDA in the spring of 1996. Phenylpropanolamine is available without prescription.

Considerable controversy exists as to the efficacy of these agents and specific indications for their use. Numerous barriers to the use of medications for obesity have been described recently by advocates for their use. These include public perception of obesity as a disease of lack of willpower, expectation that medications should "cure" obesity, hindrance by state licensing agencies, limited research on long-term efficacy, and the abuse potential of some of the medications. Numerous short-term studies of appetite-suppressant drugs (ASDs) have been conducted. A recent meta-analysis of 36 studies using mazindol and fenfluramine showed that after a median duration of 12 weeks these drugs resulted in a mean weight loss 3 kg greater than placebo. In those studies with follow-up, discontinuation of the drugs most commonly resulted in weight gain. Advocates of drug therapy point out, however, that this is true for medications for most chronic diseases, such as hypertension, cholesterol, diabetes, peptic ulcer disease; stopping a successful medication results in a recurrence of the condition being treated. In these cases as well, medications do not cure the illness. A recent long-term study with phentermine (15 mg) and fenfluramine (60 mg) showed 9.4-kg weight loss after 3 years (Of the 121 who started the study, 51 completed 190 weeks; these mean results do not include those who dropped out). Most common side effects included dry mouth, GI disturbances, somnolence, and nervousness.

Advocates of ASDs interpret these results to suggest that long-term use of such medications is safe and efficacious and merits a reevaluation in clinical practice, especially when used as an adjunct to a comprehensive weight-loss program or to prevent weight gain following successful weight loss. Medications might be particularly helpful to patients with severe obesity and medical complications of obesity. Initial experience in such patients, however, has not been encouraging. Medications seem to work best in those who need them the least, that is, motivated patients with mild obesity. Current recommendations are to use medications in selected, highly motivated patients. It is extremely important for patients to be fully informed about the limited efficacy of medications, the risk of side effects, the uncertain long-term effects, and the likely need to continue medications indefinitely before initiating their use. Such realistic information often discourages patients from selecting this approach.

SURGERY

Although generally considered to be the last resort for the treatment of obesity, over 100,000 obese patients have had surgical therapy. Few controlled trials exist, and the development of rational indications for surgery has been difficult.

Gastric operations are now the procedures of choice. Most popular are the vertical-banded (Mason) gastroplasty, in which a smaller stomach pouch is cre-

ated, and gastric bypass procedures. Although both procedures result in significant weight loss, randomized trials comparing the two tend to favor gastric bypass procedures. This is particularly true in patients who consume large amount of sweets. Perioperative mortality averages < 1% but ranges between 0–4% in different centers. Complications are common and include wound dehiscence, peritonitis, nausea and vomiting, vitamin deficiencies, and hair loss. When all necessary reversals, revisions, and patients lost to follow-up are considered, failure rates approach 50%.

Jejunoileal bypass was the first major surgical procedure popularized for the treatment of obesity. This procedure has been abandoned due to numerous complications. Jaw wiring is another surgical treatment that is not recommended. Suction lipectomy, or liposuction, permits the removal of fat from specific areas of the body. Usually performed by plastic surgeons, 5 pounds of fat can be removed with each procedure in an attempt to reshape thighs and waists resistant to more traditional weight-loss and exercise treatments. No advantageous metabolic changes are induced by the procedure.

SUMMARY

No specific behavioral technique serves as the magic bullet for the very challenging, but medically important task of weight loss. Although many of the most common problems encountered in medical practice can be treated by weight loss alone, only motivated patients should be started on weight-loss programs. Weight-loss treatments vary considerably in terms of risk, cost, and efficacy. For most patients with mild or moderate obesity, a multifactorial approach, including diet, exercise, behavior modification, and social support, can be prescribed. Close patient-provider contact and long-term follow-up with emphasis on exercise are key ingredients for success. Motivated patients with severe obesity should be considered for supervised VLCDs, again emphasizing long-term dietary change, exercise, behavior modification, and social support. The role of medications for the treatment of obesity is increasing but should still be limited to selected, highly informed patients.

SUGGESTED READINGS

Atkinson RL, Hubbard VS: Report on the NIH workshop on pharmacologic treatment of obesity. Am J Clin Nutr 1994;60:153.

Brownell KD, Rodin J: The dieting maelstrom: Is it possible and advisable to lose weight? Am Psychologist 1994;49:781.

Danford D, Fletcher SW: Methods for voluntary weight loss and control: National Institutes of Health Technology Assessment Conference. Ann Int Med 1993;119:641.

Frank A: Futility and avoidance: Medical professionals in the treatment of obesity. JAMA 1993;269:2132.

Hartman WM et al: Long-term maintenance of weight loss following supplemental fasting. Int J Eating Disord 1993;14:87.

Levy AS, Heaton AW: Weight control practices of US adults trying to lose weight. Ann Int Med 1993;119:661.

Liebel RL, Rosenbaum M, Hirsch J: Changes in energy expenditure resulting from altered body weight. N Engl J Med 1995;332:621.

Lindpainter K: Finding an obesity gene: A tale of mice and men. N Engl J Med 1995;332:679.

Nunn RG, Newton KS, Faucher P: 2.5 years follow-up of weight and body mass index values in the Weight Control for Life! program: A descriptive analysis. Addict Behav 1992;17:579.

Manson JE et. al: Body weight and mortality among women. N Engl J Med 1995;333:677.

Scott J: New chapter for the fat controller. Nature 1996;379:113.

Weintraub M: Long-term weight control study: Conclusions. Clin Pharmacol Ther 1992;51:642.

Wilson GT: Relationship of dieting and voluntary weight loss to psychological functioning and binge eating. Ann Int Med 1993;119:727.

Eating Disorders

20

Steven J. Romano, MD, & Katherine A. Halmi, MD

INTRODUCTION

The eating disorders, including anorexia nervosa and bulimia nervosa, are receiving more clinical and research attention than ever before, paralleling an increase in their prevalence over the last few decades. Such disturbances in eating behavior are, of course, not new. Historical documentation of anorexia nervosa dates back to the early Christian saints. Binging and purging, though distinct from our current concept of bulimia nervosa, took place in the lives of ancient Romans.

The eating disorders are best viewed as clinical syndromes rather than specific diseases, as they do not result from a single cause or follow a single course. As psychiatric syndromes, they are defined largely by a constellation of behaviors and attitudes that persist over time and produce characteristic complications contributing to physical and psychosocial dysfunction. Because of the complexity and breadth of contributing factors, as well as the extent of comorbid psychopathology, knowledge of the behavioral characteristics of the eating disorders can lead to improved recognition and implementation of effective treatment strategies. In light of the complicated interplay of psychiatric, psychosocial, and medical consequences, treatment beyond initial medical stabilization generally requires referral to specialists.

MULTIDIMENSIONAL MODEL

A comprehensive multidimensional model best illustrates the role various factors play in the genesis of clinically significant eating disturbances. In this schema, also referred to as a stress diathesis model, psychologic, biological, and sociocultural stressors contribute to the development of symptomatic expression.

Psychological factors include personality features, such as the anorectic's obsessive-compulsive qualities, constrained affect, and sense of ineffectiveness, and

the bulimic's impulsivity. They also include the influence of developmental stressors and family dynamics.

Biological factors are most often due to the adverse effects of starvation, malnutrition, and purging behaviors, including vomiting and the misuse of laxatives and diuretics. Restrictive dieting and subsequent malnourishment may contribute to the development of comorbid psychiatric conditions, such as anxiety and depression. A preexisting biological vulnerability may exist and is supported by preliminary findings of neurophysiologic investigations showing dysfunction of serotonin, dopamine, and norepinephrine neuromodulators; a small number of patients with anorexia develop amenorrhea preceding significant weight loss.

Sociocultural factors figure prominently in the etiology of the eating disorders. The idealization of thinness contributes to dieting behavior, often beginning in early adolescence. Of note, dieting is almost always present as a precipitant to the development of an eating disorder. Other precipitants include periods of illness leading to weight loss; in vulnerable individuals this may be followed by willful dieting.

THEORETICAL CONSIDERATIONS

Conceptual models aid in understanding the etiology and possible sustaining factors involved in the genesis and persistence of eating-disordered behavior. Important models include those derived from learning theory and neurophysiological abnormality or dysfunction.

Cognitive-behavioral theory, which is derived from learning theory, states that cognition influences behavior in a predictable manner. Cues, both internal and external, can provoke behavioral change through activation of cognitive sets. A change in negative cognition therefore influences a change from dysfunctional to healthy behavior. Overvalued thoughts about weight, food, and diet, especially the idealization of thinness, lead to the perpetuation of compromising responses, such as heroic dietary measures and abuses of substances believed effective for weight reduction. The coupling of such cognitions and behaviors affects self-esteem and may severely impair one's psychological state. Cognitive-behavioral therapy has been effective in achieving symptom reduction and improvement in both medical and psychological status.

The search for specific biological markers that may help identify patients with eating disorders has focused increasingly on neurotransmitters and other neuromodulators. Research findings suggest that dysfunction in various neurotransmitter systems, including serotonin, dopamine, and norepinephrine, as well as opioids, cholecystokinin (CCK), and others might play a role in the development and maintenance of the eating disorders. Rationale for the examination of these hormones and other substances derives from our understanding of the pathways modulating appetitive behavior, including hypothalamic regulation and the known connection between the gastrointestinal tract and the central nervous system. The complexity of these disorders, including the stress of eating-disordered behavior on physiology, however, makes it unlikely that a neurophysiological hypothesis alone can explain the etiology and maintenance of these complex syndromes.

ANOREXIA NERVOSA

Description

Anorexia nervosa is a relatively rare disorder affecting less than 1% of young women and a much smaller percentage of young men. Its most striking behavioral manifestation is the willful restriction of caloric intake secondary to an irrational fear of becoming fat, frequently in concert with a grossly distorted view of one's self as overweight, even in the presence of severe emaciation. The patient often exhibits a phobic response to food, particularly to fatty and other calorically dense items. They develop an obsessive preoccupation with food, eating, dieting, weight, and body shape and frequently exhibit ritualistic behaviors involving choosing, preparing, and ingesting meals (eg, cutting food into very small pieces or chewing each bite a specific number of times).

Early in the course of the illness, a patient begins to restrict many food items, as is typical of most dieters. As the disorder progresses, though, the anorectic's menu becomes grossly constricted and she demonstrates greater rigidity. Minor variation in meal content can produce tremendous anxiety. Unlike the average dieter, the anorectic continues her pursuit of thinness to an extreme and becomes dependent on the daily registration of weight loss. This fuels even more restrictive dieting. Extreme dieting is often complicated by other weight-reducing behaviors. Exercise is frequently compulsive, and hyperactivity in under-

weight patients is a curious but often-encountered concomitant. Weakness, muscle aches, sleep disturbances, and gastrointestinal complaints, including constipation and postprandial bloating, are common physical findings. Amenorrhea, reflecting endocrine dysfunction, is occasionally present.

Some anorectics engage in bulimic behaviors, including binging and purging. This binge-purge subtype of anorexia nervosa contrasts with the purely restricting subtype described earlier. Often, purging behavior, such as self-induced vomiting or the misuse of laxatives and diuretics, is seen in the absence of binging. The coupling of purging with self-starvation compounds the medical consequences of the disorder. Furthermore, anorectics generally minimize their symptoms and the negative consequences of their disorder and are thus rarely motivated for treatment. The characteristics of the illness are intensified with weight loss, further frustrating attempts at engaging the patient in a meaningful therapeutic process. Family and friends become increasingly anxious, angry, and at times alienated, as their loved one regresses. Superficial compliance, as is sometimes seen, belies a profound resistance. Anorectic patients can be challenging to treat as they cling tenaciously to their beliefs and behaviors.

Psychosocial dysfunction is common in patients with anorexia. Though educational performance may not be affected in adolescent patients, social relations become increasingly constricted, and sexual interest is generally diminished or absent.

Differential Diagnosis

The pathognomonic features of anorexia nervosa, namely the intense fear of becoming fat coupled with the relentless pursuit of thinness, are generally absent in other medical and psychiatric conditions. The term *anorexia,* which itself refers to absence of appetite, is a misnomer in the case of the syndrome of anorexia nervosa. True anorexia, such as that which might be seen in many medical conditions or diseases, would be accompanied by other signs or symptoms of those illnesses (as in gastrointestinal disease or many cancers).

Lack of appetite or decreased intake, with or without subsequent weight loss, is encountered in a number of psychiatric disorders. These include depression, hysterical conversion and other psychosomatic disorders, schizophrenia, and certain delusional disorders, but with each of these is associated a cluster of other substantiating symptomatology. Some patients with obsessive-compulsive disorder (OCD) may exhibit what appears to be bizarre behaviors around food, eating, or meal preparation, but, on further exploration, their behavior is in response to obsessional ideation, for example, the fear of contamination. Such patients, in contrast to those with anorexia nervosa, generally admit their discomfort with the need to perform such compelling and often excessive or senseless acts.

In summary, though comorbid psychopathology may be encountered in patients with anorexia nervosa, including symptoms of depression or OCD, the hallmark of anorexia nervosa (the morbid fear of becoming fat and the relentless pursuit of thinness) is absent in the other psychiatric syndromes. In none of these syndromes does the goal of weight loss drive the behavior.

Medical Complications & Treatment

Treatment of anorexia nervosa is initially directed at correcting the acute medical complications and is followed by supportive nutritional rehabilitation. Most medical consequences resolve with nutritional rehabilitation and the discontinuation of purging behaviors.

In most cases of anorexia associated with significant weight loss (> 15–20% of ideal body weight) a structured inpatient facility is necessary to maintain an adequate level of medical surveillance and sustain a steady rate of weight gain. On admission to an inpatient treatment facility, laboratory screening should include tests for electrolytes, liver function, amylase (elevated in patients who purge), thyroid function, a complete blood count with differential, and a urinalysis. Common laboratory findings include leukopenia with a relative lymphocytosis, metabolic alkalosis with associated hypokalemia, hypochloremia and elevated serum bicarbonate levels, and, occasionally, metabolic acidosis in those patients who abuse large amounts of stimulant-type laxatives. An electrocardiogram should also be obtained since emaciation and associated electrolyte disturbances can contribute to significant abnormalities, especially in those who purge. Hypokalemia can lead to the possibility of arrhythmia and the risk of cardiac arrest.

Acute medical conditions generally requiring immediate attention include electrolyte disturbances and dehydration, both of which are readily reversible. In most cases, initiating oral intake of fluids and food reverses minor disturbances in electrolytes and establishes adequate hydration. More severe cases may require intravenous hydration and parenteral replacement of depleted electrolytes, such as is required with significant hypokalemia. In these cases, daily electrolyte checks are necessary until the patient's condition stabilizes. Importantly, treatment must ensure prevention of purging behaviors in those with this history, as persistence of purging will, of course, alter electrolyte and fluid balance.

In patients who are significantly underweight, use of a liquid supplement, initially as replacement for solid food, helps ensure necessary caloric intake. When given in divided feedings throughout the day, it may decrease the patient's sense of postprandial discomfort and early satiety, both frequent consequences of extended caloric restriction and semi-starvation. Further, this approach to refeeding decreases the inevitable manipulations around food choices. Replacement of solid food with liquid supplement may also lessen the patient's phobic avoidance of food and the subsequent anxiety around meal choices.

Behavioral Interventions & Psychotherapy

Given the lack of motivation exhibited by the majority of patients with anorexia and their strong resistance to treatment, it is helpful to initiate behavioral strategies as soon as any acute medical condition is stabilized. Initial behavioral interventions, tied to daily weight gain in increments of no less than 0.25 lb. or 0.1 kg, include obtaining visits from family or friends, lessening physical restrictions, and increasing involvement in activities on and off the unit. It is important that all contingencies be tied to daily weight gain, which is done each morning at the same time and in like manner, as this is a quantifiable observation not open to argument or discussion. A milieu supportive of such interventions helps to motivate the patient and exert pressure toward positive change.

As the patient reaches a target weight range and establishes some degree of commitment to treatment, solid food can replace liquid supplement. The ability of the patient to maintain weight through normalization of intake marks a transition to less structured treatment, such as outpatient follow-up.

Other treatments applicable to both inpatient and outpatient settings include individual psychotherapy and family intervention. The initial focus in family therapy should be on psychoeducation and obtaining the support of family members. The dynamics that may be contributing to the patient's eating disorder should be identified and, when plausible, resolved. Such treatment often requires extensive contact beyond any acute interventions.

Individual psychotherapy is of limited value in the early stages of treatment, as the anorectic individual is generally unmotivated and, due to cognitive disturbances secondary to self-starvation, not available for meaningful therapeutic work. Supportive therapy during this acute stage is often helpful in allaying anxiety and encouraging compliance. The more focused cognitive-behavioral and interpersonal therapies are generally more effective when the patient has begun to gain weight and is beyond acute medical risk. Cognitive-behavioral therapy focuses on the particular disturbing or distorted thoughts patients have that contribute to maladaptive behaviors. It also helps the patient establish more effective behavioral alternatives. This therapy may also be effective with the central psychological features of anorexia nervosa, such as body image disturbance. Interpersonal therapy may also be helpful. It focuses on interpersonal conflicts rather than specific eating disturbances. Following stabilization and resolution of the acute crisis, including achievement of weight restoration, patients often require longer term psychotherapeutic interventions.

Pharmacotherapy

Pharmacological therapy can play an adjunctive role in the management of both primary eating symptoms and their comorbid psychiatric features, including anxiety and depression. Such treatments should focus on particular target symptoms or behaviors. No single medication is consistently effective in managing the primary psychiatric disturbances of anorexia nervosa. Antidepressants, especially the selective serotonin-reuptake inhibitors, can alleviate depressive symptoms and, due to their ability to regulate obsessive-compulsive symptomatology, may help reduce the preoccupations and ritualistic behaviors encountered in most anorectics. Low doses of antipsychotics may sometimes be employed in severely obsessional or agitated patients. Anxiolytics in general should not be given to anorectics for they are prone to develop addictions.

BULIMIA NERVOSA

Description

Bulimia nervosa affects approximately 2–3% of young women and 0.2% of young men; although bulimic behaviors may be encountered in many more patients, it is generally precipitated by periods of restrictive dieting. Bulimic individuals engage in regular episodes of binge eating, followed by compensatory behaviors in an attempt to counteract the weight gain from ingested calories. Binge eating is characterized by the rapid consumption of large amounts of food over a short time, usually 1–2 hours. It is associated with the sense of being out of control and is often followed by feelings of guilt or shame and other dysphoric affective states, such as depression or anxiety. Some report alleviation of dysphoria or even emotional numbing during or immediately following the episode, though this is short-lived. During a binge, from a few thousand up to as many as 15,000 kcal or more may be consumed. Sometimes trigger foods, often a fattening sweet such as chocolate, precipitate a binge, though the overall content of food consumed, by macroanalysis of nutritional content, varies. The bulimic individual generally binges in private; grossly overeating is humiliating. Embarrassment can lead to varying degrees of social avoidance or isolation.

Contributing further to avoidance behavior is the need to compensate for eating, frequently in the form of purging. Most bulimic individuals induce vomiting during or after a binge, and some also use laxatives or diuretics. A minority of patients employ laxatives or diuretics alone. Nonpurging compensatory behaviors include compulsive exercising and restrictive dieting or fasting between binges.

Another characteristic of bulimia nervosa is dissatisfaction with one's body shape or weight. This may evolve into a significant degree of obsessional preoccupation, overly influenced by these physical characteristics. It can have a profound affect on self-esteem and is evidenced in part by the majority of patients presenting with comorbid depressive symptomatology. Impulsive behavior is encountered in many individuals with bulimia nervosa and at times leads to substance abuse, sexual promiscuity, and theft.

Differential Diagnosis

Few medical or psychiatric disorders can be confused with bulimia nervosa. More frequently, signs of self-induced vomiting or use of diuretics or laxatives in a young woman who does not admit to binging or purging behaviors leads the primary care clinician to search for another primary medical diagnosis. Signs and symptoms associated with gastritis, esophagitis, dehydration, or electrolyte disturbances lead to primary care or emergency room visits, postponing psychiatric consultation. If the patient is underweight, amenorrheic, and is binging and purging, she has anorexia nervosa, of the binge-purge subtype.

Medical Complications & Treatment

The majority of medical complications due to bulimia nervosa are consequences of purging behaviors. Self-induced vomiting can lead to gastritis, esophagitis, periodontal disease, and dental caries. Gastric dilatation and gastric or esophageal rupture are rare medical emergencies. Metabolic alkalosis with the development of clinically significant hypokalemia in patients who vomit is not unusual, and serum electrolytes show typical indices. When present, electrocardiographic changes are significant. Arrhythmias can lead to cardiac arrest if hypokalemia and related disturbances are not effectively corrected. Use of diuretics causes similar disturbances. Metabolic acidosis can develop in those who use a significant number of stimulant-type laxatives. Dehydration, sometimes requiring intravenous hydration, can accompany each of the aforementioned purging behaviors. More often associated with bulimic behaviors are general physical complaints such as fatigue and muscle aches. Long-term use of the emetic ipecac can lead to myopathies, including cardiomyopathy.

Most patients with bulimia nervosa can be treated as outpatients or in more structured partial hospitalization programs. An individual with an acute medical condition, however, such as dehydration or symptomatic hypokalemia accompanied by electrocardiogram changes, requires hospitalization for medical stabilization. Patients who have failed outpatient treatment and continue to binge and purge frequently, and those with significant depression and associated suicidal ideation, may require inpatient treatment.

Behavioral Interventions and Psychotherapy

Helping patients to recognize the negative consequences of their behavior and dispelling myths about the efficacy of many of their dietary maneuvers, especially the usefulness of laxatives, diuretics, and self-induced vomiting, may be enough to motivate them to decrease the frequency of bulimic behaviors. Time-limited psychotherapy conducted in an individual or group format is often useful. More traditional exploratory psychotherapies, which are generally not time-limited, do not predictably affect outcome but may play a role in the treatment of underlying or persistent difficulties following resolution of bulimia.

Cognitive-behavioral therapy is an established treatment for bulimia nervosa. It targets the behavioral manifestations and challenges the cognitive distortions typically encountered in these patients. It is the mainstay of treatment for bulimic individuals. In cognitive-behavioral therapy, identifying disordered behaviors is the first step toward productive intervention, because behavioral consequences follow specific cues. In order to intervene, one must recognize the various cues and respond to them deliberately rather than automatically. Cues affecting eating-disordered patients are either internal or external. Internal cues include physiological ones, most significantly hunger, as well as emotions and thoughts. External cues encompass a broad array of experiences from sensual, such as sight or smell, to situational. Cues lead to consequences that are either positive or negative; both can be reinforcing.

Following the identification of cues, associated responses can be addressed more specifically and in greater detail. Responses consist of thoughts, feelings, and behaviors. Helping the patient to understand that thoughts and feelings affect behavioral responses to a cue is of great significance because both thoughts and feelings can be altered through cognitive-behavioral techniques. For each cue identified, patients are taught to delineate the various response components and to evaluate the appropriateness of each. Though schematically simple, many eating-associated responses are automatic, and learning to identify the cues and various responses requires much practice.

In cognitive-behavioral therapy patients have, to this point, been taught to recognize that behaviors follow cues and that responses to cues can be broken down into thoughts, feelings, and behaviors. What a patient thinks and feels about a cue dictates whether her response is adaptive or maladaptive. How she feels is influenced by how she thinks, therefore the restructuring of thoughts is of primary importance. Eating-disordered patients manifest certain patterns of distorted thinking; these patterns negatively influence feelings and fuel the maladaptive behaviors. These various styles of thinking are identified, and strategies to challenge and ultimately to alter the distortions are developed.

A simple example helps illustrate the applicability of cognitive-behavioral therapy. A common cue that frequently leads to a bulimic response is the normal sense of fullness. Rather than recognizing satiety as a normal physiologic response, the eating-disordered patient often misinterprets this cue, stating instead, "I feel fat." This distorted thought, unchallenged, is associated with negative feelings and often leads to dysfunctional behaviors. Rather than the appropriate response to fullness, understanding that it is temporary and will pass, the patient believes she must compensate for being "fat" and rids herself of the meal through purging or compensates for the caloric intake through exercise. Such a response causes the cycle to reassert itself.

Pharmacotherapy

Psychopharmacological management may play a significant role in treatment and, unlike its effect in anorexia, can more predictably affect outcome. Many antidepressants, including monoamine oxidase inhibitors (MAOIs), tricyclic antidepressants (TCAs), and selective serotonin-reuptake inhibitors (SSRIs: most notably fluoxetine), have all been effective in treating bulimia. They reduce symptoms of depression and anxiety as well as the frequency of binging and purging. Bupropion is the only antidepressant that is contraindicated, since the metabolic imbalances precipitated by purging can make the patient more prone to seizures.

SUMMARY

Eating disorders represent a broad spectrum of psychopathologic features. They are best understood in terms of multiple etiologic factors influencing the development of clinical syndromes. Understanding the complexity of these disorders, the behaviors associated with them, and their comorbid psychiatric features aids in the recognition of clinically significant cases. Focusing initially on control of these primary eating disorder behaviors helps reduce the likelihood of psychological morbidity. It also limits the medical complications that frequently develop in these conditions. Interventions to control behavior range from response prevention (for patients placed on special inpatient wards) to cognitive-behavioral therapies for more motivated patients. Behavioral control may be augmented through pharmacological management as well as other psychotherapies (psychoeductional and interpersonal) that help reduce the role that sustaining factors play in the maintenance of these disorders.

SUGGESTED READINGS

Fairburn CG, Wilson GT (editors): *Binge Eating: Nature, Assessment, Treatment.* Guilford Press, 1993.

Halmi KA: Eating disorders. Pages 857–875 in: Hales KE, Yudofsky SC, Talbott J (editors): *American Psychiatric Press Textbook of Psychiatry,* 2nd ed. American Psychiatric Association Press, 1994.

Halmi KA (editor): *Psychobiology and Treatment of Anorexia Nervosa and Bulimia Nervosa.* American Psychiatric Association Press, 1992.

Hsu LKG: *Eating Disorders.* Guilford Press, 1990.

Mitchell JE: *Bulimia Nervosa.* University of Minnesota Press, 1990.

Walsh BT, Devlin MJ: Psychopharmacology of anorexia nervosa, bulimia nervosa, and binge eating. Pages 1581–1589 in: Bloom FE, Kuffer DJ (editors): *Psychopharmacology: The Fourth Generation of Progress.* Raven Press, 1995.

Alcohol & Substance Use

21

Michael Fleming, MD, MPH

INTRODUCTION

The care of persons adversely affected by the use of alcohol and other drugs is an important clinical problem, with the prevalence of substance-use disorders exceeding 20% in ambulatory care practices. These disorders—at-risk, problem, and dependent drinking; tobacco use; illicit drug use; and prescription drug abuse—are associated with a large number of adverse health, behavioral, and social effects. Most practitioners have seen the weekend binge drinkers who are involved in high-risk sexual behavior, the steady drinkers with potentially fatal effects such as alcohol-induced liver failure, heavy cocaine users who attempt suicide, professional colleagues who smoke marijuana to relax, and anxious patients who abuse sedative drugs.

It is not only the people who use mood-altering drugs who are adversely affected; the negative influence extends to family members and friends, who may present with symptoms secondary to the other person's substance use. Young children complain of abdominal pain, headaches, and school problems or may exhibit aggressive behavior; spouses present with sleep disorders, depression, and fatigue. Family members may also present with bruises or other evidence of physical abuse. The abuse and violence induced by substance use are increasing problems at all levels—personal, community, and professional.

Although the care of patients and family members affected by these disorders is difficult, there is reason to be optimistic. The frequency of recovery from substance abuse is higher than from most other chronic illnesses, with significant recovery occurring in 30–40% of treated cases. Another 20–25% experience long periods of sobriety and improved health status. Recovering patients often credit their clinicians with being a primary factor in their recovery and with literally saving their lives. Such acknowledgment of the physician's role can be one of the most rewarding experiences in medicine. Seeing the reversal of such substance abuse effects as acute alcoholic hepatitis, heart failure, respiratory problems, family dysfunction, impaired work performance, and repeated incarcerations can be just as dramatic and gratifying as seeing patients recover from leukemia or other life-threatening illnesses. Nonetheless, many physicians view the treatment of patients with substance abuse with pessimism, believing that patients never recover and that treatment is therefore not worth the effort.

One of the primary reasons for this negativism is the physician's failure to apply the basic concepts of behavioral medicine to treating alcohol and drug disorders. Because pharmacotherapy is limited to drugs such as disulfiram, naltrexone, and methadone—and there are no appropriate surgical procedures—successful management must focus on changing behavior and health habits. Whereas 10–20% of patients become abstinent or reduce their use with brief, focused interventions, many others require multiple interventions over long periods. Caring for patients with these problems is more similar to treating those with other chronic problems, such as elevated cholesterol or arthritis, rather than patients with acute problems that respond to a single pharmacotherapeutic trial or surgical procedure.

DIAGNOSIS

Defining Substance Abuse

At-Risk Users: At-risk substance use is a relatively new term based on the observation that most persons who use alcohol and drugs have minimal or no related problems. The concept also recognizes the associated health risks and tries to establish limits above which the risks of adverse health effects become significant, much like the limits established for high blood pressure and cholesterol. At-risk and problem users constitute a much larger population than do persons who are alcohol- or drug-dependent, and primary care physicians see more of this cohort (Table 21–1).

Table 21–1. Definitions of substance abuse.

At-Risk Users

At-risk tobacco users are those who use any quantity of tobacco products, including cigars, pipes, cigarettes, and smokeless tobacco, with no symptoms of dependence or tobacco-related problems related to their use. *Any use is considered at-risk.*

At-risk drinkers are persons who drink above established cut-off limits based on epidemiologic data that find increasing levels of health risks at the following levels:

More than 14 drinks per week for men
More than 7 drinks per week for women
More than 4 drinks per occasion for men and 3 drinks per occasion for women
Adults over the age of 65, women who are pregnant, persons operating machinery, and patients on medication may be at risk below these levels.

At-risk prescription drug users are patients on mood-altering drugs for more than 3 months who may develop problems and dependence with chronic long-term use.

At-risk illicit drug users—Any illicit drug use is considered at-risk use. Adolescents are at particular risk.

Problem Users

Problem users experience problems related to their tobacco, alcohol, prescription drug, or illicit drug use, including health problems, legal problems, family dysfunction, and school or work performance problems.

Prescription drug problems or abuse—This group includes persons who use mood-altering medications (primarily sedatives and opioids) in ways other than those written on the prescription, or who try to obtain these drugs from multiple physicians. Many persons who were formerly diagnosed as substance abusers may meet the new criteria for alcohol or drug dependence.

Dependent Users

These patients have met three or more *DSM-IV* criteria for alcohol and/or drug dependence in the last 12 months, generally with loss of control, alcohol-related consequences, and physiologic dependence. The new criteria do not require tolerance or withdrawal symptoms.

Alcoholism and drug addiction are terms that are synonymous with alcohol or drug dependence; they are very powerful labels that should be used carefully.

1. At-risk tobacco users–This category includes persons who use any quantity of tobacco products, including cigars, pipes, cigarettes, and smokeless tobacco, and who have no symptoms of dependence or problems related to their use. Note that *any* use is considered at-risk use.

2. At-risk drinkers–These are defined as persons who drink above established cut-off limits. The following limits are based on epidemiologic data that have found increasing levels of health risks at greater levels of consumption. A drink is defined as 1.5 ounces of hard liquor, 5 ounces of wine, or 12 ounces of beer or wine cooler.

■ Fourteen drinks per week for men
■ More than seven drinks per week for women
■ More than four drinks per occasion for men and three drinks per occasion for women.

Some special populations may be at risk below these limits: adults over the age of 65, pregnant women, persons operating machinery, and patients on medication.

3. At-risk prescription drug use–Patients on mood-altering drugs for more than 3 months are considered to be at risk for the problems and dependence that can develop with long-term use. Although the majority of patients using long-term sedative drugs to manage anxiety disorders and persons using narcotics to treat chronic pain develop neither problems nor dependence, 10–20% do experience problems such as falls, oversedation, drug interactions, or drug overdoses or symptoms of dependence (eg, taking more medication than prescribed).

4. At-risk illicit drug use–Any use of an illicit drug is considered at-risk use. Adolescents who intermittently experiment with illicit drugs are at particular risk for the development of problems and dependent polydrug use.

Problem Users: This generic term can be very useful in a diagnostic assessment using *Diagnostic and Statistical Manual of Mental Disorders-IV (DSM-IV)* criteria. The term is more acceptable to patients than such labels as "alcoholism" or "addiction." Problem users are those who experience problems related to their tobacco, alcohol, prescription drug, or illicit drug use. These include health problems (eg, bronchitis, hypertension, hepatitis), legal problems (eg, arrests for driving under the influence), family dysfunction, and performance problems at school or work. Although most patients in this category are heavy users, some patients may experience serious problems with light to moderate use.

Prescription drug abuse is found in persons who use mood-altering medications (primarily sedatives and opioids) in ways other than those written on the prescription, or who try to obtain these prescriptions from several physicians.

Dependent Users: These persons have met three or more *DSM-IV* criteria for alcohol or drug dependence in the last 12 months. Most persons who are alcohol- or drug-dependent show loss of control, alcohol-related consequences, and physiologic dependence. The new *DSM-IV* criteria do not require tolerance or withdrawal symptoms. A large number of persons who were formerly classified as substance abusers may now be considered alcohol- or drug-dependent.

Alcoholism or Drug Addiction: These terms are synonymous with alcohol or drug dependence. They are very powerful labels with pejorative connotations and should be used with great care.

Identifying Substance Abuse

The major mood-altering drugs include tobacco products, alcohol, prescription medication (sedatives and narcotics), and illicit drugs (marijuana, cocaine, opioids, and amphetamines, etc). Clinicians may want to screen for other drugs in high-risk populations: inhalants in adolescents, anabolic steroids in weight lifters, phencyclidine hydrochloride (PCP) among young adults, and hallucinogens in polysubstance users. The primary screening methods used in clinical settings are based on patient self-report; physical or laboratory measurements are less specific and should be used with other assessment procedures for patients who report above-the-limit use.

The focus of substance abuse screening procedures needs to shift from the detection of dependence or addiction to the detection of use and risk. A number of new screening methods, assessment procedures, interventions, treatment modalities, and preventive measures are available; Figure 21–1 summarizes recommended clinical protocols based on the "Ask, Assess, Advise, and Assist" treatment model developed for the National Cancer Institute's Physician Guide.

- **Ask:** Screen for substance use with consumption questions or self-administered screening tests.
- **Assess:** Determine the presence of substance-related problems and symptoms of dependence.
- **Advise:** Use a brief intervention approach to communicate the consequences of continued substance use and to assess the patient's readiness to change.
- **Assist:** Help patients reduce their substance use through written contracts or referrals to a specialized treatment program.

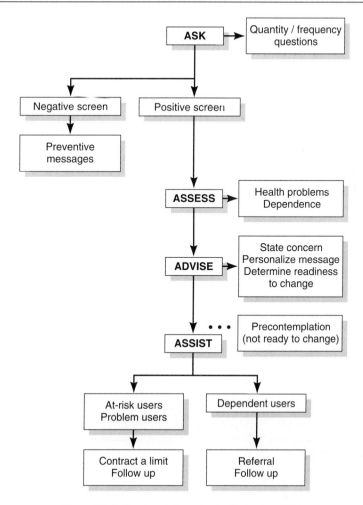

Figure 21–1 Treatment flow chart with the four "A's."

Ask

Substance abuse—consumption—questions are recommended as the initial screening procedure and are used by the majority of clinicians. Most information on substance-use sequelae is grounded on such data, forming the basis for the current standard of care and normal clinical practice. Studies on the relationship between tobacco, alcohol, and drug use and health effects primarily use self-reported quantity and frequency information, helping clinicians view alcohol and substance use in the context of other health concerns with specific cut-off limits based on health risks.

All patients seen by primary care clinicians should be asked about their use of mood-altering substances. Patients presenting with problems in which alcohol or drug use may be a contributing factor—hypertension, cardiac arrhythmia, abdominal pain, bronchitis, or depression—should be screened at the initial visit. Patients who are seen for conditions (eg, urinary tract infection) that are not likely to be secondary to substance use should be screened as soon as possible at subsequent visits. Pediatric patients should be screened for substance use beginning at about age 12—the average age of first use. Adults aged 65 and older should also participate in screening procedures, as substance use is an important and often overlooked problem in this age group (see Chapter 12).

Interview Techniques: A number of interview techniques can increase the accuracy of self-report data, including placing substance-use questions in the context of general health questions; using nonjudgmental interviewing methods; framing questions specifically and clearly; and providing a clinical environment of trust, respect, and concern. Many clinicians start by asking about exercise patterns, weight concerns, and the use of seat belts. These questions are followed with questions about the use of tobacco, alcohol, and drugs. It is important to ask about substance use in a tone of voice similar to that used with other health questions, such as a family history of heart disease. Negative inflections (especially among clinicians with unpleasant personal or professional substance-use experiences) are often discerned by patients and can result in less-than-accurate responses.

Specific, closed questions are preferable here to open-ended interview techniques. For example, asking "How many days per week did you drink alcohol last month?" provides more useful data than asking "How much alcohol do you drink?" Reassuring patients that the questions are routine and part of a regular health check-up can also provide more accurate self-reported data. Patients who are skeptical about the routine nature of the questions should be told about the health risks involved: "I need to know about how much you drink because it affects your blood pressure, your blood sugar, and your risk for heart disease." Once patients understand the relationship between use and health problems they usually become more comfortable with the questions.

Screening questions for tobacco products focus on current use: "Have you used any cigarettes, cigars, or smokeless tobacco in the past year?" Although cigarettes are the predominant tobacco product sold in the United States, other forms such as chewing tobacco and snuff are still in use. Patients who are using tobacco products should receive a brief assessment using the procedures discussed in the next section; a more extensive review of screening procedures is included in Chapter 18, which discusses smoking and smoking-cessation strategies.

Alcohol use can be determined with three consumption questions based on frequency, quantity, and binge use: "How many days per week do you drink? How much alcohol do you drink a day? How often do you have five or more drinks on a single occasion?" Exceeding the cut-off limits delineated earlier is considered a positive screening that should be followed up with assessment procedures. The assessment is necessary to determine the presence of alcohol-related problems and dependence symptoms; its goal is to help clinicians develop a treatment plan.

The CAGE questionnaire (see Chapter 1) may be helpful if the patient appears uncomfortable with direct consumption questions. The questions are "Have you ever felt a need to Cut down on your drinking?" "Have you ever felt Annoyed by someone criticizing your drinking?" "Have you ever felt Guilty about your drinking?" "Have you ever had an Eye-opener in the morning to relieve the shakes?" Two or more positive responses suggest a potential problem and should be followed up with assessment questions.

Information on the validity of specific screening questions for the detection of **prescription drug use or abuse** is limited. If answered affirmatively, straightforward questions such as "Have you used any tranquilizers in the past year?" or "Have you used pain killers in the past year?" could be followed by additional questions to determine the frequency and dose.

Screening questions for illicit drug use have not been widely tested in primary care settings. One question—"Have you used marijuana more than five times in your life?" (chosen from the National Institutes of Mental Health's diagnostic interview schedule)—can be repeated for narcotics, amphetamines, and other drugs of interest. Patients who use illicit drugs are often willing to admit to past use even though they may deny current use. The use of five times as a cut-off point is somewhat arbitrary; however, it has some validity, and the clinician is unlikely to miss persons with current drug problems. Patients who respond affirmatively should be assessed through additional questions to determine the presence of problems and addiction.

Self-Administered Tests: A number of self-administered substance-use screening tests have been well validated in primary care settings; these questionnaires can be incorporated into health-screening forms given to all new patients. These include the Alcohol Use Disorder Identification Test (AUDIT), the Health Screening Survey (HSS), and the Michigan Alcohol Screening Test (MAST). The AUDIT (the recommended screening questionnaire) was developed by the World Health Organization and has been tested in a number of countries and in diverse cultures. It includes three questions on consumption, three questions on symptoms of dependence, and three questions on alcohol-related problems. Self-administered screening tests can be conducted by interview, written questionnaire, or computer. Some data suggest that the best way to elicit sensitive information is through computer programs or pencil-and-paper tests.

The only screening test for drugs that has been tried in clinical settings is the Drug Abuse Screening Test (DAST). The DAST is a modification of the MAST and is too long to be useful as an initial screening test for large populations. There is limited information on the best screening test to use with specific populations, such as women, adolescents, older adults, and various ethnic groups. The POSIT (Problem-Oriented Substance Inventory Test), developed by the National Institute of Drug Abuse, is a long test for substance use and other problems encountered by adolescents.

Assess

Physicians need to assess patients with positive screenings for potential alcohol or drug disorders; for evidence of physical dependence, serious medical or psychiatric problems, or the use of other mood-alter-ing drugs; and family, legal, and employment issues. Table 21–2 summarizes some of the more common complaints associated with substance use. The recommended assessment procedures usually require a separate office visit. Although the length of the assessment may be of some concern, the evaluation must be placed in the context of such other chronic problems as hypertension and hypercholesterolemia, which also require a comprehensive assessment with multiple follow-up visits before an appropriate treatment plan can be developed. In fact, alcohol and drug disorders often require more complex assessment procedures than do many other medical problems.

It may be difficult within the constraints of a busy office practice to conduct a full assessment, especially with patients who are taking prescription medications such as sedatives or opioids. Clinicians who wish to refer patients with positive screenings can direct them to an addiction specialist for the diagnostic assessment. Many specialists and alcohol and drug counselors conduct the assessment in a hospital setting or in the physician's office and work with the physician, the patient, and family members in developing a treatment plan.

Persons who screen positively for any current tobacco use should be asked about the number of cigarettes used per day; the greater the number of cigarettes, the higher the rate of relapse. Patients who need a wake-up cigarette first thing in the morning often require pharmacotherapy to reduce the severity of withdrawal symptoms. The number of previous

Table 21–2. Presenting complaints of patients and family members.

Person With Substance-Use Disorder	Family Members
Respiratory	*Medical symptoms*
Asthma	Headaches
Bronchitis	Sleep disorders
Emphysema	Psychosomatic complaints
Lung cancer	
Cardiovascular	*Abuse:* verbal, physical, sexual
Hypertension	Trauma
Chest pain	Posttraumatic stress disorder
Gastrointestinal	*Psychiatric symptoms*
Chronic epigastric pain	Depression
Liver disease	Generalized anxiety disorders
Pancreatitis	Panic attacks
Diarrhea	Suicide
Musculoskeletal	*Childhood behavior*
Sprains	Diminished academic performance
Fractures	Relationship problems
Chronic pain syndromes	Sociopathic behavior
	Truancy
	Stealing
Nervous system	*Additional difficulties*
Memory loss	Legal problems
Amotivational syndrome	Commitment issues
Chronic fatigue	Court testimony about abuse
Psychiatric	*Financial issues*
Depression	Requests for sick leave or disability payments
Suicide	Inability to pay medical (or other) bills
Anxiety	
Posttraumatic stress disorder	

attempts to quit and the longest period of nonuse are also helpful data. A focused physical examination and pulmonary function testing can be invaluable in providing evidence of end-organ damage and thereby facilitating efforts to stop smoking.

Persons who drink more than the established limits should be assessed for current and potential alcohol-related problems and symptoms of dependence or addiction. Patients should be asked whether their use of alcohol has caused any problems—family, work, health—in their lives: "Have you ever been arrested for drunk driving? " "Have you ever lost a job because of your drinking? " "Does anyone in your family ever get mad at you because of your drinking? " "Has a doctor ever advised you to cut down or stop drinking?"

A review of potential medical—cardiovascular, neurologic, gastrointestinal, and sexually transmitted diseases (including risk for HIV infection)—and psychiatric effects is an important component of the assessment. A focused physical examination (eg, blood pressure, cardiac rhythm, abdomen) and appropriate laboratory tests (eg, liver function) may detect alcohol-related end-organ damage. Although most patients with alcohol abuse disorders (at-risk users, problem drinkers) have minimal or no health problems related to alcohol use, early identification of at-risk drinking may prevent further alcohol damage. This information can also serve as a powerful tool to convince patients to become abstinent.

The last area of the assessment is to ask about such symptoms of alcohol dependence as loss of control and symptoms of withdrawal: "Have you ever tried to cut down on your alcohol use? " "Have you ever been unable to stop drinking once you started? " "Do you ever drink in the morning to relieve the shakes? " Additional areas of inquiry with patients who respond positively include questions about tolerance levels ("How many drinks does it take to get high? "), their preoccupation with use (eg, planning activities around drinking), and continued use despite alcohol-related health problems. Physicians should always probe for suicidal ideation and symptoms of depression in patients with evidence of alcohol dependence.

Persons who have a history of chronic use of prescription drugs with addictive properties (sedatives, hypnotics, and narcotics) should be assessed for symptoms of dependence or addiction. Symptoms of dependence include increasing the dose without consulting the physician, obtaining additional medications from other physicians, using the medication to get high rather than for its primary purpose, purchasing extra medication from nonmedical sources, and concomitant use of illicit drugs. A history of treatment for alcohol or illicit drug use warrants further exploration. Patients with any of these symptoms should have a full assessment by an addiction specialist before the primary care clinician prescribes any additional medication.

Persons who screen positively for illicit drug use (defined as five or more times in their lifetime) should be assessed for their current level of use, problems related to use, and symptoms of dependence or addiction. Because an environment of trust and safety is essential for accurate self-reported data on illicit drug use, the patient's right of confidentiality should be emphasized. Current levels of use are difficult to determine, however, because many patients are reluctant to reveal the extent of their use and may underreport it (see next paragraph). The interviewer needs to use straightforward, nonjudgmental questions, such as how much money patients spend a week on drugs, the frequency of use, and how many days or weeks they abstained in the last 12 months. Problems can be assessed by asking about how the drug use has affected their family, friends, and employment. Patients who use drugs on a daily basis should be asked about symptoms of withdrawal, which vary by the class of drug involved.

The primary value of drug testing in ambulatory care settings is to confirm patient self-reports, which frequently understate substance use. Confirmatory drug testing is indicated in prescribing pharmacotherapies that require accurate data on the presence of mood-altering drugs. Obtaining such information is vital before recommending the use of benzodiazepines for anxiety disorders, sedative hypnotics for sleep disorders, and opioids for acute and chronic pain control.

Physicians who prescribe these medications without accurate data on the presence or absence of such drugs as marijuana, cocaine, opioids, over-the-counter sedatives, or benzodiazepines may be prescribing inappropriately. Oversedation, drug overdoses, and falls are significant potential problems. Patients should be informed that drug testing is necessary before the physician can treat them with psychoactive drugs.

Routine screening of all patients for drug use, however, is not recommended. Although some clinicians recommend routine screening in all pregnant women, false-negative and false-positive tests are common in large clinical samples in which the prevalence of use is low. Furthermore, the legal and ethical implications of ordering a drug screen are complicated. Simply ordering a drug test could be misinterpreted by an insurance company auditor or an employer as evidence of a drug problem. Although routine mass screenings are well established in workplace settings and in the armed forces, such testing is of limited value in the clinical setting unless used for a specific indication (eg, treatment of anxiety with alprazolam).

Acute-care settings, such as emergency rooms, trauma centers, and intensive care units, are other situations that may require testing patients for drug use. Accurate data on blood alcohol levels and the presence of mood-altering drugs can be critical and directly affect treatment and patient outcome. Common circumstances in which these tests are important include altered mental status, acute psychotic symptoms, chest pain, or traumatic injuries in a patient. Such testing can be done without patient consent just as other emergency tests (eg, chemistry panels, computed tomography [CT] scans) may be performed without obtaining informed consent.

A number of methods are available to assess recent alcohol use. Alcohol can be detected in the urine, blood, saliva, and breath and is metabolized at about one drink per hour for men; for women, it is one drink in about 90 minutes. Some over-the-counter drugs, such as antihistamines and sleeping aids, and prescription medications, such as benzodiazepines and opioids, can be detected in the urine for 3–7 days. The elimination rate of these drugs and their metabolites varies; short-acting drugs such as triazolam may be detectable for only a few hours, whereas diazepam (Valium) and its metabolites have detectable levels for up for up to 7 days.

Illicit drugs are readily detectable in the urine. Physicians should determine which drug panel is needed to detect the drugs of interest; the ability to identify certain drugs varies with the technique used. Drugs that may not be included in routine panels are marijuana, methadone, anabolic steroids, and short-acting designer drugs. Whereas marijuana can be detected for up to 30 days in the urine, all other illicit drugs are cleared within 72 hours. A patient who tests positively for cocaine has used cocaine within the last 2–3 days. The detection of marijuana usually indicates active inhalation. Although passive inhalation (simply being near a smoker) can produce levels of marijuana detectable by mass spectroscopy, these are below the cut-off levels (more than 100 ng) of routine drug testing.

MANAGEMENT

Case illustration: On Mary's first visit to her doctor's office, she complains about difficulty sleeping. She is married, with two young children, and works as a waitress at a small local restaurant. Her problems with sleeping began 2 months ago, when her husband lost his job at a local factory. She is taking some Valium (10 mg at bedtime) left over from a previous prescription from another physician and is requesting a refill. A screening examination reveals occasional alcohol and marijuana use, daily tobacco consumption, a history of verbal abuse by her husband when he becomes drunk, symptoms of depression without suicidal ideation, and recurring problems with sexually transmitted diseases (STDs). The physician's initial treatment plan is to discontinue the Valium and initiate treatment for depression. Mary is placed on an antidepressant and asked to return to the office for a more complete assessment and a physical examination.

On her return visit Mary reports a reasonable response to the antidepressant. A complete assessment and physical reveal an STD infection and elevated liver function tests. Further questioning reveals regular alcohol use of 12–20 drinks week. She denies any problems with alcohol withdrawal, loss of control, blackouts, legal problems, or family difficulties related to her own alcohol use. The doctor advises abstinence on the basis of the probable relationship between her depression and the abnormal liver function tests. Although Mary initially agrees with the recommendation, she is not willing to set an alcohol quit date. She does not return for her next scheduled appointment but does reschedule in response to a follow-up phone call.

The third contact with Mary reveals continued alcohol use. She is now separated from her husband, who had become increasingly abusive. She indicates that she had discontinued the antidepressant on her own shortly after her second office visit because of its side effects. At this time, she is willing to set a quit date and to sign a contract. She agrees to stop using alcohol for a period of 6 months to determine how and whether this will improve her depression, insomnia, and elevated liver function tests.

By her fourth visit, Mary has achieved abstinence and feels positive about the changes in her life since she stopped drinking. The doctor supports her efforts and encourages her to follow her abstinence contract. Mary tells the doctor about how hard it is after softball games to go out with her friends and not drink. Using traditional behavioral modification strategies, Mary and her physician discuss methods that she can use to minimize her risk of drinking. She is seen monthly for the next 6 months to follow her abstinence contract and medical and family problems. Her depression and insomnia resolve after 3 months of abstinence.

Two years later, Mary and her doctor begin to deal with her nicotine addiction; she successfully quits after two courses of medication and brief counseling. Mary continues to be followed every 6 months to support her abstinence from alcohol, tobacco, and marijuana. Eight years after her initial visit, she is still abstinent.

Advise
Brief Advice Interventions: In ambulatory care settings, the primary treatment approach is the use of brief intervention techniques—consisting of time-limited dialogues that take no more than 5–10 minutes at a single visit. Studies with tobacco and alcohol users suggest that 10–20% of persons in primary care settings reduce their substance use as a result of this approach. There is also some evidence that this technique can move patients along in the process of getting ready to change their substance use.

Although the technique has not been tested with illicit drug users, clinicians and researchers assume that those who are not dependent will also respond favorably. Information on the use of brief interventions with severely dependent persons is also limited. There are four key components of brief intervention treatment:

- State your concern as the patient's physician: "I am very concerned about how smoking and drinking are affecting your health." An empathic, nonconfrontational approach is often the most effective method. Statements should be nonjudgmental and framed in medical language. Recovering persons often state that the primary reason they became sober was because a physician asked them to stop.

- Personalize the message, using potential or real health effects associated with the substance use: "Your chronic bronchitis is caused by cigarettes." "Your hypertension is related to your drinking and may lead to a stroke." "Marijuana use may be affecting your memory." For at-risk drinkers who have not developed any consequences of their use, physicians may want to compare their alcohol-related risk with other health concerns: "Even though your drinking hasn't caused any health problems yet, you're at risk for things like liver problems, accidents, and high blood pressure."

- Discuss normative use and change patterns. A pie chart or graph shows patients how their use compares with that of others. For smokers, a pie chart can demonstrate that there are more former smokers than current smokers, with the observation that only about 25% of persons now smoke and that most smokers are trying to quit. Most at-risk and problem drinkers don't realize that fewer then 15% of adults drink as much as they do; since many of their friends are also at-risk or problem drinkers, they seem to think that everybody drinks as much as they.

- Clearly state your recommendation: "As your physician I strongly recommend that you stop smoking and cut down your drinking." "I think you have some serious medical problems because of your drinking, and I'd like you to see a specialist with more expertise in alcohol problems." "I'm concerned that you're becoming dependent on Valium, and I'd like you to participate in a treatment program." The recommendation should be as clear and specific as possible. Persons with active substance-use problems do not always think clearly or rationally; they may try to manipulate clinicians or intentionally misinterpret treatment recommendations. The statement "I would like you to consider cutting down to no more then three drinks at a time no more than 3 days a week." is more specific and less susceptible to misinterpretation than "I would like you to think about your alcohol use."

After making the recommendation, the physician may ask the patient if he or she is ready to consider making a change in substance use. Although forced interventions (eg, professionals who are told to go into treatment or lose their license, spouses who are told to go into treatment or to move out, employees who are offered the choice of treatment or loss of employment) can be effective, patients are much more likely to actively participate and change their substance use when they are in the action phase of the readiness-for-change model.

Prevention: Preventing substance abuse, especially in adolescents and pregnant women (even though their screenings are negative), is particularly important. In dealing with adolescents, the physician should discuss alternative activities and support positive choices (see Chapter 11). It is essential to talk to them about their intentions and attitudes, friends, and peer pressure, to develop a partnership and trust, and to correct any misunderstandings about the risks of tobacco, alcohol, and illicit drug use. The adolescent brain is particularly vulnerable to the adverse effects of marijuana on the central nervous system. The support of parents and other significant adults should be enlisted in assisting adolescents in setting career goals, establishing positive expectations, structuring free time, and becoming involved in school and community activities. Parents may have to be educated about the importance of their function as role models.

Women appear to be at greater risk for high-risk sexual behaviors when they are under the influence of alcohol or drugs. Clinicians may want to discuss some of these risks: sexually transmitted diseases, unwanted pregnancies, HIV infection, and sterility. Differences in metabolism that increase alcohol blood levels and associated health risks, such as liver disease, breast cancer, and hypertension, should be discussed and information presented on low-risk use. The physician should recommend abstinence for women who are considering pregnancy, as many of the severe effects of alcohol occur within the first 4 weeks of gestation.

All adults should be cautioned about the use of substances around children. Second-hand tobacco or marijuana smoke can have serious respiratory effects on young children. Drugs that are hidden—whether prescription or illicit—fascinate children, too often with fatal effects. Drug interactions are common, and persons on medications should be counseled about the possibility of serious reactions. Accidents and injury are often associated with substance use. Encouraging patients to limit substance use in potentially dangerous situations can prevent serious medical sequelae. Older adults are particularly vulnerable to the adverse effects of alcohol and other sedative drugs.

Readiness for Change

The readiness-for-change model of precontemplation, contemplation, preparation, and action can help clinicians develop a treatment plan that the patient can accept; patients who have reached the action phase are much more likely than those in the precontemplation stage to change their substance use successfully (see Chapter 16).

Precontemplation Stage: Patients should be asked whether they are interested in changing the amount of alcohol they drink (or tobacco or drugs they use) and whether they are willing to change their drinking (or smoking, etc) behavior in the next 30 days. Patients who answer no to both these questions are in the precontemplation stage and are not ready to change. For at-risk users and some problem users in this stage, it is appropriate to schedule a follow-up meeting in 1–2 months. If there are serious health problems related to the substance use, the physician may wish to push the issue further by involving the family, peers, employers, or other persons who may be able to convince the patient of the need for immediate help. Forced interventions, when done in a caring, constructive manner, can help move people to the next stage.

Contemplation Stage: Patients who are contemplating changes but aren't ready to make them in the next 30 days should be encouraged to continue to consider changing their substance use, and a follow-up appointment should be scheduled. It may take multiple visits before a patient is ready to move into the preparation and action phases. The key is to keep up the pressure. Every time the patient comes into the office, the clinician states: "I am still concerned about your marijuana use. There is more and more information that suggests serious cognitive deficits and respiratory problems with long-term marijuana use. Are you ready to make some changes in your use in the next 30 days? "

Preparation Stage: Patients who respond affirmatively to the questions are in the preparation stage. Here, clinicians can help patients develop a specific plan to change their use in the next 30 days. Patients who participate in the decision-making process are more likely to follow the plans. The physician should emphasize that it is the responsibility of the patients to change their substance use and reduce their health risks. Whenever possible, a specific date for the change should be set. For at-risk and some problem users, specific drinking goals should be based on the patient's pattern of use and health risks. In most cases, patients who are dependent users should be referred to a specialized treatment program.

Action: Patients who are ready to change their substance use are in the action stage and ready to move into the assist phase of the treatment protocol described in the following section and illustrated in Figure 21–1.

Assist

At-Risk and Problem Users: Limit Setting and Contracting: When patients are ready to change their substance use behavior, clinicians need to negotiate a use limit and set a change date. For example, the physician might suggest cutting alcohol consumption to three drinks, limited to three times a week, and ask whether the patient would like to try to decrease use to that level. If the patient hesitates, the physician should ask whether that limitation seems possible. Once a limit is agreed on, a contract might be written delineating the agreement, with both clinician and patient signing it. A change date within 30 days should be included in the contract. Weekly diary cards that list the patient's substance use can reinforce

positive changes and document the patient's progress.

In many cases, patients should be advised to abstain rather than reduce their use. Anyone using tobacco products, for example, should be advised to stop completely. Although greater use incurs greater risk, there is no safe level of tobacco use. Several categories of persons who use alcohol should be advised to abstain, including patients who have evidence of alcohol withdrawal, those who experience serious alcohol-related health effects, pregnant women, children, and adolescents. Patients on medications that interact with alcohol and other sedatives—especially those with a history of loss of control and failed attempts to limit their use, or older adults, who are especially at risk for falls and other injuries—should also be advised to abstain. Because illicit drugs are by definition illegal, anyone using these drugs should be advised to abstain.

Physicians can play a larger role in supporting changes in behavior than was previously appreciated (see Chapters 17 and 18). Follow-up visits—an essential component of office-based treatment—are necessary for the clinician to reinforce concern, support efforts, and assess behavioral changes. Clinical strategies shown to increase quit rates in smokers include follow-up phone calls by a member of the office staff, repeat office visits to encourage continued behavioral change, and repeat laboratory testing (eg, pulmonary function tests). Although the effect of follow-up visits in helping patients reduce their alcohol use has not been clearly established, such visits are part of standard medical practice, especially when there is an alcohol-related health problem.

The development of specific behavioral strategies for at-risk and problem users to help alter their substance use can supplement brief intervention techniques. Because this approach takes additional time, physicians may want to schedule another visit. Asking a family member or friend to attend the visit is helpful. The first step is to ask patients to list the positive and negative aspects of changing their substance use. The second is to ask for a list of risky situations and the triggers that often lead to substance use. The next step is to develop specific methods to cope with these situations. Patients should write the information in a diary or notebook and review the material daily; this can help them avoid high-risk situations and remind them to practice their chosen methods for changing their substance use. Once again, follow-up is important.

Physicians who want to use these techniques in their practice but do not have time may want to train a health educator, nurse, or physician's assistant in their use. An alcohol and drug counselor may be willing to provide counseling in the clinician's office rather then at a treatment center. In some cases (see later section), patients who have low levels of risk should be referred to specialized treatment programs.

Dependent Persons: Referral to Specialized Treatment Programs: Specialized treatment programs for dependent patients have become increasingly diversified over the past 10 years. Because substance-use disorders constitute a heterogeneous group of disorders and affect a wide range of persons, no single approach can be effective for the majority of patients. For example, fewer then 30% of persons with these disorders achieve abstinence with the traditional AA-based 12-step group therapy program.

1. Indications for referral–Referral to an alcohol or drug treatment program is indicated in three situations.

a. Patients who are clearly alcohol- or drug-dependent may require detoxification. Clinicians may perform the detoxification as an outpatient procedure in the office—with a treatment program available as back-up—or they may want the program's physician to monitor the patient through withdrawal. Patients at high risk for problematic withdrawal include polysubstance users, intravenous drug users, and those with medical problems. These patients include heavy smokers with emphysema who have been unable to abstain for more than 1 or 2 days, alcohol-dependent persons with a history of delirium tremens and seizures, persons using more than 5 mg of alprazolam a day, and cocaine users who are acutely suicidal after a weekend run. Once detoxification has been safely completed, patients can begin treatment for the addiction.

b. Nondependent problem users who have been unable to maintain abstinence despite the possibility of serious consequences may need referral to a treatment program. Although they may not require the intense therapy needed by persons with evidence of physical dependence, the presence of a medical or social problem suggests that continued substance use could lead to a potentially fatal condition. They should receive as much treatment as possible before their medical problems deteriorate from continued use. These users include drinkers with a history of repeated accidents, those who abuse family members when intoxicated, persons with repeated employment problems, daily users with persistent alcohol-related hypertension, and cocaine users who develop financial or legal problems.

c. Substance users who do not respond to brief intervention treatment–Patients who are unable to maintain their use at a low-risk level may require more intense therapy than can be provided in the physician's office. These are the smokers who do not respond to advice and nicotine patches, the daily drinkers who would like to cut down but who have not been successful, patients on high doses of diazepam or opioids who are unable to reduce their dose, and intermittent marijuana users who would like to stop because they now have school-age children.

2. Programs and services–The following is a summary of the major treatment approaches used by specialized treatment programs for the care of persons with alcohol and drug disorders (specialized treatment for tobacco addiction is covered in Chapter

18). Most programs use a combination of these treatment modalities.

The Minnesota model is based on the 12 steps of Alcoholics Anonymous, using group therapy and intensive confrontation techniques. Treatment is focused on breaking through the denial systems and convincing patients of the need to give up control to a higher power. This is the predominant treatment approach used in the United States.

Educational programs are aimed at helping patients understand the natural history of substance-use disorders. This approach is widely used for drunk driver programs and for persons in the contemplation stage of change.

Cognitive behavioral coping skills therapy focuses on training in interpersonal and self-management skills. Clients are taught to identify high-risk situations that may increase the likelihood of substance use. These situations include triggers that are external to the individual as well as internal events such as thoughts and emotions. Once they have identified these situations, clients are taught to cope with them.

Behavior-modification techniques involve training in the areas of stress management, the use of leisure time, communication skills, and problem solving. This patient-centered method encourages patients to accept responsibility for their substance use.

Couple and family therapy counseling methods are used to strengthen communication skills and improve interactions within the marriage and family while enlisting the spouse and family members to support the patient's efforts in treatment. The goal of couple and family therapy in the early stages of recovery is the sobriety of the identified patient. Therapy directed at family dysfunction is initiated after a stable recovery has been achieved.

Relapse-prevention techniques are intended to reduce the frequency of substance use and episodes of binge use rather than to ensure abstinence. Many patients are unable or unwilling to achieve total abstinence. This approach uses a combination of individual and group therapy techniques.

Traditional psychotherapy–Childhood trauma and the development of posttraumatic stress disorder (PTSD) are often a primary cause of substance-use disorders, especially in women. Psychotherapy can be a powerful tool to assist patients to examine these issues and to develop coping strategies to deal with the emotional trauma of these events.

Pharmacotherapy–Methadone maintenance treatment programs are the most effective treatment for opioid dependence—abstinence-based programs do not work well in this area. Nicotine replacement is an important adjunct for smoking cessation. Antabuse can be a deterrent for patients who are unable to abstain from alcohol. Other medications are in development to deal with alcohol and cocaine craving.

Detoxification–Patients withdraw from alcohol or other drugs under supervision. Many programs assist the primary care clinician in conducting detoxification on an outpatient basis (discussed further in a later section). Patients with medical problems and a history of severe withdrawal may require inpatient detoxification for 3–5 days. Older adults with mental status changes and patients with liver disease and encephalopathy may require additional time.

Residential treatment–Patients reside in a non-hospital facility for 2–4 weeks and receive a variety of treatment services. Residential treatment programs can provide a stable and structured environment for patients unable to remain abstinent long enough to benefit from outpatient treatment.

Outpatient treatment usually involves a 3- to 6-month program. Clients participate in educational programs, group therapy, and individual counseling 6–10 hours a week for 4 weeks, followed by less intensive services once they achieve an initial period of sobriety.

Half-way, or transitional, housing–An increasing number of communities have established group homes for persons trying to achieve stable recovery. Persons with limited resources can use these programs to re enter society through job-training programs, alcohol and drug counseling, and community service activities. A number of programs for impaired medical professionals use recovery houses to help clinicians achieve stable recoveries before returning to their professional careers.

Inpatient treatment is currently used for patients who have severe medical or psychiatric problems, but it has changed dramatically in the last decade. As recently as 1990, a 30-day inpatient treatment program was considered the standard of care in many communities. This practice changed as research studies demonstrated limited additional benefits from inpatient care compared with outpatient treatment. Inpatient treatment costs 3–10 times more than outpatient treatment, and the range of services provided is similar to that offered for outpatients.

Special programs for specific populations–Special populations that often require separate programs include adolescents; women; pregnant women; and patients with psychiatric disorders, substance-use problems, or both. Schizophrenic patients are a particular challenge that requires community-based approaches. Most specialized treatment programs do not work well with older adults or persons with sensory disabilities. Clients living in abusive families and broken communities also have distinct needs. Patients' attitudes toward substance use and recovery may reflect cultural differences, such as the ritual use of hallucinogenics or the acceptance of alcohol as proof of a boy's coming of age. Clinicians may need to take a broader view of recovery and tolerate some use of the substance.

Community-based mutual self-help groups, such as Alcoholics Anonymous, Narcotics Anonymous, and Cocaine Anonymous, can be an adjunct to specialized treatment programs. These organizations have also diversified and include groups specifically designed for smokers, women, older adults, cultural groups such as Native Americans, seriously mentally ill patients, and disabled persons. Many of these groups use a combination of the traditional AA 12-step program and more patient-centered and secular approaches. Mutual self-help groups for family members and friends include Al-Anon, Al-Anon-ACA (adult children of alcoholics), Alateen, and Alatot.

3. Selecting a specialized alcohol and drug treatment program–Once a clinician decides to refer patients for treatment, there are many ways to become knowledgeable about the alcohol- and drug-treatment specialists and programs in the community. It may be as simple as asking the patient's insurance carrier for a list of programs it covers; asking colleagues for the names of programs or providers they have found successful; or directly contacting a treatment specialist or program, mental health center, or hospital for consultation. The physician might also call the appropriate state agency for a list of publicly and privately funded treatment programs in the state; patients who are employed should contact the company's employee assistance program. Since many patients have limited insurance or resources to pay for alcohol or drug treatment, it is important to develop a list of publicly funded community programs. The majority of communities, even in rural areas, have county or state programs; however, the waiting list for admission or consultation with alcohol and drug counselors (especially in the cities) can be quite long.

Physicians may want to call the directors of local treatment programs to determine the range and success of services provided by their programs. They may want to inquire about the program's effectiveness: "What is your 2-year sobriety rate? " "How many patients complete your program? "; the presence of flexible treatment programs based on individual needs and family and friend participation; whether there is ongoing communication with the patient's primary care physician; the education level of the counselors; the level of physician participation in the program; and the facility's accreditation status. Referring physicians may also want to ask about the use of newer methods of treatment that are not based solely on the Minnesota model.

Clinicians should identify one or two addiction specialists within the community on whom they can call for consultation and for help in facilitating the referral process. As with other consultants, it is easier if the physician has—or can develop—a strong working relationship with the specialist.

4. Facilitating the referral process–A number of methods can increase the likelihood that patients will follow through on an alcohol or drug referral.

Tell the patient you would like a second opinion from a specialist. Emphasize the medical aspect of the referral to minimize the stereotypic response associated with referral to an alcohol treatment program. Stress the importance of the referral and emphasize that it is no different from being referred to a cardiologist for a heart condition. Set up the appointment while the patient is in the examination room or ask a member of the staff to make the appointment before the patient leaves the office.

Send a referral letter summarizing the patient's medical problems and the reason for the referral, and tell the patient you will be doing so. Patients need to sign a consent form that allows communication between the primary care clinician and the treatment program. Ask the specialist or counselor to call after the assessment or if the patient fails to show up for the appointment. Inform the consultant that you would like to participate in the treatment plan and provide long-term follow-up with visits to your office. One of the primary reasons patients do not follow through with treatment programs is the absence of communication between the referring clinician and the program staff.

Patients who lack the financial resources for private treatment can be referred to public programs as noted earlier (federal block grants and state alcohol tax revenues may provide resources for county-based programs). Another alternative is to ask the patient to attend mutual-help group meetings; in most communities several meetings are open every day to anyone interested in achieving and maintaining sobriety. Inform patients that they may need to attend several meetings in different locations to find a compatible group that fits their needs. Direct patients to specific programs likely to meet their needs. Women in particular may do better in all-female groups; such groups tend to be more sensitive to such issues as sexual and other forms of abuse. Groups that use alternatives to the 12-step approach include Rational Recovery, Women for Sobriety, and those with 116-step programs.

Outpatient Detoxification

Although the majority of patients with alcohol and drug problems can be detoxified in an outpatient setting, a number of factors must be considered.

Abstinence: Patients must agree to remain abstinent from all mood-altering agents. A clear commitment not to use drugs is essential. Patients who have ambivalent feelings and indicate they will use drugs "if things get too rough" are unlikely to benefit from an outpatient withdrawal protocol. It may be appropriate for physicians to refuse outpatient pharmacotherapy for symptoms of drug withdrawal to patients who do not meet the abstinence criteria.

Treatment: Patients should also agree to take part in a treatment program; the choice, of course, depends on personal finances and community resources. Patients must, however, commit to getting some professional help. Patients who do not agree to treatment, but insist that they can do it on their own, are unlikely to recover from their drug dependence. Such patients are likely to have a high level of denial that is difficult to overcome.

Support Systems: Patients who live alone or have no drug-free support systems are not candidates for outpatient treatment. A sober and responsible family member or friend is an integral part of outpatient medical detoxification. This person will assist the patient (and physician) in getting through the first few days of treatment. He or she can specifically aid the medical detoxification process by encouraging and assisting the patient to attend AA or NA; providing a safe, quiet, loving environment; watching for any serious withdrawal symptoms; assisting with medications; providing massages and hot baths for muscle cramps and anxiety; and minimizing the risk of relapse by helping the patient stay away from situations that may lead to relapse. It is important for the physician to discuss each of these tasks with the helper. Writing specific tasks on a prescription pad improves the likelihood of the assignments being followed through.

Physician-Patient Relationship: A trusting relationship between physician and patient is a powerful therapeutic tool; it can even help break through a seemingly impregnable denial. If the physician is also knowledgeable about the treatment of drug withdrawal, an outpatient treatment plan is more likely to work. Patients should be evaluated daily until the risk of withdrawal problems is minimal and the patient has started a treatment rehabilitation program. This may be 3 days for alcohol abuse, or 10 days for long-acting benzodiazepines, methamphetamine, opioids, and even cocaine. Weekend contact with the patient and support person is extremely important since the risk of relapse is greater on Saturday and Sunday.

Withdrawal and Pharmacology: The use of drugs for which pharmacologic intervention is often needed include alcohol, sedatives, stimulants, and opioids; cannabinoids, PCP, hallucinogens, inhalants, and anabolic steroids are seldom associated with withdrawal symptoms. Patients with a history of mild withdrawal symptoms are likely to develop similar withdrawal syndromes the next time they become abstinent. Mild tremor, anxiety, and tachycardia are a common occurrence when alcohol-, barbiturate-, and tranquilizer-dependent patients reduce or stop their use of these substances. Patients who have previously developed withdrawal seizures, delirium, or psychosis, however, are likely to develop significant withdrawal symptoms and should be admitted for observation and probable pharmacologic treatment.

Patients with a high tolerance who are taking the equivalent of more than 60 mg of diazepam a day are not candidates for outpatient treatment. Equivalent doses for other benzodiazepines are 300 mg chlordiazepoxide (Librium) = 12 mg lorazepam (Ativan) = 5 mg alprazolam (Xanax). Medical contraindications for outpatient treatment include a history of a recent head trauma or cerebrovascular accidents, acute abdominal pain, unstable liver function, pneumonia, sepsis, arrhythmias, angina, a recent history of ischemic heart disease, or severe respiratory disease.

1. Medications–The most widely used medications for the treatment of alcohol and sedative withdrawal are the benzodiazepines. Clinical trials have shown benzodiazepines to be more effective than placebo or no-drug therapy in decreasing anxiety, restlessness, tremor, and seizure and in preventing the development of stages 2 and 3 withdrawal. Phenobarbital for detoxification has several advantages over the benzodiazepines, however, particularly in polydrug abuse, hepatic dysfunction, and potential seizure.

2. Dosage–The major principle to follow in the use of these medications is to use a high enough dose in the first 24–48 hours. Medication is much less effective once major withdrawal symptoms have developed. Benzodiazepines can be administered with a high loading dose at the outset; tapering is unnecessary for long-acting benzodiazepines such as diazepam and chlordiazepoxide. A normal dosing regimen for outpatient detoxification is 10 mg of diazepam every 2 hours until the patient is sedated. Patients with low tolerance may be adequately sedated with a total of 10–20 mg, whereas others may require 60 mg in the first 24 hours. If a patient requires more than 60 mg to achieve sedation, a short inpatient stay would be indicated. Additional diazepam is usually given for 3–4 days, at doses of 10 mg two or three times a day.

Brief Counseling Methods for Ambivalent Patients

Patients who are ambivalent about changing their drinking patterns need to be approached quite differently from those who are ready to change. Physicians can help patients resolve their ambivalence by encouraging them to explore their feelings about their substance use. Motivation to change is greatly enhanced when patients can acknowledge that they are uncomfortable with their current substance-use behavior. The following can be helpful:

- **Ask about life-style and health concerns.** Clinicians who suspect that substance use is affecting the patient's life-style and health can ask such questions as "How have you been feeling since your last visit?" "Are you feeling fit?" "How do you think your drinking affects your physical fitness and health?"

- **Help patients identify both the positive and less-than-positive aspects of drinking.** The physician can help patients become more aware of personal feeling about drinking by asking, "What do you enjoy about drinking?" "What are some of the not-so-good things about your drinking?" "What personal goals are important to you (eg, family, physical fitness, career enhancement)?" "Does drinking interfere with meeting any of these goals?" The physician should summarize the patient's responses and ask whether the summary accurately reflects what has been stated. The patient's feelings and perceptions about alcohol use should be respected.

- **Help patients express their concerns.** Physicians should ask their patients to reflect on the less positive aspects of drinking by asking questions such as "What would be different about your life if you changed your drinking habits?" "What do you think might happen if you don't change them?" "Give me some examples of concerns you have about your drinking." "In what ways has drinking caused you problems?" The physician should offer information about the aspects of drinking that apply to the patient's concerns (a patient experiencing sleep problems, for example, should be reminded of the effects of alcohol on sleep) and the patient's reactions to the information elicited.

- **Help with decision making.** The patient's ideas should be sought with such questions as "Now that we've discussed some issues related to your drinking, what do you think you might do?" "Are you ready to consider a change?" Patients who are ready to consider change should be asked whether they want the physician's help to get started. The physician should make patients aware that some strategies to change behavior work better than others. It is important not to be overly concerned if commitment to change fluctuates; this is a normal part of the change process. If patients are still willing to consider a change after a relapse, the physician should offer to help when they are ready and continue to monitor the substance-use behavior at each subsequent visit.

SUGGESTED READINGS

Anderson P et al: Risk of alcohol. Addiction 1993;88: 1493.

Babor T, Stephens R, Marlatt G: Verbal report methods in clinical research on alcoholism: Response bias and its minimization. J Stud Alcohol 1987;48:410.

Bien T, Miller W, Tonigan S: Brief interventions for alcohol problems: A review. Addiction, 1993;88:315.

Fleming MF, Barry KL (editors): *Addictive Disorders.* Mosby-Year Book, 1992.

Institute of Medicine, Division of Mental Health and Behavioral Medicine: *Broadening the base of treatment for alcohol problems.* National Academy Press, 1990.

Miller WR, Rollnick S: *Motivational Interviewing: Preparing People to Change Addictive Behavior.* Guilford Press, 1991.

National Institute on Alcohol Abuse and Alcoholism: A physician's guide to helping patients with alcohol problems. United States Public Health Service, 1995.

National Institute on Alcohol Abuse and Alcoholism: *Eighth Annual Report to Congress on Alcohol and Health.* United States Public Health Service, 1993.

National Institute on Alcohol Abuse and Alcoholism: *A Clinical Guide for Therapists Treating Individuals with Alcohol Abuse and Dependence:. Cognitive-Behavioral Coping Skills Therapy Manual.* Department of Health and Human Services, DHSS # ADM 92-1895,1992.

Phelps G, Field P: Drug testing: Clinical and workplace issues. In: Fleming MF, Barry KL (editors): *Addictive Disorders.* Mosby Yearbook, 1992.

Prochaska JO, DiClemente CC: Stages of change in the modification of problem behaviors. In: Hersen M, Eisler RM, Miller PM (editors): *Progress in Behavior Modification.* Sycamore Press, 1992.

Robins L et al: National Institute of Mental Health diagnostic interview schedule. Arch Gen Psychiatry 1981; 38:381.

Solberg L, Kottke T: Smoking cessation strategies. In: Fleming MF, Barry KL (editors): *Addictive Disorders.* Mosby-Year Book, 1992.

Trachtenberg A, Fleming MF: Essentials of drug abuse for the family physician. Am Acad Fam Phys Mono Ser Summer, 1994.

Zweben A, Pearlman S, Selena L: A comparison of brief advice and conjoint therapy in the treatment of alcohol abuse: The results of the marital system study. Br J Addict 1988;83:899.

Section IV.
Mental & Behavioral Disorders

Depression

22

*Steven A. Cole, MD, John F. Christensen, PhD, Mary A. Raju, RN, MSN, &
Mitchell D. Feldman, MD, MPhil*

INTRODUCTION

Depression is common, disabling, and often unrecognized or inadequately treated in general medical practice. This chapter focuses on the diagnosis and management of major depression. Other mood disorders are briefly discussed, including chronic depression (dysthymia), minor depression (adjustment disorder with depressed mood and depression not otherwise specified [NOS]), depression secondary to general medical conditions, and bipolar disorder (Table 22–1).

DEFINITIONS

Major depression (MD), the most severe form of depression, is associated with considerable disability, morbidity, and mortality. Epidemiologic studies demonstrate that depression is associated with as much, and often more, physical and social disability as other chronic illnesses, such as diabetes, arthritis, hypertension, and coronary artery disease. The increased risk of death seen in patients with depression is only partially attributable to the increased risk of suicide. Recent studies indicate a 59% increase in mortality among nursing home patients with major depression and a threefold increased risk of mortality among postmyocardial infarction patients with comorbid major depression.

Chronic depression, or **dysthymia** is a milder but chronic form of depressive illness that is associated with significant disability. Dysthymia is diagnosed when depressed mood and at least two other symptoms of depression are present "most days" during the previous 2 years.

Minor depression, which causes functional impairment but does not meet the criteria for major depression, includes adjustment disorder with depressed mood and depressive disorder not otherwise specified (NOS). **Adjustment disorder with depressed mood**

results from an identifiable stressor, such as divorce or job loss. It presents with a level of impairment greater than is expected for most individuals and can be diagnosed within the first 6 months after a stressor has occurred. A "normal" reaction to a distressing life event should not be diagnosed as an adjustment disorder. When a stressor precipitates a depressive syndrome that meets the severity criteria for major depression, the diagnosis of major depression is made. **Depressive disorder NOS** is a condition that lasts longer than 6 months after a precipitating stressor. Depression NOS is also used to describe mixed states of anxiety-depression that do not meet criteria for other anxiety or depressive diagnoses.

Mood disorders due to a general medical condition (or substance) refers to a psychiatric syndrome judged to result from the direct physiologic consequence of a general medical condition (eg, hypothyroidism), substance use (eg, amphetamine withdrawal), or medication (eg, reserpine). Treatment focuses on resolution of the underlying general medical problem or withdrawal of the offending medication, although specific psychiatric treatment may also be required.

Bipolar disorder (also known as "manic-depressive" illness) is a common and severe mental illness that occurs in about 1% of the population and carries a strong genetic vulnerability. Patients with presumptive diagnoses of depression should always be screened for bipolar disorder.

Table 22–1. Mood disorders.

1. Major depression
2. Chronic depression (dysthymia)
3. Minor depression
   a. Adjustment disorder with depressed mood
   b. Depression NOS (not otherwise specified)
4. Depression secondary to a general medical condition
5. Bipolar disorder

EPIDEMIOLOGY

Epidemiologic studies demonstrate a lifetime prevalence of major depression in 7–12% of men and 20–25% of women. The point prevalence of major depression in a community sample is 2.3–3.2% for men and 4.5–9.3% for women. Reasons for these gender differences have not been fully elucidated, but both biological and sociocultural factors are involved. Numerous studies report a 5–10% prevalence of major depression in primary care settings with a substantially higher rate in patients with coexisting medical problems, particularly in those with diseases associated with strong biological or psychologic predispositions to depression (eg, stroke, Parkinson's disease, traumatic brain injury, pancreatic cancer, and other terminal illnesses).

Prevalence of depression varies among age groups. Recent data point to a cohort effect through which current "baby boomers" (age 35–50 years) experience the highest rates of depression of any previous generation. Although the most current epidemiologic findings show a surprisingly low 1-year prevalence rate of major depression in the elderly (1–2%), the rate of major or minor depression in elderly patients who seek treatment in primary care practices is 5%, with rates ranging from 15% to 25% in nursing home residents. Major depression is often misdiagnosed in elderly primary care patients as signs of aging, and cognitive impairment may also complicate accurate diagnosis. Some medications commonly prescribed in the elderly population may actually precipitate the onset of depression. Since the usual age of onset of depression is under 40, an apparent first episode of depression in an older patient should prompt a thorough evaluation to exclude other underlying disease and medication effects.

Depression is often mistakenly believed to be "expected" in the face of stressful life events. Studies of individuals under stress (eg, terminal cancer, natural disaster, etc) do show rates of major depression above the general population rate, but these rates rarely exceed 50%. Although sad or depressed affect is an expected accompaniment of a stressful event, the full syndrome of major depression does not necessarily emerge. Thus, there may be "good reasons" for sadness, but no good reasons to explain away a syndrome of major depression. If such a syndrome emerges following a stressful life situation, the primary care provider should strongly consider the diagnosis of major depression and treat it appropriately.

The term *reactive depression* has historically suggested a mild syndrome without a biological substrate, resulting from a psychologic precipitant and treatable with psychotherapy alone. None of these assumptions are true. A very severe depressive syndrome can result from a stressful event; a biologically predisposed individual may suffer major depression in response to a life event; a major depression resulting from a life stress may develop a biological substrate; and a major depression from a life stress may respond, as well or better, to biological therapy than to psychotherapy. Thus, the presence or absence of identifiable precipitants is irrelevant to the diagnosis of major depression, which can be treated pharmacologically whether or not the condition resulted in part from psychological stressors.

A comorbid general medical condition (such as cancer or Parkinson's disease) may seemingly "cause" many of the physical symptoms of major depression, such as fatigue, anorexia, or psychomotor retardation. These symptoms may lead clinicians to discount their relevance and thus disregard the possibility of a treatable depression. Emerging data and the revised American Psychiatric Association *Diagnostic and Statistical Manual of Mental Disorders,* 4th edition (*DSM-IV*) criteria for major depression emphasize the importance of including these symptoms in the diagnostic approach to depression in the medically ill. Although an inclusive approach might seem to overdiagnose major depression, studies in stroke, Parkinson's disease, and traumatic brain injury indicate that the problem of overdiagnosis is, if anything, quite low (around 2%).

ETIOLOGY

Major depression represents a heterogeneous group of disorders, most probably arising from a host of etiologic determinants. Since no clear anatomic, biochemical, or physiologic lesions have been found to explain major depression, most investigators agree that it is a complex psychobiological syndrome that can only be diagnosed on clinical, syndromal criteria. Some promising genetic, biological, and psychosocial studies, however, suggest etiologic possibilities as well as therapeutic interventions.

GENETIC FACTORS

Research to date identifies a combination of environmental and biological factors underlying severe mood disorders. Apparently, genetic and family experiences each play their roles, though neither are determining factors. For example, even for bipolar disorder, which has very strong genetic loading, monozygotic twins may experience a 50% concordance prevalence rate, whereas dizygotic twins show a 10% concordance rate (about the same as siblings). Recent data from twin studies on depression in women indicate that genetic factors play the strongest etiologic role in depression, followed by recent (as opposed to early environmental) negative life events. Animal studies, on the other hand, demonstrate that early environmental stress predisposes to biological abnormalities associated with depression that may not emerge until adult life.

BIOLOGICAL FACTORS

Numerous biological "markers" of depression have been identified. Although these factors may underlie major depression, they do not necessarily "cause" it. Environmental stress can lead to psychic distress precipitating a biological cascade eventuating in major depression. Several biological markers reliably and statistically differentiate groups with and without major depression, but no marker is specific enough to be used diagnostically.

Some markers include endocrine factors: elevated cortisol; inability to suppress endogenous cortisol production after receiving exogenous dexamethasone (DST); blunted response of thyroid-stimulating hormone (TSH) to thyroglobulin-releasing factor (TRF); and increased growth hormone response to prolactin. Central nervous system levels of norepinephrine (NE) and serotonin (5-hydroxytryptamine: 5-HT) may be altered, but more likely, NE or 5-HT receptor function (or both) or number are affected by depression. Platelet imipramine or platelet paroxetine binding have been identified as markers of central serotonin activity. Major depression also impairs sleep physiology, with early induction of REM sleep and overall increase of REM density. Positron emission tomography studies point to anatomically specific metabolic differences between depressed individuals and controls.

SOCIAL & PSYCHOLOGICAL FACTORS

Significant psychosocial stressors, especially those involving loss, often trigger a depression. The loss of a parent or spouse, the end of a relationship, and events involving loss of self-esteem, such as termination from a job, seem to be especially vulnerable periods for patients. It is important that the primary care provider not overlook or explain away a major depression because of the presence of a major life event. In addition, the absence or perceived lack of social supports increases an individual's vulnerability to depression in the face of life stressors.

The postpartum "blues" typically occurs in 50–80% of women within 1–5 days of childbirth and lasts up to 1 week. This "normal" reaction should be distinguished from postpartum psychosis that occurs in 0.5–2.0/1000 deliveries and typically begins 2–3 days after delivery. It is also distinct from nonpsychotic depression that occurs in 10–15% of women in the first 3–6 months after childbirth.

Table 22–2. Diagnosis of major depression.

1. Depressed mood
2. Anhedonia (lack of interest or pleasure in almost all activities
3. Sleep disorder (insomnia or hypersomnia)
4. Appetite loss, weight loss; appetite gain or weight gain
5. Fatigue or loss of energy
6. Psychomotor retardation or agitation
7. Trouble concentrating or trouble making decisions
8. Low self-esteem or guilt
9. Recurrent thoughts of death or suicidal ideation
10. Five symptoms from the preceding list, but depressed mood or anhedonia is required. The symptoms must all have been present most of the day, nearly every day for 2 weeks.

DIAGNOSIS

DSM-IV criteria for major depression (MD) require that five out of nine symptoms be present for a 2-week period (Table 22–2). One of these nine symptoms must be either a persistent depressed mood (present most of the day, nearly every day) **or** pervasive anhedonia (loss of interest or pleasure in living).

Thus, clinicians should realize that a depressed mood is not synonymous with major depression. Depressed mood is neither necessary nor sufficient for a diagnosis of major depression. Sadness (or tearfulness) does not constitute major depression (the four other symptoms described in the following paragraph are necessary), and, conversely, major depression can be diagnosed without the presence of depressed mood (if pervasive anhedonia is present).

Clinical evaluation can be facilitated by organizing these nine symptoms into clusters of four hallmarks: (1) depressed mood; (2) anhedonia; (3) physical symptoms (sleep disorder, appetite problem, fatigue, psychomotor changes); and (4) psychological symptoms (difficulty concentrating or indecisiveness, guilt or low self-esteem, and hopelessness). Physical symptoms predict a favorable response to biological intervention. For example, when middle insomnia is present (awaking at 3 or 4 AM with inability to return to sleep) and when a diurnal variation in mood is present (feeling more depressed in AM), patients are more likely to respond to biological interventions.

THE MEDICAL INTERVIEW

The medical interview is the key to the assessment of major depression. Efficient assessment involves attention to data-gathering as well as rapport-building functions of the interview. Physicians should observe nonverbal cues: for example, a sad mood may be communicated by downcast eyes, slow speech, wrinkled brow, or tearful affect. When a depressed mood is detected or emotional distress is suspected, physicians should use open-ended questions and facilitation techniques to allow patients the opportunity to discuss the issues that are troubling them (see Chapter 1).

Physicians screening specifically for depression should focus on anhedonia ("What do you do for a good time? ") or sleep ("How is your sleep? "). These questions often yield positive responses, despite the patient's focus on physical complaints or tendency to deny depressed mood. The lack of capacity for pleasure is a central hallmark of major depression.

BARRIERS TO DIAGNOSIS

Patient Barriers

Somatic Presentations: Many patients with MD present with problems such as pain (headache, backache), fatigue, insomnia, dizziness, or gastrointestinal problems. Such somatizing patients seldom state or even recognize the fact that they may be depressed. In these patients, evaluating both general medical and psychiatric problems simultaneously saves time, expense, and frustration for both physician and patient.

Stigma: Many patients and families are reluctant to accept the diagnosis of depression because of its associated social stigma. Physicians sometimes also avoid diagnosing depression because of this stigma. Physicians can help overcome this barrier by understanding and explaining to patients and families that depression is a common and treatable illness, like other medical illnesses. Depression represents a chemical imbalance that can, like diabetes and other medical conditions, be corrected or managed with adequate treatment.

Clinician Barriers

At least 50% of depressed patients are either undetected or are not adequately treated by primary care providers. Inadequate knowledge and skill, lack of time, reluctance to "open up" new domains of emotional distress, and financial discrimination all operate as barriers to recognition and treatment.

"Pandora's Box": Physicians often feel reluctant to pursue psychiatric or emotional problems for fear this will open a "Pandora's box" and take an unreasonable amount of time. Attention to emotional issues, however, can be efficient and cost-effective when physicians respond to patients' emotions and appropriately manage psychiatric disorders. Time can be conserved, while minimizing the number of extended work-ups for nonspecific physical complaints.

Financial Discrimination: Providers may avoid the diagnosis and treatment of mental disorders because coding for counseling or pharmacotherapy of depression may not be reimbursed at all or may be reimbursed at lower rates than treatment of general medical conditions.

SUICIDE

Suicide is one of the top 10 causes of death in all age groups, one of the top 3 causes in young adults and teenagers, and needs to be evaluated in all patients with symptoms of depression. Risk factors for completed suicide include gender (elderly white males are at highest risk), alcoholism, psychosis, chronic physical illness, and lack of social support. Higher risk of suicide has also been noted among adolescents (see Chapter 11) and among gay and lesbian patients (see Chapter 14). Explicit suicidal intent, hopelessness, and a well-formulated plan indicate high risk. In assessing the risk of a stated plan for suicide, clinicians can use the mnemonic **SAL.** Is the method **S**pecific? Is it **A**vailable? Is it **L**ethal? Many patients who eventually commit suicide visit a primary care physician in the month before they take their lives.

The assessment of suicidal ideation is best approached gradually, with general questions like, "Do you sometimes feel that life is not worth living? " Eventually, the patient needs to be asked directly, "Do you ever feel like hurting yourself, or actually taking your own life? " Other approaches to this issue are summarized in Table 22–3.

Physicians are sometimes reluctant to explore suicidal ideation in the mistaken belief that asking about suicide may actually increase a patient's risk. To the contrary, assessment of suicidal tendencies usually reassures patients, reduces anxiety for both patient and provider, and facilitates partnership in suicide prevention.

Once a patient reveals suicidal ideation, the physician must consider psychiatric consultation and hospitalization. This clinical judgment has no absolute decision rules. The presence of risk factors should be kept in mind, but clinical judgment remains primary. If outpatient management is considered, physicians should rely on a "no suicide contract." Although no data on the effectiveness of this technique exists, it represents the standard for practice. The no suicide contract involves asking the patient to promise the physician that he or she will contact the physician (or other appropriate caregiver) if there is a danger of losing control of a suicidal impulse. Clinicians should be cautioned, however, that having obtained a no suicide contract with a patient may give the clinician a false

Table 22–3. Questions for the suicidal patient.

1. How does the future look to you?
2. Do you ever feel that life is not worth living?
3. Do you sometimes feel it doesn't matter whether you live or die?
4. Have you ever considered taking your own life?
5. Have you developed a plan about how you might kill yourself?
6. Are you willing to promise me that you will call me (or this number) if you feel you cannot control an impulse to take your own life?

sense of security. Consequently, it is important to continue assessing suicide risk according to the indicators mentioned earlier throughout the course of the patient's depression.

SCREENING TOOLS

Studies in primary care have reported that approximately 50% of cases of depression are not diagnosed. Clinicians can miss the diagnosis if they do not perform routine screening on their patients. Screening tools for depression (eg, Zung Depression Scale and the Beck Depression Scale) and other disorders have proven useful in the past for the detection of psychiatric symptoms. These need to be followed by specific physician interviews in order the make the accurate clinical diagnosis. Studies have indicated that these instruments are highly sensitive for detecting depressive disorders but have a low specificity for the actual diagnosis of major depression.

A variety of new and potentially more valuable tools are now available for primary care physicians to help in the assessment and management of mental disorders and particularly in the assessment and management of depression. PRIME-MD was developed as a two-part instrument to assess five *DSM-IV* disorders commonly seen in primary care (depression, anxiety, substance abuse, somatization, and eating disorders). The first part is a paper-and-pencil screen completed independently by patients, followed up by a structured, brief physician interview if the patient scores positive for any of the disorders on the screening instrument. This tool has been shown to have a reliability and validity comparable to an independent psychiatric interview for the five disorders.

The Symptom-Driven Diagnostic System for Primary Care (SDDS-PC) and the DSM-IV-PC are two other screening and assessment tools for use in primary care. *DSM-IV-PC* represents an adaptation of the *DSM-IV* for use in primary care. It was developed by task groups of psychiatrists, family physicians, internists, and obstetrician-gynecologists. It focuses on the diagnostic criteria and assessment approaches (with decision trees) for nine categories of common mental disorders as well as common behavioral disturbances encountered in primary care. It has not been fully tested in clinical settings but seems to have great promise.

PHYSICAL EXAMINATION

There are no specific diagnostic signs of depression. Some nonverbal cues, however, are suggestive (eg, wrinkled brow, downcast eyes, slow speech, psychomotor retardation or agitation, hand wringing, sighing, or shoulder-shrugging). A careful medical history and physical examination is required for the evaluation of depression, at all ages, but especially in the elderly.

LABORATORY STUDIES

No laboratory studies can definitely diagnose major depression. A laboratory screen (complete blood count, chemistry profile, urinalysis, thyroid-stimulating hormone, and vitamin B_{12} levels), however, can rule out other conditions that may mimic or exacerbate depression. In treatment-resistant cases, or when indicated, a computed tomographic (CT) scan, magnetic resonance image (MRI), electroencephalogram (EEG), or lumbar puncture (LP) can be considered, but these studies do not need to be part of the standard work-up. Patients over age 40 usually require an electrocardiogram (EKG) to rule out conduction disturbances or bradycardia, especially if treatment with a tricyclic antidepressant is anticipated.

DIFFERENTIAL DIAGNOSIS

Mental Disorders
Other mental disorders also present with symptoms similar to depression and may, therefore, lead to misdiagnosis. In addition, depression often presents in combination with other mental disorders. Thus, knowledge of the other mental disorders common in primary care is essential. In general, the best way to approach the issue of psychiatric comorbidity is to evaluate the patient for major depression and treat the depression if it is present. Modifications of treatment may be necessary depending on the comorbidity present.

Anxiety Disorders
Anxiety is as common as depression in primary care. Anxiety is present in most cases of major depression, and depressive symptoms are common in anxiety disorders. The most important anxiety disorders for the primary care physician are generalized anxiety disorder (GAD), panic disorder (PD), and obsessive-compulsive disorder (OCD). Central features of these disorders include pervasive and disabling anxiety (GAD), discrete panic attacks (PD), or the presence of unreasonable and recurrent behaviors or thoughts (OCD). Treatment of major depression by itself, however, often helps to resolve or improve these other coexisting conditions (see Chapter 23).

Somatoform Disorders
Because depression often presents with unexplained bodily complaints, the differentiation between a depressive illness and a somatoform disorder can be difficult (see Chapter 24). Depressive disorders are highly treatable, but somatoform disorders can be more chronic and refractory to treatment. Somatoform disorders are usually managed conservatively with a focus on improved functioning, whereas depression should be treated aggressively with the goal of complete recovery. Any of the somatoform disorders (conversion, somatization, hypochondriasis,

body dysmorphic disorder, and somatoform pain disorder) can present comorbidly with major depression. Most patients with somatization disorder experience a major depression sometime in their lives.

Primary care physicians should focus on recognizing the symptoms of major depression. Despite the presence of a somatoform disorder, appropriate treatment of the MD usually improves the somatoform disorder. With treatment of a comorbid depression, somatoform patients typically feel somewhat better, improve their functioning, and decrease their inappropriate use of general medical services.

Substance Abuse

Patients with alcoholism or other substance abuse problems commonly present with MD. Physicians should be cautious about treating major depression in the context of substance abuse to avoid further enabling the abuse problem. Rather, the problem of the substance abuse needs aggressive intervention and treatment. Unlike anxiety disorders or somatoform disorders, treatment of MD comorbid with alcoholism does not usually alleviate the substance abuse problem. Physicians need to evaluate patients for substance abuse and design separate treatment programs whether or not MD is present. Mental health referral is usually indicated in such cases (see Chapter 21).

Personality Disorders

Personality disorders represent enduring character patterns that are deeply ingrained and not generally amenable to alteration (see Chapter 25). They often complicate the diagnosis and management of mood disorders. Because patients with personality disorders can be difficult and demanding, physicians often try to minimize contact with them. Unfortunately, this may lead to avoidance of emotional issues and failure to diagnose depression.

Effective treatment of the MD often improves functioning when the depression coexists with a personality disorder, even if the underlying disorder is not fundamentally changed. Thus, physicians should evaluate the basic symptoms of depression in all distressed individuals, whether or not they have a comorbid personality disorder.

Dementia

In its early stages, dementia can be difficult to distinguish from depression. Depression leads to reversible cognitive impairment in the form of decreased concentration, memory difficulties, impaired decision-making ability, difficulty planning and organizing, and difficulty getting started on tasks. These are also impairments that can result from an irreversible dementing process. Likewise the effect of dementia on a person's functioning can lead to depressed mood. When diagnostic uncertainty exists,

Table 22–4. General medical conditions with high prevalence of depression.

Disease/Condition
Alzheimer's disease
End-stage renal failure
Parkinson's disease
Stroke
Cancer or AIDS
Chronic fatigue
General outpatient
Chronic pain

Source: Adapted, with permission, from Cohen-Cole SA, Kaufman K: Major depression in physical illness: Diagnosis, prevalence, and antidepressant treatment (A ten-year review: 1982–1992). *Depression* 1993;9:181.

clinicians can treat the depressive component (with both medication and counseling) and observe for changes in the patient's cognitive symptom cluster.

Depression Due to General Medical Conditions or Medications

Approximately 10–15% of all depression is caused by general medical illness. The diagnosis of "depression due to a general medical condition" is recognized by DSM-IV as a psychiatric condition and is considered to be the direct physiologic result of a medical illness, such as hypothyroidism or hyperthyroidism, pancreatic cancer, Parkinson's disease, or left-sided strokes (Table 22–4). Since there are no clear criteria to help guide clinicians in their evaluation, this diagnosis is ultimately made on clinical inference, considering the timing of the depression in relation to the physical illness. The diagnosis becomes "depression due to a general medical condition, with major depressive episode" when five out of nine of the symptoms of major depression are present. Data seem to indicate that standard treatments for major depression are effective in these cases.

Similarly, depression can be caused by exogenous medications (Table 22–5). For example, reserpine has long been known to cause a severe depressive condition in 15% of patients. Of critical importance is the understanding that no medication has been noted to "cause" depression in all patients. It is, therefore, crucial to carefully evaluate the clinical history and link the onset of depressive symptoms to the initiation of new medications or changes in the current regimen.

Table 22–5. Medications that can cause depression.

- Antihypertensives
- Hormones
- Anticonvulsants
- Steroids
- Digitalis
- Antiparkinsonian agents
- Antineoplastic agents
- Antibiotics

TREATMENT

Communicating With Depressed Patients

The process of the clinician's communication with a depressed patient should take into account the patient's slower rate of cognitive processing. Since busy primary care providers are used to processing information at a high volume, the mismatch between the provider's and the depressed patient's rate of processing can be equivalent to having a 28,800-baud modem interfacing with one that is operating at 1200 baud or slower. Consequently, it is important to present information in smaller chunks and allow silences for the patient to assimilate the information. Empathy skills appropriate to the relationship-building function of the medical interview (see Chapter 1) are important here. A simple reflection by the clinician of how bad the patient is feeling enhances rapport.

Presenting the Diagnosis

After eliciting symptoms from the patient, the clinician can summarize them as a preface to stating simply that "these symptoms indicate to me that you are suffering from depression." It can be helpful to then add a couple of additional symptoms not mentioned by the patient, but which are often part of the depressed constellation, such as difficulty concentrating or making decisions. By adding these symptoms, the clinician can check out with the patient their presence or absence and, if present, enhance the patient's perception of the clinician's knowledge about this disease.

Since some patients may associate depression with a stigma, it is helpful to explain MD as a common biological disorder. Drawing a picture of a synapse and neurotransmitters may be helpful to some patients. It is often helpful to name famous people, such as Thomas Jefferson or Abraham Lincoln, who are known to have suffered from depression and yet led productive lives.

A crucial part of presenting the diagnosis is to instill hope that depression is a curable illness. The cure involves mobilizing resources in the patient (see the section on "Counseling by Physician") and sometimes external resources such as medication. Indicate that painful depressive symptoms can be relieved in time, and note that "others may notice improvements in you before you notice the change yourself" (see Chapter 6). When adverse life circumstances play a role in the cause of MD, the physician can acknowledge the role played by the stressors, but the doctor must also help the patient understand that treatment of the MD can help him or her cope better with life's adversities.

Case illustration: A 45-year-old single woman came in to see her primary care physician complaining of abdominal pain and "nervous exhaustion." In the interview her physician noted that her affect was flat and that she spoke with long latencies. She was having trouble sleeping, frequently awakening after 4 hours' sleep with perspiration, heart palpitations, and obsessive worries about her job. She had assumed a new job 4 months earlier as manager of a hospital clinic that was converting to a new data management system. After the physician ascertained that the patient was not suicidal, she summarized the patient's concerns and presented her diagnosis in the following dialogue:

DOCTOR: It's obvious that these last few weeks have been like torture for you.

PATIENT: (Tearful) When I go to bed, I dread getting up the next day, . . . and I know I have to hold it together, because the whole clinic is depending on me.

DOCTOR: It sounds like you carry a lot of responsibility. Let's talk about what I think is going on, and then I'd like to get your ideas about that. You've said that you are finding less energy during the day and that you awaken frequently at night, sometimes only getting a few hours' sleep. You tend to judge yourself harshly, and lately you feel guilty that you're not accomplishing more. You've lost interest in things you used to enjoy, and lately all you can think about is your job. You're finding it harder to concentrate, and making simple decisions feels overwhelming. Did I leave out anything?

PATIENT: No . . . I . . . just don't know what's happening to me.

DOCTOR: All these symptoms indicate to me that you're suffering from depression. This is an illness that effects our nervous system in ways that robs us of our usual ability to enjoy the pleasures of life and to have confidence in our abilities. Your depressed mood is leading you to view yourself through a distorted lens that filters out all recognition of your competence and abilities. (Pauses to check patient's response. After head nod from patient, she proceeds as follows) Fortunately, depression is a very treatable illness and there are some very effective treatment strategies you and I can work on together. This may be hard for you to believe right now, because of the hopeless feeling that accompanies depression, but I'm quite confident that within a few weeks you'll be feeling much better about yourself and about life.

Choice of Treatment

Research indicates that treatment is effective in at least 70% of cases. Treatment can include medication, counseling by the physician, referral to a mental health specialist (psychiatrist, clinical psychologist, clinical social worker, or psychiatric nurse practitioner) for psychotherapy, pharmacotherapy, and in some cases electroconvulsive therapy (ECT). Patients may need to be reminded that they deserve to feel better. They should also be told that without treatment, they will probably continue to suffer the same symptoms for a long time.

Counseling by the Physician

The importance of the doctor-patient relationship cannot be overemphasized for the recognition and treatment of depression, especially in the presence of suicidal ideation. The physician must convey feelings of concern in order for patients to discuss personal and distressing aspects of their lives. Thus, the primary care physician should be skilled at the recognition and management of emotional distress.

Office counseling by the primary care physician may be helpful to patients with milder forms of depression, including MD. The patient, however, should be notified that this interaction is not formal psychotherapy, unless the practitioner is actually trained in such treatment modalities. Psychotherapeutic situations invariably arouse strong emotions in both patients and physicians. When complex interpersonal issues or strong feelings emerge during office counseling, the physician should seek supervision from a trained therapist or consultation from a colleague.

The acronym **SPEAK** was developed by one of the authors (JFC) to help primary care physicians offer office counseling to depressed patients (Table 22–6). The five components of SPEAK (**S**chedule, **P**leasurable activities, **E**xercise, **A**ssertiveness, and **K**ind thoughts about oneself) are elements in behavioral, interpersonal, and cognitive approaches to psychotherapy. They provide a framework both for patient education and for ongoing supportive counseling by the physician. A one-page handout summarizing the SPEAK approach that can be given to patients is included in Appendix 22–A.

Following a *schedule* counteracts the motivational deficits and anergia that accompany depression. Frontal lobe functions of planning, organizing, and initiating activity are frequently impaired by depression. The physician can advise the patient to plan ahead and fill out a weekly schedule. The instructions are to follow what the schedule says, "whether or not you feel like it," thus making the patient's activities less mood-dependent and more time-contingent. The physician can present a rationale for the schedule, as well as other elements of SPEAK, perhaps using a metaphor like giving a car battery a "jump start" by getting the car moving.

The schedule should include *pleasurable activities* in order to counteract anhedonia and the tendency of depressed patients to withdraw from pleasurable activities. Although initially patients may feel they are "just going through the motions," ultimately involvement in pleasure may operate synergistically with the other elements of SPEAK in mild depression and with antidepressant medication in more severe depression to help restore neurotransmitter/neuroreceptor func-

tion. To stimulate patients' planning of these activities the physician can administer a brief "Pleasant Event Inventory" (see Appendix 22–B), in which the patients are asked to list the 15 activities they find most enjoyable. This can be given as a homework assignment to bring back to a follow-up appointment.

Exercise, depending on the medical condition and physical capabilities of the patient, is important as a short-term mood enhancer and long-term prophylaxis against depression. Exercise not only involves kinesthetic movement (breaking somatic rigidity that can play a role in maintaining a depressed mood) but also may release endorphins. The patient should be encouraged to exercise several times a week.

Assertiveness, often difficult for depressed individuals because of low self-esteem and a tendency to doubt their own judgment and opinions, is a key behavior in reversing depression. The physician can help the patient distinguish among nonassertive, assertive, and aggressive behaviors. It is helpful to describe assertiveness as "being direct with others about your feelings, opinions, and intentions." The physician can encourage the patient to make small acts of self-assertion (with significant others, friends, strangers) and to reflect on both their mood and interpersonal outcomes. Self-assertion often mobilizes and discharges affect externally, as opposed to depleting energy by inhibiting affect. It may be helpful to recommend some reading, such as Alberti and Emmons' *Your Perfect Right: A Guide to Assertive Behavior.*

Kind thoughts about oneself is perhaps the most challenging element of the SPEAK approach for depressed patients. Patients can become more aware of the self-punishing nature of their thoughts. Using an approach developed by Ellis (1977), one can teach patients to trace the origin of a depressed mood to particular recurrent thoughts and to replace the self-punishing thoughts with positive ones, ideally on a three-to-one ratio of positive-to-negative thoughts. The physician can give patients a worksheet, such as the "ABCD Method of Thought Analysis" shown in Appendix 22–C, to review their emotions, activating events, beliefs about those events, and to dispute irrational non-evidence-based beliefs giving rise to negative feelings.

There are two further considerations about the SPEAK approach to physician counseling of depressed patients. First, it is not meant to be a substitute for psychotherapy or medication when they are clearly indicated according to the criteria mentioned elsewhere in this chapter. The primary care provider may consider trying it as a first approach, however, with medication or psychotherapy to be initiated if there is no response. More commonly the SPEAK approach works synergistically with appropriate medication. Second, this approach to counseling does not require an excessive time commitment by the physician. Often the SPEAK approach can be explained to the depressed patient in about 10 minutes, with about

Table 22–6. SPEAK approach to physician counseling for depression.

S	Schedule
P	Pleasurable activities
E	Exercise
A	Assertiveness
K	Kind thoughts about oneself

Table 22–7. Considerations for acute-phase treatment with psychotherapy alone

- Less severe depression
- Prior response to psychotherapy
- Incomplete response to treatment with medication alone
- Chronic psychosocial problems
- Availability of trained, competent therapist
- Patient preference

5 minutes devoted to reviewing the relevant elements of SPEAK in follow-up visits.

Role of Formal Psychotherapy

New psychotherapeutic strategies have been generated as a result of recent interpersonal, behavioral, and cognitive approaches to understanding depressive etiology and pathology. Some of these therapies have been shown to be as effective as medication for the acute-phase treatment of mild to moderate, but not severe, depression. Considerations for choosing psychotherapy alone in the acute phase of treatment are shown in Table 22–7. Psychotherapy may be a useful adjunct to medication for the treatment of depression and may also have a role in prophylactic maintenance therapy for the prevention or delay of future depressive episodes in patients susceptible to recurrences. Consequently, psychotherapy can be useful for women with MD who want to become pregnant and bear a child in a drug-free condition or for other patients with MD who must be medication-free for limited periods.

The clinical criteria for referral to a mental health specialist depend a great deal on the experience and expertise of the primary care physician. Primary care physicians should inform patients at an early stage of treatment that consultation with a mental health specialist may be necessary if the depression does not fully remit. This can make referral at a later stage much more acceptable. Because partial remission is a common occurrence, physicians should make every effort to establish clear indications of pre-depression functioning, and if full return to baseline functioning does not occur, specialist referral should be made. In making the referral, the primary care provider should communicate with the mental health specialist the nature of the depressive symptoms; baseline premorbid functioning; other treatments, including medication, that have been tried previously or are concurrent; and patient understanding and expectations about psychotherapy.

Medication

Antidepressant medications are indicated for the treatment of major depression and possibly for dysthymia. Approximately two thirds of patients with major depression respond to pharmacotherapy within 3 weeks after reaching a therapeutic plasma level. The proportion of responders can be increased to 90% by switching initial nonresponders to another class of antidepressants or by using augmentation strategies (eg,

addition of lithium). About one third of patients with major depression (usually milder forms) improve with placebo or general support.

Once a decision is made to initiate therapy, the provider should conceptualize treatment of depression as going through three phases. The **acute phase** of treatment lasts approximately 6–12 weeks and has as its goal the reduction and removal of signs and symptoms of depression and the return to a premorbid level of functioning. A partial response at this phase is associated with a higher risk of relapse later. The **continuation phase** of treatment lasts for 4–9 months with the main goal being prevention of relapse. Medication should be continued at full dose. The **maintenance phase** of treatment, lasting 1 year or longer, aims to prevent recurrence in patients with three prior episodes of depression or other special circumstances (see AHCPR guidelines).

Regular visits are essential for the proper care of the depressed patient. Brief weekly or biweekly visits are usually indicated in the beginning of treatment to evaluate dosage, side-effects, and consequential changes in condition. Weekly phone contacts can be periodically substituted for visits, if necessary.

On initiation of treatment, patients should generally not receive more than 1 week's supply of any medication that can be lethal in overdose. Once the patient has become stabilized on a medication, monthly visits are important for support. If maintenance treatment is warranted, quarterly visits may be adequate.

Approximately 50% of patients with one episode of MD suffer a recurrence. Most experts agree, however, that patients should be slowly tapered from antidepressant medications after a first episode of depression, especially if it has not been particularly severe. Thus, 4–9 months after the first episode abates, the medication can be tapered over a period of 6–8 weeks, raising the dose only if prodromal symptoms of depression reappear.

Research now supports the use of prophylactic antidepressant treatment to decrease the likelihood of recurrence once it is recognized that a patient suffers from recurrent major depression (ie, at least three episodes). Maintenance treatment with antidepressants may also be warranted for patients with only two episodes of MD who also meet the following conditions: (1) first-degree relative with bipolar disorder or recurrent major depression; (2) history of recurrence within 1 year after previously effective medication was discontinued; (3) early onset (before age 20) of the first episode; and (4) both episodes were severe, sudden, or life-threatening in the past 3 years. For prophylaxis, full-treatment dosages of antidepressants should be used on a chronic basis.

Controversy exists concerning the extent to which antidepressants may be useful for the treatment of chronic depression (dysthymia) or of minor depression. Although most experts recommend psychotherapy as the initial treatment for dysthymia, emerging data from randomized clinical trials are pointing to the efficacy of antidepressant medications for this form of depression. Emotional support by the physician may be sufficient for the resolution of an adjustment disorder, but clinical experience indicates that when a patient experiences significant impairment in function (eg, poor work performance, poor sleep, distressed relationships), antidepressant medications may be helpful and should be considered.

Choosing an Antidepressant: Table 22–8 summarizes currently available antidepressant medications and their side effect profiles. In selecting an antidepressant medication, the patient's concurrent medical or psychiatric illnesses, history of prior response, use of other medications, patient preference, cost, and side effects should all be taken into account. In general, the various medications have similar efficacy (70–80%), so the key is to be aware of side effects and to exploit them clinically if at all possible.

First-line treatment by the primary care provider should generally be initiated with either a tricyclic antidepressant (TCA) or selective serotonin reuptake inhibitor (SSRI). They are equally efficacious, even in more severe depression, but have very different side effect profiles. Although effective, the monoamine oxidase inhibitors (MAOIs) should not be used in the primary care setting without psychiatric consultation, since they have a number of potentially serious side effects that require close monitoring and thorough patient education. If a patient fails to respond to the first-line therapy, it is usually preferable to switch to a drug from a different class, although there are anecdotal reports that suggest that some patients who fail to respond to one SSRI will respond when switched to another.

Because antidepressant medication may initially increase anxiety or insomnia, especially in patients with GAD, OCD, or PD, it is important to inform patients of this possible, but usually time-limited problem. Such medication-related anxiety or insomnia usually improves rapidly, and adjunctive low-dose sedating medication (eg, hydroxyzine, doxepin or trazodone, clonazepam, or lorazepam) may be used for a short time. Most patients are able to stop these adjunctive medications, but some benefit from continued combination therapy. Care should be exercised in the prolonged use of benzodiazepines, however, because of the possibility of habituation, tolerance, and build-up of drug levels with the use of long-acting agents.

Communicating With Patients About Medication: Patients initiating antidepressant medication for the first time sometimes are concerned about the stigma associated with medication. Some fear getting "hooked" on the medicine or that it will change their personality in some way. It is important to explain that this is a powerful but nonaddictive medicine that can restore the natural balance of neurotransmitters in the brain. It can be helpful to predict for the patient the possibility of the known side effects of the particular antidepressant and to reframe those side effects as an indicator of the drug's potency to achieve the desired results (see Chapter 6). Finally it is important to build a realistic expectation about the tempo of therapeutic effectiveness by letting the patient know that even though the symptoms of depression may persist for a week or two after starting the antidepressant, the healing process has already begun.

Heterocyclic Medications and Side Effects: Heterocyclic medications (see Table 22–8) include the tricyclics, which have been available since the 1950s. Several other agents similar in structure include

Table 22–8. Antidepressant dosages and side effects.

Antidepressants	Sedating Effect	Anticholinergic Effect	Orthostatic Effect	Effective Dosage Range
Heterocyclic Antidepressants (Tricyclics)				
Amitriptyline (Elavil and others)	+++	+++	+++	75–300 mg
Desipramine (Norpramin)	+	+	+	75–250 mg
Doxepin (Sinequan and others)	+++	+++	+++	75–300 mg
Imipramine (Tofranil and others)	++	+++	+++	75–300 mg
Nortriptyline (Pamelor and others)	++	++	+	50–150 mg
Protriptyline (Vivactil)	+	++	+	10–40 mg
Trimipramine (Surmontil)	+++	++	+++	75–300 mg
Other Heterocyclics				
Amoxapine (Asendin)	++	++	++	150–600 mg
Maprotiline (Ludiomil)	++	+	++	150–225 mg
Trazodone (Desyrel)	+++	0	++	200–600 mg
SSRIs				
Fluoxetine (Prozac)	0	0	0	20–80 mg
Paroxetine (Paxil)	0	+	0	20–50 mg
Sertraline (Zoloft)	0	0	0	50–200 mg
Other New Agents				
Bupropion (Wellbutrin)	0	0	0	150–450 mg
Venlafaxine (Effexor)	+	0	0	75–375 mg
Nefazodone (Serzone)	+	0	0	300–600 mg

0 = None; + = Slight; ++ = Moderate; +++ = Marked.

maprotiline, amoxapine, and trazodone. The heterocyclic antidepressants are similar in side effects, dosing strategies, and efficacy, however, Desipramine and Nortriptyline tend to be better tolerated by most patients. Additional visits and other medical procedures are sometimes required with the use of heterocyclics making their overall health care costs about equal to that of the SSRIs.

Heterocyclic medications are started at low doses and gradually increased to therapeutic levels. Although serum antidepressant levels are available for many of these agents, nortriptyline is the one agent with a true "therapeutic window," such that levels below and above the window are less likely to lead to remission of depressive symptoms. Physicians must assess each individual cautiously since patients with high or low blood levels may do very well clinically. For problematic situations, consultation with a psychiatric expert may be advisable. Patients need to be informed that such medications may take up to 3 weeks to reach therapeutic levels, and, therefore, patients generally will not notice immediate positive effects of treatment.

When opting for a heterocyclic antidepressant, it is generally best to use a secondary amine (desipramine or nortriptyline) and avoid the parent tertiary amines (eg, amitriptyline and imipramine) as they have more severe side effects. It is advisable to start with a low dosage and gradually titrate up as tolerated. For example, start desipramine at 25–50 mg at bedtime for 3 days and increase by 25-mg increments every 2–3 days until the patient reaches a therapeutic dose of at least 150 mg once a day. Heterocyclics can be given once a day (generally in the evening) to minimize side effects. There should be some beneficial effects after 2–3 weeks, with a full therapeutic response occurring after 4–6 weeks. If there is little or no response after an appropriate interval on an appropriate dose, check a level and increase the dose as indicated. The most common error leading to "treatment failure" with the heterocyclics is inadequate dosing. There is no reason to follow levels, however, in patients with an appropriate response and minimal side effects.

The heterocyclic antidepressants have varying degrees of problematic side effects, including anticholinergic, antihistaminic, antiadrenergic, and quinidine-like effects.

Anticholinergic Side Effects: Anticholinergic effects include urinary retention, constipation, dry mouth, confusion, tachycardia, and increased ocular pressure. These effects can be annoying, or sometimes dangerous, depending on the physical condition of the patient. Ileus and peritoneal perforation can be fatal. Increased ocular pressure may cause blindness in patients with narrow-angle glaucoma, and tachycardia can precipitate angina in patients with coronary artery disease. As can be seen in Table 22–8, Desipramine and Nortriptyline have far fewer anticholinergic side effects.

Antihistaminic Side Effects: The antihistaminic side effects cause sedation and inhibition of gastric acid secretion. The potent antihistaminic action of tricyclic agents such as doxepin have led to its use for urticaria, as well as for providing better sedation. Desipramine may have more prominent sympathomimetic effects of agitation and insomnia, and it can be used if a less sedating antidepressant is desired.

Antiadrenergic Side Effects: Antiadrenergic effects cause postural hypotension, which can be quite dangerous in the medically ill or elderly. Nortriptyline seems to be the safest of the heterocyclics in this regard.

Quinidine-like Side Effects: All heterocyclics (except trazodone) have quinidine-like effects. They delay conduction across the His bundle and increase the QT interval on an EKG. Patients with bundle branch block and increased conduction time can experience higher degrees of heart block when given these medications. A corrected QT interval of 0.44 is generally considered the maximum length for the safe use of tricyclic antidepressants. Specialty consultation should be sought when using these agents in patients with intervals greater than 0.44. In general, use of TCAs should be avoided in patients with significant conduction abnormalities.

Among the tricyclics, desipramine (a metabolite of imipramine) and nortriptyline (a metabolite of amitriptyline) are the least anticholinergic, the least sedating, and the least likely to cause postural hypotension. Among the heterocyclic medications, trazodone is notable because it does not cause anticholinergic or conduction problems and has very low lethality in overdose. Trazodone, however, is quite sedating and may also cause postural hypotension and, rarely, priapism (see Table 22–8).

New Agents and Side Effects: Selective serotonin reuptake inhibitors (SSRIs) and other newer agents have revolutionized psychiatric practice, especially for treatment of depression in the elderly and in patients with comorbid general medical illnesses. Many patients too physically ill to be safely treated in the 1960s and 1970s can now receive these antidepressants without fear of dangerous side effects. These agents have an extraordinarily low suicide risk from overdose.

The most widely used of these newer agents include the SSRIs (fluoxetine, paroxetine, fluvoxamine, and sertraline), bupropion, venlafaxine, and nefazodone. Several new SSRIs will be available in the next few years. These new agents are remarkably safe since they do not cause postural hypotension or cardiac conduction delay. Antihistaminic side effects are minimal or nonexistent, and, with the exception of paroxetine (which has very mild anticholinergic effects), none of these new agents have any appreciable anticholinergic effects.

The wide range of effective antidepressants can

make the choice of agent difficult. Fluoxetine has been the most widely used, in more than 18 million patients through 1994. Despite some speculation, all available data suggest that fluoxetine is not more highly associated with violence or suicidal tendencies than any other antidepressant or, for that matter, than with placebo.

Fluoxetine has the longest half-life (24–72 hours) of the new agents and has a long-acting active metabolite (half-life of 7 days). A long half-life may be problematic for some patients, experiencing side effects or drug interactions, but it has not appeared to be a significant problem in clinical practice. In fact, with a long-acting agent like fluoxetine, missing doses does not lead to breakthrough depressive symptoms and also permits dosing every other day, when indicated. When the drug is to be withdrawn, doses can eventually be given once or twice a week, to allow for very smooth tapering. SSRIs with half-lives of 24 hours (sertraline and paroxetine) allow the convenience of once-a-day dosing but result in rapid washout. Bupropion, venlafaxine, and nefazodone (and their metabolites) have shorter half-lives of 4–14 hours, so they must be given at least twice a day.

The starting dose of the three main SSRIs is often the effective treatment dose. This is most clearly the case for fluoxetine at 20 mg, but may also be true for paroxetine at 20 mg, and for sertraline at 50 mg. Patients not responding to the starting doses of SSRIs after 1 month should be given increased doses. Elderly patients and patients with liver disease or other general medical illness often require smaller starting dose, for example, one half of the recommended dose.

Clinicians need to be aware that SSRIs inhibit the cytochrome P-450 system, potentially causing problems with medications metabolized in the liver, such as anticonvulsants, digitalis, and warfarin (Coumadin), and may lead to increased drug levels. Reports conflict regarding which SSRIs are most or least likely to cause this problem, but paroxetine seems to be the most potent inhibitor and sertraline the least potent inhibitor of the 2D6 liver enzyme system. The SSRIs and the other new agents, however, also may have variable effects on other liver enzyme systems such as the 3A4 or 1C.

Nefazodone, in particular, seems to have little effect on any system other than 3A4, which can be a particular problem for use with other drugs metabolized by this system, such as terfenadine (Seldane), astemizole (Hismanal), erythromycin, and ketoconazole. To avoid dangerous pharmacokinetic interactions, it may be necessary to initiate treatment with very low doses, especially in the frail elderly. Side effects, blood levels, and clinical indicators of toxicity must be carefully monitored. Bupropion and venlafaxine, on the other hand, do not seem to inhibit these enzymes.

The use of bupropion in primary care is somewhat problematic because its use may be associated with a 1–4% prevalence of seizures, which may be slightly more common than with other antidepressants. Bupropion should be given in divided doses, and should not be given to individuals at risk for seizures (eg, head trauma history). It is never given in a single dose greater than 150 mg, and the starting dose (75 mg bid or tid) should be increased slowly (once a week) to therapeutic levels of 300–450 mg/day to minimize the risk of seizures. The medication should also not be given to bulimic patients (patients who gorge food and often induce vomiting) because of a possible increased seizure risk. Despite this small but potential risk, bupropion is useful because it does not cause sexual problems often associated with other antidepressants.

The SSRIs may cause side effects like anxiety, insomnia, GI distress, agitation, and sexual difficulties. These are usually mild, occur in less than 20% of patients, and usually do not lead to discontinuation of medication. Adjunctive use of a sedating antihistamine (diphenhydramine or hydroxyzine), sedating antidepressant (trazodone or doxepin), or anxiolytic (eg, clonazepam or lorazepam) can be helpful. When prescribing a sedating serotonergic antidepressant (such as trazodone) along with an SSRI, low doses of the sedating agent should be used to avoid a possible serotonergic syndrome. These adjunctive agents should usually be discontinued after a short time, but continued treatment with two agents is sometimes indicated. If a long-acting benzodiazepine is used in the elderly, care must be exercised to avoid a build-up of medication that can lead to confusion, sedation, or falls after several weeks of treatment.

Case illustration (Contd.): In the previous case of the 45-year-old clinic manager, the physician, after presenting the diagnosis, reviewed the SPEAK approach to the treatment of depression. She gave the patient the handout to read (Appendix 22-A). Discussion revealed that the patient had neglected pleasurable activities and that she engaged in negative self-judgments about her productivity, leading to a compulsive work schedule and failure to attend to the symptoms of fatigue. They decided that the P and K components of SPEAK deserved special attention, and the physician prescribed a long 4-day "strategic retreat" from work so the patient could implement a schedule that included exercise, pleasurable activities, and reflection on her thought processes, using the Pleasant Event Inventory (Appendix 22-B) and the ABCD Thought Analysis (Appendix 22-C). The physician discussed the advisability of antidepressant medication and the possibility of referral to a psychotherapist, but the patient was reluctant at this time to take these steps. The physician then negotiated an agreement that the patient would try the new schedule, that she would come back for an appointment in 2 weeks, and that if there was no improvement in sleep patterns and mood, she would undergo a trial of antidepressant medication.

The patient returned in 2 weeks, having forced herself to schedule in pleasurable activities and exercise, and limiting her work hours to a 40-hour week. Her symptoms of dysphoria and nocturnal awakening persisted. As they had agreed, the patient then began a trial of an SSRI in the morning and trazodone 50 mg at bedtime to aid in sleep. Within 4 days, a phone call to the doctor indicated that her sleep had improved dramatically. At an appointment 2 weeks later the patient showed improved affect and she reported feeling better. She indicated she was interested in pursuing psychotherapy to change her negative self-evaluations. The physician referred her to a psychotherapist for short-term therapy focused on altering these thought processes.

The patient showed complete resolution of symptoms in 6 weeks. Trazodone was discontinued, and she was maintained on the SSRI for 6 months. During that time she underwent eight sessions of psychotherapy, which resulted in increased self-awareness of her thought processes and a method to shift her thinking in a positive direction. She was seen for two additional therapy sessions in the month after discontinuing the SSRI to consolidate the gains she had made and monitor her for any recurrence of symptoms. At 9 months she reported to her primary care physician that she remained symptom-free and that she was taking a 2-week vacation to the Caribbean.

Antidepressants in the Elderly and Medically III: For many of the reasons enumerated earlier, the new agents have generally become the agents of choice in the elderly and in the medically ill. Among heterocyclic agents, the safest agents are nortriptyline and desipramine, which are still widely used because of their relatively low anticholinergic and antiadrenergic side effects. They are also widely used as second-line treatment choices and play a role in the treatment of refractory depression, either as adjunctive or alternative treatments.

Dosing strategies in the elderly and medically ill are to "start low and go slow." Pharmacokinetically, these agents are metabolized more slowly, resulting in accumulation and toxicity. Increased pharmacodynamic effects in the elderly may result from lower albumin levels, which lower protein binding.

Electroconvulsive Therapy (ECT)

ECT is still the most effective means available for the treatment of refractory depression. It is the treatment of choice for patients with psychotic depression, depression refractory to pharmacotherapy, and for some patients who are acutely suicidal. Despite prejudices and fears about ECT, new methods of administration have proven it to be a safe and effective treatment modality. In fact, ECT can be safer than antidepressant medication in the elderly. Some short-term memory loss is common, but research indicates that this reverts to normal in virtually all patients. In some cases, ECT can be life-saving and should not be denied to patients because of poor understanding or unrealistic fear. ECT does not lead to permanent remission of depression in patients susceptible to recurrence. Thus, patients with recurrent depression who receive ECT should receive either prophylactic medication after a course of therapy (as an outpatient) or maintenance ECT.

MANAGED CARE

The time and organizational pressures of managed care settings may promote even further underdiagnosis and undertreatment of depression in primary care. Health services research indicates that fee-for-service and psychiatric settings may be more effective than prepaid settings for both the recognition and the treatment of major depression. With the sustained growth of capitation and managed care, however, new systems need to be developed to align clinical and financial incentives to increase the accurate assessment and optimal management of depression in primary care. Since depression is associated with increased use of health care services, as well as increased morbidity and mortality, attention to improving the assessment and treatment of depression in primary care should become a high priority for adding value to health care and improving the quality of patient's lives.

SUGGESTED READINGS

American Psychiatric Association: *Diagnostic and Statistical Manual of Mental Disorders,* 4th ed. American Psychiatric Association, 1994.

American Psychiatric Association: *Diagnostic and Statistical Manual of Mental Disorders,* 4th ed. *Primary Care Version* DSM-IV-PC. American Psychiatric Association, 1995.

Brody DS, Larson DB: The role of primary care physicians in managing depression. J Gen Intern Med 1992;7:243.

Brody DS et al: Strategies for counseling depressed patients by primary care physicians. J Gen Inter Med 1994;9:569.

Byrne A, Byrne DG: The effect of exercise on depression, anxiety and other mood states: A review. J Psychosom Res 1993;37:565.

Cohen-Cole SA: *The Medical Interview.* Mosby-Year Book, 1991.

Cohen-Cole SA, Kaufman K: Major depression in physical illness: Diagnosis, prevalence, and antidepressant treatment (A ten year review: 1982–1992). Depression 1993;1:181.

Ellis A: The basic clinical theory of rational emotive therapy. In Ellis A, Grieger C (editors): *Handbook of Rational Emotive Therapy,* Springer, 1977.

Janicak PG et al: *Principles and Practices of Psychophar-macology.* Williams & Wilkins, 1993.

Karasu TB: *Psychotherapy for Depression.* Jason Araonson, 1990.

Kendler et al:. The prediction of major depression in women: Toward an integrated etiologic modal. Am J Psychiatry 1993;150:1139.

Rush AJ et al: *Depression in Primary Care: Clinical Practice Guideline,* Number 5. US Department of Health and Human Services, Public Health Services, Agency for Health Care Policy and Research (AHCPR Publication No. 93-0550), 1993.

Spitzer RL et al: Utility of a new procedure for diagnosing mental disorder in primary care. The PRIME-MD 1000 study. JAMA 1994;272:1749.

Weismann MM et al: Brief diagnostic interviews (SDDS-PC) for multiple mental disorders in primary care. Arch Fam Med 1995;4:220.

PATIENT BIBLIOGRAPHY

Alberti RE, Emmons ML: *Your Perfect Right: A Guide to Assertive Behavior.* Impact Publishers, 1970.

Lewinsohn et al: *Control Your Depression.* Prentice-Hall, 1978.

Seligman MEP: *Learned Optimism.* Knopf, 1991.

Appendix 22–A. Overcoming your depression: The SPEAK approach.

S   Schedule:
Make a weekly schedule for yourself, with columns for each day of the week and rows for the hours of the day. Using a pencil (so you can make changes) make a plan for activities you will do each hour. Some of the times will already be structured for you, eg, at work. Focus especially on the times that are currently unstructured. Start with things you know you usually do, eg, eating meals, preparing meals. Include on the schedule time to do household chores and errands, but also include times for fun activities and exercise. Because temporarily you may not feel the motivation or desire to do any of these things, follow what the schedule says **whether or not you feel like doing it.** Sometimes you might feel like you are just going through the motions. When the time comes to switch to another activity, do so **whether or not you have completed the previous task.** You are making progress by putting in time on all these activities, not by getting through your "to do" list. Proceeding in this way will help you move out of depression by getting yourself moving through the day.

P   Pleasurable activities:
Some of the items on your schedule should be activities that previously were fun for you before you became depressed. You might have identified some of these pleasures on the Pleasant Events Inventory. For the time being you may feel you are just going through the motions in these activities. When we are depressed the part of the brain that allows us to feel pleasure is not functioning smoothly, so it is important to have a "jump start." You should plan something each day that would normally be fun and make yourself do it.

E   Exercise:
Aerobic exercise increases oxygen and circulation to the brain and counteracts the hormonal changes caused by depression. It helps activate the natural pharmacy in your brain that will work with other parts of your treatment to help you come out of depression. Times for daily exercise should be included on your schedule. Running, swimming, bicycling, aerobic dancing, and walking are all forms of exercise that will help.

A   Assertiveness:
This involves being **direct** with other people in your communication. Practice letting others know your feelings, needs, wants, opinions, and choices. This is more difficult when we are depressed, because we tend to doubt our own judgment. Or we might hold back because we are afraid others will think poorly of us. These thoughts are a product of depression, so it is necessary to act as if you were confident, even though inside you don't feel it. It takes more energy to hold in feelings than to express them. You might find that by stating clearly what you need or by saying "No" to what you don't want will help increase your energy and confidence. Read *Your Perfect Right* by Alberti and Emmons.

K   Kind thoughts about yourself:
Since depression leads us to think self-punishing thoughts, it is very important to increase your awareness of when this is happening and to replace the negative thoughts with positive ones. Most of the time these negative thoughts are strongly held opinions that are not based on evidence. It is like carrying a negative, opinionated relative with you wherever you go. Once you become aware of this pattern of thoughts, begin to analyze them using the **ABCD** worksheet. You might write the most persistent negative thought on a 3 × 5 card. Then turn the card over and write three positive thoughts that you could replace it with. Carry this card with you and refer to it frequently. It takes about three positive statements to counteract the effect of one negative statement.

John F. Christensen, PhD.

Appendix 22–B. Pleasant Events Inventory.

Pleasant Event[1]	With Whom[2] **A** = Alone **P** = Partner **F** = Family **O** = Other People	How Often[3]	Last Time[4]	$ Amount if Costs Money[5]
1.				
2.				
3.				
4.				
5.				
6.				
7.				
8.				
9.				
10.				
11.				
12.				
13.				
14.				
15.				

[1] List the activities or events that have brought you the most pleasure over the years.
[2] Indicate with whom you like to share the pleasure.
[3] Indicate how often you do this activity.
[4] How long has it been since you engaged in this activity. If it has been months or years, perhaps you should schedule time for it soon.
[5] Make a $ sign if the pleasure costs money. You might be surprised at how many of your pleasures are free.

Appendix 22–C. ABCD method of thought analysis.

Activating Event	Belief	Consequence	Dispute
#2	#3	#1	#4
What happened before "C" ?	What am I telling myself about "A" ?	What am I feeling?	Where's the evidence for "B"?

DIRECTIONS:

1. Start your analysis in the C *(consequence)* column, by writing the negative emotion you have been feeling today. This emotion (e.g., sadness) is a consequence of something else.
2. List in the A column the *activating event* that triggered the emotion. Answer the question, "What happened before I started feeling sad?" An example might be that a close friend did not reply when you said hello.
3. Now move to the B column and write down your *belief* about the activating event. This belief is the actual cause of your negative emotion. Answer the question, for example, "What am I telling myself about my friend ignoring me?" This answer will often be an irrational judgment not based on evidence, e.g., "He's rejecting me," or more generally, "I'm a rejectable person."
4. The final step is to *dispute* the irrational belief by asking, "Where's the evidence for the statement in B?" Then write down a statement in Column D that is a more appropriate, less self-punishing belief about the activating event. For example, you might write down, "My friend was distracted because he's been under a lot of stress lately."

Anxiety

23

Wendy Levinson, MD, & Charles C. Engel, MD, MPH

INTRODUCTION

Anxiety is a common, normal emotion; virtually all people experience occasional trepidation, fear, nervousness, "jitters," or even panic. Often mild anxiety maintains one's mental sharpness as uncertainty or pressure mounts. For many individuals, however, anxiety occurs as part of an anxiety disorder, a disorder that is a prominent, persistent, and disruptive aspect of their daily lives. Among the general population in the United States, 20% of women and 8% of men experience anxiety disorders at some time in their lives; 15% of women and 7% of men are affected for 6 months or longer.

The major anxiety disorders are panic disorder (with or without agoraphobia), generalized anxiety disorder (GAD), adjustment disorder with anxiety, posttraumatic stress disorder (PTSD), acute stress disorder (ASD), specific phobia, social phobia, and obsessive-compulsive disorder (OCD). These disorders are particularly common among patients seeking primary care, since the majority of patients with anxiety disorders are initially seen in general medical settings. Because affected patients tend to complain of the prominent physical rather than the emotional symptoms of anxiety, providers must be alert and ask carefully worded questions to screen for these disorders. (Table 23–1 lists some sample screening questions.) Distinguishing

Table 23–1. Suggested screening questions for anxiety.

Disorder	Questions
Generalized anxiety disorder	Would you describe yourself generally as a nervous person? Are you a worrier? Do you feel nervous or tense?
Panic disorder	Have you ever had a sudden attack of rapid heartbeat or rush of intense fear, anxiety, or nervousness? Did anything seem to trigger it?
Agoraphobia	Have you ever avoided important activities because you were afraid you would have a sudden attack like the one I just asked you about?
Social phobia	Some people have strong fears of being watched or evaluated by others. For example, some people don't want to eat, speak, or write in front of people for fear of embarrassing themselves. Is anything like this a problem for you?
Specific phobia	Some people have strong fears or phobias about things like heights, flying, bugs, or snakes? Do you have any strong fears or phobias?
Obsession	Some people are bothered by intrusive, silly, unpleasant, or horrible thoughts that keep repeating over and over. For example, some people have repeated thoughts of hurting some one they love even though they don't want to; that a loved one has been seriously hurt; that they will yell obscenities in public; or that they are contaminated by germs. Has anything like this troubled you?
Compulsion	Some people are bothered by doing something over and over that they can't resist, even when they try. They might wash their hands every few minutes, or repeatedly check to see that the stove is off or the door is locked, or count things excessively. Has anything like this been a problem for you?
Acute stress and posttraumatic stress disorder	Have you ever seen or experienced a traumatic event when you thought your life was in danger? Have you ever seen someone else in grave danger? What happened?

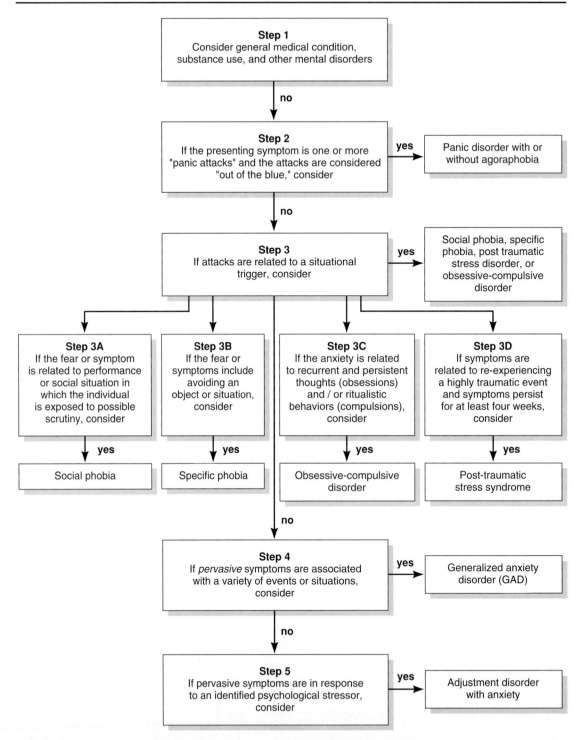

Figure 23–1. Anxiety algorithm. (Modified, with permission, from American Psychiatric Association: *Diagnostic and Statistical Manual: Primary Care Version (DSM-IV-PC).*) American Psychiatric Association, 1994.

among the various anxiety disorders is essential because of differences in their treatment, complications, and prognoses. The *Diagnostic and Statistical Manual of Mental Disorders IV-Primary Care Version (DSM-IV-PC)* suggests an algorithm for determining which anxiety disorder may be the problem (Figure 23–1). Table 23–2 summarizes this algorithm.

Table 23–2. Symptoms associated with panic disorder.

- Choking sensation or "lump in the throat"
- Skipping, racing, or pounding of the heart
- Excessive sweating
- Rubbery or "jelly" legs
- Nausea or abdominal distress
- Trembling or shaking
- Difficulty in getting one's breath, smothering sensations, hyperventilating
- Chest pain, pressure, discomfort
- Faintness, lightheadedness, or dizziness
- Feeling off balance or unsteady
- Tingling or numbness in parts of the body
- Hot flashes or chills
- Preoccupation with health concerns
- Feeling that things in the environment are strange, unreal, foggy, or detached
- Feeling outside or detached from all or part of the body, having a floating feeling
- Fear of dying or that something terrible is about to happen
- Feeling of losing control or going insane
- Agoraphobic avoidance behavior
- Feeling frightened suddenly and unexpectedly for no immediate reason

Source: Reproduced, with permission, from McGlynn TJ, Metcalf HL (editors): *Diagnosis and Treatment of Anxiety Disorders: A Physician's Handbook,* 2nd ed. American Psychiatric Press, 1991.

DIAGNOSIS

Careful use of office testing with one of a number of common screening surveys can improve the detection and treatment of anxiety and other mental disorders. These tests can also be used to serially follow patients with previously diagnosed anxiety disorders to determine whether the symptoms are improving. Before seeing the provider, patients can complete self-report measures, such as the Zung Anxiety Scale or the anxiety subscale of the Hopkins Symptom Checklist 90 Revised (SCL-90). Brief, semistructured interviews such as the Hamilton Anxiety Rating Scale (HARS) must be administered by a provider but offer the advantage of quantifying the clinical assessment of anxiety symptoms. There is a caveat, however; studies have often shown that screening alone may not improve patient outcomes. One reason may be that while screening can identify the patients most likely to suffer from treatable anxiety disorders, it also produces many false-positive results. Providers should therefore follow positive screening tests with a more careful diagnostic assessment.

A new instrument, the Primary Care Evaluation of Mental Disorders (PRIME-MD), uses this principle to improve on available screening techniques. It uses a time-efficient two-stage assessment: (1) an initial questionnaire that screens for anxiety and other mental disorders most common in primary care, and (2) a structured interview that provides diagnostic information in identified problem areas. Recently published standardization data show that the interview requires an average of 8.4 minutes per patient.

Symptoms & Signs

Anxiety disorders manifest themselves with cognitive symptoms (eg, worry, a sense of doom, or derealization) and physical symptoms (eg, muscular tension, rapid heart rate, or dizziness). One problem for primary care providers is to decide how much diagnostic investigation is both feasible and necessary to rule out important medical diseases. For example, should a patient with palpitations undergo cardiac monitoring, thyroid function studies, or even cardiac catheterization? Should a patient presenting with nausea and abdominal pain undergo upper and lower endoscopy? Understanding the signs, symptoms, and epidemiologic features of the various anxiety disorders can help the physician make an accurate diagnosis and initiate timely, appropriate treatment while avoiding invasive or unnecessary testing. Appropriate diagnosis by the primary care doctor can prevent a series of referrals to specialists—each of whom may investigate the symptoms pertaining to his or her own specialty area. Early recognition of anxiety disorders can reduce patients' discomfort, medical expenses, iatrogenic complications, anxiety-related complications (eg, inability to face others or a fear of leaving home), and mortality (eg, suicide). In addition, an appropriate diagnosis of anxiety can reduce substance abuse; as patients sometimes may self-medicate with alcohol, benzodiazepines, or other substances in an effort to ameliorate their anxiety symptoms.

Case illustration 1: Gwen is a 28-year-old woman seeking care because of episodes of shortness of breath, racing heartbeat, and a sensation that she is going to faint. The episodes have been occurring for 4 months, increasing in frequency until she was experiencing as many as four of them per week. She has seen another physician who conducted a number of tests, including thyroid function studies and use of a Holter monitor. These results were unrevealing. The patient's concerns about her symptoms are escalating, and she is fearful that she may have an attack while driving or when out with her young children. The patient's husband has been supportive and has assumed responsibility for routine household chores, such as grocery shopping and transporting the children. More detailed history revealed the patient is reluctant to perform these tasks for fear of having an episode. She is worried about her heart, since her mother had heart disease in her early fifties. She thinks her mother started experiencing her symptoms in her mid-thirties and is worried that her symptoms are cardiac in origin.

The physician recognizes the symptoms as those of panic disorder. Further historical details helped to eliminate other possibilities of medical or substance-related illness. The doctor takes another 5 minutes to explain the nature of panic disorder. He reassures Gwen that she is not alone with her symptoms and that 2–4% of all people suffer from panic disorder. He senses that the patient might be defensive about a psychological problem, so he helps her save face by emphasizing the biological basis of the disorder. Panic symptoms, he explains, originate in the stem of the brain, the part that controls the fight-or-flight response to a perceived threat. In some people, this brainstem alarm system randomly misfires and causes unanticipated surges of adrenaline, accompanied by sudden fear. The alarm system can be reset with a combination of medicines, relaxation techniques, and gradual increases in feared activities. To help Gwen learn more about panic disorder the doctor gives her a book to read on anxiety. She is started on 50 mg daily of desipramine. After a month of slowly increasing the daily dose to 150 mg and encouraging her to gradually try previously avoided tasks and situations (systematic desensitization), her symptoms have resolved, and she has returned to full function.

Differential Diagnosis

Substance intoxication from theophylline preparations, over-the-counter cold preparations, caffeine, cocaine, amphetamines, and marijuana, and others or substance withdrawal from alcohol, benzodiazepines, barbiturates, and other central nervous system (CNS) depressants can precipitate serious anxiety symptoms. *DSM-IV* classifies this as a substance-induced anxiety disorder. Anxiety symptoms can also occur as a consequence of a medical condition, for example, in a patient who experiences anxiety after a myocardial infarction. Medical problems—including endocrine disorders (such as hypo- and hyperthyroidism, pheochromocytoma, or hypoglycemia); cardiovascular problems; pulmonary embolism; arrhythmias; and neurologic conditions (such as vestibular dysfunction)—can also mimic anxiety symptoms. Historical and examination data suggest that these are substantially less likely than anxiety disorder.

Etiology

The development of anxiety disorders involves multiple factors, including biological abnormalities, past and present psychological stressors, and environmentally conditioned behaviors. Abnormalities in the central nervous system associated with anxiety disorders relate to the gamma-aminobutyric acid (GABA) receptor as well as to the locus ceruleus. Animal studies have shown that stimulation of the locus ceruleus produces hyperarousal states similar to those seen in anxious humans. GABA is an inhibitory neurotransmitter found throughout most of the CNS. It may decrease anxiety by inhibiting locus ceruleus activity and modulating the reticular activating system, another area of the brainstem thought to affect alertness and fear. Benzodiazepines, a class of medications commonly used to treat anxiety, bind specific sites on the GABA receptor. When the benzodiazepine molecule binds the GABA receptor, the effect of GABA on the GABA receptor is enhanced, reducing anxiety.

Genetic factors are also likely to play a role in anxiety disorders, as evidenced by twin studies showing a higher concordance for panic disorder and obsessive-compulsive disorder among monozygotic twins than among dizygotic twins.

Conditioned learning may play a pivotal role in the development of anxiety disorders and the resulting avoidance that often seriously compounds patients' anxiety-related functional impairment. For example, a panic attack may first occur while the patient is driving a car. He or she may associate the attack with the act of driving and feels heightened anxiety—and ultimately dread—when driving or anticipating driving. Initially, the association between driving and panic is coincidental (driving is not the event provoking the panic attack). Eventually, however, the patient may completely stop driving for fear that another panic attack will occur. This learned relationship between driving and panic may gradually become so strong that driving becomes a precipitant of panic attacks. Thus, the driver mistakenly learns to fear driving.

Stressful or catastrophic life events are also key factors leading to anxiety disorders, particularly posttraumatic stress disorder. Posttraumatic stress disorder and adjustment disorder with anxiety are examples of disorders in which these events play a specific causal role.

SPECIFIC DISORDERS

Panic Attacks

A panic attack is characterized by a discrete period of intense fear accompanied by the abrupt onset of several cognitive and somatic symptoms (see Table 23–2). Frightening physical symptoms are commonly prominent and scare many patients into seeking urgent medical care. Primary care providers can usually be reassuring, since panic attacks are generally often infrequent, self-limited, and not related to any serious mental or physical disorder. Panic attacks are categorized as:

- Unexpected (untriggered or uncued)
- Situationally bound (always environmentally or psychologically cued), or
- Situationally predisposed (sometimes, but not invariably, cued)

Panic attacks can occur in a number of anxiety disorders other than panic disorder; these include social and specific phobias, OCD, and PTSD. The presence and type of a panic trigger helps clinicians make a correct diagnosis. Uncued panic attacks are characteristic of panic disorder, whereas cued attacks suggest other psychiatric conditions such as:

- Social phobia (attack triggered by fear of embarrassment in social situations)
- Specific phobia (fear of places or things)
- OCD (triggered by exposure to the object of an obsession, such as contamination), or
- PTSD (triggered by an event resembling the original trauma)

Panic attacks are quite common; most people experience a subclinical, or limited-symptom, attack at some time. Only about 9% of people, however, ever experience a full-blown panic attack.

Panic Disorder

Diagnosis: Panic disorder is diagnosed when panic attacks are uncued, recurrent, and followed by a month or more of persistent fear of another attack or avoidance of situations out of fear of having another attack. Only about 2–4% of the population has ever had panic disorder, and about 7% of primary care patients suffer with it. Often, the dilemma for the primary care physician is whether or not to evaluate the patient's specific symptoms, since patients with panic disorder often focus on the bodily symptoms of the disorder, presenting to primary care providers with chest pain, dizziness, and other unexplained complaints (Table 23–3). Because panic disorder is so frequently missed by physicians, unnecessary procedures and treatments aimed at the physical symptoms can cause iatrogenic illnesses. A sound clinical strategy is to evaluate conservatively those symptoms that are potentially catastrophic, involve objective findings, or present as a classic constellation of symptoms. While the investigation is proceeding, the patient can be treated for panic disorder and the symptoms reassessed periodically. Effective pharmacologic treatment reduces the cognitive and physical symptoms; it also lessens the patient's' belief that the problem is an undiscovered medical condition.

Panic disorder is a potentially debilitating disease with major complications. It leads to agoraphobia in one third to one half of cases, most often within 6 months of the first panic attack. Agoraphobia is a fear of recurrent attacks, a fear that causes many patients to avoid important activities of daily living. In case illustration 1, the patient avoided tasks that required her to leave home because she was afraid of recurrent attacks. Community-based studies have shown that suicide attempts are more common among patients with panic disorder than among patients with major depression. Since panic disorder is so frequently missed by physicians, iatrogenesis can result from unnecessary procedures and treatments.

Management: In tailoring the treatment to the patient, several factors should be weighed, including the degree of avoidance present, the severity of physical manifestations of panic, and the presence or absence of overlapping psychiatric disorders (in particular, major depression and PTSD). The clinician must balance patient education and supportive counseling with patients' beliefs about the cause of their symptoms. For example, if the patient thinks panic symptoms are due to a cardiac problem, emphasizing the biological basis of the disorder may help the patient accept the diagnosis and thus improve adherence to treatment. The primary physician has a vital role to play in treatment, and many of the treatments, such as patient education and supportive counseling, can appropriately be incorporated into routine office visits. Patient education and supportive counseling are appropriate aspects of routine primary care for panic disorder, as well as other anxiety disorders, whereas extensive psychotherapy may require referral to a mental health professional.

Medications used to treat panic disorder include some antidepressants [tricyclics, selective serotonin reuptake inhibitors (SSRIs), or monoamine oxidase inhibitors (MAOIs), in order of preference] and benzodiazepines (alprazolam, clonazepam, and perhaps diazepam and lorazepam). The advantages of benzodiazepines are that they relieve symptoms rapidly, usually within the first week of treatment, and they have a relatively wide therapeutic index. Their main disadvantages are their potential for misuse and dependence, and a high incidence of rebound panic attacks when the medication is discontinued. In contrast, tricyclic antidepressants and SSRIs are not associated with dependence, but generally take 3–4 weeks or longer before reaching maximum effectiveness. In addition, antidepressants frequently exacerbate anxiety symptoms during the first 1–2 weeks of administration.

Antidepressants and benzodiazepines are frequently used in combination. A common practice is to initiate treatment with a low daily dose of a tricyclic (eg, imipramine, 25 mg orally each day), titrating the dose slowly upward to 150–200 mg per day over 2–3 weeks. If panic symptoms worsen in the initial week of therapy, alprazolam or clonazepam is started to control symptoms more quickly. After 3–4 weeks on therapeutic doses of antidepressant (eg, imipramine, 150–300 mg daily, or nortriptyline, 75–100 mg daily), the benzodiazepine can be tapered and discontinued. SSRIs can also be used to treat panic disorder.

Table 23–3. Prevalence of panic disorder in patients with medically unexplained symptoms, primary care patients, and people in the community.

Sample Source	Panic Disorder Prevalence (%)
Community	0.6–1.0
Primary care	7
Chest pain and negative angiography	33–43
Hypertensives tested for pheochromocytoma	35
Irritable bowel syndrome	29
Unexplained dizziness or syncope	13
Migraine headaches	5–15
Chronic fatigue	11–30
Chronic pelvic pain	8

Source: Reproduced, with permission, from Engel CC Jr, Kroenke K, Katon WJ: Mental health services in Army primary care: The need for a collaborative health care agenda. *Military Medicine* 1994; 159(3):203.

Treatment should be initiated at one-half the usual antidepressant dose. Although MAOIs are effective, they are seldom used in primary care because of the extensive dietary restrictions needed to minimize the risk of tyramine-induced hypertensive crisis. It is recommended that antidepressants be continued for a minimum of 6–8 months. Since panic disorder tends to be chronic, however, longer treatment is often necessary; the length of treatment often depends on patient preference and ability to tolerate relapse.

Whereas pharmacologic intervention improves the physical manifestations of panic, avoidance behaviors should be dealt with using behavior modification. Once their physical symptoms are controlled, patients should be helped to gradually face their feared situations and activities. For example, Gwen in case illustration 1 would be encouraged to drive, shop, and manage other tasks outside her home. If patients are at first overwhelmed by the prospect of doing this, it can help to initiate exposure mentally, using relaxation techniques and guided imagery. The patient should be instructed to imagine a frightening but tolerable aspect of the activity (in this case, driving) while doing a relaxation exercise and to repeatedly visualize herself successfully facing it. Eventually, using successive small exposure steps, the patient will be able to drive without anxiety.

All patients benefit from a clear understanding of their problem. This eases anxiety, increases the strength of the therapeutic alliance, and increases the likelihood that the patient will follow the treatment plan. It is essential to emphasize the biological nature of panic disorder and to refer patients to the appropriate self-help books and support groups. Most patients find it reassuring and destigmatizing to know that they have a recognized, treatable syndrome. As shown in case illustration 1, explaining the biological nature of symptoms reduces the sense of guilt, shame, and self-doubt many patients with panic disorder feel. Self-help books and support groups are widely available (see suggested readings).

Phobias
Diagnosis: **Specific phobias** and **social phobias** are characterized by episodic anxiety in response to specific precipitants. Typically, affected individuals are aware that their fears are exaggerated or unreasonable; nonetheless, when exposed to a precipitant, patients experience intense, excessive fear and subsequently avoid the situation or thing. Stimuli for specific phobias are places, things, or events, such as airplane flights, heights, insects, snakes, or rodents. Social phobia involves excessive fear of embarrassment, failure, or humiliation before others. This sometimes becomes evident as a fear of speaking, performing, eating, or writing in public. Most often, social phobia involves a single focus such as fear of public speaking; occasionally it presents as a general-ized type that disables the patient in a wide range of social situations. Marked anticipatory anxiety can cause avoidance behaviors that significantly disrupt patients' functioning. It is important to differentiate phobias, in which the panic attacks are anticipated and occur in a predictable situation, from panic disorder, in which panic is unpredictable and uncued.

Case illustration 2: Charlie, a man in his mid-thirties, presents to his primary care provider complaining of severe palpitations, sweating, and tremulousness. The symptoms occur when he is waiting in customs lines. As he approaches the front of the line, fear of talking with the customs official intensifies until the symptoms occur. The patient then flees to the end of the long line just before reaching the customs agent. Charlie realizes this cycle is silly and laughs anxiously as he describes it. This symptom is a major problem for him, however, since his occupation is writing travel books. He has begun avoiding travel and is increasingly worried about his ability to meet writing deadlines—and to continue working. A conservative medical work-up is unrevealing, and the primary care provider makes the diagnosis of social phobia and prescribes a trial of beta-blockers to be used a short time before standing in the customs line. He also gives Charlie a self-help book and tape on relaxation techniques and the use of guided imagery as a way of visualizing success in the customs line. Charlie uses these treatment approaches successfully on his next trip and realizes that the problem is controllable. He incorporates them into his routine work schedule, and within 2 months has returned to full occupational functioning.

Specific phobias are perhaps the most common but least disabling anxiety disorder. Although many patients have them, most experience only minor related dysfunction, and they seldom seek care for them. When care is sought, the diagnosis is usually evident from the history and requires no further testing.

Management: Treatment of phobias almost always involves some form of behavior modification (systematic desensitization using in vivo or guided imagery exposure, relaxation techniques, or biofeedback) entailing gradual introduction of small amounts of the feared stimulus or a related but less feared situation. Although pharmacologic treatment is currently being used, generally accepted pharmacotherapy guidelines have not been established. As noted in case illustration 2, patients are often prescribed beta-blockers to be taken prior to an anticipated exposure to the phobic stimulus. Benzodiazepines are often given for exposures to infrequent events that have no complex performance requirements (eg, traveling by commercial airliner on an annual vacation trip). Patients should be informed of the risk of anterograde amnesia, or blackouts, associated with some of these drugs. Preliminary data suggest that SSRIs may be effective for treating social phobia, but they tend to be reserved for refractory patients who cannot tolerate other medications.

Obsessive-Compulsive Disorder

Diagnosis: Patients with obsessive-compulsive disorder (OCD) experience regular intrusive thoughts—called obsessions—or are driven to repeatedly perform seemingly unnecessary or bizarre rituals—called compulsions. Aggression, sex, and religion are common obsessional themes. Compulsions may involve mental tasks such as counting or praying, or they may involve physical rituals such as repeatedly hand-washing or checking the state of an object. Patients may become so preoccupied with their obsessions and compulsions that they become extremely anxious, slow, and disabled. In one instance, a patient wrung her hands so constantly she could not cook, work, or sleep. Another washed his hands every 10–15 minutes, which interfered significantly with his normal business and social activities. Although patients' level of insight is typically high—they generally experience obsessions and compulsions as intrusive, upsetting, and silly—such insight may diminish acutely when they are faced with the focus of an obsession. (eg, the patient with a contamination obsession who soils his clothing).

Until the introduction of effective pharmacotherapies for OCD, the disorder was markedly under-recognized in both primary care and psychiatric practice. About 1–3% of the general population develops OCD during their lives. The disorder has been found to have a distinct biological component, a finding supported by the efficacy of biological therapies that selectively inhibit the reuptake of serotonin at CNS neurosynapses. Twin studies have shown a significantly higher fraction of monozygotic twins with diagnostic concordance than is the case for dizygotic twins. Additionally, there is a distinct and reciprocal association between OCD and Tourette's syndrome. Tourette's syndrome is a neurologic disorder involving persistent motor and verbal tics. It is often treated with centrally acting dopamine antagonists, such as haloperidol and pimozide. Consequently some have suggested that dopamine may also play a role in OCD.

Management: The FDA-approved pharmacologic treatment of OCD includes two medications: clomipramine and fluoxetine, the latter in relatively high doses (40–80 mg per day) compared with those used for major depression. Clomipramine is a tricyclic with relatively selective effects on serotonin reuptake. It is commonly prescribed for depression in Europe but is FDA-approved in the United States only for OCD. Clomipramine shares the usual tricyclic antidepressant profile of anticholinergic, sedative, and orthostatic side effects. Sertraline, another SSRI antidepressant, has surpassed placebos in controlled trials.

Psychotherapy for OCD may involve a range of strategies. A frequently discussed approach, called cognitive-behavioral therapy, broadly speaking, holds that behavior is driven by underlying beliefs, or *cognitions.* Mental disorders affect cognitions in characteristic ways; depressed and anxious patients often base their behaviors on unrealistically pessimistic beliefs. For instance, "learned helplessness" could be viewed according to this model as excessively passive behavior based on the often-mistaken assumption that there is no way to escape a punishing outcome. Compulsions can also be seen as behaviors occurring in response to faulty beliefs. A common normal childhood compulsion illustrating this is the urging, "Don't step on the crack (the behavior), or you'll break your mother's back" (the faulty belief). In cognitive-behavioral therapy, the provider guides the patient to identify the faulty belief and assists the patient into testing the belief. Continuing with the example, the individual who can be convinced to step on a crack soon discovers that Mom's back does not break. Another cognitive-behavioral technique often used for OCD patients with prominent obsessions is called *thought stopping.* Patients are instructed to block intrusive ruminations by crowding them out with the repeated silent mental command for obsessions to stop.

Posttraumatic Stress Disorder & Acute Stress Disorder

Diagnosis: Posttraumatic stress disorder (PTSD) and acute stress disorder (ASD) are the common mental sequelae of catastrophic trauma. ASD involves symptoms that occur within the first month after trauma. PTSD is essentially the same syndrome, but beginning or persisting beyond a month. Severe trauma of either ASD or PTSD entails an observed or experienced serious injury (actual or threatened). By definition, the trauma experience is accompanied by feelings of intense fear, helplessness, or horror. Patients subsequently develop a mix of flashbacks, nightmares, persistent avoidance of stimuli resembling (concretely or symbolically) the precipitating event, numbing of general responsiveness (restricted range of affect, feelings of interpersonal estrangement, anhedonia), and persistent signs and symptoms of physiologic arousal. Secondary depression, panic attacks, substance abuse, unexplained physical symptoms, and aggressive behavior may also be present.

Overall, the lifetime prevalence for PTSD is 1–14% for the general population. The prevalence for Vietnam combat veterans is about 15–20% (veterans wounded in action are at relatively high risk). Recent epidemiologic studies suggest that about one third of the population suffers some trauma, placing them at risk for PTSD, and one fourth of those at risk develop PTSD over the ensuing year.

Case illustration 3: Jacques was a successful accountant with no psychiatric history until he had aortic valve surgery at the age of 42. Subsequently, he became totally dysfunctional, losing jobs and clients. He finds that he is always angry and suffers flashbacks about the postoperative period of pain and confusion. Jacques gradually became depressed, and his obnoxious, angry behavior alienated both friends and providers.

His primary care physician developed a trusting relationship with Jacques, helping him to disclose the painful information about his personal failures. The doctor identifies the onset of symptoms as associated with the surgery and helps Jacques recognize the role of the traumatic event in his life. The doctor explains the potential for improvement with psychotherapy and treatment for depression and encourages him to enter an established multidisciplinary treatment program.

Management: Treatment of PTSD is multifaceted and usually best accomplished with a multidisciplinary team. Typical team members include the primary care physician, a mental health professional, an addiction specialist, a social worker, and possibly community-based referral resources such as theme counseling groups (eg, veterans groups, abuse-survivor groups, etc.). It is helpful to label the problem as PTSD and thus legitimize the manifestations, since patients often blame themselves. The physician might say to the patient, "The kinds of feelings, thoughts, and problems you're having are not unusual—they're fairly common among people who have gone through a catastrophe." Aggressive treatment of substance abuse, using addiction specialists, is essential to maximize the patient's occupational and other functions. Support groups of persons who have suffered similar trauma help patients feel understood; they share their experiences and solve problems together.

There is little evidence of efficacy in using pharmacologic agents for treating flashbacks and nightmares. The best pharmacologic strategy is to diagnose and treat coexisting major depression, panic disorder, or substance abuse. Some practitioners advocate the use of clonidine or beta-adrenergic antagonists for treating aggression and other psychophysiologic arousal symptoms. Care should be taken to avoid benzodiazepine use in patients with a substance-abuse history.

Generalized Anxiety Disorder

Diagnosis: Generalized anxiety disorder (GAD) consists of constant, nonepisodic worry and anxiety that affects patients for more than 6 months and interferes with normal functioning. The worry and anxiety are difficult for the patient to control and are associated with edginess or restlessness, easy fatigability, difficulty concentrating, irritability, muscle tension, or sleep disturbance. Worries are typically about routine life circumstances, with the magnitude of worry being out of proportion to the severity of the situation. Symptoms must not be due to the physiologic effects of a medical problem like hyperthyroidism or abuse of a medication or drug. Patients with GAD usually complain of feeling "up tight" or constantly nervous. Physical symptoms such as muscle aches, twitching, trembling, sweating, dry mouth, headaches, gastrointestinal symptoms, urinary frequency, and exaggerated startle often accompany the disorder (Table 23–4).

Table 23–4. Specific symptoms associated with generalized anxiety disorder.

Symptom	Manifestation
Motor tension	Trembling, twitching, feeling shaky Muscle tension, aches, soreness Restlessness Easy fatigability
Autonomic hyperactivity	Shortness of breath, smothering sensations Palpitations, accelerated heart rate Sweating, cold clammy hands Dry mouth Dizziness, lightheadedness Nausea, diarrhea, other types of abdominal distress Flushes (hot flashes), chills Frequent urination Trouble swallowing, "lump in throat"
Vigilance and scanning	Feeling keyed up or on edge Exaggerated startle response Difficulty concentrating or "mind going blank" because of anxiety Trouble falling or staying asleep Irritability

Source: Reproduced, with permission, from McGlynn TJ, Metcalf HL (editors): *Diagnosis and Treatment of Anxiety Disorders: A Physician's Handbook,* 2nd ed. American Psychiatric Press, 1991.

The 1-year prevalence of GAD in the community is approximately 3%; the lifetime prevalence, approximately 5%. About two thirds of affected individuals are women. The disorder tends to have a chronic, fluctuating course that worsens under stress. Secondary depression is common and predicts a better outcome.

Management: Benzodiazepine therapy at lower doses than those required for panic disorder is usually rapidly effective with few adverse effects. Sedation is the most common side effect but diminishes over time. Tolerance to therapeutic effects is minimal. Minimum effective doses should be used, but care must be taken not to undertreat patients out of fear of making them drug-dependent. As with benzodiazepine treatment for other anxiety disorders, rebound anxiety symptoms are the rule as medication is discontinued. Often a lengthy (a month or more) taper is required. Buspirone is a nonsedating, nonbenzodiazepine anxiolytic specifically indicated for patients with GAD. Buspirone is not associated with tolerance, withdrawal, or dependence. Its onset of action is about 3–4 weeks. There is some evidence that buspirone is most effective for less chronic patients who have never tried benzodiazepines. Tricyclic antidepressants are also often effective for patients with GAD, especially those with coexisting depressive symptoms. There is no consensus yet about the appropriate length of treatment.

Short-term supportive psychotherapy can also be helpful. Many patients with GAD have focal life conflicts or stressors for which psychotherapy may be helpful. Basic primary care strategies include empathic listening; encouragement; and assisting patients to identify problems, discuss possible solutions, and solve the problem. Cognitive-behavioral techniques can be used to help patients examine the catastrophic beliefs that underlie their unrealistic worries. Biofeedback and relaxation techniques are useful for improving patient control over muscle tension and other physiologic signs of anxiety.

Adjustment Disorder With Anxiety

Diagnosis: Adjustment disorder with anxiety should be considered in patients who are responding with maladaptive anxiety to a recent situational stressor but do not meet the criteria for another mental disorder. The stressor may be a medical event (eg, surgery, hospitalization, onset of an illness), but most often is a personal crisis like a divorce, financial problems, or a job change. Symptoms usually begin within 2 months of the onset of the stressor and significantly impair social or occupational functioning. If symptoms persist for more than 6 months, then another diagnosis, such as GAD, is usually more appropriate. Sleeplessness and the physiologic aspects of anxiety predominate, and the patient may seek care for somatic complaints. Eliciting the history of the stressful life event and ascertaining the relationship of symptoms to that event help to establish this diagnosis.

Management: The fundamental management of adjustment disorder with anxious mood is supportive counseling, in which the patient discusses the stressful event and the provider helps the patient actively identify and solve problems (as described earlier for GAD). Patients with adjustment disorder are generally well cared for by a primary care physician who has learned the details of the precipitating event and can incorporate brief supportive strategies into the office visit. Structured relaxation exercises and group instruction in stress management may also be helpful. Support groups of patients with similar stressors (eg, patients with breast cancer) is often helpful. Sometimes a brief benzodiazepine trial (less than 3 weeks) can help improve patient coping by reducing the debilitating stress-related symptoms (eg, insomnia, or overwhelming fear). Referral to mental health professionals may help if patients do not respond quickly, are severely incapacitated, or specifically request a therapist.

Many studies suggest that there is a substantial group of primary care patients who present with relatively minor complaints of anxiety and depression. Although they do not satisfy criteria for a mental disorder, they do experience associated poor functioning. Often psychosocial stressors or chronic medical problems exacerbate the emotional symptoms. Generally speaking, effective management should emphasize supportive psychosocial rather than pharmacologic interventions.

MANAGEMENT OF ANXIETY: GENERAL PRINCIPLES

Most of the treatments for anxiety disorders were described previously along with the disorders they characteristically treat. Some general principles pertaining to the primary care treatment of anxiety disorders are worthy of note, however, and are therefore described here.

Pharmacotherapy

Pharmacologic treatment (Table 23–5) is appropriate when the patient's symptoms are severe enough to significantly interfere with functioning and the

Table 23–5. Pharmacotherapy for anxiety disorders.

Disorder	Examples of Treatment Options	Comments
Panic	(1) Imipramine, 25 mg qd; increase up to 150–200 qd; maximum 300 mg Add alprazolam or clonazepam for 3–4 weeks while increasing antidepressant. (2) Paroxetine, 20 mg qd (smaller doses may be effective, especially in the elderly)	Panic often increased in initial treatment
Phobias	(1) Beta-blocker: propanolol 10– to 40 mg prior to anticipated exposure (2) Benzodiazepine as needed prior to anticipated, infrequent exposure	
OCD	(1) Clomipramine, 25 mg qd; increase to 100 mg qd over 2 weeks; maximum daily dose 250 mg (2) Fluoxetine 40–80 mg qd	Treatment often chronic
GAD	(1) Low-dose benzodiazepine (eg, lorazepam), 1–5 mg qd, divided (2) Buspirone, 5 mg tid; increase in 5-mg increments; maximum daily dose 60 mg	Tolerance develops to initial sedation Nonsedating, no dependence
Adjustment disorder	Brief benzodiazepine use as sedative or anxiolytic	Main treatment is support; medication treatment is time-limited

benefits of medication outweigh its risks for a given patient. The treatment must be carefully individualized, based on the patient's particular constellation of symptoms, complicating medical or substance-abuse problems, vulnerability to various side effects, and willingness to collaborate in a psychopharmacologic approach to treatment.

When medications are prescribed, it is important to recognize, track, and document specific target symptoms. The dosage of medication should be titrated so as to minimize both the target symptoms and bothersome side effects. Lower than normal doses of psychoactive agents are recommended for the elderly, since these drugs have longer half-lives in this age group, accumulation can easily occur, and sensitivity to unwanted cognitive and other toxic effects is greater (see Chapter 12).

Although monotherapy is almost always preferable to medication combinations, one common exception to this rule is prescribing both antidepressants and minor tranquilizers together for patients with panic disorder. This strategy achieves rapid reduction of symptoms, avoids the intensification of anxiety typical of early antidepressant treatment of anxiety disorders, and allows discontinuation of benzodiazepines before dependence occurs. Benzodiazepines should seldom be used in patients with a history of substance abuse.

Psychosocial Therapies

Primary care providers should not underestimate the importance of basic supportive measures that can easily be performed in the general medical setting. The relationship between the doctor and patient usually plays a pivotal role for anxious patients. Patient-provider trust is especially important for anxious patients, enhancing timely and accurate history-taking, physical exam, diagnosis, and treatment compliance. An accurate history and diagnosis help avoid unnecessary testing.

Anxiety symptoms are extremely distressing to patients, who often fear that occult disease is driving their symptoms. Clinicians must try to view the symptoms through the eyes and perceptions of the affected patient—what seems trivial to a provider may be overwhelming for the patient. Listening to patients, expressing empathy for their feelings and concerns, and providing information about anxiety disorders are crucial ways to improve patient rapport (see Chapters 1 and 2) and should be routine in the course of care.

Equipping patients with basic information about anxiety disorders is essential (Table 23–6). Patients often present as very fearful, thinking something terrible is wrong with them. Patients with anxiety are common enough that providers should be prepared with standard explanations such as the example described in the section on panic disorder. Most patients find such explanations, and suggestions for appropriate lay publications, reassuring.

INDICATIONS FOR REFERRAL

Patients should be considered for referral to a mental health professional under the following circumstances:

1. The treatment does not lead to improvement in the patient's symptoms within the expected timeframe.
2. The physician is confused about the primary diagnosis. It is particularly important to differentiate patients who have depression with symptoms of anxiety, or who are alcoholics, from those with anxiety disorder. Mental health consultation is appropriate if the primary care doctor is uncertain and the distinction has therapeutic implications.
3. Complicating substance abuse is suspected.
4. The patient has suicidal thoughts, or plans, or exhibits or intended suicidal behavior.
5. The provider has questions about appropriate administration or tapering of benzodiazepines and questions regarding possible dependence.

In some circumstances, the primary care physician may be uncertain about whether a patient has another medical illness and feels a specialist is necessary to consider that possibility. It is helpful to pick a spe-

Table 23–6. Nonpharmacologic management of anxiety disorders

Type of Treatment	Description	Indication
Education	Provides basic information and reassurance	Appropriate in all disorders Lay publications useful
Behavior therapy, eg, systematic desensitization	Gradually increases exposure to feared stimulus using relaxation techniques	Particularly helpful in panic disorder Useful in treating agoraphobia, specific and social phobia
Cognitive therapy	Helps patient reorganize way of thinking about symptoms	Useful in all disorders.
Relaxation techniques	Uses muscle-relaxation therapy, including hypnosis, biofeedback, meditation	Particularly useful in panic disorders, GAD, adjustment disorder with anxious mood

cialist who understands anxiety disorders and will work with the referring physician to explain the nature of the specific anxiety disorder to the patient. It is imperative that the specialist bring a conservative approach to diagnostic studies, an understanding of the many physical manifestations of anxiety, and a respectful approach to treatment of the anxiety disordered patient.

The primary care physician who is knowledgeable and skilled in the diagnosis and management of anxiety disorders can make an important contribution to the quality of patient care and to the appropriate use of health resources, particularly in the managed care environment. The accurate and prompt diagnosis of anxiety disorders can prevent unnecessary diagnostic testing, which could lead to further distress and expense for the patient—and be wasteful of health-care resources.

SUGGESTED READINGS

American Psychiatric Association: *Diagnostic and Statistical Manual of Mental Disorders: Primary Care Version (DSM-IV-PC).* American Psychiatric Association, 1994.

Katon W J: *Panic Disorder in the Medical Setting.* American Psychiatric Press, 1991.

McGlynn TJ, Metcalf HL (editors): *Diagnosis and Treatment of Anxiety Disorders: A Physician's Handbook,* 2nd ed. American Psychiatric Press, 1991.

Myers JK et al: Six-month prevalence of psychiatric disorders in three communities: 1980–1982. Arch Gen Psychiatry 1984;41:959.

Roy-Byrne PP: Integrated treatment of panic disorder. Am J Med 1992;92(suppl 1A):49S.

Shader RI, Greenblatt DJ: Use of benzodiazepines in anxiety disorders. N Engl J Med 1993;329(19):1398.

Sheehan DV: *The Anxiety Disease.* Bantam, 1983.

Spitzer RL et al: Utility of a new procedure for diagnosing mental disorders in primary care: The PRIME-MD 1000 study. JAMA 1994;272:1749.

REFERENCE BOOKS FOR PATIENTS

Leaman TL: *Healing the Anxiety Diseases.* Plenum Press, 1992.

Sheehan DV: *The Anxiety Disease.* Bantam, 1983.

24

Somatization

Craig B. Kaplan, MD, MA

Case illustration: Beatrice, a 57-year-old woman, makes an appointment with a new physician. She presents with a 10-year history of multiple, unexplained symptoms. She has seen many physicians over the past decade, including several primary care physicians and numerous subspecialists. Her principal complaints today include abdominal pain, chest pain, headache, palpitations, fatigue, and intermittent dizziness. She brings with her a thick stack of records from some of her prior physicians. These records include multiple laboratory tests and diagnostic procedures, none of which have identified any cause for her symptoms.

DOCTOR: How can I help you today, Ms. Arthur?

PATIENT: *(sighing)* I don't know, doctor. A friend of mine saw you a few months ago and said you were very good. I hope you can help me. I've had these problems for years now, and no one seems to be able to figure them out. Maybe you can. I know there's something wrong. I've been so sick.

DOCTOR: Why don't you tell me about your symptoms?

PATIENT: Well, it all began about 10 years ago. . . .

INTRODUCTION

Most physicians have encountered frustrating patients who repeatedly present with unexplained physical complaints that defy their best diagnostic and therapeutic efforts. Although these patients are seen in most medical practices, they seem to be particularly common in primary care settings, where they are significant users of medical care, are frequently subjected to repeated diagnostic tests and invasive procedures—and often frustrate and anger their physicians. Many of these patients, who seem unable to use emotional language to describe their distress, are expressing psychological illness or social distress in the physical language of somatic symptoms, an entirely unconscious process known as *somatization*.

Somatization

This term is used throughout this chapter to indicate a general illness process rather than the more specific disorders included in the *Diagnostic and Statistical Manual of Mental Disorders (DSM-IV)* category of somatoform disorders (described later in the chapter). Conceptualized thus broadly, somatization includes many more individuals than do the more restrictive diagnoses of the somatoform disorders. In fact, although most patients in this category are suffering from significant psychosocial distress, many somatizers do not have a specific psychiatric diagnosis

Mechanisms of Somatization: Somatization may be understood from four theoretical perspectives: neurobiological, psychodynamic, behavioral, and sociocultural. Note that no single perspective is "right" or "correct" for all patients; each offers a specific viewpoint from which to understand a patient's somatizing behavior. Although one of these perspectives alone may enable us to understand why a given patient somatizes, more often a deeper understanding results from considering multiple perspectives.

1. Neurobiological—In this perspective, somatization results from defective or deficient neurobiological processing of sensory and emotional information. For example, somatization might occur as a consequence of deficient central inhibition of incoming sensory information or of impaired right-to-left hemispheric communication.

2. Psychodynamic—From the psychodynamic perspective, somatized physiological sensations occur as expressions of underlying emotional conflict. They may also enable patients to meet latent needs for nurturing and support—which they obtain from the medical community.

3. Behavioral—In this perspective, somatization is viewed as behavior that is brought about and reinforced by others in the patient's environment. "Illness-maintenance systems" are constellations of environmental reinforcers that sustain somatizing behavior in any given patient. These systems consist of desirable (from the patient's point of view) responses of family members or others (supervisors, friends), disability payments, or medical care, which are brought about by and reinforce the patient's medical complaints. To modify abnormal illness behavior, these illness-maintenance systems and the individuals who participate in them must be identified and influenced. For example, a lonely elderly woman who complains of unexplained abdominal and chest pains might be rewarded inadvertently by her children's tendency to visit only when she is "feeling bad." Encouraging the family to visit instead when the patient states she is feeling well reinforces her well behavior rather than her illness behavior:

> DOCTOR: (*talking to the patient's son on the phone*) I know it sounds insensitive, Mr. A., but you might consider *not* visiting your mom when she calls you and says she's sick. You can tell her you're sorry she's sick and that you wouldn't want to disturb her when she's feeling bad. Say you'll call in a few days to see if she's feeling better. But then, be sure you do visit her when she says she's all right.

4. Sociocultural–According to this perspective, people learn from their culture "correct" behaviors for dealing with emotions and feelings. Direct expression of emotions is permissible in some cultures; in others it is highly stigmatized. When a culture does not allow direct communication of emotional content, one (possibly the only) means available to express emotions is through physical symptoms. In effect, somatization serves to notify others of emotional stress or mental illness in ways that are acceptable and not stigmatizing. The condition of "nerves" common in rural Appalachia is an example. Patients with "nerves" are understood by others in the Appalachian culture to be less capable of tolerating the stresses of daily living, even though they are not looked on as having a psychiatric illness. Another example may be chronic fatigue. It has been postulated that some (certainly not all) patients with chronic fatigue are communicating their distress at a cultural level, and that the diagnosis is an acceptable means of allowing them to decrease their overachieving behavior.

Significance of Somatization: Data from the United States and England suggest that somatizing patients are an important problem for primary care physicians, accounting for an average of 40-75% of visits to outpatient clinics. These patients are suffering from mental disorders such as depression and anxiety, which are among the most common problems seen in primary care settings. Many of these depressed or anxious patients visit their physicians with such predominantly physical complaints as fatigue, dizziness, headache, and abdominal or extremity pain, accompanied by requests for "check-ups."

Because of the frequency with which they visit their physicians—added to the many diagnostic tests ordered to evaluate their complaints—somatizing patients have a significant economic impact on health-care costs. Analyses done in the early 1980s suggested that somatizing patients are a substantial economic burden to HMOs. For example, among the top 10% of health-care users in one large Pacific Northwest HMO, half had a current psychiatric diagnosis such as depression, anxiety, or a somatoform disorder. Despite its pervasiveness, this costly pattern can be significantly improved by treating these patients using relatively simple principles.

Somatizing patients are also costly in terms of our own professional satisfaction, evoking among physicians a wide variety of negative feelings, including frustration, anger, a sense of impotence, and demoralization. A better understanding of this phenomenon, together with reasonable expectations and a proper approach to management, can help doctors to avoid—or at least cope with—these feelings.

DIAGNOSIS

Presentation of Somatizing Patients in Primary Care Settings

Many somatizers are unaware of the psychological disorders that underlie their symptoms. Even when they perceive anxious or depressed feelings, they rarely understand or acknowledge a connection between these feelings and their physical complaints. Consequently they choose to visit primary care physicians or the "appropriate" subspecialists, who in their turn frequently refer these somatizers back to primary care physicians (a phenomenon that has been termed "reverse referrals").

Given that somatizing patients are common, how can clinicians detect this phenomenon and be comfortable with this diagnosis? Clearly, there are no absolute diagnostic tests. There are, however, clues that, when taken together, increase the diagnostic suspicion of somatization (Table 24–1).

Some of the terms used by experienced providers to describe somatizers are an indication of how their patients present. One such term is "thick-chart syndrome." Somatizing patients' charts are often stuffed with progress notes, telephone-call records, and letters from referring physicians, as well as multiple laboratory and diagnostic tests. Such a thick chart, particularly when filled with multiple, unexplained (but persistent) physical complaints, should be an obvious

Table 24–1. Clinical clues to somatization.

1. "Thick-chart" syndrome
2. Marked change in utilization pattern with increasing unexplained complaints, office visits, and hospitalizations
3. Vague, confusing, or bizarre symptoms
4. Resistance, often angry, to psychological inquiry or explanations
5. Specific complaints such as dizziness, fatigue, or insomia
6. Physician's "heartsink" response

clue to somatization. Somatization should also be suspected in previously stable patients who suddenly begin to make repeated visits with unexplained symptoms—a clue can be the marked change in the pattern of health-care use that occurs when patients develop psychiatric disorders or psychological distress. These developments of a psychiatric disorder significantly change patients' health-care use patterns, as evidenced by increasing unexplained complaints, office visits, and hospitalizations.

The symptoms described by somatizers can be vague, confusing, or even bizarre. Although they are certainly not limited to this patient population, repeated complaints that seem vague or confusing or do not fit with known neuroanatomic structures may indicate somatization.

An important clue can be the patient's often-dramatic resistance to psychological inquiry or explanations. Most patients are willing to consider psychological explanations, even though they may not agree with them. On the other hand, many somatizers, particularly those with the somatoform disorders, angrily resist the suggestion that their symptoms are linked in any way to psychological distress. They often become angry even when questioned about their psychological or social lives. The more they protest, the more likely it is that somatization is present.

Yet another clue may lie in the particular complaint(s) offered by the patient. Symptoms such as dizziness, fatigue, or insomnia are especially common as presenting complaints in somatizers. Finally, the physician's own feelings and emotional responses to patients can be valuable diagnostically. Some somatizing patients have been referred to as "heartsink" patients: the provider sees the patient's name on the daily list and his or her heart sinks. It can be useful to recognize these feelings and treat them as data indicative of somatization.

No one of these clues is sufficient by itself to establish somatization as the explanation for a patient's symptoms. If a number of these diagnostic clues are present, however, the likelihood of somatization increases. It is important to avoid diagnosing somatization negatively, that is, solely through the absence of physical disease. Without at least several of the positive clues described here, such a diagnosis may be premature. In these cases it may be best simply to follow the patient's symptoms with an open mind, simultaneously considering both somatization and medical illnesses.

Differential Diagnosis

Most people perceive but ignore minor pains or sensory disturbances in the course of daily activity. Psychiatric disorders or significant psychosocial stress increase the likelihood that patients will pay more attention to these physiological sensations and label them as abnormal—a phenomenon known as "symptom amplification" (see Chapter 6). Stress and

psychiatric disorders can also directly produce disturbing physiological symptoms.

Transient, or Acute, Somatization: This occurs when symptoms result from transient stress that temporarily overwhelms a person's usual means of coping and is probably the most common form of somatization. At such times, these individuals may experience disturbing bodily sensations and seek care for them. Rarely is there a history of prolonged symptoms, and health-care–seeking is not usually a dominant aspect of their lives. These patients usually do not have diagnosable psychiatric illnesses and fairly readily accept stress as a cause of their symptoms.

Chronic Somatization: On the other hand, chronic somatization is a long-lasting process that occurs in the context of often specific psychiatric disorders: depressive, anxiety, somatoform, personality, and factitious. Depressed or anxious patients may minimize or not perceive mood symptoms, instead presenting with the physical symptoms associated with these disorders. With depressed patients, this form of presentation has been referred to as "masked depression."

Somatoform Disorders: Unlike somatization associated with depression and anxiety, the somatoform disorders are psychiatric illnesses for which somatization is the *sole* manifestation. *DSM-IV* describes six specific somatoform disorders (Table 24–2). Common to these disorders is the long-standing "presence of physical symptoms that . . . are not fully explained by a general medical condition, by the direct effects of a substance, or by another mental disorder." These disorders are grouped together, not because of a common pathophysiological mechanism, but because of the need to exclude medical or substance-induced illness before making the diagnosis. The category now includes the addition of "undifferentiated somatoform disorder." This diagnosis recognizes the patients without other psychiatric disorders who, particularly in primary care settings, have several persistent somatic symptoms but not the very large number of symptoms required for the diagnosis of full-blown somatization disorder. Because of this distinction, more of the somatizing patients seen in primary care settings can now be described under the somatoform disorder category.

It is generally not fruitful for primary care physicians to make a specific *DSM-IV*–based diagnosis of one of the somatoform disorders. Although a specific diagnosis can facilitate communication with mental-health-care providers, none of the disorders is amenable to pharmacological therapy; neither has any form of psychiatric treatment been found more beneficial for some patients than others. The natural history of most of these disorders, particularly those in the newer classifications, is not clear. The category of somatoform disorders is useful primarily because it recognizes that there are indeed patients who somatize throughout their lives in the absence of other psychiatric disorders such as depression or anxiety. These pa-

Table 24–2. *DSM-IV* Somatoform disorders.

Somatization Disorder: A polysymptomatic disorder that begins before age 30 years, extends over a period of years, and is characterized by a combination of pain, gastrointestinal, sexual, and pseudoneurologic symptoms.

Undifferentiated Somatoform Disorder: Unexplained physical complaints, lasting at least 6 months, that are below the threshold for a diagnosis of somatization disorder.

Conversion Disorder: Unexplained symptoms of deficits affecting voluntary motor or sensory function that suggest a neurological or other general medical condition. Psychological factors are considered to be associated with the symptoms or deficits.

Pain Disorder: Pain as the predominant focus of clinical attention. In addition, psychological factors are considered to have an important role in its onset, severity, exacerbation, or maintenance.

Hypochondriasis: Preoccupation with the fear of having, or the idea that one has, a serious disease, based on the person's misinterpretation of bodily symptoms or bodily functions.

Body Dysmorphic Disorder: Preoccupation with an imagined or exaggerated defect in physical appearance.

Source: Based on definitions from American Psychiatric Association: *Diagnostic and Statistical Manual of Mental Disorders,* 4th edition. American Psychiatric Association, 1994.

tients, as a group, are among the most difficult to treat and therefore have the worst prognosis of all of the psychiatric disorders associated with somatization.

Malingering and Factitious Disorders: These are rarely encountered in the primary care setting. Malingering is seen predominantly in military populations and in patients involved in legal proceedings. Of note, malingering is the only disorder associated with somatization in which the patient intentionally produces the symptom and consciously attempts to gain by it. In all the other disorders the gain, when present, is unconscious.

Evaluation

Even when a psychiatric disorder is apparent, to what extent should medical disorders be excluded as possible causes of unexplained, persistent symptoms? Are providers being negligent if they do not perform extensive diagnostic testing to rule out every uncommon illness (eg, pheochromocytoma, Cushing's disease, vasculitis, heavy-metal toxicity, and many, many others)? The core issue here is *uncertainty.* These symptomatic patients, particularly when they angrily demand physical explanations for their symptoms, heighten our discomfort with the uncertainty inherent in all of medical practice. Can any amount of testing enable us to be certain the patient does *not* have one of these rare diseases or, alternatively, is that they are indeed a somatizer? In fact, we can never be absolutely certain. Each patient deserves careful and empathic listening, a thorough physical examination, review of previous records and, for some, limited diagnostic testing.

The laboratory evaluation should be directed by patient-specific symptoms and, more important, physical signs. Rarely is more than a complete blood count, liver and renal function tests, a thyroid-stimulating hormone (TSH), and sedimentation rate needed. Often these tests have been performed recently enough by other physicians that there is no need to repeat them. Without specific indications, more diagnostic testing increases the likelihood that false-positive results will appear—and may also indirectly

reinforce the patient's belief that a physical disease is present.

It is often beneficial to explicitly acknowledge this inherent uncertainty, both to ourselves and to the patient:

> PATIENT: I don't know, doctor. A friend of mine had a disease called Cushing's. Do you think I might have that?
>
> DOCTOR: That's a good question, Ms. A. There are a great many diseases that can present with symptoms like yours. I want you to know that, as I've listened to you and examined you, I've tried to think of rare diseases. I don't believe any of them are very likely, especially since you've had your symptoms for so long. I do want to be honest with you, though. There's no way to be absolutely certain. There are so many different diseases that it would cost a fortune to get tests for all of them. Even then it would be impossible to rule out all possibilities since there are no laboratory tests available for some of them. Let's get a few laboratory tests done, though. If they're normal, let's not do any more tests, but I'll keep an open mind as to these possibilities as we get to know each other during the course of the next few months. If you develop symptoms later that suggest one of these rare diseases to me, I'll certainly order more tests. How does that sound to you?

In this brief dialogue the physician acknowledges uncertainty while communicating a sense of honesty and trustworthiness. By reinforcing the continuity of the relationship and the willingness to entertain different possibilities in the future, the physician helps the patient feel cared for without the need for multiple, and most likely unnecessary, diagnostic tests. See Chapter 7 in this text for a discussion of patient requests in a managed care setting.

MANAGEMENT

The most important aspect of managing somatizing patients is the development of an empathic, trusting physician-patient relationship. Establishing this therapeutic relationship is critical to both diagnosis and treatment. Table 24–3 lists the specific communication skills that can be used in building such relationships (see Chapter 2).

This is not to say that relationships with somatizing patients are easy to establish. Physicians sometimes have to work at viewing them positively. It helps to remember that somatizing patients are reacting in the best and—without help—only way available to them. It also helps to listen to the frequently very moving life stories these patients tell. Hearing the neglect, abuse, and other painful events in many patients' lives, physicians may often find themselves admiring how these patients have survived. Finally, somatizing patients are often intellectually challenging. They often push physicians to consider unusual medical illnesses and to draw on all of their interpersonal skills and knowledge of psychology.

Transient somatizers generally have a good prognosis. They are often willing to consider or accept psychological or psychophysiological explanations for their symptoms:

> DOCTOR: Your fatigue is due to all of the energy required by your body to deal with the stress you've been under lately.

Often it is necessary only to tell these patients that the experience of stress as physical symptoms is a common and normal occurrence, reassuring them that you have considered their symptoms thoroughly. When stress is severe or likely to be prolonged, these patients often readily accept suggestions for stress management or referrals for therapy (see Chapter 29).

Chronically somatizing patients require a somewhat more complex management strategy. Because these patients consider their symptoms to be physical problems, they strongly resist psychological explanations and usually refuse psychiatric referrals. Primary care providers can treat these patients, however. Effective management strategies in the primary care setting can reduce costs and improve both patient and physician satisfaction with the quality of care (Table 24–4).

Do Not Dispute the Reality of Symptoms: It never helps to dispute the reality or severity of patients' physical complaints; their symptoms are very real to them. For the vast majority, somatization is an unconscious process. Most symptoms are subjective in nature and not objectively verifiable. When physicians imply that they don't believe their patients are sick, these patients may feel they are not being taken seriously. In fact, it helps to acknowledge their suffering explicitly:

> DOCTOR: I can see how much you've suffered with all of these symptoms, Ms. A.
>
> PATIENT: (*tearfully*) Oh, doctor. You're the only one who seems to understand that. . . .

Paying close attention to and fully clarifying patients' illness stories, their underlying beliefs, and their expectations for care will also convince them they are being taken seriously and help establish a therapeutic relationship.

Use Mutually Acceptable Language: Try to use understandable and mutually acceptable language to explain the patient's symptoms. Avoid the use of psychological labels (eg, depression, anxiety, or stress). Also, avoid such statements as "There's nothing physically wrong with you." Do not try to convince the patients that their symptoms are psychological in origin. Many patients actually believe the opposite: that their mood symptoms, if present, are caused by their physical symptoms.

> DOCTOR: Have you ever considered that you might be depressed, Ms. A.?
>
> PATIENT: Oh, I know I'm depressed. Wouldn't you be depressed if you had all of this pain and no one could help you?

Table 24–3. Empathic communication skills used to establish effective relationships with patients.*

Skill	Example
Empathy	*That must have been a very sad event for you.* *I can see how angry you were after you'd heard the diagnosis.*
Legitimization	*I think anyone in your circumstances would have felt the way you did.* *Feeling sad about something like this is perfectly normal and natural.*
Partnership	*I want you to know that you and I will be working on this together as a team.*
Support	*Whatever else happens, I'll always be in your corner.*
Respect	*I'm impressed that you've been able to maintain all your obligations at home and at work in spite of your pain. I respect your commitment.*

* See Cohen-Cole SA. *The Medical Interview: The Three-Function Approach.* Mosby-Year Book, 1991.

Table 24–4. Suggestions for managing chronic somatizers.

1. Don't dispute the reality or severity of the patient's physical complaints.
2. Use understandable and mutually acceptable language to explain the patient's symptoms.
3. Establish appropriate goals and expectations for both yourself and the patient.
4. Schedule follow-up visits at regular intervals, independent of symptoms.
5. Set limits on phone calls and drop-in visits.
6. Respectfully evaluate each symptom, with a careful interview, physical examination, and judicious use of diagnostic tests.
7. Use medications to treat defined disorders (eg, depression, anxiety, etc) or to reduce (not remove) specific target symptoms, particularly chronic pain.

Although it may seem somewhat counterintuitive, the physician should begin each visit with a discussion of the somatic complaint. Descriptive physiological explanations such as "abnormally tense muscles in your chest that go into painful spasm" tend to be more acceptable to patients and to their families. As they learn to trust their physicians, patients may eventually (over months to years!) begin to explore the relationship between their psychosocial issues and their symptoms.

> PATIENT: I don't know, doctor. Maybe I am crazy . . . that's what everyone else seems to think.
>
> DOCTOR: Let me assure you that you're not crazy. I hear your concern, Ms. A. Why don't we talk about this a little bit? I think it's possible that depression may be taking its toll on your body and your sense of well-being. Now, you tell me: What is the worst thing that would happen if these symptoms were caused by depression?

Since it is the patient who is bringing up the topic, this represents a golden opportunity to begin cautiously discussing psychological explanations.

Establish Appropriate Goals and Expectations: Although somatization is rarely curable, physicians often find themselves fantasizing that one more pain medication will help, or that a mental health referral will bring about an epiphany for the patient. When these fantasies become the goals of the relationship, they inevitably lead to disappointment and worsening frustration for both physician and patient. Rather than aiming for a dramatic insight or complete resolution of symptoms, it is better to set less global, more realistic goals. For physicians such goals might be reducing the number of urgent telephone calls and unscheduled visits, decreasing doctor-shopping, and avoiding unnecessary hospitalizations or invasive procedures. For patients, positive, realistic goals might include improved coping with symptoms, increased feelings of control of themselves or their symptoms, or improved social or occupational functioning.

These goals should be explicitly negotiated:

> DOCTOR: Today I would like to talk about what we should expect from each other in this relationship, Ms. A. From your perspective, I suspect that the best of all things I could do would be to figure out what's causing these symptoms and make them go away. Given all of your years of suffering and the many doctors you've seen, however, I'm sad to say that I don't think that is very realistic. What do you think?
>
> PATIENT: Well, of course I was hoping that you could find a cure. (*long pause*) So—does this mean you can't help me?
>
> DOCTOR: No, I didn't mean to imply that. I do think I can help. First, I'd like to work on helping you learn to cope more effectively with your symptoms. We could also work to improve how you function from day to day. Whether you get better or not, I'm committed to being your doctor and helping you in the best way I can.

Schedule Regular Follow-up Visits: Appointments should be scheduled at regular intervals, every 2–4 weeks, for example, whether the patient's symptoms have improved, gotten worse, or remained the same. Basing the frequency of visits on the number or severity of symptoms merely reinforces and maintains the behavior. Follow-up appointments that are independent of symptoms stress the importance of the doctor-patient relationship and de-emphasize the physical complaints. Physicians should consider asking the patients when they want to return. Often patients, given time and a sense of control, will themselves suggest lengthening the visit interval. Unless the patient suggests it, however, attempting to lengthen the times between appointments may actually lead to worsening symptoms.

Establish Limits: Once the physician and the patient commit to regular follow-up appointments, it is appropriate to set limits on phone calls and drop-in visits. Rules for these behaviors should be set early in the relationship. One helpful rule is that the patient will reserve all but emergency complaints for regularly scheduled sessions. If the patient calls between scheduled visits, the discussion should be limited to ascertaining that there is no objective emergency or psychological crisis requiring immediate action. If there is none, further discussion should be gently deferred until the next scheduled appointment.

> DOCTOR: (*picking up telephone*) Hi, Ms. A. What can I do for you?
>
> PATIENT: Oh, doctor. My chest has been hurting again. I thought it might be gone, but it's back.
>
> DOCTOR: (*after several pertinent questions about the chest pain*) Ms. A, it sounds like this is the same pain you've had before, although I do understand that it's a little worse. I don't think we should do anything different from the plan we've agreed on. I see that you have an appointment next Tuesday. Let's continue to discuss it then.

Although this scenario may occur several times (with the physician or members of the office staff), patients eventually realize that these "urgent" telephone calls will not result in more caring behavior from the physician. Surprisingly, most patients also ultimately accept these arrangements if limits are enforced in the context of regular visits and a caring relationship.

Evaluate Symptoms: Each symptom should be respectfully evaluated with a careful interview, physical examination, and judicious use of diagnostic tests. Do a physical examination, no matter how unusual the symptom. Patients often judge how seriously they are taken by whether or not the doctor actually examines them. Not all complaints merit diagnostic tests, however. When necessary, tests should be used in a conservative, stepwise fashion. Physicians should try negotiating about diagnostic tests (especially the expensive ones) if patients ask for them. In return for ordering diagnostic tests, the physician can frequently ask patients to agree to accept the proposed conservative management strategy if the test results are negative.

Use Medications: Medications, if used, should be prescribed to treat defined disorders (depression, anxiety, etc) or to reduce (not remove) specific target symptoms, particularly chronic pain. Severe somatizers often warrant an empiric trial of tricyclic antidepressants because of the frequency with which they deny depression. Anxiolytics may help if they are used specifically for anxiety or panic disorder. It should be noted that treatment with narcotics, hypnotics, or sedatives is ineffective, and the dangers of addiction are real in this patient population.

Referral and Consultation

When discussing referrals or consultations with patients, it is wise to remember that most of them have, at some point in their lives, experienced referral as the first step in rejection or termination by a physician. Although acute somatizers may accept referral, chronic somatizers are hard to refer to mental health providers because these patients resist the psychological labeling required to justify the referral. Even when successful referrals are made, patients with somatoform disorders rarely respond to insight-oriented therapy and frequently return to primary care physicians for chronic management. A consultation model, in which patients are asked to see mental health providers for one or a few visits in order to "advise and help the primary care provider do a better job," is often better accepted. When possible, consultation can help by confirming the presence of an underlying mental disorder or by advising on the use of psychotropic medications. To reinforce the relationship between the primary care provider and the patient, the follow-up appointment should be made first, before the referral is discussed.

> DOCTOR: I'd like to see you in a month, Ms. A. In the meantime, I'd like you to consider seeing Dr. R., the psychiatrist we've talked about. I know you don't think that your chest pain is caused by your depression. But we've both agreed to try to treat the depression. I still don't know if we've found the right antidepressant, and I'd really value Dr. R.'s opinion. What do you think?

It is helpful to ask if the patient has any concerns about the request for referral or consultation. There are still many negative beliefs and significant stigma associated with mental health care. Unless these factors are discussed, they can decrease the likelihood

that the patient will actually make it to the mental health provider's office.

TIPS FOR SURVIVAL

Survival in treating somatizing patients lies primarily in resisting the temptation to try to cure them. It is important for physicians to set reasonable expectations for themselves and their patients and follow the management principles outlined here. Survival may also depend on the doctor's own willingness to acknowledge and accept the sometimes disturbing feelings that can arise in the course of caring for somatizers. Discussing these feelings with sensitive colleagues can be extraordinarily valuable.

Although difficult and frustrating at times, somatizing patients can be effectively treated in a primary care setting. In fact, a well-trained primary care provider may well be the ideal person for such treatment. A combination of empathic listening, conservative evaluation, and gentle limit-setting can greatly improve the lives of patients while increasing physicians' personal satisfaction with these relationships.

> ***Case illustration (Contd.):*** Beatrice continues to come for regular visits. Her symptoms continue, varying in severity and character, although her unscheduled visits and requests for diagnostic tests gradually diminish in frequency. As months pass and the doctor's relationship with her develops, she is more willing to cautiously discuss some of the psychosocial problems in her life. She does not, however, admit to a relationship between them and her symptoms. Her visit with the psychiatrist does not result in a therapeutic relationship with him, but he concurs with the primary care physician's suspicion that Beatrice is chronically depressed. The psychiatrist makes some helpful suggestions with respect to her antidepressant regimen and agrees to be available to the primary care doctor for periodic telephone consultation.

In time, both the physician and patient grow more comfortable with their inability either to establish a precise etiology for her symptoms or eliminate them. Although she still occasionally wonders aloud what might be causing them, she does not seem to expect her physician to cure them. For his part, the doctor stops hoping for a dramatic response to treatment or for sudden psychological insights. As he comes to know Beatrice better, he discovers aspects about her that he actually likes and respects. She seems to appreciate his caring and accepting attitude, and periodically says so. Providing care for Beatrice will never be easy, but it does have its rewards.

SUGGESTED READINGS

American Psychiatric Association: *Diagnostic and Statistical Manual of Mental Disorders: Primary Care Version.* American Psychiatric Association, 1994.

Cohen-Cole SA: *The Medical Interview: The Three-Function Approach.* Mosby, 1991.

Ford, CV: *The Somatizing Disorders: Illness as a Way of Life.* Elsevier, 1983.

Kaplan CB, Lipkin ML: Somatization in primary care. In: Branch WT (editor): *Office Practice of Medicine,* 3rd ed.), Saunders, 1994, pp 1027–1035.

Smith GR, Monson RA, Ray DC: Psychiatric consultation in somatization disorder. N Engl J Med 1986:314:;1407.

25   Personality Disorders

Adriana Feder, MD, & Seth Wigdor Robbins, MD, MPH

INTRODUCTION

Establishing successful relationships with patients who are suffering from personality disorders can be quite challenging for health-care providers, yet these patients are common in medical practice. Patients with personality disorders may over- or underuse medical care, and they often have more difficulty complying with treatment. In addition, these patients are more likely to be hospitalized. An understanding of personality disorders allows physicians to anticipate the challenging interpersonal and behavioral problems that can arise in working with these patients. This knowledge can help physicians to work through the negative emotions that working with such patients may arouse, thereby facilitating the development and implementation of appropriate treatment plans.

The current edition of the *Diagnostic and Statistical Manual of Mental Disorders (DSM-IV)* defines personality disorder as

> . . . an enduring pattern of inner experience and behavior that deviates markedly from the expectations of the individual's culture, is pervasive and inflexible, has an onset in adolescence or early adulthood, is stable over time, and leads to distress or impairment.

People suffering from personality disorders are affected in their view of themselves, their ability to establish and maintain relationships with others, and their ability to function at work and to experience pleasure in life. These patients have difficulty negotiating complex situations and coping with stress and anxiety. The sick role and the demands of medical care can be particularly problematic for them. The stress of illness is often extreme and sets into motion defensive and inflexible emotional processes, cognitions, and behaviors—with negative consequences for their medical treatment. In addition, these patients' difficulties in relating to others manifest themselves

in the doctor-patient relationship. They may be quite demanding or disrespectful of the needs of others, or they may experience such anxiety when needing to trust or confide in others that they may avoid building relationships.

Personality theorists have long debated how best to understand and classify personality disorders. The debate has centered on two models. The **categorical model,** adopted by *DSM-IV,* views personality disorders as entities that are distinct from one another—that is, classified in separate categories—and also distinct from normalcy. This model blends more easily with traditional medical diagnosis than does the **dimensional model,** which views personality disorders as overlapping with each other and with normalcy, so that the maladaptive traits of patients with personality disorders represent normal traits that are exaggerated.

In fact, both models hold some truth. Some personality disorders, such as schizotypal and paranoid, may belong to a spectrum of illness that includes psychotic Axis I disorders and are thus better explained by a categorical model. Other personality disorders, such as histrionic and obsessive-compulsive personality, may depict exaggerated normal traits, reinforcing the concept of a dimensional model.

Diagnostic Classification of Personality Disorders

DSM-IV classifies personality disorders on a separate axis, Axis II, and groups them into three clusters based on descriptive similarities. Cluster A includes paranoid, schizoid, and schizotypal personality disorders—individuals who often appear odd or eccentric; cluster B includes antisocial, borderline, histrionic, and narcissistic personality disorders—individuals who often appear dramatic, emotional, or erratic; and cluster C includes avoidant, dependent, and obsessive-compulsive personality disorders—individuals who often appear anxious or fearful. Given the unique nature of any individual personality, a patient can exhibit nature of any individual personality, a patient can exhibit traits of two or more personality disorders, or meet the full diagnostic criteria for more than one disorder.

Diagnosing a personality disorder can be a difficult task. In order to make an accurate diagnosis, it is usually necessary for the physician to get to know the patient over time, to find out how the patient reacts in other situations, and to obtain collateral information from family and friends. Clinicians should attend to three key issues.

First, it is important to differentiate a true personality disorder from personality traits that become exaggerated under stress. The stresses of illness on the patient often cause patients to behave in a more childlike manner; because of this, many patients, at one time or another, seem to have a personality disorder. Patients who do not suffer from a true personality disorder, however, are usually capable of more adaptive functioning. In these cases, the physician can successfully intervene by supporting and strengthening the patients' own natural coping skills.

Second, it is also important to differentiate personality disorders from such Axis I disorders as major depression or generalized anxiety disorder. For example, a patient with panic disorder may—out of sheer terror—become extremely dependent on her physician. If her panic disorder is diagnosed and treated, she may reveal an underlying independent and self-sufficient personality. When patients who do have a personality disorder are evaluated, looking for Axis I disorders is particularly important, since the latter are more frequent and difficult to treat if patients actually have a personality disorder. Treating an episode of major depression in a patient with borderline personality disorder, however, can alleviate suffering and lead to better coping with illness.

Third, the primary care provider must distinguish personality disorders from personality changes caused by general medical conditions, such as head trauma, stroke, epilepsy, or endocrine disorders. Patients with one of these problems may exhibit many of the characteristics of a personality disorder. These behaviors can be distinguished from a true personality disorder, however, in that they typically represent a change from baseline personality characteristics. Medical conditions such as these at times may also exacerbate preexisting personality traits (eg, obsessive mannerisms). Treatment of the underlying medical problem may bring about reversal of the personality changes.

Finally, personality disorder diagnoses, like other mental disorder diagnoses, are often misunderstood and may serve to stigmatize the patient. These diagnoses should therefore be made carefully, deferred in cases of uncertainty, and noted in medical records and correspondence only when they are likely to be helpful in enhancing patient care.

Doctor-Patient Relationship Issues

The primary care provider may find many challenges in working with patients with personality disorders. Personality disorders often significantly impair the quality of interpersonal relationships. Since the doctor-patient relationship requires effective communication about important health issues of a personal nature, tensions, and—at times—overt conflict, may develop between patients with personality disorders and their providers. These tensions may also affect other members of the health-care team and may be especially pronounced in the context of acute illness or crisis situations. In fact, the first diagnostic clues suggesting personality dysfunction, or disorder, may appear as difficulties in the doctor-patient relationship.

For patients with personality disorders, physical illness can cause exaggerated degrees of emotional distress, which is not always expressed to the provider. Although some patients do tell their providers about their emotional distress, others may instead exhibit the distress as noncompliance with the agreed-upon plan of evaluation or treatment, or it may appear as changed, unexpected, or undesirable behavior (as judged by the physician) toward the physician. Alternatively, expression of emotional distress may manifest as noncompliance with the agreed-on plan of evaluation or treatment.

Physicians are likely to become aware of patients' expression of distress, whether through the patients' actions or statements. This expression of distress may result in physicians having a significant emotional reaction to these patients, possibly leading to changes in their behavior toward the patients. Even when they experience no subjective distress from a medical condition or the doctor-patient relationship, patients with personality dysfunction may have such aberrant expectations of others that their statements or behavior are troubling or burdensome to the physician. Physicians must be aware of their own emotional responses to such patients so as to avoid reacting inappropriately. Physicians who deny their negative feelings toward the patients may fail to recognize a personality disorder or other psychiatric diagnosis, or fail to address the diagnostic and treatment needs of the patient with the necessary vigor and thoroughness. When clinicians recognize and deal with their negative feelings, they are better able to make thoughtful and appropriate responses to these patients' psychologic symptoms and behavior, minimizing the emotional strain for both patient and doctor and optimizing the quality of the medical outcome.

A clear understanding by both patient and doctor of the role each expects the other to play can aid in identifying problematic behaviors and can help to maintain the necessary degree of cooperation and collaboration, even when the patient has significant personality dysfunction. In this regard, it is important to understand how patients with different personality disorders vary in their needs and expectations

Table 25–1. Common personality disorders and typical manifestations

Personality Disorder	Paranoid	Schizoid	Antisocial	Borderline
Prominent features of disorder	Distrust and suspiciousness of others, such that their motives are interpreted as malevolent	Pattern of detachment from social relationships and a restricted range of emotional expression	Disregard for and violation of the rights of others, beginning in adolescence	Pattern of instability in interpersonal relationships, self-image and affects, and marked impulsivity
Patient's experience of illness	Heightened sense of fear and vulnerability	Threat to personal integrity; increased anxiety because illness forces interaction with others	Sense of fear may be masked by increased hostility or entitled stance	Terrifying fantasies about illness; feels either completely well or deathly ill
Problematic behavior in the medical care setting	Fear that physician or others may harm them. Misinterpretation of innocuous or even helpful behaviors. Increased likelihood of argument or conflict with staff	May delay seeking care until symptoms become severe, out of fear of interacting with others. May appear detached and unappreciative of help	Irresponsible, impulsive, or dangerous health behavior, without regard for consequences to self or others. Angry, deceitful, or manipulative behavior	Mistrust of physicians and delay in seeking treatment. Intense fear of rejection and abandonment. Abrupt shifts from idealizing to devaluing caregivers; splitting. Self-destructive threats and acts
Common problematic reactions to patient by caregiver	Defensive, argumentative or angry response that "confirms" patient's suspicions. Ignoring the patient's suspicious or angry stance	Overzealous attempts to connect with patient. Frustration at feeling unappreciated	Succumbing to patient's manipulation. Angry, punitive reaction when manipulation is discovered	Succumbing to patient's idealization and splitting. Getting too close to patient, causing overstimulation. Despair at patient's self-destructive behaviors. Temptation to punish patient angrily
Helpful management strategies by caregiver	Attend to and be empathic toward patient fears, even when irrational in appearance. Carefully detail care plan for patient with advance information about risks of procedures/treatments. Maintain patient's independence when possible. Professional, but not overly friendly stance	Appreciate need for privacy and maintain a low-key approach. Focus on technical elements of treatment; these are better tolerated. Encourage patient to maintain daily routines. Do not become personally overly involved or too zealous in trying to provide social supports	Carefully, respectfully investigate patient's concerns and motives. Communicate directly; avoid punitive reactions to patient. Set clear limits in context of medically indicated interventions	Don't get too close to patient. Schedule frequent periodic check-ups. Provide clear, nontechnical answers to questions to counter scary fantasies. Tolerate periodic angry outbursts, but set limits. Be aware of patient's potential for self-destructive behavior. Discuss feelings with coworkers and schedule multidisciplinary meetings

(continued)

in this relationship. Table 25–1 outlines typical responses to illness by patients with each of the most common personality disorders, details troublesome reactions by physicians, and suggests strategies to avoid further problems with these challenging patients. (Avoidant and schizotypal personality disorders are not included in the table—or discussed in this chapter—because of their relative rarity in primary care practice.)

Management of Patients With Personality Disorders

In most cases, a stable therapeutic alliance with patients who have personality disorders can be maintained by implementing the behavioral strategies suggested in the following sections. Sometimes other factors must also be addressed. As mentioned earlier, comorbid Axis I diagnoses must be treated. The most common examples of this would be treatment of de-

Table 25–1. Common personality disorders and typical manifestations. *(cont.)*

Personality Disorder	Histrionic	Narcissistic	Dependent	Obsessive-Compulsive
Prominent features of disorder	Pattern of excessive attention-seeking and emotionality	Pervasive pattern of grandiosity, need for admiration, and lack of empathy for others	Pervasive and excessive need to be taken care of that leads to submissive and clinging behavior, and fears of separation	Pattern of preoccupation with orderliness, perfectionism, control
Patient's experience of illness	Threatened sense of attractiveness and self-esteem	Illness may increase anxiety related to doubts about personal adequacy	Fear that illness will lead to abandonment and helplessness	Fear of losing control over bodily functions and over emotions generated by illness; feelings of shame and vulnerability
Problematic behavior in the medical care setting	Overly dramatic, attention-seeking behavior, with tendency to draw caregiver into excessively familiar relationship Inadequate focus on symptoms and their management, with over-emphasis on feeling states May provide answers they believe physician wants to hear Tendency to somatize	Demanding, entitled attitude Excessive praise toward caregiver may turn to devaluation, in effort to maintain sense of superiority Denial of illness or minimization of symptoms	Dramatic and urgent demands for medical attention Angry outbursts at physician if not responded to Patient may contribute to prolong illness or encourage medical procedures in order to get attention May abuse substances and medications	Anger about disruption of routines Repetitive questions and excessive attention to detail Fear of relinquishing control to health-care team
Common problematic reactions to patient by caregiver	Performing excessive work-up (when patient is dramatic) or inadequate work-up (when patient is vague) Allowing too much emotional closeness, thereby losing objectivity Frustration with patient's dramatic or vague presentation	Outright rejection of patient's demands, resulting in patient distancing self from caregiver Excessive submission to patient's grandiose stance	Inability to set limits to availability, thus leading to burnout Hostile rejection of patient	Impatience and cutting answers short Attempts to control treatment planning
Helpful management strategies by caregiver	Show respectful and professional concern for feelings, with emphasis on objective issues Avoid excessive familiarity	Generous validation of patient's concerns, with attentive but factual response to questions Allow patients to maintain sense of competence by re-channelling their "skills" to deal with illness, obviating need for devaluation of caregivers	Provide reassurance and schedule frequent periodic check-ups Be consistently available but provide firm realistic limits to availability Enlist other members of the health-care team in providing support for patient Help patient obtain outside support systems Avoid hostile rejection of patient	Thorough history taking and careful diagnostic work-ups are reassuring Give clear and thorough explanation of diagnosis and treatment options Do not overemphasize uncertainties about treatments Avoid vague and impressionistic explanations Treat patient as an equal partner; encourage self-monitoring and allow patient participation in treatment

pression or anxiety disorders. Pharmacotherapy and psychotherapy (and their integration) are often more complex for patients with comorbid Axis I and II disorders. This difficulty is particularly evident when patients with personality disorders have concurrent substance-abuse problems or psychotic symptoms (eg, hallucinations, delusions, paranoid ideation). In such cases, mental health consultation can be particularly helpful.

When a provider feels unable to continue productive work with a patient with a personality disorder, it may be appropriate to transfer the patient to another clinician. Although such transfers of care may be both necessary and helpful, they require consideration of the impact of the transfer on the well-being of the patient. Patients with certain personality disorders may experience such transfers as rejection or abandonment, perceptions that may exacerbate their emotional distress and may potentially disrupt their medical treatment. Prior consultation with a mental health provider can be useful in determining whether such a transfer might be helpful and can aid in carrying it out smoothly.

The remainder of this chapter discusses eight personality disorders commonly encountered in the primary care setting.

PARANOID PERSONALITY DISORDER

Symptoms & Signs

Patients with paranoid personality disorder (Table 25–2) have a long-standing pattern of distrust and suspiciousness. They perceive the behavior and motives of others as malevolent in nature and expect, in many situations, to be disappointed or taken advantage of. They may perceive seemingly benign or innocuous statements or behavior by others as threatening, insulting, or hurtful. In order to defend against their perceived vulnerability, they usually adopt a rigid, distanced, or guarded position. In general, persons with this personality structure find intimate relationships undesirable and difficult, which often leaves them without any significant social supports.

Differential Diagnosis

Long-standing psychotic symptoms, such as delusions and hallucinations, suggest a diagnosis of paranoid delusional disorder or paranoid schizophrenia. Although persons with paranoid personality disorder usually do not have frank paranoid delusions, at times of extreme stress they may develop such symptoms. Brief paranoid ideation may be associated with medical causes or with alcohol or substance abuse or withdrawal.

Illness Experience & Illness Behavior

Illness is difficult for individuals with paranoid personality disorder, because having to communicate personal information to the physician may challenge the self-protective, rigid way they approach social interactions. Patients may experience a heightened sense of vulnerability and fear of harm by the physician. In their fearful state, they may perceive innocuous or even overtly helpful behavior as threatening. They may then question or challenge the physician about the content of an intervention or the motives behind it. This can lead to possible conflict and argument between patient and doctor.

The Doctor-Patient Relationship: Physicians confronted with such a paranoid stance may react in ways that exacerbate the situation. Physicians who feel that their intentions are inappropriately suspect might argue with the patient or become defensive, perhaps using an angry tone. This kind of reaction may frighten the patient and may be perceived as confirmation of the patient's suspicion. Although such a response should be avoided, ignoring the patient's distrustful or angry behavior can also be problematic; the patient's concerns, however irrational, may increase if not addressed.

Table 25–2. Diagnostic criteria for paranoid personality disorder (301.0).

A. A pervasive distrust and suspiciousness of others such that their motives are interpreted as malevolent, beginning by early adulthood and present in a variety of contexts, as indicated by four (or more) of the following:
  1. suspects, without sufficient basis, that others are exploiting, harming, or deceiving him or her
  2. is preoccupied with unjustified doubts about the loyalty or trustworthiness of friends or associates
  3. is reluctant to confide in others because of unwarranted fear that the information will be used maliciously against him or her
  4. reads hidden demeaning or threatening meanings into benign remarks or events
  5. persistently bears grudges, that is, is unforgiving of insults, injuries, or slights
  6. perceives attacks on his or her character or reputation that are not apparent to others and is quick to react angrily or to counterattack
  7. has recurrent suspicions, without justification, regarding fidelity of spouse or sexual partner
B. Does not occur exclusively during the course of schizophrenia, a mood disorder with psychotic features, or another psychotic disorder and is not due to the direct physiologic effects of a general medical condition.

Source: Reprinted, with permission, from American Psychiatric Association: *Diagnostic and Statistical Manual of Mental Disorders: DSM-IV.* American Psychiatric Association, 1994.

Specific Management Strategies

It is essential to address the patient's concerns and fears empathically, however irrational they seem. Although the physician may see the patient's concern as unrealistic, to the patient the fear is real. Dismissing these patients' concerns or calling them paranoid will not address their emotional needs and may instead create distance in the doctor-patient relationship. A professional stance is most reassuring to these patients. Excessive friendliness or reassurance may be misinterpreted and may intensify their paranoia. It is important to give these patients detailed information about their proposed treatment plan, allowing them to feel they are in control of the treatment and can make independent decisions. Provide factual information about risks associated with the treatment, whenever possible, before any major procedures or changes in treatment.

Case illustration 1: Simon, a 42-year-old, single, male parking lot attendant, presents to his primary care provider, complaining of 3 months of tension headaches and fatigue in the context of what he calls "job stress." The only notable finding in the physical examination is a new, but mild, elevation of blood pressure. The physician also observes that Simon seems angry and anxious, in contrast to his previously distant and somewhat guarded demeanor. When asked about his job stress, Simon reveals anxieties about not being able to trust two new coworkers, along with fears that his supervisors are conspiring to dismiss him from his job. He also mentions, hesitantly, that he had not sought evaluation of his headaches sooner, because he worried that the physician would dismiss his fears as unfounded or "crazy." Additional social history reveals difficulty with close relationships and recurrent problems adjusting to changes in the workplace.

The physician responds by listening in a nonjudgmental and empathic manner. She prescribes an over-the-counter analgesic for the headaches and lorazepam, 0.5 mg every 4–6 hours for occasional anxiety and agitation. She plans follow-up measurements of the blood pressure and suggests that Simon see a psychiatrist for further evaluation of his very stressful job situation.

Simon feels that his concerns have been taken seriously. He finds the referral to a psychiatrist acceptable because it has been proposed in a way that offers support and does not dismiss his fears as pathological. The physician's matter-of-fact responses to Simon's somatic complaints help increase the patient's trust in his physician.

SCHIZOID PERSONALITY DISORDER

Symptoms & Signs

Individuals with schizoid personality disorder (Table 25–3) remain detached from social relationships and exhibit a restricted range of emotional expression in their interactions with others, often appearing cold or indifferent. Because patients with this disorder find emotions, intimacy, and conflict threatening, they tend to isolate themselves and avoid close or sexual relationships. They prefer dealing with technical or abstract concepts to contact with people, and so they may devote their time to pursuits such as mathematical games. Work can be problematic if it involves interactions with others, but many individuals can perform quite well if they work with some degree of independence.

Differential Diagnosis

Patients with schizoid personality disorder do not exhibit prolonged psychotic symptoms. They may, however, suffer a brief psychotic decompensation during times of extreme stress. In addition, schizoid personality disorder may in some cases precede the development of psychotic Axis I conditions, such as schizophrenia or delusional disorder. It can also co-exist with schizotypal, paranoid, or avoidant personality disorders.

Illness Experience & Illness Behavior

Illness can be especially stressful for these patients because it gives rise to strong emotions that they are not prepared to deal with. The necessity of interacting with caregivers when ill, often around quite personal issues, forces them to do the very thing they systematically avoid. They may therefore delay seeking care until their symptoms become more serious. When

Table 25–3. Diagnostic criteria for schizoid personality disorder (301.20).

A. A pervasive pattern of detachment from social relationships and a restricted range of expression of emotions in interpersonal settings, beginning by early adulthood and present in a variety of contexts, as indicated by four (or more) of the following:
  1. neither desires nor enjoys close relationships, including being part of a family
  2. almost always chooses solitary activities
  3. has little, if any, interest in having sexual experiences with another person
  4. takes pleasure in few, if any, activities
  5. lacks close friends or confidants other than first-degree relatives
  6. appears indifferent to the praise or criticism of others
  7. shows emotional coldness, detachment, or flattened affectivity
B. Does not occur exclusively during the course of schizophrenia, a mood disorder with psychotic features, another psychotic disorder, or a pervasive developmental disorder and is not due to the direct physiologic effects of a general medical condition.

Source: Reprinted, with permission, from American Psychiatric Association: *Diagnostic and Statistical Manual of Mental Disorders: DSM-IV.* American Psychiatric Association, 1994.

they finally present for medical attention, they may appear indifferent or detached as a way of protecting themselves from overwhelming emotion. They may show little facial expression and may not respond in kind to caregivers' empathic nods or comments—which may make establishing a therapeutic relationship difficult.

The Doctor-Patient Relationship: Since these patients often appear cold or indifferent, physicians may consider them as unappreciative of help. They may also be puzzled or frustrated by their patients' delay in seeking medical care and their apparent passivity in the face of illness. As a result, caregivers may make overzealous attempts to connect with patients by trying to be especially empathic, a tactic that may instead frighten them away. On the other hand, providers may themselves draw back and lose their enthusiasm for helping patients who seem so unappreciative or uninvolved in their own treatment.

Specific Management Strategies

Understanding that individuals with schizoid personality disorder have difficulty tolerating emotions and intimate interactions is important. Physicians should appreciate their patients' need for privacy and should maintain a low-key approach, avoiding attempts to reach out by becoming too close or by insisting on providing social support. It is helpful to focus on the more technical aspects of treatment, since these are better tolerated, and encourage patients to maintain daily routines. Caregivers should remain available and provide steady but nonthreatening help.

> *Case illustration 2:* Ben, a 44-year-old computer programmer, presents to a university outpatient clinic for evaluation of nausea, anorexia, and a 30-pound weight loss occurring over the previous several months. When asked why he hadn't sought treatment before, Ben states that he has always been healthy and thought he would probably regain the lost weight.
>
> Throughout the interview, Ben makes poor eye contact and gives brief answers to questions. He appears to dislike being interviewed by both a medical student and a resident. He becomes more uncomfortable when asked questions about his personal life and how he likes spending his time. Ben states that he usually keeps to himself, with the exception of visiting his sister about once a month. He spends much of his time programming and playing with his computer.
>
> Ben appears visibly anxious when the resident recommends a consultation with a gastroenterologist. He asks whether this is truly necessary, since it will be hard for him to take time off from work. The resident emphasizes the importance of this consultation, and Ben seems to calm down a bit when the conversation focuses more on the possible tests that might be done to evaluate his symptoms, thereby distracting his attention from his concerns about having to see yet another doctor.

The resident later explains to the medical student that it is important to minimize the number of doctors Ben sees over time and to avoid an overfriendly style—which might frighten him.

ANTISOCIAL PERSONALITY DISORDER

Symptoms & Signs

Persons with antisocial personality disorder (Table 25–4) demonstrate a disregard for others and behavior that violates others' rights. The diagnosis can be made only in persons over age 18, and it requires a history of conduct disorder prior to that age. Characteristics include lack of conformity to social norms and laws, using lies or other deceitfulness for personal gain, and impulsiveness and irresponsibility in many settings. These individuals may be threatening, manipulative, or harmful to others, and they are generally not remorseful. Their tendencies toward aggressive behavior may not be immediately evident, but contact with collateral sources frequently reveals a criminal record. These character traits affect relations with both strangers and family alike, as persons with antisocial personality disorder may engage in

Table 25–4. Diagnostic criteria for antisocial personality disorder (301.7)

A. There is a pervasive pattern of disregard for and violation of the rights of others occurring since age 15 years, as indicated by three (or more) of the following:
  1. failure to conform to social norms with respect to lawful behaviors as indicated by repeatedly performing acts that are grounds for arrest
  2. deceitfulness, as indicated by repeated lying, use of aliases, or conning others for personal profit or pleasure
  3. impulsivity or failure to plan ahead
  4. irritability and aggressiveness, as indicated by repeated physical fights or assaults
  5. reckless disregard for safety of self or others
  6. consistent irresponsibility, as indicated by repeated failure to sustain consistent work behavior or honor financial obligations
  7. lack of remorse, as indicated by being indifferent to or rationalizing having hurt, mistreated, or stolen from another
B. The individual is at least age 18 years.
C. There is evidence of conduct disorder with onset before age 15 years.
D. The occurrence of antisocial behavior is not exclusively during the course of schizophrenia or a manic episode.

Source: Reprinted, with permission, from American Psychiatric Association: *Diagnostic and Statistical Manual of Mental Disorders: DSM-IV.* American Psychiatric Association, 1994.

inconsiderate, angry, or harmful behaviors. These individuals may present themselves in a superficially grandiose manner, and they can also initially appear somewhat charismatic, until others recognize their charm as manipulative.

Differential Diagnosis

Antisocial personality disorder can overlap significantly with other personality disorder traits, most commonly narcissistic, histrionic, or borderline personality disorder. Because substance abuse is a frequent comorbid diagnosis, it is important to distinguish between the problems when making the diagnosis.

Illness Experience & Illness Behavior

In order to mask the fear that illness may cause, patients with antisocial personality disorder may unconsciously adopt an excessively self-assured, entitled, or hostile stance. Irresponsible, impulsive, or dangerous health behavior may help these patients deny their vulnerability to illness. This behavior can occur without regard for medical consequences, and many patients show blatant disregard for the health-care personnel and resources from which they have benefited. Patients may assume a privileged, self-deserving stance and can become antagonistic if they fail to obtain the desired response. They may attempt to manipulate their physician, malingering to obtain things such as drugs or inappropriate disability benefits. This behavior can be an embellishment of a real illness, or it can occur when they are not ill.

The Doctor-Patient Relationship: Since these patients often behave in ways that are noncompliant, ungracious, or dishonest, they are frequently irritating to health-care providers. Physicians may become angry with these individuals or reject them if they see that the treatments in which they have invested their knowledge and energy have not been followed, or if they discover they have been manipulated by these patients.

Specific Management Strategies

Managing manipulative patients can be particularly challenging. If the patient tricks the physician, the outcome is usually detrimental to the patient's overall health (broadly defined). On the other hand, although recognizing the manipulative behavior may avert a detrimental health outcome, the physician's confrontation can alienate the patient. The more authoritarian the physician's stance, the more likely it is that the patient will become oppositional, reducing the possibility for development of an effective therapeutic alliance.

The key here is to maintain an objective, thorough, nonauthoritarian, and respectful approach to investigating patient's presenting complaints. If the patient's presentation or motives are suspicious, the provider should gather corroborating data from collateral sources (other providers or family members) when

needed. It is important to avoid becoming angry, punitive, or rejecting toward the patient; these behaviors may recapitulate behavior the patient experienced earlier in life that contributed to the development of the antisocial personality disorder. Such behavior by the physician can cause the patient to become hostile, with additional deterioration in the doctor-patient relationship. If confrontation or disagreement is necessary, it is essential to avoid humiliating the patient while identifying the attempted manipulation. Communication should be direct and factual with these patients, based on what is medically indicated, and set clear limits on the diagnostic or treatment plan.

> *Case illustration 3:* On her return from vacation, the doctor's first patient is Randy, an angry 42-year-old man, well known to her for his problems with long-standing recurrent low back pain. Although his back pain is generally well controlled with back exercises and as-needed nonsteroidal analgesics, Randy frequently takes long motorcycle trips with friends, during which he does not exercise or take his analgesics. While the physician was away, Randy went on a motorcycle tour and had a recurrence of acute back pain. He then telephoned the clinic and became angry and abusive toward the on-call nurse practitioner, who would not submit to his demands for narcotics.
>
> The physician, who has seen similar behavior from Randy in the past, listens carefully to his story, acknowledges his anger, and reflects empathically on how painful his back must be. She inquires, nonjudgmentally, about the reasons for his failure to exercise. She then explains the benefits of a more preventive approach—using exercise and avoiding pain-inducing behaviors—compared with the long-term risks of relying on narcotics and failing to exercise. Finally, she offers him referral to a physical therapist for a review of the exercise plan, along with a refill of his nonsteroidal analgesic, emphasizing her view that this would offer the best long-term outcome. Though with some bitterness, Randy acknowledges the benefits of the physician's recommendations and agrees to try to follow through with them.

In dealing with Randy, the physician uses her past experience with him to guide her. Randy's self-destructive behavior, hostility, and disregard for others are met with clear limit-setting by the physician, who responds in a calm and nonpunitive manner, emphasizing her concern for the patient's long-term well-being.

BORDERLINE PERSONALITY DISORDER

Symptoms & Signs

Patients with borderline personality disorder (Table 25–5) exhibit instability in their self-image, their affect, and their relationships with others. They can be

Table 25–5. Diagnostic criteria for borderline personality disorder (301.83).

A pervasive pattern of instability of interpersonal relationships, self-image, and affects, and marked impulsivity beginning by early adulthood and present in a variety of contexts, as indicated by five (or more) of the following:
1. frantic efforts to avoid real or imagined abandonment; *Note:* Do not include suicidal or self-mutilating behavior covered in criterion 5.
2. a pattern of unstable and intense interpersonal relationships characterized by alternating between extremes of idealization and devaluation
3. identity disturbance: markedly and persistently unstable self-image or sense of self
4. impulsivity in at least two areas that are potentially self-damaging (eg, spending, sex, substance abuse, reckless driving, binge eating); *Note:* Do not include suicidal or self-mutilating behavior covered in criterion 5.
5. recurrent suicidal behavior, gestures, or threats, or self-mutilating behavior
6. affective instability due to a marked reactivity of mood (eg, intense episodic dysphoria, irritability, or anxiety usually lasting a few hours and only rarely more than a few days)
7. chronic feelings of emptiness
8. inappropriate, intense anger or difficulty controlling anger (eg, frequent displays of temper, constant anger, recurrent physical fights)
9. transient, stress-related paranoid ideation or severe dissociative symptoms

Source: Reprinted, with permission, from American Psychiatric Association: *Diagnostic and Statistical Manual of Mental Disorders: DSM-IV.* American Psychiatric Association, 1994.

quite impulsive and may engage in self-destructive behaviors, such as substance abuse, self-mutilation, and suicide attempts. These behaviors reflect a deep sense of emptiness and an intense fear of abandonment by others. On the other hand, patients with borderline personality are often also fearful of closeness. They experience many contradictory emotions and feelings that are not integrated into a stable sense of who they are and that may be associated with rapid shifts in mood. This instability can cause rapid changes in goals and values. These patients usually have difficulty differentiating reality from fantasy and tend toward all-or-nothing thinking in their view of themselves and others, alternating between overidealization and devaluation.

Differential Diagnosis

Some patients with borderline personality disorder may suffer brief psychotic episodes when under stress. They may, for example, become very anxious or experience auditory hallucinations. Such episodes are distinguishable from Axis I psychotic disorders by psychotic symptoms of brief duration. In addition, patients with borderline personality disorder also often suffer from a concurrent Axis I mood disorder, such as major depression, which should, of course, be treated. Other personality disorders (eg, histrionic, or narcissistic) may be confused with borderline personality disorder. Some patients, however, may have traits of more than one personality disorder.

Illness Experience & Illness Behavior

Patients with borderline personality disorder have difficulty distinguishing reality from fantasy, and they may have terrifying fantasies about illness. The complex and contradictory feelings engendered in response to illness can feel intolerable to these patients, so they may try to cope by pretending that they are completely well and denying the presence of illness. Alternatively, they may become convinced that they are deathly ill, even when suffering from a mild illness. Having felt wounded in earlier relationships, individuals with borderline personality disorder mistrust and fear caregivers. In an attempt to cope with their simultaneous intense wish for, and fear of, closeness, they tend to conceptualize caregivers as all-good or all-bad—a mechanism called "splitting." To complicate things further, these conceptualizations are not stable. Even an overidealized caregiver can abruptly be devalued if a borderline patient becomes angry and disappointed or feels abandoned. In addition, patients with borderline personality disorder may respond to feeling overwhelmed by engaging in impulsive and self-destructive acts, such as self-mutilation, substance abuse, and suicide gestures or attempts. They may also be noncompliant with treatment as a way to remain ill and thus maintain an ongoing relationship with the caregiver.

The Doctor-Patient Relationship: A common mistake clinicians make in treating patients with borderline personality disorder is getting too emotionally close. This occurs when clinicians feel intensely drawn to help the patients through their suffering and spend a great deal of time with them. This usually causes overstimulation of the patient's emotions, leading to increased instability and acting out. It should be noted that the patient's emotional behavior can cloud the clinician's judgment, causing him or her to succumb to the patient's idealization and splitting. The borderline patient's self-destructive or often-provocative behaviors can cause despair and helplessness in caregivers. The caregivers may also feel tempted to punish the patient, for example by becoming verbally hostile or withholding needed pain medication.

Specific Management Strategies

While providing basic support and reassurance, clinicians should be careful not to become emotionally overinvolved with the borderline patient. It is appropriate to counter the patient's frightening fantasies about illness by scheduling frequent periodic checkups and providing clear, nontechnical answers to questions. Caregivers may have to tolerate periodic angry outbursts, but it is appropriate to set firm limits on both the patient's disruptive behavior and on the caregiver's response. When a multidisciplinary team of clinicians is involved, meetings of all providers should be arranged, to allow them to vent their feelings about the patient and to reach consensus on a treatment plan. It is helpful to select a small number of caregivers to interact with the patient directly and to present the same clear and consistent plan. This approach often prevents splitting. Finally, it is essential to remain aware of these patients' potential for self-destructive behavior and not to retaliate for their disruptions by displaying anger at them when setting limits.

Case illustration 4: A primary care resident expresses concern about her patient Amanda to her clinic's attending physician. She is scheduled to leave the clinic in 3 months and believes that Amanda will find transferring to a new doctor difficult.

Amanda is a 35-year-old temporary clerical worker with a long-standing history of migraine headaches. She often delays taking medication until her migraine headaches become severe, and then calls the resident, complaining of unbearable pain, and sometimes stating that the pain is so intolerable that she wishes to die. She sometimes comes to the clinic without a scheduled appointment, demanding to be seen right away. On the other hand, she often misses regularly scheduled appointments. During her visits, she expresses a fear of becoming homeless; she house-sits at other people's homes, but doesn't have a stable place of her own.

The resident asks for a psychiatric consultation to help her work with Amanda. She is particularly concerned about Amanda's periodic statements that she wishes to die.

Following the psychiatrist's recommendations, the resident continues to schedule regular, brief follow-up appointments, and encourages Amanda to keep these appointments. She explains that this is not a walk-in clinic, and that Amanda will have to seek treatment for acute pain in the emergency room. She also reminds Amanda that taking medication early will likely keep the headache from becoming very intense.

Other helpful interventions include providing increased support to Amanda by referring her to a psy-

chotherapist and asking the team social worker to assist her in finding a stable residence. It is also important to monitor Amanda for suicidal ideation. If she expresses a wish to die, the resident assesses her suicidal ideation and intent. One afternoon, Amanda drops in at the clinic expressing suicidal ideation, and a nurse practitioner calls for an urgent psychiatric consultation. After talking to the psychiatrist, Amanda gradually calms down and denies any suicidal intent; however, she refuses a referral for ongoing psychiatric treatment.

Over time, Amanda continues to miss some appointments, and occasionally becomes demanding or complains bitterly about the resident to the nurse practitioner. When both the resident and the nurse practitioner, however, firmly and supportively continue to reiterate their treatment plan—to meet with the doctor for regular appointments, to treat migraines early, and to go to the emergency room for acute pain—Amanda's unpredictable visits and noncompliance diminish. Periodic meetings between the resident and the nurse practitioner help them both present the same coherent plan to Amanda, thus minimizing splitting.

In planning ahead for her departure from the clinic, the resident and the attending physician discuss some helpful strategies to facilitate this transition, such as introducing the new resident to Amanda ahead of time and involving the nurse practitioner—who is staying at the clinic—in the process.

In this case, regular meetings of the resident, the attending physician, and the nurse practitioner allow them to present the same coherent plan to the patient, minimize the splitting, and reduce the patient's anxiety and unpredictable behavior. This approach successfully combines increased support and limit-setting.

HISTRIONIC PERSONALITY DISORDER

Symptoms & Signs

Histrionic personality disorder (Table 25–6) is marked by excessive attention seeking and emotionalism. These patients may present with dramatic, theatrical shows of feeling, or they may dress or behave in a sexually provocative fashion in an unconscious effort to engage others and draw attention to them-

Table 25–6. Diagnostic criteria for histrionic personality disorder (301.50).

A pervasive pattern of excessive emotionality and attention seeking, beginning by early adulthood and present in a variety of contexts, as indicated by five (or more) of the following:
1. is uncomfortable in situations in which he or she is not the center of attention
2. interaction with others is often characterized by inappropriate sexually seductive or provocative behavior
3. displays rapidly shifting and shallow expression of emotions
4. consistently uses physical appearance to draw attention to self
5. has a style of speech that is excessively impressionistic and lacking in detail
6. shows self-dramatization, theatricality, and exaggerated expression of emotion
7. is suggestible, ie, easily influenced by others or circumstances
8. considers relationships to be more intimate than they actually are

Source: Reprinted, with permission, from American Psychiatric Association: *Diagnostic and Statistical Manual of Mental Disorders: DSM-IV.* American Psychiatric Association, 1994.

selves. The emotions they express may be shallow and inconsistent, but the patients may still believe that the sharing of those feelings creates a special closeness (which they often exaggerate) with the physician. These patients have a tendency to prefer subjective and intuitive impressions over objective, linear, logical thinking. They often have somatic complaints, with impressive—but inconsistent—presentations.

Differential Diagnosis

Histrionic personality disorder may be difficult to distinguish from narcissistic or borderline personality disorder, and patients in each of these categories may exhibit traits common to patients in the others. Patients with histrionic personality disorder are deeply affected by perceived frailties in relationship bonds, as are patients with borderline personality. The latter, however, display less emotional stability and are more impulsive and self-destructive. Patients with histrionic personality disorder may crave attention—as patients with narcissistic personality disorder crave admiration—but the former tend to be less grandiose, arrogant, and self-absorbed.

Illness Experience & Illness Behavior

Medical illness represents a particular threat to the emotional well-being of patients with histrionic personality disorder, who derive much of their sense of self-worth and personal desirability from their sense of physical attractiveness. To reduce the fear of being deemed less desirable by others, these patients may attempt to bolster their physical appearance or embellish their abilities.

As a result, patients of either gender may engage in flirtatious or seductive behavior. When they feel weak and vulnerable, they may express their emotions with more intensity, in an attempt to strengthen their bond with the physician. In addition, since these patients focus on feelings, rather than on carefully observed physical symptoms, they may present with a collection of loosely connected somatic complaints. Their descriptions of the symptoms may reflect their desire to capture the physician's interest.

The Doctor-Patient Relationship: In working with the histrionic patient, the physician may be drawn in by the patient's dramatic and somewhat dependent style, become overly involved, and perhaps embark on an excessive work-up. As the physician becomes increasingly engaged by the patient's style, the patient may then become anxious, distant, or noncompliant, puzzling and frustrating the physician. Alternatively, the physician then may instead pursue too cursory an evaluation, because of a lack of objective information, or out of frustration with the patient's emotional and vague style.

Specific Management Strategies

Because the patient with histrionic personality disorder has an emotional (rather than a logical) style

and may display contrasting behaviors—that range from excessive anxiety about potentially minor symptoms to inappropriate indifference about significant medical problems—it is essential that the physician maintain an objective stance. The physician must offer a supportive and logical approach to the patient's problems. This requires being both sensitive to the patient's emotional concerns and sufficiently distanced to avoid any degree of closeness that the patient might misperceive as intimate or sexual.

> ***Case illustration 5:*** Rita is 38-year-old, single, unemployed actress with lupus. She is excessively friendly and flirtatious with her 45-year-old male physician, calling him frequently with questions about her medical problems and dressing somewhat seductively for office visits. During these visits she asks for examinations of a variety of somatic complaints. Over time, the physician becomes increasingly uncomfortable. Finally, Rita complains that she would like more time to discuss her problems at each office visit, and asks the physician if he thinks her problems "deserve more time."
>
> After reflecting on the chronicity of this pattern of behavior, the physician responds that Rita's medical problems are significant and deserving of attention. He states that he intends to evaluate each of them carefully, allocating time on the basis of his impression of their medical necessity. He also says that he understands that she would like more time to discuss her concerns, but that as a busy doctor he cannot make additional time available to her. He suggests, gently, that if he cannot provide adequate emotional support to her, he could refer her to a local clinic's health psychologist. Although she is rather disappointed, Rita is able to accept this limit-setting and continues to work with this doctor.

This approach is successful because the physician shows positive regard for the patient and her problems—while clearly setting the limits of the doctor-patient relationship.

NARCISSISTIC PERSONALITY DISORDER

Symptoms & Signs

Narcissistic personality disorder (Table 25–7) is characterized by a long-standing pattern of grandiosity, with a need for praise and admiration that stands out in contrast to a lack of sensitivity to the feelings of others. These persons may have an exaggerated sense of self-importance and social status. They may be driven toward attaining an idealized position in terms of social, personal, romantic, or career accomplishment. In this regard, they may be envious and potentially devaluing of others whose accomplishments they perceive as exceeding their own.

Differential Diagnosis

Narcissistic personality disorder may be difficult to distinguish from borderline, antisocial, histrionic, or

Table 25–7. Diagnostic criteria for narcissistic personality disorder (301.81).

A pervasive pattern of grandiosity (in fantasy or behavior), need for admiration, and lack of empathy, beginning by early adulthood and present in a variety of contexts, as indicated by five (or more) of the following:

1. has a grandiose sense of self-importance (eg, exaggerates achievements and talents, expects to be recognized as superior without commensurate achievements)
2. is preoccupied with fantasies of unlimited success, power, brilliance, beauty, or ideal love
3. believes that he or she is "special" and unique and can only be understood by, or should associate with, other special or high-status people (or institutions)
4. requires excessive admiration
5. has a sense of entitlement, ie, unreasonable expectations of especially favorable treatment or automatic compliance with his or her expectations
6. is interpersonally exploitative, ie, takes advantage of others to achieve his or her own ends
7. lacks empathy: is unwilling to recognize or identify with the feelings and needs of others
8. is often envious of others or believes that others are envious of him or her
9. shows arrogant, haughty behaviors or attitudes

Source: Reprinted, with permission, from American Psychiatric Association: *Diagnostic and Statistical Manual of Mental Disorders: DSM-IV.* American Psychiatric Association, 1994.

obsessive-compulsive personality disorders, and in many cases it may overlap with these disorders. When the differentiation is unclear, identifying a high degree of grandiosity and a need for admiration can help clarify the diagnosis. In contrast to persons with borderline personality disorder, persons with narcissistic personality disorder have a more stable self-image and display less impulsiveness and sensitivity to relationship losses. In addition, persons with narcissistic personality disorder are generally less aggressive and deceitful than are persons with antisocial personality disorder, who also display evidence of childhood conduct disorder. Persons with histrionic personality disorder, in contrast, may be relatively more dramatic and emotional than are those with narcissistic personality disorder. Although persons with narcissistic personality disorder, like those with obsessive-compulsive personality disorder, may both be perfectionistic, the former often have a higher self-assessment of their accomplishments.

Clinicians must also be careful not to misdiagnose a person with transient hypomanic or manic grandiosity as having narcissistic personality disorder. Similarly, it is important to distinguish between narcissistic personality disorder and transient substance-related personality changes (eg, from central nervous system stimulants) or personality changes caused by a general medical condition.

Illness Experience & Illness Behavior

Health problems are a particular blow to patients with narcissistic personality disorder. Illness threatens these patients' unconscious attempts to maintain an intrapsychic and external image of untarnished well-being and resiliency. Medical problems and physical limitations may disrupt this image, threaten their public personas, and leave them fearing disruption of their (unrealistically unchallengeable) sense of self. In an attempt to defend against this threat, patients may minimize the significance of symptoms or deny the presence of the illness. More commonly, as patients try to recapture their admired, idealized status, they may demand special treatment or ridicule the physi-

cian caring for them. These patients may devalue, criticize, or question the behavior or credentials of the treating physician, or they may fail to comply with treatment recommendations.

The Doctor-Patient Relationship: Narcissistic patients' arrogant and grandiose behavior, combined with demands for special treatment, can be extremely irritating to physicians. Reactions to these patients can take many forms. Sometimes, in an attempt to avoid conflict, physicians submit to the demands. With particularly critical patients, providers may feel frustration, resentment, and even anger. Frustration may be especially great if the physician expends special energy on behalf of a charismatic or demanding patient, only to later become the butt of unfair criticism. Physicians may reject or avoid the patient, withhold treatment, or respond in an angry manner—responses that can harm both the patient and the doctor-patient relationship.

Specific Management Strategies

The most effective strategy for dealing with narcissistic patients is to be respectful and nonconfrontational about their sense of specialness and entitlement and to help them use their self-perceived talents in the service of their treatment. If narcissistic patients feel vulnerable and threatened by the illness, they are more likely to criticize and devalue the physician. Providers can appeal to the patients' narcissism by explaining that they chose a particular course of action because they believe it represents the best possible care—a course of action they feel the patients deserve. Physicians can further support the patients by validating their concerns about the illness and pointing to their patients' ability to respond competently to its challenges. This approach helps the patients feel more secure and able, allowing them to ally confidently with—rather than defensively attack—their physicians.

Case illustration 6: Maggie is a 44-year-old married female lawyer, who is quite prominent in the community and an unusually demanding patient. She becomes very angry with her male physician, whom she accuses of not responding adequately to her complaints about menopausal symptoms. In fact, the physician has done all the necessary laboratory tests, has conferred extensively with the patient's gynecologist, and has answered numerous phone calls by the patient over a period of several months.

The physician, aware of Maggie's long-standing sense of entitlement and her extreme sensitivity to slights, responds by reviewing her concerns, discussing the treatment plan and rationale, and encouraging her to discuss some of her emotional reactions to this unexpectedly early menopause. He then emphasizes the special consideration he has put into her evaluation and treatment plan. He arranges more frequent office visits, and tells Maggie that he predicts a relatively good response to treatment, given her active involvement in her own care.

This response is reassuring to the patient, because it validates her concerns and satisfies her narcissistic feelings of entitlement.

DEPENDENT PERSONALITY DISORDER

Symptoms & Signs

Patients with dependent personality disorder (Table 25–8) have a pervasive and excessive need to be taken care of. They experience intense fear of separation and abandonment and feel great discomfort when they are alone. This leads to submissive and clinging behavior in their interpersonal relationships. These patients have difficulty making independent decisions without a great deal of advice and reassurance, and they are afraid of disagreeing with others.

Differential Diagnosis

It is important to distinguish dependent personality disorder from the dependency that arises from panic disorder, mood disorders, or agoraphobia. Patients suffering from medical illnesses may also become very dependent on others, without having this disor-

der. Dependent personality disorder can sometimes be confused with other personality disorders, and dependent personality traits may be the result of chronic substance abuse.

Illness Experience & Illness Behavior

Patients with dependent personality disorder fear that illness will lead to both helplessness and abandonment by others. In their interactions with caregivers, they may become very needy and make dramatic demands for urgent medical attention. If the response is not what they wish, they may display angry outbursts at the physician. They may also blame their physical discomfort on others, including their physician. In addition, they may use addictive substances or overuse medications in a desperate attempt to obtain immediate relief from their suffering. Because receiving medical care may fulfill their wishes for attention from others, some dependent patients may unconsciously contribute to prolonging their illness, or—in some extreme cases—they may encourage unnecessary medical procedures.

The Doctor-Patient Relationship: Clinicians treating patients with dependent personality disorder may initially react with aversion to their patients' clingy and demanding behavior. Alternatively, clinicians may find it difficult to set limits on their availability and may try to provide reassurance by attempting to meet every demand, which ultimately leads to burnout or feelings of inadequacy. Eventually, the caregivers may react in a hostile fashion and openly reject these patients.

Specific Management Strategies

Effective ways to provide reassurance to dependent patients and allay their fear of being abandoned include scheduling frequent periodic check-ups and being consistently available. It is nonetheless important to provide firm, realistic limits to this availability early on in treatment or as soon as the patient's dependent traits become apparent. To prevent burnout, enlist other members of the health-care team in providing support for the patient. In addition, physicians

Table 25–8. Diagnostic criteria for dependent personality disorder (301.6).

A pervasive and excessive need to be taken care of that leads to submissive and clinging behavior and fears of separation, beginning by early adulthood and present in a variety of contexts, as indicated by five (or more) of the following:

1. has difficulty making everyday decisions without an excessive amount of advice and reassurance from others
2. needs others to assume responsibility for most major areas of his or her life
3. has difficulty expressing disagreement with others because of fear of loss of support or approval. *Note:* Do not include realistic fears of retribution.
4. has difficulty initiating projects or doing things on his or her own (because of a lack of self-confidence in judgment or abilities rather than a lack of motivation or energy)
5. goes to excessive lengths to obtain nurturance and support from others, to the point of volunteering to do things that are unpleasant
6. feels uncomfortable or helpless when alone because of exaggerated fears of being unable to care for himself or herself
7. urgently seeks another relationship as a source of care and support when a close relationship ends
8. is unrealistically preoccupied with fears of being left to take care of himself or herself

Source: Reprinted, with permission, from American Psychiatric Association: *Diagnostic and Statistical Manual of Mental Disorders: DSM-IV.* American Psychiatric Association, 1994.

should help these patients find outside support systems to lessen fears of abandonment. They must also be alert to the patients' potential contribution to prolonging their illness or to their possible abuse of substances or medications.

> *Case illustration 7:* Terry, a 50-year-old divorced secretary repeatedly presents to her primary care physician complaining of various somatic symptoms, including dizziness, headaches, blurred vision, and leg pains. Repeated work-ups of her symptoms are negative, and her evaluation for major depression is negative. Further inquiry into Terry's life reveals that after her divorce 6 years ago, her daughter became the focus of her life. Even though her history of occasional somatic symptoms goes back to her teenage years, there had been no appreciable change until 2 years ago, when her daughter got married and left her home.
>
> Terry makes frequent phone calls to her doctor. She usually sounds nervous, expresses concern about some new symptom, and asks for medication. The doctor decides to schedule regular follow-up appointments to address Terry's concerns. Terry often complains during office visits that there is not enough time to evaluate all her symptoms and laments that her daughter no longer has much time for her. Her doctor listens in a supportive manner and acknowledges that the available appointment time is limited, explaining how he will ultimately cover all the complaints. He also underlines the importance of continuing to meet for regular appointments. In addition, the doctor acknowledges Terry's increased sense of isolation after her daughter's marriage. He also evaluates Terry for possible major depression. He further suggests a referral to the clinic's social worker as a means of helping her pursue a volunteer activity and increase her social interactions.

This approach usually helps diminish the patient's anxiety and decreases the frequency of phone calls. If the patient's distress were not to improve with such interventions, a referral for psychotherapy and evaluation for a possible underlying anxiety disorder would be indicated.

OBSESSIVE-COMPULSIVE PERSONALITY DISORDER

Symptoms & Signs

Individuals with obsessive-compulsive personality disorder (Table 25–9) are preoccupied with orderliness, perfectionism, and control. They are excessively concerned with details and rules, tend to be overly moralistic, and are usually focused on work to the exclusion of leisure. They find it difficult to adapt themselves to others and instead insist that others follow their plans. Their general inflexibility and restricted emotional expression betray an underlying fear of losing control. Because they can be indecisive, they feel distressed when faced with the need to make decisions.

Differential Diagnosis

Obsessive-compulsive disorder (see Chapter 23) is distinguished from obsessive-compulsive personality disorder by the presence of actual obsessions (repetitive intrusive thoughts) and compulsions in the former. Sometimes, however, both disorders coexist in one patient, and obsessive-compulsive personality disorder can also be confused with other personality disorders.

Illness Experience & Illness Behavior

Illness is threatening to persons with obsessive-compulsive personality disorder because it generates an intense fear of losing of control over bodily functions and emotions. Patients may experience extremely unsettling feelings of shame and vulnerability. They may also feel anger at the disruption of their usual daily routines by medical appointments and treatments. They may fear having to relinquish control to health-care providers. In the physician's office, their intense anxiety tends to drive them to ask repetitive questions and to pay excessive attention to detail.

The Doctor-Patient Relationship: Caregivers may react to patients with obsessive-compulsive personality disorder by becoming impatient at their

Table 25–9. Diagnostic criteria for obsessive-compulsive personality disorder (301.4).

A pervasive pattern of preoccupation with orderliness, perfectionism, and mental and interpersonal control, at the expense of flexibility, openness, and efficiency, beginning by early adulthood and present in a variety of contexts, as indicated by four (or more) of the following:
1. is preoccupied with details, rules, lists, order, organization, or schedules to the extent that the major point of the activity is lost
2. shows perfectionism that interferes with task completion (eg, is unable to complete a project because his or her own overly strict standards are not met)
3. is excessively devoted to work and productivity to the exclusion of leisure activities and friendships (not accounted for by obvious economic necessity)
4. is overly conscientious, scrupulous, and inflexible about matters of morality, ethics, or values (not accounted for by cultural or religious identification)
5. is unable to discard worn-out or worthless objects even when they have no sentimental value
6. is reluctant to delegate tasks or to work with others unless they submit to exactly his or her way of doing things
7. adopts a miserly spending style toward both self and others; money is viewed as something to be hoarded for future catastrophes
8. shows rigidity and stubbornness

Source: Reprinted, with permission, from American Psychiatric Association: *Diagnostic and Statistical Manual of Mental Disorders: DSM-IV.* American Psychiatric Association, 1994.

repetitive questions, cutting their answers short. They may feel their competence challenged by their patients' insistence on knowing every single detail and reason for choosing a particular treatment. Clinicians may also inadvertently attempt to control treatment planning rather than making it a joint effort, without realizing how important it is for these patients to remain in control.

Specific Management Strategies

Helpful strategies in working with patients with obsessive-compulsive personality disorder include taking a thorough history, performing a careful diagnostic work-up, giving patients a clear and thorough explanation of their diagnosis and treatment options, and providing and explaining laboratory test results. It is important not to overemphasize uncertainties about treatments or the patient's possible response to treatment. Patients find it reassuring when clinicians cite literature reports and avoid vague and inexact impressionistic explanations. It is helpful to treat these patients as equal partners, encourage self-monitoring, allow their participation in treatment, and give them recognition for their clear reasoning and high standards.

Case illustration 8: Sam, a 42-year-old biochemist, requests an appointment with his primary care physician for evaluation of an uncomfortable lump in his left groin. The physician is familiar with Sam's mild nervousness during routine medical check-ups and his tendency to ask detailed questions about his health. After a physical examination, the doctor diagnoses an inguinal hernia and recommends a surgical consultation for further evaluation and possible surgery. Sam, in his usual formal and somewhat restricted manner—but this time appearing visibly more anxious—repeatedly asks several questions about surgical repair, whether the literature discusses any alternative treatments, and what guidelines physicians follow to recommend one treatment over another. He then asks questions about the risks of general anesthesia and whether this procedure can be performed under local anesthesia.

When the physician tries to reassure him that this is a routine procedure, Sam asks him whether he is sure of his diagnosis; he also asks him to list the criteria he used in diagnosing the inguinal hernia. Sam also talks at length about his responsibilities at work and expresses concern that surgery might disrupt ongoing projects at his laboratory, since several people depend on him for ongoing supervision. He also wants to know how long his doctor has known the recommended surgeon, and whether they have worked together in the past.

Reassurance is essential here. The doctor explains that the surgeon is both trustworthy and well known to him. He praises Sam for his thoroughness and initiative in finding out about treatment alternatives before making a decision. He answers basic questions in a precise manner and defers some answers to the surgeon, explaining that these will be better answered by a specialist. He reassures Sam that he will not wait for a written report but will personally contact the surgeon after the consultation to discuss treatment options. The physician also suggests a follow-up appointment to help Sam with his decision.

Although Sam continues to express concern that the surgery will disrupt his work, his anxiety decreases somewhat after the physician takes his concerns seriously. His questions are answered precisely, and the physician further suggests an article in the literature that he can read to learn more about the treatment of inguinal hernias.

SUGGESTED READINGS

American Psychiatric Association: *Diagnostic and Statistical Manual of Mental Disorders: DSM-IV.* American Psychiatric Association, 1994.

Cohen-Cole SA: Difficult interviews: Personality disorders, psychosis, delirium, and dementia. In: *The Medical Interview: The Three-Function Approach.* Mosby-Year Book, 1991.

Fogel BS: Personality disorders in the medical setting. In: Stoudemire A, Fogel BS (editors): *Psychiatric Care of the Medical Patient..* Oxford University Press, 1993.

Geringer ES, Stern TA: Coping with medical illness: The impact of personality types. Psychosomatics 27: 1986;27(4):251.

Groves JE: Taking care of the hateful patient. N Engl J Med 1978;298:883.

Gunderson JG, Links PS, Reich JH: Competing models of personality disorders. J Pers Disord 1991;1:60.

Kahana R, Bibring G: Personality types in medical management. In: Zinberg N (editor): *Psychiatry and Medical Practice in the General Hospital.* International Universities Press, 1964.

Lipkin M: The medical interview and related skills. In: Branch WT (editor): *Office Practice of Medicine,* Saunders, 1987.

Livesley J: Classifying personality disorders: Ideal types, prototypes, or dimensions? J Pers Disord 1991;5(1):52.

Marmar C: Personality disorders. In: Goldman H (editor): *Review of General Psychiatry.* Appleton & Lange, 1995.

Oldham JM: Personality disorders: Current perspectives. JAMA 1994;272:1770.

Putnam SM et al: Personality styles. In: Lipkin M, Putnam S, Lazare A (editors): *The Medical Interview: Clinical Care, Education, and Research,* Springer-Verlag, 1995.

Dementia

26

David M. Pope, PhD, & Alicia Boccellari, PhD

INTRODUCTION

Dementia is characterized by progressive loss of memory and other cognitive skills, leading to an inability to function independently. Eventually, individuals with dementia fail to recognize family members, are unable to express themselves clearly and meaningfully, and often undergo dramatic personality changes. Depression is common in the early stages, and psychotic symptoms may occur during more advanced stages.

This definition of dementia is narrower than that used in the *Diagnostic and Statistical Manual of the American Psychiatric Association (DSM-IV)*. According to the manual, dementia is characterized by multiple cognitive deficits, including memory, that are due to the direct physiological effects of a general medical condition. The specific condition that produces the impairment is included in the diagnosis. The definition does not necessarily imply a progressive course; for example, the persistent cognitive deficits that can follow a head injury, which typically improve or remain static over time, would meet these criteria. The most common and generally accepted use of the term **dementia,** however, refers to conditions such as Alzheimer's disease and vascular dementia, in which deficits do worsen over time and death is the eventual result. Therefore, to avoid confusion, the term *dementia* is used here to refer to disorders with such a progressive and deteriorating course. Other conditions that result in cognitive impairment are here referred to more generally as **organic brain syndromes.**

The main tasks for the primary care provider working with individuals with dementia are to correctly diagnose the condition, to rule out any reversible or treatable disorders, to treat any associated complications such as psychosis, to ensure that the patient is as comfortable and safe as possible, and to work with family and other caregivers to help them understand and care for the patient.

Cortical & Subcortical Disorders

Dementia may be caused by a number of medical disorders or conditions (Table 26–1). They can be divided into two general types based on the areas of the brain that are affected.

Cortical Areas: Alzheimer's disease, and less common disorders such as Pick's disease, primarily affect the cortical areas of the brain. In addition to the prominent memory deficits that are the hallmark of all dementias, patients present with deficits associated with these cortical areas, such as aphasia or visual-spatial and visual-motor impairment. Speed of mentation, motor, and sensory functions are relatively spared.

Subcortical Areas: Other dementias, including HIV-1–related dementia and dementia associated with Parkinson's disease or Huntington's chorea primarily affect subcortical areas and present somewhat differently. The differences are most apparent in the early and middle stages of the disorders. In the early stages, individuals with subcortical dementia often present with motor slowing, tremor, loss of coordination, and changes in reflexes. These are frequently accompanied by a prominent mental sluggishness and inertia, distractibility, and general lack of spontaneity. Specific cognitive deficits such as aphasia are less common at this stage, although word-finding difficulty may be present. Subcortical dementia is more commonly associated with affective disorders such as depression or manic states in the early and middle stages. In the later stages, cortical and subcortical dementias tend to lose their distinctive characteristics as impairment becomes global and profound.

TYPES OF DEMENTIA

Alzheimer's Disease

Alzheimer's disease is the most common form of dementia, causing an estimated 50–80% of dementia cases. The age of onset varies considerably, but the disease rarely presents prior to the fifth decade of life.

Table 26–1. Common causes of dementia.

Alzheimer's disease
Chronic vitamin B$_{12}$ deficiency
Korsakoff's syndrome
AIDS
Huntington's chorea
Hydrocephalus
Multiple infarcts
Parkinson's disease
Prolonged severe alcohol abuse

Many cases occur between ages 50 and 60, but for most patients, common age of onset is during their seventies or eighties. Women are two to three times more likely to develop the disorder than are men.

Alzheimer's disease usually follows a slow, but progressive and insidious, course (Table 26–2). Life expectancy following the appearance of the disorder ranges from 5–7 years, but considerable variation may occur, and survivals of up to 20 years have been reported. Memory deficits are prominent in all dementias, but especially so in Alzheimer's disease. Typically the first and most obvious manifestation of the disorder, these deficits often become quite pronounced. It appears that Alzheimer's disease affects both the encoding and retrieval of new information to a profound degree; these patients, unlike those with subcortical dementias, do not appear to benefit from

cueing and prompting of memory. Alzheimer's disease is a so-called cortical dementia in which the areas of the brain associated with specific cognitive functions and the integration of these functions are directly affected. Diagnosis is one of exclusion; AD should not be diagnosed until other causes or medical conditions have been ruled out. A CT or MRI scan often shows cerebral atrophy and ventricular dilatation; the EEG may show diffuse slowing.

Case illustration: Gertrude is 74 years old. She is brought by her family to a medical clinic for evaluation. Since the death of her husband 2 years ago, Gertrude has become increasingly absent-minded, withdrawn, and sedentary. Her family assumed at first that she was grieving and would eventually readjust. Gertrude's condition has continued to deteriorate, however, until she is now obviously confused and disoriented and has difficulty recognizing family members. Physical examination and routine laboratory tests are essentially normal, but Gertrude shows clear signs of cognitive deficits on the mental status examination. For example, given three words to remember she is unable to recall any of them after several minutes. She cannot give the correct month and year and thinks she is in the city where she had lived many years ago. Asked to repeat several sentences, she makes a number of verbal slips. When she is given a geometric design to copy, her drawing is distorted and unrecognizable. Other causes of the patient's deficits are ruled out, and a diagnosis of Alzheimer's disease is eventually made.

Table 26–2. Stages of Alzheimer's disease.

Stage	General Changes	Specific Changes
Early	Patients show relatively subtle changes in memory, along with declining clarity of thought and ability to perform everyday tasks. These changes may go largely unnoticed by the patient and significant others. Patients typically retain some ability to compensate for the cognitive changes.	• Mild memory problems such as missed appointments, failure to pay bills • Occasional mild and transitory confusion and disorientation • A "slowed-down" quality to thinking, personality, and lifestyle • An increase in personal rigidity and intolerance of changes • Social isolation, loss of interest in usual activities • Possible increase in restlessness and impulsivity
Middle	Cognitive deficits become more prominent during this stage and the loss of functioning becomes obvious to others.	• Severe memory impairment • Frank and persistent confusion and disorientation • Aphasia, apraxia, and visuospatial disturbances • Serious difficulties in the ability to manage everyday activities • Agitation, simple paranoia, other delusions
Late	In the third, and terminal, stage of the disorder, the patient becomes very inactive, is extremely withdrawn, and loses nearly all ability to engage in purposeful activities.	• Profound loss of short- and long-term memory • Severe confusion and disorientation • Bladder and bowel incontinence • Patient eventually is bedridden and nonresponsive • Primitive reflexes such as grasping, rooting, and sucking • Seizures • Signs of gross neurologic impairment, such as hemiplegia, tremor, pronounced rigidity • Bodily wasting in the face of adequate nourishment just prior to death

Note: The signs and symptoms of dementia include the progressive loss of cognitive abilities, especially memory, and a decline in everyday functioning. Dementia is generally a deteriorating condition, and its progression is best described in terms of several stages. The stages outlined above are based on the most common form of dementia, Alzheimer's disease.

In retrospect, her family recalls that Gertrude had been having some mild difficulties in memory and functioning prior to her husband's death and had been dependent on him for helping her to manage things. Recognition of Gertrude's emerging dementia had been made more difficult by her depression and grief after her husband's death.

The physician spends some time with family members discussing the nature of Gertrude's condition and options for future care. She inquires about immediate concerns such as agitation, coordination and balance, and any tendency to wander—none of which are currently present. The physician then refers the family to a social worker specializing in geriatric issues and indicates the availability of groups such as the Family Caregiver Alliance for education and support. She reassures them that Gertrude will continue to receive appropriate medical care.

Vascular Dementia

This dementia is the second most common cause of dementia, accounting for 15–20% of cases among older adults. Previously known as **multi-infarct dementia,** the condition is characterized by the development of multiple areas of infarction in both cortical and subcortical areas. Patients with a history of hypertension and atherosclerotic cerebrovascular disease are at increased risk for the disorder, and many patients who go on to develop vascular dementia have a previous history of stroke. A patchy and inconsistent pattern of deficits is seen initially, with relative preservation of some cognitive areas. As strokes accumulate, impairment becomes more widespread and generalized in nature. A so-called stepwise course is typical, with fairly stable periods of functioning interrupted by sudden deteriorations and the establishment of a more impaired level of functioning.

Focal neurological signs are more common in vascular dementia, and lateralized motor and sensory signs may be seen. CT and MRI scans frequently reveal multiple areas of infarction in the brain, often with diffuse white matter changes. Later in the course of the disorder atrophy from loss of brain tissue may be seen.

HIV-1–Associated Dementia

The emergence of AIDS as a major health crisis has unfortunately included the appearance of a new form of dementia, HIV-1–associated dementia (HAD) (see Chapter 31). As a result, substantial numbers of younger adults are now affected by a disorder that, until recently, was seen almost exclusively in older patients. HAD is caused by the direct infection of the brain by the HIV-1 virus. It is associated with late-stage AIDS and is generally seen in individuals whose T-cell count has fallen below 200.

In diagnosing HAD, care must be taken to rule out opportunistic infections such as toxoplasmosis and cryptococcal meningitis, drug toxicity, and other causes of cognitive impairment. HAD is a subcortical dementia, primarily affecting the white matter of the brain. CT and MR imaging studies often show cortical atrophy, ventricular enlargement, and diffuse or patchy white matter abnormalities.

Lumbar puncture can be helpful in ruling out other central nervous system infections. Individuals with a diagnosis of HAD often have an elevated cerebrospinal fluid (CSF) total protein, with low or normal glucose concentrations. Elevated levels of CSF neopterin have been associated with severity of HIV-1 neurological disorders, and CSF beta$_2$ microglobulin (β_2-M) has also been reported to be elevated in such individuals with a diagnosis of HAD. Although both CSF neopterin and β_2-M are associated with the presence and severity of HAD, they are considered to be nonspecific markers and should be used in addition to the other procedures to rule out different HIV-1–related opportunistic infections.

Peripheral neuropathy and the new onset of clumsiness and balance problems often accompanies or precedes the development of the disorder. The course is fairly rapid, with cognitive deficits intensifying over a period of several months. Advanced HAD is characterized by several typical signs and symptoms, including personality changes, poor judgment, and impoverished speech (Table 26–3).

Other Causes

A number of less common degenerative neurological disorders, such as Huntington's chorea, Parkinson's disease, Pick's disease, and Creutzfeldt-Jakob disease, also cause dementia. Chronic alcohol abuse can also result in dementia if it is severe and prolonged; in this case, further cognitive deterioration can be avoided if the patient can stop drinking. Severe head trauma can also result in permanent cognitive impairment that represents a kind of static dementia. The cognitive effects of mild brain trauma typically decrease over time, and many individuals return to their previous level of functioning, but this is not invariably the case.

Reversible Conditions

A number of medical conditions can result in primary and secondary organic brain syndromes. These may be treatable and partially or completely reversible. Assessing the patient for these conditions is one of the most important parts of the dementia workup. Reversible brain syndromes are usually the result

Table 26–3. Signs and symptoms of advanced HIV-1–associated dementia.

- Impaired attention and difficulty learning new information.
- Slow, soft, and impoverished speech.
- Ataxia, decreased manual dexterity, and motor slowness.
- Poor judgment.
- Flat and unspontaneous facial expression with fixed gaze.
- Personality changes that may include apathy or increased impulsivity.

Table 26–4. Possibly reversible organic brain syndromes.

Hydrocephalus	Chronic hematoma
Metabolic disease	Toxic states
Thyroid	Medication toxicity
Adrenal	CNS infections
Renal failure	Meningitis
Hepatic failure	Encephalitis
Deficiencies	Neurosyphilis
Vitamin B_{12}	Cerebral abscess
Folate	Mild head trauma
Niacin	
Thiamine	

Table 26–5. Delirium versus dementia: Signs and symptoms.

Delirium	Dementia
Rapid onset; short duration	Insidious onset; progressive deterioration
Heightened autonomic arousal	No impairment in autonomic arousal
Clouded consciousness or gross confusion	Confusion less prominent
Prominent waxing and waning	Consistently impaired mentation except in late stage dementia
Often restless or agitated	Agitation less prominent; varies with stress
Gross perceptual distortions and hallucinations common	If psychotic, usually vague paranoid symptoms

of a toxic or metabolic disorder. The most common types of primary and secondary organic brain syndromes are listed in Table 26–4.

Differential Diagnosis

Persons suspected of having dementia are encountered in a number of medical settings. For example, a patient who presents to the emergency department with confusion, disorientation, and hallucinations should be evaluated for psychotic disorders such as schizophrenia, delirium from alcohol withdrawal or other drug intoxication or withdrawal, or dementia that may be complicated by another medical disorder. To take another example, an older adult seen in private practice, who has a history of recent bereavement, withdrawal, and increased forgetfulness, may be demented or may be suffering from cognitive deficits related to major depression.

Normal Aging

As people age, some degree of decline in cognitive functioning is common. The presence of mild memory impairment among older adults has been reported to occur among a very wide range (11–96%) of participants in various research studies. The prevalence of dementia among 75-year-old adults is 2–8%; and among 85-year-olds is 10–20%. Normal aging often brings increased forgetfulness and some changes in the speed and efficiency of thought. These changes, however, typically do not cause significant problems in everyday functioning or produce confusion or disorientation, which are signs of impaired cognition (see Chapter 12).

Dementia Versus Delirium

Both delirium and dementia involve cognitive deficits, often severe, that are the result of an underlying medical problem. They are often described as **dichotomous conditions,** although this term is rather misleading. Although there are many important differences, the conditions are best conceptualized as existing on a continuum. Dementia is frequently complicated by delirium, and a patient in a delirium is often found to suffer from an underlying dementia. Relatively "pure" cases of delirium and dementia, although probably not as common as believed, are distinctive; and these are the forms considered here.

Delirium is a rapidly evolving state of cognitive impairment in which gross distortions in attention, perception, and clarity of thought are prominent. It is most often caused by toxic states or metabolic derangement.

Problems in differentiating between delirium and dementia (Table 26–5) are particularly common with older adults. These patients are at greatest risk for dementia and are also more susceptible to medication toxicity and to the development of delirium as a consequence of illnesses such as pneumonia. Illness or injury can serve to "unmask" a developing dementia by overtaxing resources that are already compromised. To compound the problem, it is not uncommon to find delirium superimposed onto a preexisting dementia. In such cases, taking a careful history and getting reliable information from families and caregivers are essential. It is important to ask about the patient's level of functioning prior to the onset of the immediate situation. Were there any indications of a gradual deterioration in the patient's level of activity and functioning over the past 6 months or year?

In determining the cause of the patient's more acute mental status changes, the clinician should ask about all the patient's regular and new medications and examine the possibility of accidental overdose or adverse drug interactions. Medication toxicity is especially common among individuals whose cognitive problems do not allow them to monitor their drug use safely. In addition, alcohol and drug abuse should not be overlooked as a possible causes of delirium.

Dementia Versus Depression

Especially among older adults, symptoms of depression may masquerade as dementia (Table 26–6) making it difficult to distinguish between dementia and **dementia syndrome of depression (DSD),** once referred to as **pseudodementia.** One of the reasons for the change in terminology is that there is nothing "pseudo" about the cognitive problems seen in these

Table 26–6. Differentiating between dementia and dementia syndrome of depression (DSD).

Dementia	DSD
History	
• Slow, insidious onset	• Rapid onset
• Stress not necessarily present	• Recent stress, loss
• No history of depression	• Previous depression
• Family complains of problem	• Patient complains of problem
Evaluation	
• Often indifferent or anxious	• Sad, withdrawn, hopeless
• Willing to put forth good effort on mental status examination	• Little motivation, poor effort on mental status examination
• Excuses or denies deficits	• Complains of deficits
• Vague, shifting paranoia	• If psychotic, has depressive quality

individuals. They may be quite profoundly impaired, even confused and disoriented, and at times it can be very difficult to tell them apart from patients with genuine dementia. Cognitive deficits of this magnitude are generally seen only among the severely depressed. Individuals with milder depression—even when they are elderly—usually have mild, if any, cognitive deficits.

It is important to note that individuals with histories of depression and recent losses do become demented, just as individuals with early-stage dementia can be depressed. It is also sometimes difficult to distinguish between the withdrawal and apathy that can accompany depression and the withdrawal and apathy that may be seen with dementia. Both depressed and demented patients may appear quite impaired cognitively. In some cases, an empiric trial of antidepressant medication may provide the best means of distinguishing between dementia and DSD.

Dementia Versus Psychotic Disorders

The symptoms of psychotic disorders such as schizophrenia or bipolar disorder may resemble the disorganization, confusion, delusions, and agitation that sometimes accompany dementia (Table 26–7). The typical presence of more consistent and systematized delusions and the increased likelihood of previous psychosis and a family psychiatric history among

Table 26–7. Differentiating between dementia and psychotic disorders.

Dementia	Psychotic Disorders
Vague, shifting paranoia	Systematized and stable delusions
Manic symptoms in HIV-1 dementia	
No history of psychosis	Previous psychosis
"Sundowning" effect: symptoms worsen at night	No sundowning effect
Prominent cognitive deficits	Cognitive deficits less prominent

individuals with non–dementia-related psychotic disorders are important in making this differentiation.

DIAGNOSTIC WORK-UP

A dementia work-up should include a careful history (Table 26–8) and physical, neurological, and mental status examinations. In many cases additional tests and procedures may be helpful; these are discussed later.

History

As noted earlier, the history should be elicited from both patients and their families. In many cases it is helpful to ask both about the same topics, when appropriate. Although many demented individuals are unreliable historians, they may still be able to give much useful information, including symptoms of which family members are not aware. In addition, observing the ability of patients to provide a coherent and organized account of their complaints and recent history can often tell you much about their conditions.

A complete social and family history that includes place of birth; significant family members; and educational, marital, and employment background can also be useful. An educational and occupational history, for example, may provide information about a patient's previous level of functioning. Obvious memory problems may quickly become apparent, as when, for example, patients cannot name all their siblings or children. A quality of vagueness in patients' reports or inconsistency in the information supplied may suggest less blatant memory deficits. Particular attention should be paid to patients' accounts of more recent events. Individuals with mild or moderate dementia often show intact recall for older, overlearned information (eg, family, education, work) but cannot provide accurate information about the immediate past.

Ask patients about their regular activities, appetite, and sleep habits, as well as any physical or cognitive complaints. Information about their mood can be gained by inquiring directly, but also by asking about things that they enjoy and look forward to, any worries or concerns they may have, and their plans for the future.

Family members may be able to supply a more complete and balanced impression of the patient's

Table 26–8. Dementia work-up: history.

• Time course and nature of symptoms
• Slow and insidious versus more sudden/dramatic changes
• Current ability to function
• Accompanying mood or personality changes
• Presence or absence of confusion, agitation, and disorientation
• Psychotic symptoms
• Complicating factors, such as alcohol or substance abuse

Table 26–9. Dementia work-up: potential safety issues.

- Ambulation and balance
- Dizziness
- Ability to live independently
    - Ability to drive
    - Leaving stove or running water unattended
    - Wandering behavior
    - Confusion/agitation
- Level of supervision available

symptoms and level of functioning. Individuals with dementia typically lack insight into their cognitive problems and minimize or deny any difficulties. In fact, it is the family that most frequently raises concerns about the patient. Because family members may feel more comfortable discussing their observations away from the presence of the patient, they should be interviewed separately. It is especially important to inquire about both current and potential safety issues (Table 26–9).

Physical and Neurological Examinations

In addition to a routine physical examination, a complete neurological examination should be done, although the results of the latter are generally unremarkable in cases of mild-to-moderate dementia. Parkinsonian signs may be apparent during the later course of the disorder. Individuals with a developing vascular dementia may show focal signs on the neurological examination.

The Mental Status Examination

Because cognitive impairment is the hallmark of dementia, it is necessary to add additional screening items to the traditional mental status examination. Several brief dementia screening instruments offer the

advantages of both a structured format and a scoring system. These instruments must be used with caution, however, for the reasons discussed here.

The Mini-Mental State Examination (MMSE), which takes about 5 minutes, is probably the most commonly used dementia-screening instrument and is recommended for use by the primary care provider. It samples a wide range of functions, including orientation, immediate and delayed memory, concentration, basic language and reading functions, and visual construction abilities (Table 26–10). Patients are asked to count backward by 7, write a sentence, follow concrete directions, and copy geometric figures. A maximum score of 30 is possible; a score lower than 23 (some clinicians recommend 27) is suspicious for dementia. The clinician should be aware that the test is a gross screening instrument and that a significant number of false-negative results occur among individuals with mild dementia. Conversely, low scores may be obtained from individuals who are not demented but who show marked psychiatric symptoms, who are uncooperative, or whose first language is not English. Consequently, results should be interpreted cautiously. Other brief dementia-screening instruments include the Blessed Dementia Scale and the Neurobehavioral Cognitive Status Examination.

Other Tests

Laboratory tests are an important part of the dementia evaluation, as they can aid the clinician in identifying infectious or metabolic processes that may be causing or exacerbating the patient's cognitive problems (Table 26–11).

No clear consensus exists on the routine inclusion of a brain CT scan in a dementia work-up, and many physicians believe it is not essential in the absence of focal neurological signs. A brain CT scan is an im-

Table 26–10. Dementia work-up: Mini-Mental State Examination.

Function	Question or Task	Maximum Score
Orientation	What is the year, season, date, day, month? (5 points) Where are we: state, county, town, hospital, floor? (5 points)	10
Registration	Name three objects and ask the patient to repeat the names of the objects (correct response = 1 point). Repeat the names of the three objects until the patient learns them.	3
Attention and calculation	Ask the patient to recite serial 7s backward from 100. Stop the patient after five responses (correct response = 1 point).	5
Recall	Ask the patient to repeat the names of the three objects learned above (correct response = 1 point).	3
Language	Show the patient two common objects, eg, a pencil and watch, and ask the patient to identify them (2 points). Ask the patient to repeat "no ifs, ands, or buts" (1 point). Instruct the patient to follow the three-stage command: "take a paper in your right hand, fold it in half, and put it on the floor" (3 points). Ask the patient to read and obey the following: "close your eyes" (1 point). Instruct the patient to write a sentence (1 point). Ask the patient to copy a design (1 point).	9

Source: Reprinted, with permission, from Folstein MF, Folstein SE, McHugh PR: "Mini-Mental State": A practical method for grading the cognitive state of patients for the clinician. J Psychiatr Res 1975;12:189.

Table 26–11. Dementia work-up: recommended laboratory tests.

Urinalysis: urinary tract infection, diabetes	
Blood tests:	
Complete blood count	Blood urea nitrogen
Liver function	Calcium
Rapid plasma reagin	Phosphorus
Magnesium	Electrolytes
Glucose	B_{12} and folate
Thyroid	

Blood serum levels for any medications taken by the patient that might cause confusion if taken improperly.
Toxicology screens for alcohol and other abused drugs if indicated.

portant means of ruling out conditions such as chronic subdural hematomas and hydrocephalus, but it is probably not required without a history of falls or ataxia with incontinence. Scans should be ordered, however, in the case of rapid onset of mental status changes, or when lateralized neurological signs or seizure, such as tumor or cerebrovascular accident, raise the question of a structural brain lesion. Scans can also sometimes aid in differentiating between the dementia of Alzheimer's disease and that secondary to cerebrovascular disease.

At times it may be necessary or advisable to request additional tests and procedures. Although these procedures are not a routine part of the dementia work-up, they should be considered in certain situations.

An MRI scan may be advisable when the CT scan results are inconclusive, or when enhanced visualization of the white matter of the brain is needed. This may be helpful in assessing patients for multiple sclerosis or HIV-1–associated dementia.

An EEG can be helpful when seizures have occurred or subtle or equivocal signs of brain impairment are present. For example EEG changes are often present even in the early stages of Alzheimer's disease and may be helpful in the diagnosis of delirium. On the other hand, a normal EEG cannot be taken as definitively indicating the absence of dementia or other brain pathology.

Lumbar punctures are indicated when there is a question of an infectious process or when a rapidly progressing condition is present.

Neuropsychological Testing

Often the single most useful tool in the assessment of subtle or questionable dementia, neuropsychological testing involves the use of psychometric tests designed to detect and characterize a wide variety of cognitive problems. Test batteries, such as the Halstead Reitan and Luria Nebraska batteries, are available, but they take several hours to administer and are beyond the tolerance of many patients. Lezak has developed a flexible battery of tests using the Wechsler Adult Intelligence Scale (WAIS) as its foundation. Shorter sets taking 1–2 hours are frequently used, particularly with older adults. The tests themselves are similar to many of the tasks used in the brief cognitive screens discussed earlier but are more sophisticated and comprehensive. Consider referring a patient for neuropsychological testing in the following circumstances:

- When the reported deficits are subtle or equivocal and the impairment is mild.
- When the differential diagnosis is difficult to resolve (eg, distinguishing between dementia and depression).
- When a baseline is needed to measure the degree of cognitive deterioration over time.
- When a greater understanding of the patient's everyday level of functioning, limitations, potential safety issues, and the appropriate level of supervision is needed.
- When problem behaviors are present and management strategies must be worked out.
- When deficits or competency issues must be documented, such as in conservatorship proceedings.

Neuropsychological testing does require the patient to be able to attend for a minimum of 20–30 minutes, and some patients may be too agitated, withdrawn, or resistant to comply. Assess the patient's ability to participate in testing before a referral is made. An individual who can cooperate with a physical examination, for example, can probably be tested. Keep in mind that although serious perceptual impairments in hearing and vision limit testing, they do not necessarily rule it out.

TREATMENT & MANAGEMENT ISSUES

Treatment of dementia has usually been limited to identifying and addressing a treatable basis for the underlying condition (if one exists), treating secondary disorders such as anxiety or depression, educating patients and their families as to the nature of the condition, and assisting caregivers with safety and management issues. More recently, clinical trials have focused on agents, such as vasodilators, neuropeptide-related substances, and cholinergics, that may directly improve cognition and functional capacity, or at least slow their decline. Tacrine (tetrahydroaminoacridine, or THA) has received attention as a possible means of inhibiting or even reversing the cognitive deterioration of Alzheimer's disease. Unfortunately, although studies with tacrine and other drugs have sometimes demonstrated modest improvement on tasks such as the MMSE, no demonstrable improvement has been made in the level of function.

Management

Management of patients with dementia involves issues of self-care, safety, and communication. Individuals with dementia are disorganized, forgetful, and inefficient in many of their activities. They have difficulty following directions, in managing everyday activities, and in expressing themselves clearly. They are frequently impulsive, may have limited insight into their abilities, and generally do not learn well from experience. Emotionally, they may be changeable and unstable, irritable, or anxious; they may be fearful, easily frustrated, or apathetic and withdrawn. Because of circadian rhythm disturbances, patients with Alzheimer's disease may tend to be awake and wandering during the night, leading to sleep deprivation in caregivers.

These traits create special problems in managing and caring for patients with dementia, and many interactions with family and caregivers therefore focus on day-to-day management issues and behavioral problems. The following sections provide some general guidelines for addressing these issues. It may be useful in many situations to refer patients and their families to groups that can provide counseling, home evaluations, and case management.

1. Self-care: This area includes dressing, grooming, and hygiene. The best approach is to provide sufficient structure and guidance so that the patient can manage, while allowing some preservation of independence and choice. Individuals with mild cognitive impairment often get by with prompts and reminders. For individuals with more severe impairment, caregivers should offer a limited choice of clothing, food, or activities; use signs or pictures to identify important objects and locations; and emphasize routine and predictability.

2. Safety issues: Individuals with dementia are at increased risk for accidents because of their problems with attention, perception, and judgment. The following guidelines are designed to minimize the risk of household accidents:

- Carefully supervise use of medications.
- Keep things simple: reduce clutter; keep passageways clear.
- Install railings and other safety equipment, such as shower chairs and tub rails.
- Use a night light where necessary.
- Remove stove and oven controls if necessary.
- Use safety gates or install keyless locks on exterior doors if wandering is a problem.
- Make sure patients wear medical and personal identification bracelets.

Another important safety issue concerns driving and dementia. Deficits in attention, reaction time, visual spatial abilities, and judgment typically impair the ability of individuals with marked cognitive deficits to operate a motor vehicle safely. Individuals with advanced dementia who continue to operate a car seriously endanger others as well as themselves. Unfortunately, patients with dementia may insist on driving because of

their lack of insight into their problems, and caregivers may be reluctant to press the issue. Because driving is symbolic of independence, this often becomes an emotional issue for everyone involved.

Health-care providers need to be aware of the ethical ramifications of this problem. Confidentiality must be weighed against issues of competency, safety of the public, and the duty to warn. Legal responsibilities may also be involved. For example, in California physicians are required by law to report patients who are unable to operate a motor vehicle because of "Alzheimer's or other related dementias." In the case of accident or injury, physicians who have failed to make such a reports may be legally liable. Primary care providers should therefore inform themselves of the legal requirements in their own state regarding this issue.

3. Communication: Individuals with brain impairment may have specific deficits in language comprehension and expression similar to the various forms of aphasia that occur in stroke patients. More common may be a generalized difficulty in communication secondary to a short attention span, memory problems, or confusion. In these cases, there is a significant risk that the patients may not understand much of what they are being asked or told. Conversely, caregivers may not be receiving important information from patients regarding their needs and symptoms, which can result in increased anxiety, depression, or agitation on the part of patients. Some guidelines for communicating with the cognitively impaired are presented in Table 26–12.

4. Emotional and behavioral problems: These can include confusion, anxiety, agitation, depression, and anger. More severe psychiatric symptoms, such as delusions and hallucinations, may also occur. If patients become upset or agitated, it is better to distract them than to try to reason or argue with them. Attempts should be made to divert their attention to other topics or activities. Patients' medications should be carefully reviewed to determine whether they are causing these or other problems.

Overstimulation can cause restlessness, agitation, and confusion. If this occurs, it is important to have patients move to a less noisy or busy environment, for example, have them spend some time alone in their rooms.

Table 26–12. Tips for communicating with the cognitively impaired.

- Make sure you have patients' attention when you speak with them. Keep distractions, such as television, radio, or other conversations, to a minimum by meeting with patients in a quiet place.
- Keep communications brief, simple, and concrete. Break more complex information down into smaller pieces.
- Give patients several options to choose among, or phrase questions in multiple-choice format.
- Have patients paraphrase back the information to make sure they have understood what was said.

Disorientation can lead to anxiety and depression. Posting orientation information, for example clocks and calendars, in an easily visible location may help reduce this problem. Understimulation can also result in agitation and anxiety. When patients must spend long periods in their rooms because of immobility or safety issues and regular contact is not possible, it may be helpful to have a radio playing softly in the room or to provide some other such source of mild stimulation.

The depression and anxiety that coexist with dementia are not generally amenable to traditional psychotherapy. Nonetheless, many individuals benefit from the opportunity to verbalize their fears and concerns and appreciate the presence of a sympathetic listener. In general, cognitively impaired individuals do best with frequent brief interactions, rather than longer ones. For example, family members or home health aides might be advised to spend 1–2 minutes with the patient every 15 or 30 minutes. Patients often find it reassuring to be given orientation information and to be reminded of upcoming events during these check-ins.

Psychotropic Medication

When more serious psychiatric symptoms occur, such as severe depression, agitation, or psychosis, psychotropic medications may be indicated. Some general guidelines should be followed:

- Because these medications have the potential to further disrupt cognitive processes and worsen the problem, use considerably lower doses than those used for younger or nondemented individuals. Older adults in particular are particularly susceptible to side effects from these medications, especially when there are concurrent medical problems.
- Avoid benzodiazepines, especially for more than brief periods, as they have significant potential for causing sedation, confusion, and ataxia.
- Haloperidol (Haldol) is often a good choice for addressing symptoms of psychosis and agitation, as it does not promote anticholinergic effects and is a high-potency medication. An initial dosage of 0.5 mg is often used, gradually increasing up to 10 mg a dose if symptoms persist. If the problem continues, consider another agent or obtain consultation with a psychiatrist, particularly one specializing in geriatrics. Buspirone hydrochloride (BuSpar) has received some attention in this area but is not the drug of choice with agitation. It may be effective in controlling context-specific panic (eg, anxiety associated with a move) and might be used in conjunction with other medications.
- Methylphenidate hydrochloride (Ritalin) may sometimes be effective in increasing alertness and the level of arousal and improving food intake in patients with advanced dementia. It may also be helpful in reversing symptoms of depression in HIV-1–associated dementia.

Caregivers

Caring for cognitively impaired individuals is a demanding, often exhausting, very stressful undertaking. Primary care providers should ensure that caregivers also attend to their own needs and guard against fatigue and burnout. A number of support services, such as the Family Caregiver Alliance, offer education, support groups, and information about resources. Specialized case management and home consultation services can also be very helpful in assessing patient and family needs and locating additional services. Respite-care and day-activity programs may be invaluable in allowing stressed families and caregivers time off and providing needed stimulation and increased structure for the patient.

Nursing Home Placement

Inevitably in the management of demented patients, the issue arises of whether the patient can continue to be managed at home. This is an area fraught with strong feelings on the part of patient and caregiver alike, and it is often difficult to make objective decisions. Some of the important issues are listed as follows:

- Can the necessary level of supervision and care required by the patient be realistically and dependably supplied at home? Such issues as wandering and the potential for neglect and abuse should be considered here.
- Is sufficient assistance available to caregivers for them to continue to care for the patient without becoming overstressed and burnt out?
- What financial resources are available for the patient's care?

All things being equal, allowing patients to remain in their own homes is desirable. In many cases, however, doing so creates other significant problems, and however desirable this goal, it must be carefully weighed against issues of safety and practical limitations. In the advanced stage of dementia, when the patient becomes mute, bedbound, and incontinent, very often the services of a skilled nursing facility are required to ensure that the patient receives proper care. Nursing facilities should be chosen carefully; obviously, cost must be considered, but the quality of care must also be investigated. Information about both complaints and compliance with state regulations can be found through government agencies, advocacy groups, published reviews, and organizations (eg, geriatric-care programs) that frequently place patients in such facilities.

SUMMARY

The dementias have a variety of etiologies, but all are characterized by a progressive loss of cognition and functioning. When patients present with these symptoms, the primary care provider must consider differential diagnoses including dementia, delirium, depression, and psychosis. Diagnostic work-up includes a careful history from both patient and family, physical examination, labwork, mental status examination, and, on occasion, referral for CT, EEG, LP, or neuropsychological testing.

Treatment and management consists of ruling out any treatable condition, treating secondary disorders such as anxiety or depression, providing information to patients and families, and assisting caregivers with safety and management issues. Use of medications is appropriate when severe psychiatric symptoms occur, but interventions most frequently consist of adjusting the environment to make the patient as comfortable and safe as possible.

SUGGESTED READINGS

Beyer J, Moser S, Antuono P: Alzheimer's disease and driving: The role of the health care professional and caregiver. In: Nicolini M, Zatta PF, Corain B (editors): *Alzheimer's Disease and Related Disorders. Proceedings of the IIIrd International Conference on Alzheimer's Disease and Related Disorders,* Padua, Italy, July 1993. Pergamon, 1993.

Blessed G, Tomlinson BE, Roth M: The association between quantitative measures of dementia and of senile change in the cerebral grey matter of elderly subjects. Br J Psychiatry 1968;114:797.

Boccellari A, Zeifert P: Management of neurobehavioral impairment in HIV-1 infection. Psychiatr Clin North Am 1994;17:183.

Brock CD, Simpson WM: Dementia, depression, or grief? The differential diagnosis. Geriatrics 1990;45:37.

Coffrey CE, Cummings JL: *Textbook of Geriatric Neuropsychiatry.* American Psychiatric Press, 1994.

Folstein MF, Folstein SE, McHugh PR: "Mini-Mental State": A practical method for grading the cognitive state of patients for the clinician. J Psychiatr Res 1975;12:189.

Freeman M, Stuss D, Gordon M: Assessment of competency: The role of neurobehavioral deficits. Ann Intern Med 1991;115:203.

Hackett TP, Cassem NH: *Massachusetts General Hospital Handbook of General Hospital Psychiatry.* PSG, 1987.

Mungas D: In-office mental status testing: A practical guide. Geriatrics 1991;46:54.

Lezak M: *Neuropsychological Assessment,* 3rd ed. Oxford, 1995.

Lishman W: *Organic Psychiatry,* 2nd ed. Blackwell, 1987.

Schwamm LH et al: The neurobehavioral cognitive status examination: Comparison with the Cognitive Capacity Screening Examination and the Mini-Mental State Examination in a neurosurgical population. Ann Intern Med 1987;107:486.

Terry R. Katzman TR, Bick K (editors): *Alzheimer's Disease.* Raven, 1994.

Weiner M (editor): *The Dementias: Diagnosis and Treatment.* American Psychiatric Association, 1991.

White JC, Christensen JF, Singer CM: Methylphenidate as a treatment for depression in acquired immunodeficiency syndrome: An n-of-1 trial. J Clin Psychiatry, 1992; 53(5):153.

Sleep Disorders

27

Clifford Singer, MD, & Robert Sack, MD

INTRODUCTION

Thirty-five percent of adults in the United States experience sleep-related symptoms over the course of a year; of this group, half consider the problem a serious one. These figures place insomnia and daytime sleepiness among the most common symptoms seen in primary care practice. Sleep disorders are more than just a large part of clinical practice, however; they represent a major public health problem. Sleepiness impairs work performance and is a major factor in traffic and industrial accidents; sleep-related breathing problems lead to hypertension, cardiovascular disease, and sudden death. In addition, sleep medications themselves carry significant morbidity risks, including falls, daytime anxiety, and worsened sleep apnea. Diagnosis is based on the duration and nature of the symptoms: depression, restless legs, periodic leg movements, substance abuse, circadian-rhythm disturbance, or poor sleep habits that perpetuate the insomnia. Treatment depends on the underlying disorder. Physicians clearly need to be knowledgeable about sleep to treat patients effectively and advocate sound public policy.

Normal Sleep Physiology

Adulthood: The sleep-wake cycle is a complex electrophysiologic process consisting of alternating periods of wakefulness, non-REM (rapid eye movement) sleep, and REM sleep. Each of these periods has characteristic electroencephalogram (EEG), peripheral muscle, and autonomic nervous system patterns. These sleep periods can be documented with a polysomnographic recording (PSG), a procedure that allows sleep clinicians to make specific diagnoses based on electrophysiologic monitoring of EEG; electroculogram; electromyogram of submentalis and anterior tibialis muscles, respiratory muscles, nasal airflow, ear oximetry; and electrocardiogram.

Sleep has a structure, or architecture, that consists of four stages of non-REM and REM sleep cycles.

The awake EEG consists of low-voltage high-frequency waveforms that become dominated by alpha waveforms as the person becomes drowsy. Stage 1 sleep is defined by the disappearance of the alpha pattern and the establishment of theta waves and slow, roving eye movements. Stage 2 is defined by the appearance of low-frequency high-amplitude discharges and brief high-frequency variable-amplitude discharges on a background of theta waves. Slow waves (high-amplitude low-frequency delta waveforms) herald stage 3 sleep when they make up at least 20% of sleep time and stage 4 sleep when they constitute more than 50% of sleep time. These two stages are known as the deep stages of sleep, since they are associated with high arousal thresholds. REM sleep is a distinct state of sleep characterized by a wake-pattern EEG; skeletal muscle paralysis; and rapid, conjugate eye movements.

With the initiation of sleep, the healthy adult descends through the non-REM stages of sleep within 45–60 minutes before beginning the first REM cycle, which tends to be brief. As the night progresses, less time is spent in slow-wave sleep, and the REM cycles are longer in duration; overall, REM sleep makes up 20–25% of total sleep time. The non-REM–REM cycle typically lasts 90–110 minutes, so there are usually four complete cycles per night.

The timing and duration of sleep are controlled by many factors. Although most adults have some control over when they go to sleep and when they wake up, there is less control over how much sleep they need and when they feel sleepy. Although stimulants such as caffeine and habituation to a state of chronic fatigue can help people cope with inadequate sleep, they must ultimately pay the price of diminished mental efficiency and physical energy. The human range of sleep requirements is enormous, ranging from 3 to more than 12 hours, but the vast majority of people need 6–9 hours.

The body clock, located in the suprachiasmatic nucleus of the hypothalamus, functions as the circadian pacemaker. It superimposes a rhythm of sleepiness and alertness to days and nights and determines whether specific persons are night owls, morning larks, or somewhere in between. The light-dark cycle and nightly rhythm of melatonin secretion by the pineal gland act synergistically to keep the body clock synchronized with the day-night cycle, allowing alertness during the day and sleepiness at night.

Childhood: Newborns spend about 70% of each day asleep, with a high proportion of REM sleep. Circadian patterns do not develop for at least several weeks—or even months. Sleeping through the night is one of the first maturational milestones. Sleep continues to be polyphasic, with daytime naps, until the child is 5 or 6. From ages 5–10, children are normally consummate sleepers with few arousals. Total sleep time decreases gradually though childhood, but for hormonal as well as psychosocial reasons, the quality and quantity of sleep drop sharply with puberty. Sleep can be erratic—brief on some nights and long "recovery" periods on others.

There has been some renewed interest in household arrangements for children's sleep. Anthropologists point out that isolating a newborn in a separate bedroom is almost unique to western cultures and that cosleeping with infants is more natural and may be beneficial. Sleeping alone is a desirable mark of independence, but at what age this should occur varies considerably, depending on the child and the family.

Old Age: As people age, sleep tends to be lighter, with more arousals and near disappearance of slow-wave sleep. Sleep onset and final awakening come earlier. Many people experience this change in early midlife; it may progress as they grow older, and waking at 4:00 in the morning is normal for many older persons. Severe insomnia also increases with age, and excessive daytime sleepiness is extremely common as well, possibly the result of a high prevalence of sleep apnea and periodic leg movements, both of which disrupt nighttime sleep.

CLASSIFICATION OF SLEEP DISORDERS

Sleep disorders are generally grouped into three categories: disorders of initiating and maintaining sleep (insomnias), disorders of excessive daytime sleepiness (hypersomnias), and abnormal sleep behaviors (parasomnias) (Table 27–1).

Every clinician's review of systems should include screening patients for daytime sleepiness and nighttime sleep. Three basic questions give physicians a head start in diagnosing sleep disorders and determining whether they are severe enough to warrant treatment.

- How are you sleeping?
- How much sleep do you get in a typical night?
- How sleepy are you during the day?

Table 27–1. The sleepless patient: disorders of initiating or maintaining sleep.

Category	Disorder
Insomnias	Transient and persistent insomnia Chronobiologic disorders Restless legs syndrome Periodic leg movements Mental illness Alcohol and drugs Medical disorders affecting sleep
Hypersomnias	Sleep apnea syndrome Narcolepsy
Parasomnias	Pavor nocturnus (sleep terrors) Nightmares Somnambulism (sleepwalking) REM behavior disorder

Follow-up questions should sharpen the differential diagnosis of specific insomnia disorders.

The Sleepless Patient: The Insomnias

Transient and Persistent Insomnia: These insomnias are among the most common complaints presented to the primary care clinician. It is best to think of insomnia as a symptom rather than a disease or diagnosis. Many factors combine to produce insomnia, which often occurs when a delicate balance is tipped; for example, a constitutionally light sleeper may be fine until he or she enters a period of stress or uses a medication (eg, aminophylline) that has alerting effects. It may be necessary to deal with several causative factors concurrently in order to restore a natural sleep cycle.

Temporary insomnia caused by stress, environment (cold, noise, a new baby), acute illness, or pain is easy to identify and usually needs no special intervention. A brief course of sedative-hypnotic medication is occasionally warranted and may reduce the risk of developing long-term insomnia. Travel across time zones brings about a mismatch of the body clock and social clock and induces the transient insomnia known as "jet lag," which can ruin the first few days of a trip. Shift workers whose shifts change experience the same phenomenon and can suffer severe health and social consequences because of it.

In a large multicenter study, the diagnosis of chronic insomnia accounted for 40–88% of patients in medical, psychiatric, and sleep clinics who presented with a primary complaint of insomnia. Chronic insomnia goes by many names: psychophysiologic insomnia, conditioned insomnia, learned insomnia, and primary insomnia. These terms all imply what is known about this condition: it is a chronic ailment that develops over time by operant conditioning to an arousal state that is incompatible with deep, sustained, restful sleep. Chronic insomnia is a diagnosis of exclusion and must be differentiated from the many other causes of persistent sleep disruption (see later discussion). It may develop after a period of sleep disruption caused by stress, infant care, medical illness, or pain. Unfortunately, after the inciting cause disappears, the insomnia can take on a life of its own. Conditioning mechanisms have been inferred from the observation that patients may have difficulty initiating sleep in the bedroom but sleep normally in the sleep laboratory, a hotel, or even their own living room.

Long-term dependence on sedative-hypnotics is often one result of chronic insomnia, as is incessant sleep deprivation with daytime fatigue and dysphoria. Psychophysiologic insomnia requires a holistic approach that can include medication; sleep-hygiene measures (especially avoiding caffeine, alcohol, and excessive time in bed while awake); and cognitive therapy. Cognitive-behavioral treatment approaches are successful with motivated patients. Such treatment involves techniques to reduce anxiety and initiate behavioral changes that improve sleep hygiene (Table 27–2). Short-term use of sedative-hypnotic medications is appropriate to break the cycle of anxiety, arousal, and insomnia (see the section "Medical Treatment,"). In some patients, the symptoms suggest another disorder that can be targeted separately (eg, depression, restless legs syndrome).

Before initiating treatment, it is helpful to have the patient keep a sleep diary for 2 weeks, documenting sleep onset and wake-up times, rating both sleep quality and daytime fatigue and sleepiness. The sleep diary helps determine the frequency of insomnia and its daytime significance. Many patients report dissatisfaction with their sleep but still function well during the day. These patients should be reassured that nighttime wakefulness is a problem only if daytime somnolence results. Polysomnography is unenlightening for most cases of insomnia and should be reserved for the more refractory cases.

Chronobiologic Disorders of the Sleep-Wake Cycle: Disturbances in the circadian timing

of sleep may be only transient, as in jet lag and shift-work syndromes; or chronic, as in delayed-sleep-phase syndrome, advanced-sleep-phase syndrome, and free-running-sleep syndrome. The last is most common in blind persons, who lack the critical input of the light-dark cycle in regulating circadian rhythms. Diagnosis of chronobiologic sleep disorders is based on the understanding that—except for its timing—sleep itself is normal in these conditions. Given the freedom to choose sleep times based only on internal cues of sleepiness, persons with chronobiologic insomnias usually sleep well on weekends or while on vacation. A mismatch between the body clock and the hours during which a person tries to sleep, however, may cause insomnia. Successful treatment can require strategically timed exposure to light that is bright enough to reset the body clock and thus shift the timing of the sleep cycle. The timing of light exposure is critical, based on the fact that bright light in the morning advances the body clock and bright light in the evening delays it. Commercial light boxes are recommended for this purpose (see "Chronobiologic Treatment" later in this chapter). The pineal hormone melatonin, currently sold over the counter in health food stores as a food supplement, may achieve this same goal with greater convenience. For example, a person with delayed-sleep-phase syndrome might take synthetic melatonin (0.5—3 mg) early in the evening, at 8:00 or 9:00 PM—hours before endogenous melatonin secretion begins—to reset the body clock to an earlier hour.

Case illustration 1: Greg is a 27-year-old man who presents with a complaint of insomnia. He describes having great difficulty getting up in the morning, which is placing his job in jeopardy because he is chronically late to work. No matter what time he goes to bed, Greg cannot fall asleep until about 2:00 AM and then sleeps through the alarm set for 6:00. His wife has given up trying to wake him, and he has arranged for an answering service to call him, but the ringing telephone does not awaken him either. He is often tired and sleepy during the day, but in the evening gets his second wind just as his wife goes to bed. He craves weekends and vacations, when he sleeps until noon and feels rested.

Greg has delayed-sleep-phase syndrome. Persons with this disorder are extreme night owls—they lack the chronobiologic flexibility to adjust their sleep times according to school, work, and social demands. Origins of delayed-sleep-phase syndrome are probably multifactorial. Sleep timing is delayed, and there are surges of energy in the evening, late sleep onset, and severe morning hypersomnia.

This syndrome is extremely common in teenagers and young adults, in whom the insomnia complaint is usually prolonged sleep onset, with an inability to fall asleep until several hours past midnight. Parents or spouses may describe their frustration with getting the patient out of bed in the morning. Treatment can

Table 27–2. Cognitive-behavioral treatment for insomnia.

Essential Cognitive Techniques	Essential Behavioral Changes
Talk about the frustration of not falling asleep and put this into perspective; ie, "decatastrophize" being awake at night.	Bed restriction (out of bed if awake for more than 30 minutes; no television, reading, or eating in bed); gradually increase time in bed as sleep improves.
Education about sleep requirements (not everyone needs 8 hours) and daytime napping (all right if midday and less than 1 hour).	No caffeine, alcohol, or nicotine late in the day.
Discuss patients' belief that they are defective in sleep and will always be poor sleepers; reframe concept in hopeful way.	Bright light exposure (especially in the morning) and exercise in afternoon.

involve bright light exposure in the morning (to phase-advance the body clock) and short-term use of a sedative-hypnotic medication to facilitate earlier sleep onset and to make getting up for bright light treatment manageable. Properly timed melatonin intake may also be helpful. Successful management calls for fairly strict adherence to a lifestyle that avoids late-night activity. This last requirement is difficult, especially for teenagers and young adults, with deviations from the early-to-bed schedule resulting in relapses into the delayed-sleep cycle.

Restless Legs Syndrome (RLS): This condition comes on with rest and produces an irresistible need to move, stretch, or rub the lower extremities. Severe dysesthesia, sometimes described as "creepy-crawly" sensations, aching, tension, tingling, or prickling, may occur. Most people with RLS also have periodic limb movements during sleep, leading to further sleep disruption. RLS can interfere with plane travel, desk work, reading, and, especially, sleep onset. The syndrome is common, affecting at least 5% of the population, and may be even more common in periodic or subclinical form. It sometimes first appears in females during pregnancy, can run in families, and tends to worsen with age. Many physicians do not think to ask about this symptom and hence fail to recognize it as a source of discomfort and insomnia for their patients.

There is no definitive treatment, although avoidance of caffeine and nicotine, moderate late-afternoon exercise, stretching before bedtime, opioids, L-dopa, and sedative-hypnotics may all be helpful. Carbamazepine and clonidine may also be effective. The syndrome is so distressful for some of its sufferers that there is now a national support group and newsletter (see "Resources" at the end of the chapter).

Periodic Leg Movements During Sleep (PLMS): These are repetitive myoclonic movements of the lower extremities that come in bursts lasting from a few seconds to many minutes; they are more common in, but are not limited to, the first half of the night. The movements are usually associated with brief arousals and can lead to nonrestorative sleep and daytime somnolence. The prevalence of PLMS increases with age—5% in people 30–50 years of age, 29% in those 50–65, and 44% in those over 65—and is often seen in metabolic and neurodegenerative diseases. PLMS should be distinguished from nocturnal leg cramps, which are painful, prolonged muscle spasms in the legs; these cramps are often treated with quinine sulfate. Tricyclic antidepressants, lithium carbonate, and withdrawal from benzodiazepines and alcohol can induce or worsen PLMS. It is often asymptomatic, but in its severe form, patients may have sleep-onset insomnia, nonrestorative sleep, or frequent arousals during the night from the more robust myoclonic movements. Not infrequently, the bed partner is the one complaining about the jerking leg movements at night.

Whereas RLS is primarily a symptomatic diagnosis, PLMS is best documented by polysomnography at home or in a sleep laboratory. A PLMS index greater than 5 (muscle jerks per hour) is considered definitive. PLMS responds to some of the same treatments as RLS. Benzodiazepine sedative-hypnotics can improve sleep continuity in PLMS patients, but it does not reduce the number of leg movements. L-dopa may be the treatment of choice, but rebound in the second half of the night or during the following day may make dosing a challenge. Opioids, such as a bedtime dose of codeine, work well in PLMS (as in RLS) but should be reserved for patients with severe symptoms.

Mental Illness and Insomnia: Sleep disturbances are among the most common symptoms of mental illnesses, particularly mood disorders. Major depression must always be considered in patients who complain of frequent nighttime awakenings and early morning arousal, particularly when those arousals are accompanied by anxiety and worry. On the other hand, many depressed patients complain of hypersomnia, with fatigue and difficulty waking and getting started in the morning. This change in sleep pattern is especially characteristic of seasonal affective disorder and so-called atypical depression. Both are rather common in young and middle-aged adults.

Mania is frequently accompanied by a reduced need for sleep, making a change in sleep patterns a cardinal diagnostic symptom of the disorder; patients usually do not complain about this change, however. Depressed patients, on the other hand, find their sleep changes very distressing. Sedating, antidepressant medication is the treatment of choice. Doxepin, nortriptyline, trazodone, or nefazodone are all reasonable choices for treating insomnia in depressed patients. Nonsedating antidepressants can also be used, in conjunction with a brief course of a sedative-hypnotic drug for temporary help with sleep. The benzodiazepine can be stopped as the insomnia improves with the resolution of the depression (see Chapter 22).

Severe anxiety disorders, including posttraumatic stress disorder, can present with severe insomnia. Nightmares frequently complicate the picture. Treatment is often challenging and may require intensive psychotherapy as well as polypharmacy. Antidepressant medication and clonidine may be helpful with the sleep-related symptoms. (see Chapter 23).

Bereavement is usually accompanied by anxiety and insomnia. Short-term use of benzodiazepines may be very helpful for patients struggling to get through long nights.

Case illustration 1: Francine is 47 years old and is seeking her physician's help in dealing with anxiety. She feels restless and fidgety during the day, but she is also tired. She has difficulty concentrating, making decisions, and getting things done, all of which are out of character for her. Although quite fatigued, it can take her an hour to fall asleep. When sleep does come, it is restless and interrupted by many awakenings, filled with worried thoughts.

Francine has major depression, presenting with prominent symptoms of anxiety and insomnia. All patients with these symptoms need to be screened for depression, with a few questions regarding their mood, sense of the future, appetite, and libido. Education, emotional support, and medical treatment with antidepressant medication, perhaps with short-term adjunctive use of a sedative-hypnotic, provide enormous benefit for most patients.

For example, treatment for Francine might start with either a selective serotonin reuptake inhibitor (SSRI) such as sertraline (50 mg every morning) or one of the nonspecific reuptake inhibitors, such as venlafaxine (25 mg three times a day with meals) or nefazodone (100 mg twice a day), with dosage adjustments according to clinical response. For the first few weeks of therapy, a sedative-hypnotic (temazepam, 15 mg at each bedtime, or zolpidem, 5 or 10 mg at each bedtime) should also be prescribed to facilitate sleep until the underlying depression has improved. Some patients get sleepy while taking nefazodone and do not need additional medication for sleep. Fluoxetine and nefazodone can slow the clearance of alprazolam and triazolam, so these drugs should be coadministered with care, although a longer half-life for these benzodiazepines can be beneficial in some cases, such as in patients with end-of-dose rebound insomnia.

Alcohol and Drugs: Alcohol has variable effects on sleep patterns, but it generally causes decreased alertness. Like other sedatives, however, alcohol suppresses slow-wave sleep, making sleep lighter. With its short half-life, alcohol also tends to produce a rebound arousal effect in the second half of the night and thus produces less sleep overall.

Other drugs also bring about characteristic sleep changes. Amphetamines and cocaine cause a marked reduction in sleep during acute intoxication and profound hypersomnia during the withdrawal phase. Opioids have variable effects on sleep; they can, of course, improve sleep when used for analgesia. Caffeine causes longer sleep latency (time needed to fall asleep) and increased wakefulness during the night. Some persons may not perceive the effects of caffeine on sleep even when they are documented on sleep EEG; others are very much aware of these effects. Caffeine can even affect sleep when ingested several hours before bedtime.

Both prescription and over-the-counter sedative-hypnotic medications can contribute to rebound cycles of insomnia in the latter part of the night and anxiety the next day. Daytime drowsiness and worsened sleep apnea are other potential problems. Confusion, ataxia, and unexplained falls should cue the physician to consider the presence of alcohol or sedative-hypnotic dependence, especially in elderly patients.

Education about the effects of these substances on sleep may motivate patients to reduce their intake, particularly at times when use may affect sleep. Patients with more severe dependency and abuse problems need referral to specific treatment programs (see Chapter 21).

Medical Disorders: Pain, rheumatologic disorders, neuromuscular disease, cardiac disease, pulmonary disease, dyspepsia, inflammatory bowel diseases, and nocturia are all common medical causes of insomnia. Another classic medical syndrome affecting sleep is fibrositis, a condition in which sleep is characterized by alpha-wave intrusion into non-REM sleep. This syndrome produces nonrestorative sleep, in which patients complain of feeling tired despite sleep duration within the normal range. Acquired immunodeficiency syndrome (AIDS) has been associated with daytime sleepiness; a decrease in total slow-wave sleep, with alpha-wave intrusions; increasing arousals; night sweats; and frequent nightmares. Patients with chronic disease are often desperate for good sleep, making adequate nighttime analgesia and sedating antidepressants very welcome.

Acute illnesses often cause diffuse cerebral dysfunction in the frail elderly. The resulting delirium is almost always accompanied by disruption of the sleep-wake cycle and alertness. In many patients, the confusion and sleepiness of delirium are the first clues of illness.

Medications can also cause insomnia and daytime drowsiness. Bronchodilators, activating antidepressants, and steroids, for example, often interfere with sleep; many psychotropics, opioid analgesics, and clonidine can cause daytime drowsiness.

Neurodegenerative Disease and Sleep: There is no localized sleep center in the brain; rather, there are several neuronal circuits that function in maintaining sleep or alertness. Diseases that affect diffuse brain functions invariably affect sleep and alertness; Alzheimer's disease (AD) and Parkinson's disease (PD) have been studied more than most others. AD causes the same kinds of changes in sleep as normal aging does, but they are more severe: less clear day-night difference with more daytime and less nighttime sleep. The classic day-night reversal is probably rare, but the trend to many nighttime awakenings is common. This is very stressful for caregivers, who must continue to supervise their charges for safety during these nocturnal wanderings. Sleep disruption is among the most stressful aspects of caring for a demented person at home.

PD patients also have severe sleep problems. Akinesia causes physical discomfort over pressure points that would, in a healthy person, be relieved by tossing and turning in sleep. Parkinsonian medication itself can cause arousal. Furthermore, the intrinsic neurotransmitter and neurodegenerative changes PD causes in the neuronal circuits that are important for sleep can also induce insomnia.

The Sleepy Patient: Disorders of Excessive Somnolence

Patients are more likely to complain to physicians about insomnia than about hypersomnia, or excessive daytime sleepiness. This is rarely a primary complaint of patients, and uncovering symptoms of excessive daytime sleepiness may take some intuitive detective work on the physician's part. Two questions that can lead to the critical diagnosis of sleep apnea or narcolepsy should be part of every review of systems:

- Do you struggle to stay awake while driving, reading, watching television and movies, or listening to lectures during daytime hours?
- Do you feel tired, fatigued, and lacking in energy during the day, especially in the morning?

If the answer to either question is yes, follow-up questions should be directed at determining if the problem is inadequate nighttime sleep from insomnia, drowsiness from medications, or one of the two serious sleep disorders described in the following section.

Sleep-Related Breathing Problems

1. Snoring–Apart from being a nuisance to bed partners, snoring may herald serious respiratory obstruction during sleep along a continuum of partial to complete airway closure. Males snore more than females do, although postmenopausal females snore almost as much as men do. Aside from gender, other factors associated with snoring include anatomic narrowing of the airways, body habitus and sleep position (obese, supine), the use of alcohol and sedative-hypnotics, endocrinopathy (hypothyroidism, acromegaly), smoking, and possibly genetic factors. The view of snoring as a mild form of obstructive sleep apnea is supported by the transient drop in blood oxygen saturation and increases in pulmonary and systemic pressure that can occur in snoring. Losing weight, avoiding sedating medications or alcohol, and using appliances to prevent sleeping on the back (eg, a tennis ball sewn to the back of the nightshirt) are warranted in severe cases. Laser surgery to enlarge the oropharynx is increasingly popular, but the long-term effects are not well documented. Because surgery can eliminate the noise of snoring without affecting an associated obstruction, PSG evaluation prior to an operation should be performed to rule out obstructive sleep apnea.

2. Sleep apnea syndrome–Obstructive sleep apnea (OSA) is a major cause of cardiovascular morbidity and daytime somnolence in adults. Originally thought of as a relatively rare disturbance in severely obese patients with the classic "Pickwickian syndrome" of somnolence, hypoventilation, and polycythemia, OSA is now known to represent a wide range of severity in upper airway narrowing during sleep that begins earlier in life and is more prevalent than previously thought. In midlife, 2% of women and 4% of men have OSA, with serious daytime sequelae. Nighttime symptoms of OSA include loud snoring (often beginning early in adulthood and worsening progressively with age and increased weight), snorting and gagging sounds, tossing and turning, night sweats, abrupt awakenings with a feeling of choking, and profound sleep disruption. The arousals triggered by the apneic episodes cause such daytime symptoms as fatigue and excessive sleepiness. In mild cases, subjective insomnia may be the chief complaint. Patients are often unaware of the severity of the sleep disruption and may attribute their sleepiness to some other cause, such as working hard. The degree of sleepiness is variable, but it is a key symptom. People may be so accustomed to living with fatigue that they are not fully aware how sleepy they are. Questions about dozing while reading or watching television, nodding off at the wheel, or poor concentration must be directly posed to patients. Untreated OSA leads to hypertension and is probably a significant risk factor for lethal cardiovascular events, including myocardial infarction and stroke. Clinical assessment by PSG either at home or in a sleep laboratory confirms the diagnosis and helps determine the proper setting for positive airway pressure devices, which are the major form of treatment. Surgical uvuloplasty, tracheostomy, and dental appliances designed to keep the tongue from falling back and occluding the airway are other forms of treatment available for those who cannot tolerate continuous or two-stage positive airway pressure therapy (CPAP or bilevel positive airway pressure [BIPAP]). The diagnosis of OSA is an important one to make in terms of both improving the patient's quality of life and preventing serious accidents and cardiovascular disease.

Obstructive apneas also occur in children. Enlarged tonsils and adenoids are usually responsible, but craniofacial abnormalities and obesity can be the underlying causes. As in adults, loud snoring, restless sleep, and observed pauses in breathing make up the picture. Children with obstructive apnea may not complain of sleepiness; instead, they may manifest daytime irritability, decreased concentration, or declining school performance. Some children have even been misidentified as intellectually impaired. Nocturnal enuresis may be another symptom of OSA in children. Parents should be asked about snoring and breath-holding during sleep. Consultation with an ear, nose, and throat specialist is advised whenever OSA is suspected. Tonsillectomy (if the underlying cause) is usually completely curative. Other causes of obstructive apnea can be treated with CPAP. Surgical approaches such as tracheostomy or craniofacial reconstruction may be necessary in rare cases.

Central apnea is defined as the cessation of airflow for at least 10 seconds with no ventilatory effort. Patients with predominantly central apnea tend to complain more of insomnia with frequent awakenings than of the hypersomnolence that is so typical of patients with obstructive apnea. Arterial oxygen desaturation usually occurs in central apneas, but serious cardiovascular sequelae are less common than in obstructive apnea. Predisposing factors to central sleep apnea are congestive heart failure (mechanism unknown), nasal obstruction, and neurodegenerative diseases that can affect the central nervous system's respiratory control or induce profound hypoventilation from respiratory muscle weakness.

Central apneas are often seen in sleeping neonates, especially premature infants and can be fatal (eg, sudden infant death syndrome [SIDS]). The cause of SIDS remains a tragic mystery; obstructed breathing has long been suspected as an important etiology in at least some cases, but it is far from proven. There is currently an ongoing public information campaign to encourage mothers to avoid placing infants face down (prone), especially in soft bedding. Epidemiologic assessments will determine whether this public health intervention is effective.

> *Case illustration 3:* Jim, who is 64, visits his primary care physician for a follow-up of his hypertension treatment. His wife has accompanied him to the office to ask whether there is any medical explanation for her husband's fatigue. Close questioning reveals that the fatigue predates the hypertension treatment and is not clearly attributable to the medication. The tiredness is accompanied by true sleepiness; Jim can fall asleep anytime during the day while reading or driving. He minimizes the problem, yet he acknowledges having difficulty with concentration and memory. He falls asleep easily after getting into bed at night, but his wife describes him as a restless sleeper who snores loudly.

Jim has obstructive sleep apnea. The clinical clues are his snoring, daytime sleepiness, and hypertension. Referral to a sleep disorders specialist should help confirm the diagnosis and provide a review of the best treatment options.

Narcolepsy: Narcolepsy is a syndrome consisting of four primary symptoms: excessive daytime sleepiness, cataplexy and, less frequently, sleep paralysis and hypnagogic hallucinations. It occurs in approximately 1 in 2000 people. Narcolepsy often begins in the teens or early twenties but mid- and late-life onset can occur. Males are affected more commonly than are females. A formal diagnosis is frequently not made until 5 or 10 years after the onset of symptoms. If the syndrome is not diagnosed, patients are typically perceived as lazy and unmotivated. Genetic factors play an important role in the disorder, with at least two genes involved, one of them HLA (human leukocyte antigen)-related. The cardinal symptom is sleepiness that comes on suddenly and irresistibly in what are called "sleep attacks." Low-grade, persistent sleepiness that affects concentration, thinking, and memory may also occur. Sleep episodes may be brief (several minutes to an hour), but the person usually awakens feeling more alert, and the next sleep episode usually does not come on for at least an hour. When unrecog-

nized, the disorder leads to poor school and work performance, social stigma, and accidents.

Cataplexy, the brief, sudden loss of muscle tone leading to slurred speech, clumsiness, leg weakness, or complete collapse, is triggered by strong emotional reactions such as laughter or anger. **Sleep paralysis** is transient immobility on awakening, often accompanied by the vivid hallucinations of REM dreaming, all while the patient is lying in bed perfectly alert. The spells are brief, lasting several minutes at most. Narcolepsy can impair nighttime sleep with frequent awakenings, vivid nightmares, and intense, realistic (hypnagogic) hallucinations that precede sleep onset. The hallucinations are usually visual but can involve any sensory modality.

Patients should have a formal evaluation by a sleep disorders specialist before treatment for narcolepsy is initiated. The diagnosis usually requires documentation of sleep-onset REM by PSG. Excessive daytime somnolence is treated with scheduled daytime naps and medication. CNS stimulants, most commonly dextroamphetamine (5–60 mg a day), methamphetamine (20–25 mg/day) or methylphenidate (10–90 mg/day), improve daytime function. Cataplexy and sleep paralysis can be treated with REM-suppressant drugs such as tricyclic antidepressants. Joining a narcolepsy support group can help patients cope with the disorder's psychologic sequelae, which result from the social and occupational stigma of having little control over sleep onset.

Patients With Bizarre Nighttime Behavior: The Parasomnias

Parasomnias are perhaps the least common sleep disorders and their diagnosis can be difficult, although they should be considered whenever bizarre nighttime behavior is present.

Pavor Nocturnus: Sleep terrors (pavor nocturnus) are very disconcerting to parents but are usually quite benign. The child (usually aged 3–6) awakens with a scream and appears terrified, with signs of autonomic arousal: eyes bulging, heart racing, sweating. Although episodes usually last a few minutes, they can go on for half an hour. Attempts at comfort are to no avail. Finally, the child falls asleep. In the morning, the child is typically amnestic about the episode or may have a fragmentary memory of a bad dream. Sleep terrors involve partial arousals from stage 4 (deep) sleep. Reassurance of the parents is the usual treatment; in persistent night terrors, however, benzodiazepines may be justified.

Nightmares: True nightmares occur in REM sleep and involve a narrative story people can often relate. Nightmares are usually a transient problem, presumably triggered by stressful personal events. Persistent nightmares are a serious concern, however, and may require referral to a mental health specialist.

Somnambulism: Like sleep terrors, sleepwalking is a partial arousal from stage 4 sleep. Occasional sleepwalking is very common in childhood and may follow a period of stress or sleep deprivation. The main concern is accidental injury, and protective measures, such as placing gates in front of a stairwell, may need to be taken.

REM-Behavior Disorder (RBD): In this syndrome, loss of the normal REM sleep muscle atonia leads to dream-enactment behavior. The diagnosis is made in patients with sudden bursts of excited, intense, sometimes violent, activity during sleep. The syndrome may be subtle, in the form of leg movements and talking, or dramatic, in the form of punching, kicking, grabbing, strangling, running, and moving about the bedroom. Dreams of an intense, violent nature are typical. RBD is seen frequently in toxic or metabolic delirium, but most persistent forms of the syndrome occur in old age and are presumed to be idiopathic, ischemic, or neurodegenerative in etiology. Lesions or dysfunction in the pons are responsible for the loss of inhibition to spinal motor-neurons. Treatment of RBD with clonazepam is highly effective.

TREATMENT

Managed health-care systems vary considerably in their coverage of sleep disorder evaluations. The routine use of expensive polysomnographic evaluations for most cases of insomnia is unwarranted and is appropriately limited by most insurance plans. Nonetheless, the timely and accurate diagnosis of sleep apnea syndrome and other severe sleep disorders can have powerful effects in maintaining health, and physicians should advocate for their coverage. The optimal assessment and treatment of sleep disorders can also decrease unnecessary office and emergency department visits and reduce drug use.

Medical Treatment

Treating insomnia with medication should involve specific target goals, such as shorter sleep latency, delayed wake-up, or fewer nocturnal awakenings. Insomnia of recent onset should be treated with the expectation that short-term therapy will be effective. Sedative-hypnotic drugs should be used in conjunction with a sleep-hygiene program to maximize efficacy and reduce both the dosage and the duration of treatment (see Table 27–1). These medications should not be used in pregnancy. Patients with insomnia secondary to depression, pain, substance abuse, medication, or circadian-rhythm disorder should also receive treatment for the primary cause of the insomnia.

Benzodiazepines: These are the most commonly prescribed sleeping medications.

1. Efficacy and safety–All benzodiazepines have sleep-promoting effects, although only five are currently marketed as sedative-hypnotics. These drugs work well for short-term treatment of insomnia; tolerance to their sleep-promoting effects can develop

quickly, and some authorities recommend avoiding long-term use. Some patients, however, especially those with an anxiety component to their insomnia, may benefit from long-term use. Benzodiazepines alter sleep structure, reducing both REM and slow-wave sleep, but the clinical significance of this is uncertain. They are generally safe for younger adults, even in overdose, although combining them with alcohol and other depressants can produce potentially catastrophic synergistic effects. In older individuals, the safety profile is less benign; amnesia, ataxia, confusion, and worsening sleep apnea may develop.

2. Pharmacokinetics–Choosing a benzodiazepine on the basis of half-life involves ranking the target goals. Short-acting drugs such as triazolam are useful for the treatment of sleep-onset insomnia, but many individuals have rebound insomnia in the second half of the night or anxiety the following day. Longer-acting drugs such as flurazepam may work better for middle-of-the night insomnia, but some persons have morning hangover effects. Longer-acting drugs can be particularly troublesome in the elderly, in whom drug accumulation magnifies toxic effects. Temazepam and estazolam have an intermediate half-life and represent reasonable compromises for patients with sleep-maintenance insomnia who get hangover effects from longer-acting drugs.

Patients with sleep apnea, severe respiratory disease, gait and balance problems, or alcohol abuse should not be given these drugs. Doses should be kept low for the elderly and for patients with hepatic insufficiency. Rebound insomnia can complicate withdrawal from these drugs, causing patients to return to their use.

Zolpidem: An imidazopyridine, this drug is structurally unrelated to benzodiazepines but shares some characteristics with them. Its short half-life (1.4–3.8 hours) makes it most suitable for patients with sleep-onset or initial sleep maintenance problems. Zolpidem preserves the natural sleep architecture, providing at least a theoretical advantage. The dose is 5–10 mg at bedtime, and patients should be cautioned to get into bed shortly after taking the drug because of its quick onset. Precautions similar to those for the benzodiazepines apply to zolpidem, although tolerance and withdrawal problems may be less likely.

Sedating Antidepressants: Many clinicians believe drugs such as trazodone, nefazodone, doxepin, and amitriptyline are better choices for long-term treatment of severe insomnia than are benzodiazepines, although this has not been well studied. The theoretic advantages include less impairment of nighttime breathing and slow-wave sleep. Treatment of underlying depression in many insomnia patients provides another advantage. Tolerance to the sedating effects of these drugs develops in many patients, but some clinicians believe this is slower to develop than with benzodiazepines. Side effects of these drugs are numerous, and special care must be taken in elderly patients, especially with amitriptyline and its potent anticholinergic effects.

Barbiturates: Similar to benzodiazepines in mechanism and efficacy, these drugs are extremely dangerous in overdose, and tolerance develops quickly.

Antihistamines: Diphenhydramine is sedating and is found in many over-the-counter preparations. It is generally safe and effective for short-term use, although tolerance develops very quickly after nightly ingestion. Diphenhydramine has some anticholinergic properties and can cause confusion and urinary retention in elderly persons.

Alternative Substances: Since L-tryptophan was taken off the market because some preparations were found to cause eosinophilic myalgia syndrome, various homeopathic and folk remedies have become popular. Teas and capsules containing valerian root extracts may be the most effective of these alternative substances, but safety and efficacy studies have not been done. The pineal hormone melatonin, which is secreted at night in decreasing amounts as people age, clearly has sleep-promoting effects in many people. It is currently under intensive investigation. Although considered an experimental drug by the FDA, it is marketed as a food supplement at health food stores and has attracted a large following. Patients should be cautioned that melatonin remains an experimental drug and is a naturally occurring hormone with potential neuroendocrine, immunologic, and reproductive effects, although it appears to be remarkably benign in short-term use. Commercial preparations may contain 0.5–5 mg of melatonin per capsule (sometimes in combination with vitamins). The most effective dose is unknown and may vary from person to person. Doses in the 0.5–10 mg range are reasonable, although doses above 0.5 mg produce plasma levels greater than would occur naturally and thus engender more concern as to long-term effects. Preparations containing "pineal extracts" should be avoided in favor of synthetic melatonin.

Chronobiologic Treatment

Sleep-wake-cycle disorders can be treated with scheduled exposure to bright natural or artificial light. Patients with advanced-sleep-phase syndrome need a corrective phase delay with exposure to bright light in the evening. Bright light exposure must be carefully timed so that the circadian pacemaker is phase-shifted to move sleep propensity to a later time. For the more common delayed-sleep-phase syndrome, patients need to force themselves awake in the early morning (between 6:00 and 7:00 AM) to receive appropriately timed light exposure. The first few mornings are very difficult, but after several 30- to 60-minute light exposures, patients can begin falling asleep before midnight and wake up in time for morning classes or work. Light fixtures for treating these syndromes are available from numerous commercial vendors. The

Society for Bright Light and Biological Rhythms (see "Resources" at the end of the chapter) can provide a list of vendors and more details about using bright light exposure in treating sleep disorders and winter depression. Melatonin may also be useful in treating these disorders; this remains an experimental modality for the time being.

Psychosocial Treatment

Sleep problems in children and adolescents usually affect the rest of the family, causing sleep loss in parents and siblings who may suffer—in some respects—as much as the patient. Because misinformation and inappropriate blaming may confound the problem, the disturbed sleep of such patients needs to be addressed as a problem for the whole family.

Modifying family routines may be helpful. Good sleep hygiene, including well-maintained bedtime rituals such as bathing, story-telling, and rocking a small child can facilitate the winding-down process that is an important prelude to sleep. Occasionally a child becomes overdependent on a particular routine (eg, repeated drinks of water every time he or she wakes up), and parents must set limits. After an expected period of protest, most children relinquish unnecessary attention. These benign disruptions must be differentiated from the more serious panic that some children experience with separation. For this latter kind of anxiety, parental access through the night may be necessary, at least for a time.

In adolescence, sleep is often shortened at both ends. In the evening, there are the demands of homework, telephone socializing, and family life. In the morning, high school schedules often begin quite early, sometimes preceded by an even earlier bus ride. For many teenagers, the morning includes a formidable grooming routine. Add to this the increasing tendency for teenagers to take part-time jobs after school, and the result is an epidemic of chronic sleep deprivation that is an increasing societal concern. Weekend sleeping may recover some of the lost sleep, but it tends to produce a phase delay in circadian rhythms that makes it more difficult to fall asleep during the week. In one experiment, high school students increased their IQ scores by 20 points after a week in which they systematically extended their sleep times.

In counseling teenagers, some flexibility and compromise are usually most effective. Adding naps during the day may improve alertness. A warning about the dangers of driving while sleepy, intoxicated—or both—is important. Chronobiologic interventions, such as light therapy, may be needed to counteract extremely delayed sleep. Outside the office, informed and politically active physicians may be able to influence public policy to help alleviate the problem, such as adopting sensible work rules for teens and scheduling school activities at reasonable hours.

Adults with sleep complaints need to feel that their health-care providers take the problem seriously and understand the effect the disorder has on their lives. At the same time, clinicians can reassure the insomnia patient without severe daytime sleepiness that the problem of nighttime awakenings is more a nuisance than a serious health problem. Educating patients about appropriate sleep hygiene and cognitive measures helps them regain some sense of control over their symptoms (see Table 27–2). Persons with more persistent insomnia or those who appear to have severe psychologic distress as a result—or cause—of the sleep disturbance may warrant evaluation by a mental health specialist.

Sleep disorders in adult patients can, of course, affect others. Partners or caregivers of patients with severe sleep disorders may need both emotional support and education about the nature of the sleep disturbance. Understanding the problem can help them reduce their frustration and enable them to support the patient in following treatment recommendations.

Resources

The National Sleep Foundation, at 122 South Robertson Boulevard, third floor, Los Angeles, CA 90048, publishes an outstanding newsletter for physicians and other health-care providers.

The RLS Foundation, at 1904 Banbury Road, Raleigh, NC 27608, offers support, including a newsletter, for persons with RLS.

The Society for Bright Light and Biological Rhythms, at 10200 West 44th, Suite 304, Wheat Ridge, CO 80033 [Telephone (303) 424-3697; fax (303) 422-8894], offers information on treating chronobiologic sleep disorders and seasonal affective disorder. Names of vendors of clinical bright light fixtures are also available through the organization.

SUGGESTED READINGS

Carskadon MA, Dement WC: Normal Human Sleep: An Overview. In: Kryger MH, Roth T, Dement WC (editors): *Principals and Practice of Sleep Medicine,* 2nd ed. Saunders, 1994.

Czeisler CA, Richardson GS, Martin JB: Disorders of Sleep and Circadian Rhythms. In: Isselbacher KJ et al (editors): *Harrison's Principals of Internal Medicine,* 13th ed. McGraw-Hill, 1992.

Gillin JC, Byerly WF: The diagnosis and management of insomnia. N Engl J Med 1990;322:239.

Hla K et al: Sleep apnea and hypertension: A population-based study, Ann Intern Med 1994;120:382.

Kryger MH: Management of Obstructive Sleep Apnea: An Overview. In: Kryger MH, Roth T, Dement WC (editors): *Principals and Practice of Sleep Medicine,* 2nd ed. Saunders, 1994.

Lack P, Morin CM: Recent advances in the assessment and treatment of insomnia. J Consult Clin Psychol 1992; 60: 586.

Mitler MM et al: Catastrophes, sleep, and public policy: Consensus report. Sleep 1988;11:100.

Young T et al: The occurrence of sleep disordered breathing among middle-aged adults. N Engl J Med 1993; 328:1230.

Sexual Problems

28

David G. Bullard, PhD, & Harvey Caplan, MD

Sex is a problem for everyone . . . Indeed, for a couple of weeks or a couple of months, or maybe even for a couple of years, if we are lucky, we may feel that we have solved the problem of sex. But then, of course, we change or our partners change, or the whole ballgame changes, and once again we are left trying to scramble over that obstacle with this built-in feeling that we can get over it, when actually we never can. However, in the process of trying to get over it, we learn a great deal about vulnerability and intimacy and love. . . .

(Peck, 1993, *Further Along the Road Less Traveled*)

INTRODUCTION

The primary care provider is in an optimal position to evaluate sexual problems, since he or she often has the most comprehensive and long-lasting relationship with the patient. In contrast to most other medical diagnoses, however, it is the patient who usually defines when a sexual problem exists. Although referral to medical or mental health specialists (or both) may be indicated in certain situations, many problems can be diagnosed and treated by the primary care practitioner. When questions about sexuality are approached in an open, matter-of-fact manner, most patients are relieved and respond positively. They appreciate the affirmation that these issues are valid and important, whether or not they have current sexual concerns or are sexually active (Table 28–1).

CHALLENGE FOR PRIMARY CARE PROVIDERS

Providing patients with helpful responses to their sexual health concerns requires that health professionals have:

- Willingness and ability to discuss sexual topics comfortably.
- Awareness of the range and diversity of human sexual practices and concerns, as well as the importance of the circumstances or conditions under which individuals function best.
- Ability to separate one's own personal beliefs and values from those of patients. Unless the practitioner encounters information indicating objective harm to someone involved, it is important to maintain a nonjudgmental demeanor.
- Skill at taking a sex problem history in appropriate detail.
- Knowledge of simple interventions, such as permission-giving, transmittal of accurate information, specific suggestions (eg, for making sex less pressured and more pleasurable), and making referrals to other resources, when appropriate.

Health professionals may have limited sexual experience, as well as questions and problems of their own, and a consequent discomfort in discussing particular sexual material. Time, thought, and experience, however, can build confidence and expertise in talking about sexual problems. Providers can increase their comfort level by examining their own attitudes, beliefs, assumptions, and experiences; reading in the literature (see Patient and Professional Bibliographies at the end of this chapter); discussing these issues with friends and colleagues; and routinely incorporating sexual health questions into the general health assessment of patients.

Of course, no one—patients *or* caregivers—should be forced to talk about sexuality. It is important for all of us to recognize the limits of our own interest, comfort, and competency. Sexual health is an integral part of health care, however, and all who deal with patients should be alert to the possibility of sexual concerns and at the minimum be able to respond with nonjudgmental listening and reassurance or by referring to a colleague who is comfortable and competent in discussing sexual issues.

Table 28–1. Sexual concerns of patients.

- **Common sexual worries about normalcy,** such as: *Am I O.K.? What is a "healthy" sex life? How do I compare? Is my sex life satisfactory?*
- **Sexual identity questions** relevant to life-style, orientation, and preference.
- **Developmental issues of sexuality** for children, adolescents, parents, and the elderly, including the development of gender identity, masturbation, genital exploration, child sex play, sexuality and the single life, marriage, divorce, and death of a partner.
- **Reproductive concerns** covering infertility, family planning, contraception, pregnancy, and abortion.
- **Sexual desire, satisfaction and dysfunctions,** such as a couple's differing levels of desire, and problems with vaginal lubrication, erections, orgasm, and pain.
- **Sexual changes** due to physical disability, medical illness, and treatment.
- **Sexual trauma** resulting from molestation, incest, and rape.
- **Safe sex practices:** AIDS and sexually transmitted diseases.
- **Paraphilias and sexual compulsions.**

PERSPECTIVES ON HUMAN SEXUALITY

Although a knowledge base of human sexual response is developing, even the most scholarly sexual research is rarely value-free. Sexuality encompasses an enormous range of behaviors, beliefs, desires, experiences, and fantasies that patients may discuss with their health care providers. Sexuality can also have legal, medical, moral, political, and religious aspects. It is difficult to find a more controversial area of human experience!

Motivations for human sexual expression are complex and numerous, existing throughout the life cycle in times of illness as well as health, varying from culture to culture and from individual to individual. They include the need to express love, and the need for physical release, reproduction, recreation, and to increase self-esteem. Conversely, sexuality can also be used to coerce, control, or degrade others.

Sexual worries or difficulties are probably experienced by all of us at some periods in our lives and may result from developmental growth and changes in life circumstances rather than from pathology alone. Sexual problems are sometimes a blessing, such as when they compel a person to get help for symptoms that indicate underlying problems with self-esteem or with a relationship. For some people, seeking help for an erection or orgasm problem may be more acceptable than for self-esteem issues such as not liking themselves.

Since the language of sex is broad and varied, it is helpful to become familiar and comfortable with the vernacular and to be able to discuss calmly and in detail such matters as masturbation, sexual positions, oral sex, anal sex, penis size, and breast size. The following section discusses a few of the areas in which misconceptions can be resolved.

COMMON MISCONCEPTIONS

From a medical viewpoint, **masturbation** is "normal," universal, and physically harmless at all ages. It is highly correlated with self-acceptance and sexual adjustment, and is often used to further sexual self-awareness in sex therapy. Some people freely choose not to masturbate, perhaps following personal or religious tenets. Guilt about masturbation, however, continues to affect many patients. Less frequently, one may encounter patients who use masturbation compulsively to avoid authentic relationship issues, or sex offenders who reinforce their antisocial fantasies via masturbation.

There is no standard for what constitutes acceptable **sexual frequency.** Individuals who are celibate may still consider themselves sexual beings, whereas others may have sex rarely but find it satisfying and enjoyable when they do. Compulsively frequent sex can become unrewarding for some, whereas others thrive on a frequent and active sex life. What is "right" for a particular individual or couple must be determined by them based on the various meanings and expectations they associate with sex.

Sexual fantasies are limited only by human imagination and may be enjoyed for their own sake. They may be exciting to a person who would never want to experience them in real life, or they may be yearned for. Obsessive and intrusive images that cause discomfort may need to be addressed therapeutically.

The majority of women enjoy and need direct **clitoral stimulation** manually or orally to reach orgasm. Unfortunately, many men assume that their female partners only enjoy intercourse. A result of this overemphasis on intercourse is that many women and men are uncomfortable with genital caressing alone. Couples can benefit from encouragement and permission to learn about and enjoy noncoital sex.

Most gay, lesbian, or bisexual patients do not wish to have their **sexual orientation** changed or challenged and may present the same concerns as heterosexuals about normalcy, dysfunction, and intimacy (see Chapter 14).

Normal changes in sexual response with **aging** include the following:

1. More direct genital stimulation and more time is needed for arousal (lubrication or erection).
2. Women may experience irritation and pain with intercourse after periods of abstinence.
3. Erections may become less rigid.
4. Orgasm may not occur with each sexual encounter and the urge to ejaculate may become less intense.

5. The refractory period (the time interval between a man's ejaculation and his next erection) lengthens.

Many adults in their 70s, 80s, and even later years are willing to experiment in response to changes in their interest, sexual physiology, and partner status. Some older men and women become less focused on intercourse, finding increased enjoyment in petting, oral sex, and masturbation. Others may be happy to have retired from an active sexual life, or may be comfortable with relatively fixed beliefs as to what is sexually appropriate.

DISCUSSING SEXUALITY IN THE GENERAL MEDICAL EXAMINATION

Some patients may be more reluctant to discuss their diet or exercise patterns than the details of their sexual life, while others feel they risk disapproval or judgment when talking with a medical authority about sexuality.

It is often helpful to introduce the topic of sexuality and acknowledge that the patient might feel some embarrassment. Routinely asking questions about sexual health in an initial history-taking can accomplish many important things. By introducing the subject, a caregiver shows acceptance of sexual health as an integral part of a person's well-being and removes much of the "charge" around sexuality.

The following is a potential opener for a discussion about sexuality:

> DOCTOR: One area of health care that is often neglected is sexual health, yet it can be important to people. Do you have any questions about your sex life that you would like to discuss?

A "no" response can be accepted, without ruling out possible future discussion.

> DOCTOR: If you have any questions later on, I'd be glad to talk with you or help you find someone with whom you would be comfortable talking.

When providers are uncomfortable about a sexual topic, they can make comments such as: "I feel somewhat awkward bringing this up . . . ," "I haven't had that experience, but let me find out . . . ," or "Can you educate me about that . . . ?" These phrases are acceptable to most patients and can extricate the clinician from some difficult situations, as well as foster patient rapport.

As part of the psychosocial component of the general medical examination, a brief sex history should cover the following:

- "Are you sexually active now? " "How many current partners do you have? " If none, "When was the last time you had sex?" "Is that O.K. for you at this point in your life?"
- "Are you sexually active with men, women, both, or neither?" To encourage the confidence of lesbian, gay, or bisexual patients, ask about the patient's "partner" rather than using the gender-specific terms "wife," "husband," "boyfriend," or "girlfriend." And ask about "sexual encounters" rather than "intercourse."
- "How satisfied are you with your sexual experiences and functioning?" (Frequency, variety, who initiates, etc)
- "Do you experience any problems with lubrication, orgasm, erection, or ejaculation?"
- Before assessing type of contraception and consistency of use, ask "Do you have a need for contraception?" rather than assuming contraception is necessary.
- History of STDs and their treatment.
- "Have you ever been tested for HIV, and if so do you know if you are positive? " "Are you aware of safer sex precautions?"
- "Have you ever had a difficult, disturbing, or abusive sexual experience?"

Use questions that show openness to other than the modal heterosexual preferences. Making assumptions about a person's sexuality based on age, gender, race, marital status, or sexual orientation may be diagnostically misleading and send damaging messages to the individual (eg, an elderly patient assumed to be sexually inactive may in fact have multiple sexual partners, and important risk factors for STDs and AIDS may be missed; a monogamous gay male may feel stereotyped or misunderstood if it is assumed he has multiple partners). Make sure that the terminology is *mutually understood.* Overly general or euphemistic terms, such as "having sex," "getting it on," "making out," "making love," or "losing one's nature" may obscure important details. Terms that are too technical ("coitus," "copulation," "cunnilingus") or too colloquial ("cunt," "cock," "fucking") may be inappropriate for use in the professional relationship.

Avoid words that convey *moral judgments or indicate little* about what an individual is actually experiencing (eg, "adultery," "frigid," "impotent," "nymphomaniac," "perversion"). Clinicians can help patients discard demeaning labels by substituting behavioral descriptions such as "having sex outside of your primary relationship," "difficulty getting erections or getting aroused," or "trouble learning to have orgasms." Again, time and experience with a variety of patients provides a sense of what terms are most useful in conveying information to a given patient.

Patients may bring up vague or psychosomatic-like complaints (eg, insomnia, fatigue, musculoskeletal aches, indigestion, headaches, or any specific symptoms of depression or anxiety) as a veiled request to talk about sexual concerns. Others mention a sexual concern at the end of a visit in an offhand manner, when there is no time for the problem to be adequately evaluated. The provider may then choose to assess the problem briefly and validate the importance of investigating this as soon as a new appointment can be scheduled.

Since sexual problems are often the result of a distressing gap between the patient's expectations and experiences, the effective sexual interview aims to elucidate both sides of the equation: if expectations are unrealistic, the treatment is education; if the experience fails to meet realistic expectations, intervention or referral is indicated. Often education and other clinical interventions are combined.

Case illustration 1: One couple sought help from a sex therapist because, after 30 years of enjoyable and satisfying sex (involving intercourse that would last less than 5 minutes), they had read an article extolling the virtues of extended intercourse and began to feel inadequate. When encouraged to value their own unique sexual patterns, versus what might be right for someone else, they were relieved and decided they didn't have a problem after all.

SEX PROBLEM INTERVIEW

As with any other medical problem, five basic areas need to be addressed for the patient presenting with a sex problem (Table 28–2):

1. Explicit symptom or question
2. Onset and course of the symptoms
3. Patient's perception of the cause and maintenance of the problem
4. Medical evaluation, including medical history, past treatment, and outcome
5. Current expectations and goals for treatment

Answers to the preceding inquiries can help guide the clinician to specific interventions.

PHYSICAL EXAMINATION

The detailed examination of the genitourinary system should include checking for signs of androgen or estrogen deficiency or excess, neurological dysfunction, genital abnormalities, and vascular disease. For men, this includes examination of the penis (to ex-

Table 28–2. Sex problem interview.

Description of Current Symptom in Detail
- Signal that you are glad the patient brought up the problem (to give approval, counteract shame, and encourage the patient).
- Help the patient specify exactly what the problem is, being careful to use understandable language—low desire, not getting wet or lubricating, difficulty getting or losing a "hard-on" or erection, difficulty "coming" or having orgasm, "coming too quickly" or rapid ejaculation, etc.
- *I'd like to ask a few questions to help us sort it out.*
- *Tell me what happens.*
- *How is that a problem for you?*
- *Anything else that has changed?*

Onset and Course
- *Does it happen alone with self-pleasuring or masturbation, with a specific partner, or with any partner?*
- *How does your partner respond when the problem occurs?*
- *Was there a time it was more enjoyable and then changed?*
- *Any situations when it's not a problem?*

Patient's Perception of Cause and Maintenance of Problem
- *Anything you **think** might be causing it or that you **worry** might be causing the problem or keeping it going?*

Medical Evaluation, Past Treatment, and Outcome
- *Do you smoke or use prescription or over-the-counter medications, drugs, or alcohol?*
- *Do you have any medical illnesses or treatments, depression, anxiety, or relationship problems?*
- *For women: Are your menses normal, regular? Have you had any children? Were any problems associated with pregnancy, delivery, breast-feeding?*
- *For men: Do you notice morning or nocturnal erections? Are they firm enough for penetration?*
- *Do you have a need for birth control; if so, what methods do you use?*
- *Are you concerned you might have gotten a sexually transmitted disease?*
- *Any history of physical, emotional, or sexual abuse?*
- *What have you already tried to help to change the problem?*
- *Have you ever had psychotherapy, couple or sex therapy? If yes, was this sexual problem addressed in the treatment?*
- *Have you discussed this problem openly with your partner?*

Current Expectations and Goals for Treatment
- *How important is it to you to get help with this problem and are you interested in trying to change it now?*
- *What would be the minimum improvement you would need in order to feel it was worth your time and effort in dealing with this problem?*
- *Most everyone has sexual concerns at one time or another. Talking about them is the most important first step. I'm glad you've felt comfortable talking with me and I suggest . . . (or will suggest some things after I've had a chance to review the best resources for you). Many people have been helped with these issues.*

clude conditions such as Peyronie's disease, penile discharge, and hypospadias); testes and scrotum (for masses, atrophy, hernia, or varicoceles); skin, prostate, and rectum; and testing for evidence of gynecomastia, peripheral vascular disease, and neuropathy. Testicular self-examination should also be taught.

For women, the examination should look for evidence of atrophic vaginitis; vaginal atresia; defective vaginal repair; pelvic inflammatory disease; endometriosis; and signs of cystitis, vaginitis, urethritis, and vulvitis. For dyspareunia, the patient can use a mirror to help identify painful areas. Breast self-examination should also be taught.

When pathology can be excluded, patients can be reassured that their genitals look "quite healthy" and are in the normal range. This can help counter the shame that many people feel about these vulnerable areas of the body. Naming specific genital parts, such as the foreskin and glans of the penis and clitoris and labia, may give increased permission for the patient to ask any questions or express any concerns they may have about them. Men concerned about the size of their penis or women with worries that their genitals are somehow abnormal are more likely to voice these concerns after the clinician has comfortably used these words.

LABORATORY TESTS

In general, few laboratory tests are necessary for patients presenting with the most common sexual problems. For complaints of low sexual desire, patients should be screened for depression and tested for anemia, endocrine, liver and renal disease, or any other debilitating medical problems suggested by the history and physical examinations.

Tests for women with sexual problems might include measurement of serum estradiol (<35 ng/mL is predictive of low sexual frequency), follicle-stimulating hormone (FSH), prolactin, luteinizing hormone (LH) levels, and androgen.

Some authorities recommend evaluation of serum testosterone and prolactin levels in all male patients with erectile failure or low libido. Elevated prolactin levels can be the result of many medical conditions, including pituitary tumors; renal dysfunction; sarcoidosis; thyroid disease; trauma; pelvic surgery; or use of medications such as cimetidine, haloperidol, and phenothiazines. If any of these tests are abnormal or other endocrine problems are suggested by the history or physical examination, the additional relevant tests should be performed.

Depending on the problem, additional diagnostic studies for men with erectile dysfunction may be conducted by a urologist and include monitoring of nocturnal penile erections (NPT) in a sleep laboratory or, more commonly and less expensively, with a home monitoring unit or simple snap-gauge. Increasingly, urologists have been using intracavernosal injection of local vasodilators such as prostaglandin E_1 (PGE_1) to assess penile tumescence. In the future, oral vasodilators and those delivered intraurethrally may also be used diagnostically as well as for treatment.

ORGANIC & PSYCHOGENIC FACTORS

Rather than describing sexual problems with a simple differential diagnosis of either organic *or* psychogenic etiology, it is useful to identify *both* categories of causal factors. These can be assessed with the psychosocial history, sex problem interview, physical examination, and laboratory testing. A symptom that is generalized (occurring in all circumstances) may indicate major organic or psychogenic involvement, whereas situational symptoms tend to be psychogenic (Table 28–3).

ORGANIC FACTORS

Organic factors may be suspected when a man reports an absence of nocturnal or morning erections or is unable to get erect with masturbation. For painful intercourse, important situational variables to identify include whether the woman has been adequately stimulated and aroused prior to penetration, whether she feels pain with masturbation or when having sex with another partner, and whether she is able to direct the extent and timing of thrusting or is passive. Also, organic factors should be considered when a patient has not responded to an adequate course of sex therapy.

Medical Conditions & Treatments

Medical conditions and treatments affecting sexuality are listed in Tables 28–4 and 28–5.

Table 28–3. Symptom patterns and etiology.

Symptom Patterns Suggestive of Principally Organic Etiology
- Generalized (especially for absent desire, erectile disorder, secondary premature ejaculation and painful intercourse. Even when generalized, however, primary rapid ejaculation and primary female orgasmic disorder in otherwise healthy individuals are rarely organic)
- Gradual onset
- Rapid onset when associated with certain medications

Symptom Patterns Suggestive of Principally Psychological Etiology
- Situational
- Rapid onset (unless medications are suspected)
- Sexual phobia and aversion

Table 28–4. Medical conditions commonly associated with sexual disorders.

- Arthritis/joint disease
- Diabetes mellitus
- Endocrine problems
- Injury to autonomic nervous system by surgery or radiation
- Liver or renal failure
- Mood disorders, including depression, anxiety, and panic
- Multiple sclerosis
- Peripheral neuropathy
- Radical pelvic surgery
- Respiratory disorders (eg, COPD)
- Spinal cord injury
- Vascular disease

COPD = chronic obstructive pulmonary disease.

Medications

Medications of many kinds have been implicated in sexual dysfunction (Table 28–6). Older antidepressants such as amitriptyline (Elavil) and doxepin (Sinequan) have anticholinergic properties that undermine sexual arousal. The newer and widely used selective serotonin-reuptake inhibitors (SSRIs)—antidepressants such as fluoxetine (Prozac), sertraline (Zoloft), and paroxetine (Paxil)—may inhibit orgasm for women and ejaculation and orgasm for men. Strategies to alleviate such dysfunction include (1) reducing the dosage; (2) taking a weekend "holiday" in which the last dose for the week is taken on Thursday morning and the medication is resumed at noon on Sunday; (3) switching to another medication; or (4) *co*administering other medications, such as neostigmine (Prostigmin), cyproheptadine (Periactin), bethanechol (Duvoid), and yohimbine (Yohimex) 1–2 hours prior to sexual activity. Newer antidepressants will hopefully become available in the future with effects equal to the SSRIs yet with fewer sexual problems.

PSYCHOLOGICAL FACTORS

Psychological factors often play a causal role in maintaining the sexual dysfunction even when there has been identification of a medical condition or medication commonly known to cause problems (Table 28–7). For example, a female patient experiencing

Table 28–5. Reversible and irreversible organic causes of sexual disorders.

Potentially reversible medical conditions
1. *Low desire due to endocrine deficiencies:* testosterone deficiency (common in older males); thyroid deficiency (rare). (*Treatment:* hormone replacement)
2. *Low desire due to endocrine secreting tumors:* prolactin-secreting tumors of the pituitary (relatively common); estrogen-secreting tumors of the testes and adrenals (rare). (*Treatment:* medical, surgical, and radiologic treatment of the tumor)
3. *Low desire due to depression and stress* (common). (*Treatment:* psychotherapy, antidepressant medication)
4. *Low desire due to substances* (common): centrally acting beta-adrenergic blockers, centrally acting antihypertensive agents, excessive alcohol and narcotics. (*Treatment:* substitution of alternative medications; treatment of substance abuse)
5. *Vaginal dryness or atrophy* and discomfort on intercourse due to estrogen deficiency (very common in postmenopausal women). (*Treatment:* estrogen replacement, oral or local, dilation, and use of lubricants and vaginal moisturizers)
6. *Erectile disorder due to antihypertensives or other medications* (very common). (*Treatment:* reversible only if blood pressure can be controlled by diet, relaxation, and physical exercise, lifestyle changes, or substitution of other medications with lesser sexual side effects)
7. *Erectile disorder* due to blockage of large vessels supplying the penis (rare). (*Treatment:* vascular surgery)
8. *Organic erectile disorders due to other organic factors.* (*Treatment:* PGE₁ penile injections, penile implants, oral vasodilator medications under clinical study and possibly available in 1998)
9. *Vaginal obstructions* due to vaginal agenesis, imperforate or rigid hymen. (*Treatment:* stretching, dilation, surgery)
10. *Female dyspareunia* due to vaginal infections, bladder infections, PID. (*Treatment:* antibiotics) Endometriosis. (*Treatment:* hormonal, surgical) Painful hymenal tags, episiotomy scars. (*Treatment:* surgery)
11. *Male dyspareunia* due to prostate infections, vesicular infection, urethral infection and tumors, hernia, chordee, penile infections, herpes. (*Treatment:* antibiotics, surgery)
12. *Arousal and orgasm disorders* due to reversible neurologic conditions caused by (a) vitamin deficiencies. (*Treatment:* vitamin replacement); (b) neurotropic viral infections. (*Treatment:* supportive management)
13. *Delayed or absent orgasm* due to SSRI and MAOI antidepressant medication. (*Treatment:* periodic drug "holiday," lower dose, substitution of other medication, or coadminister other medication)

Medical conditions that are not reversible but that should be actively managed or treated in order to prevent further progression of the disease and further deterioration of sexual functioning
1. *Diabetes,* attention to glucose control
2. *Hypertension,* with its high risk of arteriosclerosis of the small blood vessels
3. *Vaginal atrophy,* secondary to pelvic irradiation and surgery. (*Treatment:* dilation and frequent sexual intercourse; estrogen cream when not medically contraindicated)

Common conditions not reversible or controllable with present methods
1. *Small vessel arteriosclerosis* of the penile vessels and corpora cavernosa (very common)
2. *Diabetic damage* to vessels and nerves involved in the erection and orgasm reflex (very common)
3. *Degenerative neurologic diseases* and injury to the central nervous system and surgical trauma to the nerves and anatomic structure involved in the genital reflexes (rare)
4. *Erectile disorder* and diminished libido associated with renal dialysis
5. *Drug-related erectile disorder* when no effective substitute without sexual side effects is available

Source: Adapted, with permission, from Kaplan HS: *The Evaluation of Sexual Disorders,* Brunner/Mazel, 1983.

Table 28–6. Medication and drug categories commonly associated with sexual disorders.

- Alcohol
- Anticancer drugs and hormones
- Anticonvulsants
- Antihypertensives, including beta blockers (at high dosage), excluding ACE inhibitors
- Carbonic anhydrase inhibitors
- Cytotoxic drugs
- Digitalis family
- Diuretics
- H2 receptor antagonists
- Nonsteroidal anti-inflammatory agents
- Opiates
- Pain medications
- Psychedelic and hallucinogenic drugs
- Psychiatric medications (benzodiazepines, tricyclic antidepressants, monoamine oxidase inhibitors, selective serotonin reuptake inhibitors, antipsychotics, lithium carbonate)
- Recreational drugs (tobacco, alcohol, and opiates)
- Sleep medications
- Tranquilizers

difficulty reaching orgasm since being treated with an SSRI antidepressant may continue to have this problem even after switching to a lower dosage or different medication, because of a conditioned performance anxiety.

Following hysterectomy, some women report increased sexual enjoyment because of the relief from uncomfortable physical symptoms and bleeding, whereas others find the surgery difficult and have a psychological response to the loss of these organs and to their reproductive capacity. These women may then experience a decrease in sexual desire, arousal, or orgasmic responsiveness. The research is mixed as to the effects of hysterectomy on orgasm in women; it has been proposed that women differ in the extent to which they perceive uterine and cervical contractions during orgasm, with differing sense of loss after the

Table 28–7. Psychological conditions commonly associated with sexual disorders.

I. Immediate causes (of most concern for the general medical practitioner)
  A. Performance anxiety—fear of inadequate performance
  B. Spectatoring—critically monitoring one's own sexual performance
  C. Inadequate communication with partner regarding sex
  D. Fantasy—absence of fantasy, antifantasy incompatible with sexual arousal, or distracting thoughts
II. Deeper causes (for referral)
  A. Intrapsychic issues—early conditioning, sexual trauma, depression, anxiety, guilt, fear of intimacy, or separation
  B. Relationship issues—lack of trust, power and control issues, anger at partner
  C. Sociocultural factors—attitudes and values, religious beliefs
  D. Educational and cognitive factors—Sexual myths or expectations (gender roles, age and appearance, proper sexual activity, performance expectations), sexual ignorance

Source: Adapted, with permission, from Plaut SM, Lehne GK: Sexual dysfunction, gender identity disorders, and paraphilias. In: Goldman HH (editor): *Review of General Psychiatry,* 4th ed. Appleton & Lange, 1995.

surgery. There is similar variability in men after prostatectomy. For many, orgasm may feel satisfactory even with a "dry" or retrograde ejaculation, with semen going into the bladder, but others may complain of a loss of orgasmic sensation.

> *Case illustration 2:* Juan, a 38-year-old male patient, complained of erectile dysfunction with a possible organic component (type II diabetes) and performance anxiety. When he quit smoking cigarettes and tried noncoital caressing to decrease his pressure to perform, he was able to experience satisfying erections firm enough for intercourse. In this case, the diabetes by itself was not the determining factor in maintaining the problem.

Some medical illnesses and treatments are believed to decrease sexual desire or to cause sexual dysfunction *directly.* Psychosocial adaptations to virtually any medical condition, however, can *indirectly* affect sexual desire or functioning. For example, fears of rejection by a sexual partner because of a stoma or mastectomy, or concerns about sexual functioning may lead to a suppression of sexual feelings and avoidance of sexual opportunities. Of course, many medically healthy men and women either choose to be sexually inactive or refrain out of a sense of inadequacy. The capacity to enjoy one's sexuality cannot therefore be predicted on the basis of medical diagnosis alone.

Psychological problems such as depression or anxiety can either be the *cause* or the *effect* of diminished sexual desire or functioning. Both may be true to some degree. In other instances, depression and sexual problems may both be the result of a third underlying factor, such as an endocrine disorder.

Sexual problems might have remote psychological causes, such as childhood trauma or prohibitions about sexual pleasure, but almost all such problems can be seen as having current maintaining variables of anxiety or depression. In general, psychological etiology is primarily suggested when the problem is situational; seems related to performance anxiety, depression, or guilt; or is associated with significant relationship and communication problems.

PSYCHOLOGICAL MANAGEMENT & BRIEF SEX COUNSELING

A paradigm shift occurred in the treatment of sexual dysfunctions with the publication in 1970 of Masters and Johnson's signal work on sex therapy. The previous emphasis on the diagnosis and treatment of individual psychopathology, with somewhat poor treatment results for the sexual dysfunctions, gave way to an understanding of the importance of the **conditions** (internal variables such as attitudes, expectations, and lack of knowledge, as well as external factors related to the partner or the situation) under which people attempt to function sexually. Education and suggestions for focusing on pleasure rather than on performance were found to lower anxiety and to promote improved sexual functioning and enjoyment.

Anxiety is seen as one of the major psychological causes of the sexual dysfunctions, whether stemming from individual or relationship issues. Are patients comfortable, at ease, and feeling close to their partners? Or are they anxious due to lack of information, strained relationships, unrealistic attitudes about and focus on sexual performance goals, or other conditions? In these cases, modern sex therapy commonly provides anxiety-reduction interventions, many of which can be adapted for use by primary care providers. These include validating that sexual problems probably occur at some time or another to all of us and that such problems are often an understandable response to stress, worry, and concerns about performance; encouraging open communication between partners; dispelling maladaptive beliefs about sex; suggesting ways that patients can increase their level of comfort and safety and their ability to relax during sex; and encouraging the view that noncoital sex can be very satisfying and does not have to be considered "second-best."

THE P-LI-SS-IT MODEL

Annon's P-LI-SS-IT model is a useful hierarchical guide to anxiety-reduction approaches to sexual problems and can be used by primary care practitioners. The letters in the acronym stand for different levels of intervention:

P = Permission: The fundamental intervention is to give permission to patients to discuss their sexual concerns. **Empathic listening**, including verbal and nonverbal reassurance, helps give patients permission to talk openly about sexual issues and may encourage and enable them to discuss the problem more directly with a partner. **Reassurance and permission** can help to normalize and validate that having a sexual problem can be part of being human, rather than pathological. **Inquiry into positive exceptions:** patients can describe those areas of sex that they do feel good about; for example, a woman can appreciate her ability to become aroused despite difficulty reaching orgasm, and a man can be a skillful lover despite his erectile disorder. Permission to choose **not** to be sexually active may be very helpful for patients who feel pressured to have sex or who feel inadequate if they don't care to be sexually active.

LI = Limited Information: Facts can add to the effectiveness of reassurance and can be at the disposal of any clinician who has done basic reading about sexuality and keeps up through the literature or review courses. Keeping responses focused and limited to the expressed concern saves time and does not overwhelm the patient with extraneous information (Table 28–8). Such information gives the patient the choice of maintaining or changing sexual practices or attitudes. A simple explanation of the psychophysiology of sexual arousal and the importance of conditions for relaxation helps "normalize" the symptom and refocuses the problem as stemming from conditions that can possibly be changed rather than from something that is wrong with the patient. This can be conveyed by the following "rhinoceros" story about sexuality:

> Imagine you are lying on a blanket in a secluded meadow with a loving partner after having had a wonderful picnic lunch on a beautiful sunny day. You start kissing and feel arousal in your genitals, when, all of a sudden, a rhinoceros charges out of the jungle straight for you. What happens to your arousal (lubrication or erection)? The fight-or-flight response causes a rapid redirection of blood to the brain and large-muscle groups, with a corresponding loss of erection or genital arousal. The rhinoceros represents worrisome thoughts and anxieties about having erections, arousal, or orgasm, or fears that you won't please your partner or be seen as a good lover. Some simple suggestions can help you keep the rhinoceros out of your bedroom!

SS = Specific Suggestions: Where permission and limited information do not suffice, the patient may benefit from specific suggestions to help overcome a sexual problem. Most sex counseling interventions are designed to help the patient (and partner, if available) communicate better about sex and enjoy increased sexual pleasure by reducing performance anxiety about attaining the goals of arousal, lubrication, erection, and orgasm. Helpful interventions taken from sex therapy include (1) temporary agreement not to have intercourse; (2) suggestions for focusing on pleasurable touch, genital caressing, Kegel exercises (tensing and relaxing the pubococcygeal muscles) and progressive muscle relaxation methods; (3) correction of cognitive distortions ("self-talk"); and (4) suggestions to improve emotional and sexual communication.

Even for couples who initially enjoyed previous patterns of lovemaking, the predictable repetition of this sequence over time can lead to sexual boredom. Suggesting that a couple agree, for example, to temporarily forego intercourse or otherwise change their usual sexual pattern often helps them to focus on moment-to-moment pleasure. Rather than making assumptions about what the other wants, the couple can communicate about their likes and dislikes. Many people remember how arousing and exciting it was when they were younger and were "making out" (sexual petting) without intercourse. If agreeable to both, they can take turns exploring other ways of caressing and pleasuring each other. The **sensate focus** exercise, from Masters and Johnson, is done for the interest of the person doing the touching, rather than for the pleasure of the receiver. In order to minimize performance anxiety, each is encouraged to take turns "sa-

Table 28–8. Maladaptive ideas and therapeutic responses to them.

Maladaptive Idea	Therapeutic Response
My sexual problems are because I'm too old.	For those who are interested and willing to be creative, sex can be an enjoyable part of life in their seventies, eighties, and beyond!
I should only be interested in survival, not sex (for someone with terminal or chronic illness).	If sex was important to you before your illness it can remain so or become so again.
I am *asexual* because I don't have an active sex life.	We are *all* sexual beings. You can be aware of and enjoy your sexual feelings without being sexually active.
Sex equals love.	Many people have very loving relationships without being sexually active, and, of course, some people have sex without having loving feelings.
Sex equals intercourse.	There is no one *right* way to be sexual, and many people enjoy touching and caressing more than intercourse.
Having sex is the same as *enjoying sex*.	Many people have to learn to enjoy their sexuality.
It is not proper to talk about sex, either with your partner or a health care provider.	It is often a great relief when people can talk confidentially about their sexual feelings and concerns.
You shouldn't talk about sex because it will destroy the mystery.	Most people find that talking about their important feelings deepens intimacy, and trust develops when you know you can be vulnerable with another. You can create more mystery from deeper sharing.
You should be interested in having sex with any willing partner.	It is most important to be able to respect yourself. Your sexuality is a gift that you share only with those you truly want to share it with.
You should be able to enjoy sex with a partner even when you are tired, angry, or feel hurt.	We all have our own conditions for what makes a sexual encounter enjoyable, and feeling close to and loved by your partner is important to most of us.
I try not to masturbate and feel guilty when I give in because I have a partner and shouldn't need to do that.	Most married people continue to masturbate and find it does not interfere with the pleasure they have with their partner.
Sex is a performance, and it would be grim and catastrophic to "fail."	Sexual sharing can be playful, with the goals of giving and receiving feelings of pleasure and caring. If things don't go as planned, there is always next time!
A new partner will not like the size of my (breasts/penis).	Most men and women enjoy having sex with a person, not a body part. Most men compare themselves to other men when their penises are soft . . . size differences are usually not as great when erections are compared. Vaginas accommodate different penis sizes, with the outer third and the clitoris the most responsive areas for many women.
Sex should result in orgasm every time.	Does *not* having dessert ruin a fine meal? Orgasm is only one of the pleasurable aspects of a sexual encounter. Many people find it a relief to not have "should's" in their sex life.
Sex should never be a problem. Experiencing a problem is not normal.	Sex is perfectly natural, but not naturally perfect. Probably everyone has "problems" with sex at some time or another.

voring" the experience of touching and exploring the other's body, in contrast to worrying about "turning on" or performing for the partner. For many people, permission for **genital caressing** in this way increases sexual pleasure and satisfaction.

Arranging for follow-up after giving specific suggestions keeps the health care provider informed as to their effectiveness, helps the patient stay focused on problem-solving, and informs the clinician about the necessity for further intervention.

IT = Intensive Therapy: This is the last step in the hierarchy and involves referral to the appropriate specialist when the previous three levels of intervention have not been effective (see later section).

ADDITIONAL PATIENT EDUCATION

Pamphlets detailing approaches for safe sex for the prevention of AIDS can supplement discussion and should be made readily available for patients. Many good self-help books dealing with common sexual disorders enable patients to move at their own pace. Often people who are reluctant to enter counseling or who are hesitant about discussing their problems in depth are willing to read in the privacy of their home where they can be relaxed and comfortable. Several books are recommended at the end of this chapter (see the Patient Bibliography).

INDICATIONS FOR REFERRAL

Refer to an appropriate medical specialist if the brief treatment suggestions in this chapter fail to help or if the history and physical examination suggests primarily an organic component. Refer to a mental health specialist trained in sex therapy if the problem is situational, occurring only with a certain partner; if functioning is adequate under certain conditions; or if significant emotional distress is present.

Primary care clinicians can develop a resource list of providers for sex-related problems. Colleagues, teachers, friends, and clinical societies can be asked for recommendations. Identify medical and mental health specialists with expertise in treating sexual issues. Practitioners can be licensed in psychiatry, psychology, social work, psychiatric nursing, or marriage and family counseling. Most states do not license "sex therapists" or "sex counselors."

COMMON SEXUAL DISORDERS

LOW OR ABSENT SEXUAL DESIRE & SEXUAL AVERSION

The range of sexual desire issues is wide (Table 28–9). Some people simply put a low priority on sex, some are inhibited or find sex aversive, and some are clinically phobic. These problems can be of recent origin or reflect a long-standing pattern. Lack of desire may pertain only to certain sexual partners or practices (such as oral sex). Couples with a desire discrepancy may disagree about which partner's level of desire is "abnormal." In this situation, each side has valid feelings, and it is important not to stigmatize the patient with the lower desire level. Most couples deal occasionally with periods of desire discrepancy or of mutually low desire and feel they should have sex more often than they do. Demands of family, career, and friends often take precedence over sex.

Desire problems or sexual aversion can derive from deeper relational power struggles or reflect childhood sexual, physical, or emotional abuse that require couple counseling or individual psychotherapy for resolution. The following case example, however, demonstrates how permission and encouragement to talk about sex directly, together with specific suggestions, can have a powerful influence.

Case illustration 3[*]: Alice, a healthy 33-year-old primary school teacher, reported having lost her desire for sex. Her sex problem history established that she had enjoyed sexual activity with her husband for the first 2 years of their marriage, although in the past year it had become a chore that she never put on her extensive "to do" list. Since sex was seen as a bedtime activity, when she was usually tired, their sexual frequency dropped from weekly to once every several months. While not addressing the problem directly, Alice and her husband's feelings of estrangement from each other were growing.

When asked what steps they had taken to address these problems, Alice disclosed that she and her husband had never had an open discussion about sex. Her primary care physician validated for her that this was frequently true for couples and that most people have to learn to talk more comfortably about their sexual needs (**Permission** and **Limited Information**). She also explained that everyone has certain conditions that need to be met in order to be interested in sexual activity (**P and LI**) and encouraged Alice to think about her conditions and then, with her husband, to "set some private time aside outside of the bedroom and let yourselves have a discussion about this, even if it is awkward" (**Specific Suggestions**).

DOCTOR: It can be good for relationships when people risk a bit of uneasiness. You don't have to have the same perspective. You are each entitled to your own separate feelings about the situation, but together you can talk it out, try to understand each other, and see what other choices you have. (**P, LI, SS**).

The physician also recommended a self-help book (**SS**) and offered to refer them to a therapist who treats couples, should their attempts to communicate falter (**Intensive Therapy**).

Case illustration 3 (Contd.): At her 1-month follow-up appointment, Alice reported significant progress. When the couple set time aside to discuss their sex life, they had a very meaningful and tender talk. The husband was relieved to learn about the major sources of Alice's lack of desire while she acknowledged her resentment that he seemed unresponsive to her needs. He admitted that he had taken her lack of desire very personally, secretly and painfully interpreting the problem as her lack of desire for *him*. With these hidden resentments expressed, they could set aside their power struggles and cooperate in addressing these issues. Recognizing how they had both felt lonely and uncared for allowed them to take specific actions, such as planning a regular evening each week just for the two of them to talk and nurture their intimacy.

---

[*] Cases 3–10 described in this chapter were of actual patients seen in primary care settings as reported in consultation with the first author. Although some identifying characteristics of the patients have been changed to ensure confidentiality, the essential clinical issues presented are accurately portrayed. We thank all the patients and their health providers who helped us gather these examples.

Table 28–9. DSM-IV sexual disorders and treatment approaches.

Disorder	Diagnostic Criteria	Treatment Approaches
Hypoactive Sexual Desire Disorder (302.71)	Persistently or recurrently deficient (or absent) sexual fantasies and desire for sexual activity. The judgment of deficiency or abscence is made by the clinician, taking into account factors that affect sexual functioning, such as age and the *context of the person's life.*	After organic causes ruled out or if situational: **Permission and Limited Information:** (a) Restate problem in behavioral terms, (b) Explore patient conditions for good sex (rhinoceros story), including whether patient receives adequate direct stimulation, (c) Validate patient's right to say "no" to sex. (d) May be secondary to depression, anxiety, panic, or phobic disorder (occasionally related to childhood sexual abuse), or (e) May be symptomatic of hidden arousal or orgasmic disorder (if so, treat appropriately). **Specific Suggestions:** (f) Listening exercises to increase *communication* with partner, (g) Suggested *readings* (Barbach, 1976 and 1978; Gottman, 1994; Schnarch, 1989 and 1997; Zilbergeld, 1992). **Intensive Therapy:** Refer to mental health professional trained in sexual therapy.
Sexual Aversion Disorder (302.79)	Persistent or recurrent extreme aversion to, and avoidance of, all (or almost all) genital sexual contact with a sexual partner.	
Female Sexual Arousal Disorder (302.72) Male Erectile Disorder (302.72)	Persistent or recurrent inability to attain, or to maintain until completion of the sexual activity, an adequate lubrication-swelling response of sexual excitement (female) or erection (male).	**Permission and Limited Information:** (a–d), above, (h) Give brief explanation of the physiology of arousal and the need for relaxation. (i) Is sexual desire present? (If not, treat as desire disorder). **Specific Suggestions:** (f–h), above, and (j) Enough and desired kind of direct stimulation by partner? (k) Use of lubricants (Astroglide, K-Y, etc) or vaginal moisturizers (Replens), (l) Suggest temporary intercourse ban, (m) sensate focus, (n) Genital caressing, (o) Progressive relaxation and Kegel exercises, (p) Explore ways other than intercourse of pleasuring partner, (q) Hormonal therapy, (r) Low-dose beta blocker (10 mg Inderal) if high performance anxiety, (s) Vacuum device, especially if organic and older male, (t) Intracorporeal penile injection or intraurethral application of PGE_1, (u) Penile implant, (v) Future: vasodilator oral medications will be available.
Premature Ejaculation Disorder (302.75)	Persistent or recurrent ejaculation with minimal sexual stimulation before, on, or shortly after penetration and before the person wishes it. The clinician must take into account factors that affect duration of the excitement phase, such as age, novelty of the sexual partner or situation, and recent frequency of sexual activity.	**Permission and Limited Information:** as above, and explore masturbation patterns—may have conditioned himself to ejaculate rapidly. Explain connection between rapid ejaculation and anxiety versus relaxation and longer lasting erections. **Specific Suggestions:** (l–p), above, (w) Increase frequency of ejaculation, (x) Stop-start exercises (Zilbergeld, 1992), (y) SSRI antidepressant medication, (z) Prilocaine-lidocaine cream with condom, (v), above.
Female and Male Orgasmic Disorder (302.73)	Persistent or recurrent delay in, or absence of, orgasm following a normal sexual excitement phase. Women exhibit wide variability in the type or intensity of stimulation that triggers orgasm. The diagnosis of female orgasmic disorder should be based on the clinician's judgment that the woman's orgasmic capacity is less than would be reasonable for her age, sexual experience, and the adequacy of sexual stimulation she receives. For the male, the clinician should take into account the person's age, and judge the stimulation to be adequate in focus, intensity, and duration.	**Permission and Limited Information:** (a–e), above. **Specific Suggestions:** For primary preorgasmic woman, recommend Barbach (1978); for male, Zilbergeld (1992). If orgasmic disorder is secondary (at one time patient was orgasmic), then evaluate and treat for desire or arousal disorder or relationship problems. (f) (j), (l–p), above.

(continued)

Table 28–9. DSM-IV sexual disorders and treatment approaches. *(cont.)*

Disorder	Diagnostic Criteria	Treatment Approaches
Dyspareunia (302.76) Vaginismus (306.51)	Recurrent or persistent genital pain associated with sexual intercourse in either a male or a female (dyspareunia). Recurrent or persistent involuntary spasm of the musculature of the outer third of the vagina that interferes with sexual intercourse (vaginismus).	**Permission and Limited Information:** (a–e), above. **Specific Suggestions:** (f–k), (m–p), above, (aa) Encourage explicit communication with patient's partner about her need to have enough stimulation prior to penetration, give control to the woman to choose when penetration occurs and timing of thrusting. **Intensive Therapy:** Sex therapy may be necessary for long-standing dyspareunia and vaginismus, due to conditioned expectation of pain.

Management

Permission and Limited Information: Some couples can learn to accept that low desire may be understandable given their immediate circumstances (eg, the months after childbirth) and that their previous levels of desire can be expected to return over time. Validate the patient's right to say no to sex.

Specific Suggestions: A "prescription" to go away on a weekend or to arrange a sleep-over for children with relatives may help couples "break the ice" and reexperience intimacy. Suggest that patient and partner set time aside to talk and listen to each other's feelings and conditions for more enjoyable sex, with each taking an uninterrupted amount of time for self expression. Self-help books may also be recommended.

Other Medical Interventions: Hormonal replacement therapy, especially testosterone, may be helpful for those with low levels. For example, vaginal application of testosterone cream may be useful to some women who experience a loss of desire following chemotherapy for breast cancer, unless otherwise contraindicated.

FEMALE SEXUAL AROUSAL DISORDER

Symptoms & Signs

Problems with female arousal are primarily manifested as vaginal dryness and are reported less often than lack of desire, difficulty reaching orgasm, or pain with intercourse. The most common cause in older women is estrogen deficiency with resulting signs of vulvar irritation and atrophic vaginitis. Medication side effects also may inhibit arousal and should be explored (see Table 28–6).

Case illustration 4: Betty, a 78-year-old woman patient brought in her 82-year-old husband for her appointment with her female physician because she wanted to discuss what she called her "sexual problems." Betty said she did not care about sex, that her husband was often angry with her lack of enthusiasm, and that this pattern had existed throughout the 50 years of their marriage. She believed she was not "a sexual person" because she had never been very excited by intercourse. She did enjoy kissing and caressing and mentioned that on several occasions she had been able to have orgasm when he stroked her labia and clitoris, but that she had never had orgasm from the "real sex" (intercourse) that he preferred. The physician responded that there really is no *one* way to be a "sexual person," that many people cherish the sensual and emotional aspects of sex, and that Betty did not need to consider herself asexual just because she preferred different aspects of sexual intimacy than her husband (**P and LI**). The physician further explained that the majority of women reach orgasm more often from manual caressing than from coitus, and that many couples enjoy bringing each other to orgasm without intercourse (**P and LI**). The couple was relieved and admitted to having curiosity about trying this petting alone. They were given brief instructions to take turns at home touching and stroking each other without the goal of orgasm (sensate focus), to get reacquainted with each other's body, and to refrain from any attempts at intercourse for two weeks (**SS**).

A follow-up telephone call confirmed that they were enjoying taking turns caressing each other, that orgasm often happened for each, and that they occasionally progressed to intercourse. A 1 ¹/₂ -year follow-up was especially poignant—the husband reported that Betty had recently died from a stoke, and, while grieving her loss, he expressed profound appreciation for having gotten help for their sexual conflicts from the physician.

HUSBAND: Settling those old battles over sex made our last year together more loving and caring than ever before in our marriage.

Management

Permission and Limited Information: Is the patient getting stimulation in the best way that works for her?

Specific Suggestions: Homework may be suggested for her to identify what stimulation works best. The goal is to experience the pleasure of arousal in that mode—not to reach orgasm. Inquiry should be made into the quality of the patient's relationship. Commercial lubrication (Astroglide, KY Jelly, etc) and vaginal moisturizers such as Replens can be suggested. Recommend self-help books.

Intensive Therapy: Recommend couple or individual therapy.

MALE ERECTILE DISORDER

Symptoms & Signs

Generally, a man with a significant psychological component is aware of nocturnal or morning erections, is able to maintain his erection for a reasonable time and then ejaculate with masturbation, or has good erections in some situations but not in others. He may be able to get a firm erection but lose it after penetration or may not get an erection with a partner at any time. The original cause of the problem is often distinct from the maintaining variable, which is generally anxiety. Consider possibilities such as performance anxiety, lack of direct physical stimulation of the penis, conscious or unconscious guilt (eg, "widower's syndrome"), anger at his partner or other relationship issues, and childhood sexual abuse.

> *Case illustration 5:* Carl, a 58-year-old HIV-negative gay male, confided to his physician that he had been "impotent" since the death of his lover of 17 years, with whom he had had an active and monogamous sexual life. Attributing this problem to aging and worries about HIV infection, Carl nonetheless asked for any help the primary care physician could provide. A full session was scheduled for talking only. His partner had died suddenly from cardiac arrest a year ago. In the past month Carl had attempted sex on four occasions with two different men and was unable to get an erection. After a thorough sociosexual history, Carl was seen to fit the "widowers' syndrome." Clearly, he was still grieving the loss of his lover but attempted to control his tears with statements such as "I should be over this by now" and "Life has to go on; he wanted me to go on." Carl then revealed that he was very scared of feeling such loss, fearing that he would never be able to come out of the sadness. His grieving was acknowledged and validated (**P**), and it was explained to him that temporary sexual problems were common after such loss because of a number of factors: performance pressure of being with a new partner, continuing feelings of loyalty to a deceased partner, subsequent guilt at having sex with new people, and concerns about HIV infection with a new partner (**LI**). The physician encouraged Carl to join a grief support group or to contact a psychotherapist comfortable with gay sexuality (**SS**). In addition, the doctor referred Carl to a book on male sexuality, with suggestions for how he could talk with a potential partner about both safe sex practices and ways they could reduce the pressure to have erections (**LI and SS**). At a follow-up visit 4 months later, Carl reported he had been able to cry more about his loss and was enjoying sex and intimacy with a new friend who had also lost a partner.

Management

Permission and Limited Information: Many patients over 40 years old report previous successful sexual encounters when they were younger in which they became erect without direct physical stimulation of the penis. If their pattern for sexual interaction has rarely or never included direct touching by a partner, it might help them to learn that such touching becomes more necessary as men age, and that it can be an enjoyable part of sex.

Specific Suggestions: Institute a temporary ban on penetration and suggest sensate focus, progressive relaxation, and Kegel exercises. The couple should agree to *not* attempt penetration or intercourse even if the patient gets an improved erection.

> DOCTOR: For every minute you are relaxing with your partner and have an erection, your body is remembering just what it needs to do to get and maintain an erection. Your mind can be free to enjoy the pleasurable feelings and sensations of being caressed and kissing your partner. You might even *allow* your erection to go away. If you stay relaxed, it will likely return again with resumed stimulation.

Other Medical Interventions *Testosterone replacement therapy.* For men with demonstrated low levels of serum testosterone, hormone replacement therapy may be helpful. This does not benefit men whose serum testosterone is within normal limits. Side effects can be serious, including increase of any existing prostatic cancer, enlargement of the prostate, retention of fluids, and liver damage. Careful monitoring and follow-up prostate-specific antigen (PSA) screening and prostate examinations are necessary.

Yohimbine tablets. Given in 5.4-mg doses three times a day for 4–6 weeks, this medication tends to stimulate desire and improve erections. Often suggested for men with suspected psychogenic etiology, yohimbine may help 15–20% of such patients. Side effects may include headaches, dizziness, and nausea. It is generally contraindicated for men with ulcers or hypertension.

Antidepressant medication. Antidepressants, especially trazodone, can be effective treatment for some, but other patients may find SSRI antidepressants to hinder erection and ejaculation.

Low-dose beta blocker therapy. Prescribed for men whose performance anxiety is very high, 10 mg of propranolol (Inderal) as needed has been effective with some patients.

External penile vacuum device. A tension ring is placed around the base of the penis after it has become erect with the aid of a vacuum cylinder. These devices may work better for men who clearly have a major organic component to their erectile problem, such as severe diabetes, multiple sclerosis, or spinal cord injury. Although this device can create erections functional for intercourse, men with a more psychogenic etiology may be disappointed when the results are not as firm as they had been expecting. Side effects may include bruising of the penis.

Intracorporeal penile injections or intraurethral delivery of prostaglandin E_1 (PGE$_1$). Originally used diagnostically in urologists' offices, patients can now be taught to inject themselves prior to sexual encounters, resulting in firmer erections that often do not disappear at orgasm or ejaculation and last about an hour. Side effects are priapism in less than 3% of patients, and pain. In addition, scarring may be a concern with repeated injections over time.

Penile implant surgery. A variety of implants with semirigid silicone rods or inflatable cylinders are available. Total costs are high, ranging from $6,000 to $15,000. Complications include device failure (requiring additional surgery) and infection.

Future oral pharmacologic agents. Among the drugs currently undergoing phase III clinical research trials, the phosphodiesterase inhibitor, sildenafil (Viagra), taken as needed, shows promise for helping men attain and maintain erections with minimal side effects.

RAPID EJACULATION (PREMATURE EJACULATION)

Symptoms & Signs

Terms such as *rapid,* or *early ejaculation* are clinically preferable to the established *premature ejaculation,* since they highlight the subjective nature of the problem and are less pejorative. No absolute measure—either in number of minutes or thrusts—is applicable to the diverse numbers of men presenting with this problem. Factors to be assessed include a patient's subjective evaluation, degree of sexual satisfaction, and sense of control.

Case illustration 6: Donald, a 45-year-old divorced male reported ejaculating after 1 minute or less of intercourse. This had been his pattern ever since becoming sexually active in his late teens. He reported proudly that he never masturbated but had a high sex drive, which led him to multiple sexual partners including prostitutes. His primary care physician gave Donald a supportive talk about how he could teach himself to last longer with certain physical exercises (**P,LI,** and **SS**). The patient was willing to do "self-stimulation" or "self-pleasuring" exercises for this "medical reason" and was comforted that, as with the physical fitness regimen that he valued, he could tone up his pubococcygeal (p.c.) muscles and learn to relax the pelvic muscles during sexual stimulation. Donald was advised to increase his frequency of ejaculation, was told about the importance of relaxation for maintaining erection, and was encouraged to read Zilbergeld's self-help section on "stop-start" exercises for lasting longer (**P,LI,** and **SS**). As his confidence grew through the solo exercises, and as he increased the frequency of ejaculation, Donald was able to try the stop-start exercises with a partner with increasing success. He said that it also helped him to read about the experiences of other men (getting validation from the universality of sexual concerns) and about how many women enjoy a variety of forms of sexual stimulation in addition to intercourse.

Management
Permission and Limited Information: Point out that early ejaculation is a very common problem—one study found 35% of married males reported that they ejaculated too quickly. Tell the patient that men with this problem have a high success rate when they try one or more specific suggestions that will be given to him for this problem. Give a *brief explanation of the psychophysiological mechanism.*

> DOCTOR: Men aren't supposed to be able to have long-lasting erections if they are too nervous or distracted. The fight-or-flight response generally makes men more likely to ejaculate. Most men have trained themselves through rapid masturbation to get erect and ejaculate quickly; so it makes sense that they would continue to ejaculate quickly when with a partner.

Assure the patient that men often report more intense orgasms after they have learned to last longer and that it is highly likely that he will gain greater ejaculatory control by following these suggestions.

Specific Suggestions: The patient may need to *increase his frequency of ejaculations,* alone or with a partner, perhaps masturbating to orgasm earlier on a day that a sexual encounter with a partner is anticipated. Discuss *other ways he can please his partner,* so he doesn't feel pressure to do it all with an erect penis. Discuss the role of muscle relaxation as necessary to a prolonged erection. Suggest *breathing exercises and progressive muscle relaxation exercises,* targeting the p.c. muscles or those in the buttocks.

Suggest that, in contrast to common attempts by men to diminish the sensations in the hope of lasting longer, they actually need to *increase their tolerance for the good sensations and feelings* and can best do this by concentrating on their feelings and getting more "turned on." Focusing on these feelings in a relaxed "practice" atmosphere can lead to increasing the threshold of enjoyment before ejaculation and orgasm.

He and his partner can read about and practice the *"stop-start technique."* Encourage the patient to change positions and to go from intercourse to oral or manual stimulation of his partner, and then back to intercourse (following the desires of his partner); changing positions and pleasuring a partner to orgasm without intercourse helps many men last longer.

Other Medical Interventions: *SSRI anti-depressants and clomipramine* (Anafranil, 25 mg as needed) help men prolong their erections prior to ejaculation.

Prilocaine-lidocaine cream applied to the penis and then used with a condom has been recommended by some clinicians (although "numbing" of the genitals may detract from enjoyment for both partners).

New vasodilators, currently in Phase III clinical trials, show promise for helping men attain and maintain erections with minimal side effects.

FEMALE & MALE ORGASMIC DISORDER

Symptoms & Signs

Many women do not learn to have orgasms until they are in their 20s, 30s, or even later. A **primary anorgasmic** or **preorgasmic** woman is not yet able to reach orgasm reliably either with a partner or by herself. A woman with **secondary orgasmic disorder** was previously able to reach orgasm but is no longer able to do so. **Situational orgasmic disorder** refers to a condition in which a woman can have orgasm with masturbation but not with a partner, or with one partner but not another. She may reach moderate to high levels of arousal without experiencing the pleasure and release of climax. If no arousal or interest is present, she should be evaluated for a desire or arousal disorder.

Case illustration 7: Ethyl's complaint of low sexual desire and difficulty feeling aroused led the physician to do a brief sex problem interview. With this more open discussion, Ethyl revealed that she had never been able to climax, but *had* been highly aroused in the first year of her 5-year marriage. Their lovemaking style was focused on intercourse, and Ethyl's husband didn't seem to understand why she didn't enjoy it as much as he did. She had not faked orgasm but had never told him about her feelings of frustration about not reaching orgasm. Ethyl had never masturbated and remembered vague attitudes conveyed by her parents and her church that masturbation was not a correct thing to do. The physician then validated that many women first learn about self-pleasuring as adults and that the information she could get about how her own body worked would then be useful in her sexual relationship with her husband. It was suggested that Ethyl read a self-help book for women who want to learn to have orgasms. (**P,LI,** and **SS**). At a visit 3 months later Ethyl reported that she had proudly experienced her first orgasm by herself and felt so encouraged by this that she was able to talk more openly with her partner, who then agreed to go with her to see a marital/sex therapist to discuss ways they could bring more pleasure into their own lovemaking.

For males, this *American Psychiatric Association Diagnostic and Statistical Manual,* 4th ed. (DSM-IV), category primarily refers to delayed or absent ejaculation despite prolonged intercourse or other stimulation. Some report ejaculation without the sensation of orgasm (see Table 28–9).

Case illustration 8: Frank, a 24-year-old man, confided that he had never reached orgasm with a partner. A sex problem history revealed that he had never ejaculated during intercourse and that his partners had never tried to bring him to orgasm manually or orally. Frank was able to ejaculate with masturbation, describing a vivid sexual fantasy (which he did not allow himself to have when with a partner) and a lifelong pattern of stimulation in which he rubbed his penis back and forth against a pillow without using his hands. He was congratulated for bringing this problem to his physician's attention (**P**) and was told that anxiety was often a cause of this problem, together with a masturbation pattern that did not simulate the type of sensations he would have during intercourse (**LI**). The physician encouraged Frank to take a stepwise approach to the problem by enlisting the help of a willing partner and starting with those elements that had been successful for him. He was also encouraged to expand on the kind of physical stimulation he received during masturbation by gripping his penis with his hand and stroking it. With his partner, Frank was to focus on the goal of having high arousal while his partner stimulated his penis manually, and he was imagining his "tried-and-true" fantasy. The next step was to reach higher levels of arousal in this manner and to stimulate an orgasmic response (**SS**). Frank was also referred to a self-help book (**P, LI, SS**). Follow-up indicated that Frank had successfully reached orgasm with manual stimulation with a partner in 3 weeks and was following suggestions in the book on his goal toward ejaculation during intercourse.

Management

Permission, Limited Information, and Specific Suggestions: Both men and women may present with orgasm difficulties because of a repeated pattern of masturbation that does not approximate the stimulation they receive from a partner. Although physical arousal may be apparent (erection or lubrication), these patients may not be feeling excited if they have to forego the fantasies or kinds of stimulation that had worked for them in masturbation. Encouraging them to incorporate the conditions under which they can reach orgasm alone into their sexual play with a partner is the first step in their expanding their sexual enjoyment. In some instances, use of a vibrator may be recommended to provide more intense stimulation needed for some people.

Other Medical Interventions: Currently, *oral vasodilator medications* being tested for managing male erectile dysfunction and premature ejaculation are also being considered for treating arousal and orgasm difficulties in women.

SEXUAL PAIN: DYSPAREUNIA, VAGINISMUS, & MASTURBATORY PAIN

Symptoms & Signs

Female dyspareunia—pain associated with penile-vaginal intercourse or other forms of vaginal penetration—may be one of the most common and perhaps most underreported of the female sexual dysfunctions. **Vaginismus,** the involuntary spasm of muscles around the vagina, may cause dyspareunia and is highly curable with psychological and physical interventions. The etiology of dyspareunia has had little if any systematic, controlled research. Manual-visual examination is of course important, but Meana and Binik warn against assuming that observed pathology causes the pain. Also factors that originally caused the pain may not be the maintaining variables. Psychological causes of vaginismus vary and may include fears of penetration because of confusion about genital anatomy and physiology, or be the result of other trauma or irrational fears, causing a conditioned response of involuntary spasm of the vaginal muscles.

> *Case illustration 9:* Nineteen-year-old Gina complained to her primary care provider that she had dyspareunia, was losing interest in sex, and was worried that her boyfriend was becoming impatient with her avoidance of sex. The physician then encouraged her to describe this problem behaviorally and in detail (**P**). Gina said that she had enjoyed intercourse since age 17 and always used latex condoms, but on one occasion 6 months ago she suddenly felt as if her vagina "was being rubbed with sandpaper" when her partner penetrated her. Although the physical pain had not actually returned in subsequent lovemaking sessions, Gina's *fear* of the pain recurring diminished both her interest in and her enjoyment of sex. When asked what she would do if the pain happened again during intercourse, Gina replied that she "would have to ask him to hurry up, but sometimes he lasts longer then." The physician asked how she would feel about telling him to stop all movement immediately and to withdraw when she felt discomfort or pain. Gina expressed concern that an abrupt withdrawal from intercourse might result in her boyfriend having testicular pain. She was reassured that this would create no lasting discomfort for him, and that there were alternatives for reaching ejaculation and orgasm, either with her or alone (**P, LI,** and **SS**). She was also offered some suggestions for reading about how couples learn to increase their enjoyment of sex (**SS**). The physician also praised Gina for having shown the courage to discuss this personal issue and encouraged her to bring up any future concerns (**P, LI**).

Management

Specific Suggestions: These issues can be approached gradually, by encouraging the woman to speak with her partner about her needs and to be a full participant in the sexual encounter, educating her and her partner about the need both for sufficient stimulation and arousal prior to attempted penetration, and for her to be in control of the sexual movement, so that she can be assured that she can stop instantly if pain is felt. Instruction in Kegel's pubococcygeal muscle exercises increases the woman's awareness and control of her vaginal muscles. Vaginal self-dilatation can be accomplished with graduated cylinders or with fingers, from the little finger to multiple fingers, while practicing muscle relaxation and calming mental imagery. The patient should be encouraged to be the one in control by bearing down on the finger(s) or penis as if pushing something out of the vagina, then relaxing. It helps for some women to imagine "capturing" the penis or other object in this manner, instead of being "penetrated."

Other Medical Interventions: Other medical suggestions include the use of artificial lubricants, such as Astroglide, Gyne-Moistrin, or KY Jelly; vaginal moisturizers, such as Replens; vaginal and vulvar application of estrogen creams; surgical repair of the vulvar region; and excision of abnormal growths in the genital area. Diseases thought to cause the pain, such as vaginitis, condylomata, endometriosis, pelvic inflammatory disease, and other gynecologic or pelvic diseases, all may be treated directly. When painful intercourse has been a long-standing problem, however, medical intervention alone is seldom adequate and should be followed by sex therapy directed at the probable fear and expectation of pain that have been conditioned.

SEXUAL DISORDERS DUE TO A GENERAL MEDICAL CONDITION

> *Case illustration 10:* When Hannah was 22, she was diagnosed with clear cell adenocarcinoma of the vagina and had surgery that removed one ovary, her uterus, tubes, the upper two thirds of her vagina, and her bilateral pelvic lymph nodes. None of her health care team was able to comfortably discuss sexuality with her. She was completely unprepared for the first attempts at intercourse several months following the surgery and was shocked and distraught to discover how little genital sensation she had left. She sought help from a male psychiatrist who listened as she expressed her grief and fears that she would never find a man because of her sense of diminished sexual self-worth. After rapport was established, he acknowledged her fears by saying that she might never have a "clitoral" orgasm again, but that there were other routes to orgasm and sexual pleasure. He discussed with her ideas that have been helpful to others who have sustained the loss of genital sensation: that her brain knew how to feel pleasure and have orgasms, that men and women can learn to focus on sensations from other, nongenital parts of the body, such as breasts, neck, ears, and lips, and that with or without accompanying fantasy, one can thus relearn to enjoy a sense of orgasmic release and pleasure. Twelve years after her surgery, Hannah wrote, "The growth in my ideas and experiments with sexuality have increased manyfold since my surgery. What was most helpful was being able to share my experiences with people who could understand and be accepting, and finding people who were trained and had accurate information on how I could help myself. Health professionals don't have to have all the answers, but they should know of their own limitations and be able to refer when necessary."

OTHER SEXUAL PROBLEMS NOT OTHERWISE SPECIFIED

It would take a full textbook to describe and give treatment suggestions for the wide variety of additional sex-related human problems. A patient with truly **compulsive sexual behavior**—sometimes described as **sexual addiction**—may be suffering from a form of obsessive compulsive disorder and may require intensive psychotherapy, use of support groups, and medications such as the SSRI antidepressants. **Gender identity disorders** require referral for specialized treatment, as do issues of **spousal abuse, incest,** and **rape,** and patients troubled by **paraphilias.**

CONCLUSION

For every human being, sexuality—like health—is a challenge at some point. Feelings of personal vulnerability are inherent in sexual interactions and help to make sexuality a powerful and unique part of life. Problems of sexual desire, arousal, or functioning can lead us to confront and overcome our fears of not being lovable and to seek better communication and increased intimacy with others. The deepest expressions of love often result from just such a sharing of our vulnerabilities or problems.

Acknowledgments: The authors would like to thank Linda Perlin Alperstein, LCSW; Jean M. Bullard, RN, MS; Lisa Capaldini, MD; Deborah Grady, MD, MPH; and William B. Shore, MD, for reviewing earlier drafts of this paper. Our appreciation especially goes to the coeditors of this book for their valuable comments and suggestions.

SUGGESTED READINGS

Berkovitch M, Keresteci AG, Koren G: Efficacy of prilocaine-lidocaine cream in the treatment of premature ejaculation. J Urol 1995;154:1360.

Bullard D: The treatment of desire disorders in the medically ill and physically disabled. In *Sexual Desire Disorders.* Leiblum SR, Rosen RC (editors). Guilford Press, 1988.

Caplan H: An effective clinical approach to vaginismus: Putting the patient in charge. West J Med 1988;149:6.

Fooken I: Sexuality in the later years—the impact of health and body image in a sample of older women. Patient Educ Coun 1994;23:227.

Graysen S: Adjust medication to alleviate effects on sexual functioning. Psychopharmacol Update 1994;5:1.

Kligman EW: Office evaluation of sexual function and complaints. Clin Geriatric Med 1991;7:15.

Masters WH, Johnson VE: *Human Sexual Inadequacy.* Little, Brown, 1970.

Meana M, Binik YM: Painful coitus: A review of female dyspareunia. J Nerv Ment Dis 1994;182:264.

Merrill JM, Laux LF, Thornby JI: Why doctors have difficulty with sex histories. South Med J 1990;83:613.

Mohr DC, Beutler LE: Erectile dysfunction: A review of diagnostic and treatment procedures. Clin Psychol Rev 1990; 10:123.

Peck MS: *Further Along the Road Less Traveled.* Touchstone, 1993.

Rosen RC et al: Prevalence of sexual dysfunction in women: Results of a survey study of 329 women in an outpatient gynecological clinic. J Sex Marital Ther 1993;19:171.

Schiavi RC et al: Healthy aging and male sexual function. Am J Psychiatry 1990;147:766.

Schover L, Youngs DD, Cannata R: Psychosexual aspects of the evaluation and management of vulvar vestibulitis. Am J Obstet Gynecol 1992;167:630.

Segraves RT: Hormones and libido. In: Leiblum SR, Rosen RC (editors): *Sexual Desire Disorders.* Guilford Press, 1988.

Segraves RT et al: Clomipramine versus placebo in the treatment of premature ejaculation: a pilot study. J Sex Marital Ther 1993;19:198.

Shahar E, Lederer J, Herz MJ: The use of a self-report questionnaire to assess the frequency of sexual dysfunction in family practice clinics. Fam Prac 1991;8:206.

Solstad K, Hertoft P: Frequency of sexual problems and sexual dysfunction in middle-aged Danish men. Arch Sex Beh 1993;22:51.

Spector IP, Carey MP: Incidence and prevalence of the sexual dysfunctions: A critical review of the empirical literature. Arch Sex Beh 1990;19:389.

Waldinger MD, Hengeveld MW, Zwinderman AH: Paroxetine treatment of premature ejaculation: a double-blind, randomized, placebo-controlled study. Am J Psychiatry 1994;151:1377.

PATIENT BIBLIOGRAPHY

Barbach L: *For Yourself.* Signet, 1976.
(A classic that empowers women to enjoy their own sexuality, with suggestions for women who want to learn to become orgasmic).

Barbach L: *For Each Other.* Signet, 1978.
(Encouragement and suggestions for couples wanting to enhance their sexuality and intimacy).

Barbach L: *Falling in Love Again.* 1990.
(A video and workbook self-help program for men and women).

Dackman L: *Up Front: Sex and the Post-Mastectomy Woman.* Viking, 1990.
(Moving and insightful account of one woman's experiences).

Gottman J: *Why Marriages Succeed or Fail . . . And How You Can Make Yours Last.* Simon & Schuster, 1994.
(Results of over 20 years of research pointing out the danger signals for troubled marriages, with suggestions to help marital communication).

Heiman J, LoPiccolo J: *Becoming Orgasmic: A Sexual and Personal Growth Program for Women.* Simon & Schuster, 1988.
(Available from LoPiccolo & Pridal, PO Box 7562, Columbia, MS 65205; tel. 573-474-4733; price $11 plus $3 shipping.)
Schover LR: *Prime Time: Sexual Health for Men over Fifty.* Holt, 1984.
(Provides validation and useful suggestions for men and their partners).

Schnarch DM: *Passionate Marriage: Sex, Love, and Intimacy in Emotionally Committed Relationships.* W. W. Norton & Co., 1997.
Zilbergeld B: *The New Male Sexuality.* Bantam, 1992.
(A common-sense, practical, and sane antidote to media pressures on males to be sexual superstars. Excellent discussion of the fantasy model of sex and myths of male sexuality, the importance of an individual's conditions for good sex, and specific self-help chapters dealing with common male sexual problems).

PROFESSIONAL BIBLIOGRAPHY

Annon J: *Behavioral Treatment of Sexual Problems.* Harper & Row, 1976.
Bancroft J: *Human Sexuality and its Problems,* 2nd ed. Churchill Livingstone, 1989.
Butler RN, Lewis MI: *Love and Sex After 60* (revised). Ballantine, 1993.
Leiblum SR, Rosen RC: *Sexual Desire Disorders.* Guilford Press, 1988.
Leiblum SR, Rosen RC: *Principles and Practice of Sex Therapy—Update for the 1990s,* 2nd ed. Guilford Press, 1989.
Leiblum SR, Rosen RC: *Case Studies in Sex Therapy.* Guilford Press, 1995.

Person E: *Dreams of Love and Fateful Encounters.* Norton, 1988.
Schnarch DM: *Constructing the Sexual Crucible: An Integration of Sexual and Marital Therapy.* Norton, 1991.
Weinberg M, Williams C, Pryor D: *Dual Attraction: Understanding Bisexuality.* Oxford University Press, 1994.
Wincze JP, Barlow D: *Enhancing Sexuality: A Problem-Solving Approach. Client Workbook.* The Psychological Corporation. 1996. (A new workbook for patients based on empirically supported systematic treatment including exercises and self-assessment measures).

OTHER RESOURCES

The SaferSex Page (World Wide Web Site: http:/www.safer-sex.org/)

Videotapes
Becoming Orgasmic. 1993. (Available from the Sinclair Institute, Chapel Hill, NC.)
Treating Vaginismus. 1984. (Available from the Sinclair Institute, Chapel Hill, NC.)

Section V.
Special Topics

Stress & Disease

29

Jeffrey L. Boone, MD, MS, & John F. Christensen, PhD

INTRODUCTION

Human history is replete with stories of the connection between mental stress and disease. In the biblical Book of Acts (5:1–11) Ananias and his wife Sapphira both succumbed to stress-related sudden death. Confronted by the apostle Peter, Ananias "fell down and died" on hearing the words, "You have not lied to men, but to God." Sapphira died instantly 3 hours later when judged by Peter to be a willing accomplice in "testing the Spirit of the Lord."

More recently, a review of coroner's records in Los Angeles in 1994 revealed a sudden increase in deaths, including sudden death, related to atherosclerotic cardiovascular disease on the day of the 1994 Northridge earthquake. Less dramatically, research since the late 1960s has demonstrated correlations between significant changes in individuals' lives and the subsequent onset of various types of illness. A consistent relationship has even been found between daily hassles and the onset of illness.

The interrelationship between mental stress and physical disease is complex and multifactorial. As a result, the study of stress and disease embraces a wide range of sophisticated behavioral, emotional, cognitive, physical, medical, hormonal, biochemical, cellular, environmental, and even spiritual interconnections not easily understood or encapsulated in the controlled clinical trial.

It has been estimated that up to 70% of visits to primary care physicians are for problems related to stress and life-style. Most clinicians, however, have not been trained to extend their diagnostic work-up and treatment interventions into the psychosocial context of these illnesses. Yet adequate treatment and prevention requires that primary care providers regard their patients' illnesses and suffering in the context of their life struggles. This broader perspective allows the clinician to intervene at multiple points along the continuum from mind to molecule.

This chapter offers a framework for clinicians to think broadly and clinically about the stress-illness connection and suggests some approaches to assessing and treating stress-related illness. It offers a brief background of the research base for this new perspective; provides a conceptual framework to guide diagnosis and treatment; suggests methods for communicating with patients about stress; and offers some options for stress assessment, prevention, and intervention.

DEFINITIONS

The concept of stress was borrowed by physiology and psychology from physics, where it generally refers to a force acting against some resistance. Hooke's law of elasticity states that "stress = $K \times$ strain," where K is a constant (the modulus of elasticity) that depends on the nature of the material and type of stress used to produce the strain. This constant K (ie, the stress-strain ratio), is called Young's modulus. In materials science, stress is what is imposed on a material by the outer world; strain is the reaction of the material to the stress.

Hans Selye is generally credited with introducing the concept of stress into physiology. He defined stress loosely as "the rate of wear and tear in the body" and more rigorously as "the state manifested by a specific syndrome which consists of all the non-specifically induced changes within a biologic system." In this specific syndrome, termed by Selye the **general adaptation syndrome (GAS),** glucocorticoids are secreted by the adrenal cortex in response to adaptational demands placed on the organism by such disparate stressors as heat, cold, starvation, and other environmental insults—hence the expression "non-specifically induced changes."

Various other definitions of stress have been offered by researchers. Some, like Selye's, refer to a state of the organism; others refer to the stressful stimuli; and still others refer to a combination that includes stimuli, organismic responses, and intervening variables. Currently, a distinction is usually made between stress and stressors. Although **stress** is sometimes loosely used to refer to the environmental sources of threat to the organism, the term **stressor** is more appropriate in reference to these agents.

More recent definitions of stress in humans emanate from a transactional model that takes into account the interactions between persons and their environment. In this view stress occurs when a situational demand presents a call for action that the individual perceives as exceeding available resources. Christensen proposed the following working definition: "Stress is a process of interchange between an organism and its environment that involves self-generated or environmentally induced changes that, once they are perceived by the organism as exceeding available resources (internal or external), disrupt homeostatic processes in the organism-environment system." This definition includes the traditional notion of stress as originating with an external demand (environmentally induced change) that exceeds the coping resources of the organism. It also includes, however, those expectations of events that arise from within, that are seen as essential to one's life project, and that cannot be accommodated by the environment (exceeding external resources). The disruption of homeostasis in the organism-environment system can have its primary manifestation as a pathological end-state in the organism (illness or tissue damage) or as a destructive alteration of the environment (domestic violence as a stress response).

RESEARCH BACKGROUND

Stressful Life Events

In the 1930s Adolf Meyer advocated the use of a life chart in medical diagnosis. Data were entered on date of birth, periods of disorders of various organs, and various life situations and the patient's reactions to them. In 1954, a program of studies in life changes and illness patterns was initiated at Cornell University. These studies found that illnesses appeared to be associated with definite periods of life change, although illness patterns varied among those who had been through major life changes. In 1967, Holmes and Rahe published a scale of 43 life events, along with a method of quantifying life changes according to the amount of readjustment they require for the average person. This scale allowed greater quantitative precision in life change and illness studies and provided a pivotal methodological leap that broke through the circularity in which the stressful life changes had been measured in terms of illness outcome, rather than in terms of the inherent magnitude of the stressor. Questionnaires based on this and similar scales have gathered data on several populations globally. Retrospective studies have shown a relationship between recent life change and a host of pathologic outcomes, such as sudden cardiac death, onset of myocardial infarction, occurrence of fractures, pregnancy and birth complications, aggravation of chronic illness, tuberculosis, multiple sclerosis, diabetes, onset of leukemia in children, and onset of mental disorders such as depression and schizophrenia. Prospective studies, particularly those conducted on US Navy populations while deployed at sea, predicted future illness based on life change scores prior to deployment and subsequently verified the accuracy of those predictions by inspection of medical records.

Although a consistent relationship has been found between stressful life events and illness patterns, this does not account for why some individuals who undergo significant change develop illnesses but others undergoing equally intense changes remain healthy. A typical correlation between life change and illness reported in these early studies was 0.30, which leaves 91% of the variance unexplained. Recent attention has focused on individual and situational variables that may mediate the relationship between life change and illness. Among the psychological variables that seem to mediate the stress response are locus of control (including the extent to which individuals prefer control in their lives and how much control they perceive having over specific life events), need for stimulation, openness to change, stimulus screening, self-actualization, the use of denial, the presence of social supports, and emotional self-disclosure. In one study of Illinois Bell executives during the divestiture of AT&T, those executives who experienced high stress while remaining healthy differed from those with high stress and high illness on a dimension of "hardiness." This personal characteristic consisted of a strong commitment to self, work, family, and other important values; a sense of control over one's life; and the ability to see change as a challenge rather than a threat.

Circadian Occurrence of Cardiac Events

Data from the Framingham study, the Massachusetts Death Certificate Study, and other large epidemiologic studies provide information regarding the timing of cardiovascular events such as angina and sudden cardiac death. Such events tend to occur with a greater frequency during the morning hours before noon with a second peak in the early evening hours. From the perspective of stress medicine, this circadian frequency data may be an objective description of the stress response as it affects the presentation of serious cardiovascular events.

A closer look at the data reveals that the death rate during the daytime work hours plummets over the noon hour to less than half the rate seen at 9:00 AM. The stress model suggests this may be more than coincidence. The peak death rates occur in the early hours of the work day and in the early evening hours when workers return home. These peaks are substantially blunted during the corresponding hours of the weekend days when people are moving toward recreation. Furthermore, circadian peaks in cardiac events are steeper and more deadly on Monday than on other days of the week. Employed workers die more frequently on Monday, whereas age-matched unemployed workers die on random days of the week.

The death patterns of tourists are markedly different from patterns of sudden cardiac death found in workers. For example, one study of vacationers on the island of Kauai, Hawaii, showed a sudden death rate elevated in the late afternoon hours. The sudden death rate of the local Kauai population was similar to that of working people in other locations with a peak in the hours from 6:00 AM to 12:00 noon. These data suggest that the stress of moving into the workday (for the local island population) is related to the circadian occurrence of cardiac events, just as it is in Massachusetts, but that vacationers show a different pattern that is consistent with the absence of work stressors.

Psychoneuroimmunology

Psychoneuroimmunology (PNI) involves the study of the interactions of consciousness, the central nervous system (CNS), and the immune system (involving the body's defense against infection and aberrant cell division). The compelling evidence of these studies is that the CNS influences immune function and that, conversely, the immune system can influence the CNS. It is likely that the brain is normally part of the immunoregulatory network. Specifically, stimulation of the hypothalamic-pituitary-adrenal (HPA) axis leads to down-regulation of immune system function in response to stress. Stressful thoughts and emotions may reach the hypothalamus by axons projecting from the limbic system or from the forebrain. Corticotropin-releasing factor (CRF), produced in the hypothalamus under conditions of stress, acts on the anterior pituitary to form adrenocorticotropin hormone (ACTH), which in turn stimulates the production of corticosteroids in the adrenal cortex. Corticosteroids have immunosuppressive effects on the lymphoreticular system and marked antiallergic and anti-inflammatory effects.

In addition, CRF leads to release of catecholamines, which themselves may produce changes in lymphocyte, monocyte, and leukocyte functions. Opiates are also elevated with stress, and they are generally reported to be immunosuppressive. Finally, growth hormone and prolactin, which are immunoenhancing factors, are initially elevated at the onset of stress, but under conditions of prolonged stress their secretion is inhibited. Thus the combined effect of elevated corticosteroids, catecholamines, and opiates, along with inhibition of growth hormone and prolactin, is to down-regulate the immune system.

A STRESS MODEL FOR PRIMARY CARE

The etiology of illness and its waxing and waning course is multifactorial. Any given illness episode is determined by many circumstances. The complex pathway by which stress influences the outcome of illness is subject to the ongoing accumulation of data and elaboration of heuristic and clinical models. A model of stress that can aid diagnosis, prevention, and intervention is shown in Figure 29–1. Adapted from an optical model first proposed by Rahe and Arthur (1978), it depicts stressors as light rays filtered through successive lenses representing the individual's perception (threat appraisal), coping, physiological processes, and arousal reduction activities, and then projected onto illness outcome screens. Each lens either augments or diminishes the intensity of light (heavy bold lines or dotted lines, respectively) on its pathway to illness outcome, and represents a potential focal point for the clinician's diagnosis of a stress influence or risk factor for patient illness. Each lens also represents a potential focus of preventive health care or intervention.

Perception refers to the person's appraisal of the threat involved in various stressors. Several personal variables that may affect the degree of perceived threat are shown in the figure. For example, the degree of a person's openness to change or the extent to which he or she values change influences whether a particular life change, such as a child leaving home, is perceived as a threat to the self or an opportunity for growth. The degree of control individuals prefer to have in their lives, as well as the amount of control they perceive they have over specific stressors, also influence their perception of threat. Thus a parent with a high need to control an adolescent child's outside activities experiences more stress when the child struggles toward emancipation than does a parent who has less of a need for control and who trusts the child's judgment.

Coping refers to methods an individual uses to mitigate the influence of stressors perceived as threatening. One approach to coping is "exposure management," or attempts to increase or decrease the amount and intensity of stressors encountered. Thus an overworked, overcommitted manager might attempt to mitigate stress by withdrawing from some commitments and by reducing work hours by delegating more responsibility to subordinates. Social supports are an important stress buffer, and successful coping with stressors may involve both developing confiding relationships and increasing the amount of one's self-disclosure about the effect of stressors in one's life. There is some research evidence that emotional self-disclosure about stressors enhances immune functioning. "Stimulus screening" involves techniques to focus attention on relevant stimuli and to regulate the overall flow of stimulation to one's optimal level of functioning.

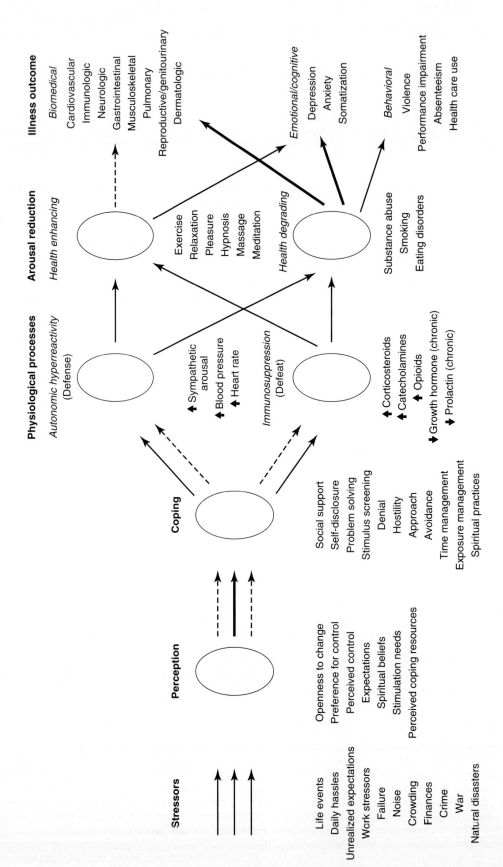

Figure 29-1. An optical model of stress pathways.

Stressors

Life events
Daily hassles
Unrealized expectations
Work stressors
Failure
Noise
Crowding
Finances
Crime
War
Natural disasters

Perception

Openness to change
Preference for control
Perceived control
Expectations
Spiritual beliefs
Stimulation needs
Perceived coping resources

Coping

Social support
Self-disclosure
Problem solving
Stimulus screening
Denial
Hostility
Approach
Avoidance
Time management
Exposure management
Spiritual practices

Physiological processes

Autonomic hyperreactivity (Defense)

↑ Sympathetic arousal
↑ Blood pressure
↑ Heart rate

Immunosuppression (Defeat)

↑ Corticosteroids
↑ Catecholamines
↓ Opioids
↓ Growth hormone (chronic)
↓ Prolactin (chronic)

Arousal reduction

Health enhancing

Exercise
Relaxation
Pleasure
Hypnosis
Massage
Meditation

Health degrading

Substance abuse
Smoking
Eating disorders

Illness outcome

Biomedical

Cardiovascular
Immunologic
Neurologic
Gastrointestinal
Musculoskeletal
Pulmonary
Reproductive/genitourinary
Dermatologic

Emotional/cognitive

Depression
Anxiety
Somatization

Behavioral

Violence
Performance impairment
Absenteeism
Health care use

Two major classes of **physiologic response** to stressors that lead to target organ pathology are autonomic hyperreactivity and immunosuppression. Both are cortically mediated through the individual's perceptions and methods of coping. **Hyperreactivity** in the presence of stress, sometimes called the **defense reaction,** has been shown to be a factor in disease processes specific to vulnerable organ systems in persons with established disease. Thus exaggerated pressor responses in hypertensives, increased EMG responses in those suffering from tension headaches and chronic back pain, disturbances in glucose metabolism in insulin-dependent diabetics, and bronchoconstrictive responses in asthmatics are all examples of hyperreactivity in the presence of a definable stressor. In the case of hypertension, hyperreactivity is present in normotensives at risk for the disorder and in some studies has predicted future blood pressure levels. Other examples are increased levels of serum cholesterol seen in studies of tax accountants in the 2 weeks prior to April 15 and of fighter pilots landing on aircraft carriers compared with pilots on long commercial airline flights.

One of the adaptive functions of sympathetic activation is to prepare the organism for large-muscle movement in order to attack or flee a threat. In 20th century human society, these somatomotor responses are often voluntarily suppressed or sublimated, leading to delayed elimination of released glucose and fatty acids and often bringing more powerful and prolonged blood pressure increases. In addition, the relative absence of skeletal muscle exertion in affluent societies (without compensatory aerobic exercise) prevents the endorphin activation that normally accompanies muscle exertion. Since these endorphins have the effect of dampening mental arousal and sympathetic activity, in the absence of skeletal muscle exertion these arousal and activation states are prolonged.

Immunosuppression, as discussed previously, occurs through the mechanisms of increased levels of circulating corticosteriods, catecholamines, and opioids, in addition to the decrease in levels of growth hormone and prolactin under conditions of prolonged stress. Sometimes referred to as the **defeat reaction,** this response pattern occurs when patients are exposed to long-term stressful situations that tend to overwhelm ordinary coping mechanisms, thus leading to despair or deep sorrow in situations that appear to be beyond all hope and rescue. Rather than working directly on target organ systems as in the case of hyperreactivity, down-regulation of the immune system in the defeat reaction increases vulnerability to external invasive organisms and endogenous neoplasms.

Several **arousal reduction** strategies are available to individuals to mitigate physiologic activation and disruption of homeostatic processes in conditions of stress. These include both **health-enhancing** and **health-degrading** activities. Among the health-enhancing arousal-reduction strategies are exercise, which expends accumulated corticosteriods and dampens sympathetic activation through the release of endorphins, and various approaches to stimulating the parasympathetic nervous system. This latter category includes relaxation exercises, abdominal breathing, self-hypnosis, meditation, soothing music, massage, and contact with nature.

Health-degrading activities, which may be attempts at physiological arousal reduction but that actually magnify the stress response and lead to target organ disease, include substance abuse, tobacco use, and eating disorders. Intensification of all of these behaviors may coincide with stressful life episodes. An example is the mediating role of increased alcohol intake in the relationship between occupational stress and hypertension seen in studies of air traffic controllers.

Various **illness outcomes** of stress include **biomedical disease** manifested in specific organ systems, such as cardiovascular, immune, and neurological disorders; **emotional and cognitive disorders,** such as depression, anxiety, and somatization; and **behavioral disorders,** such as violence, performance impairment, absenteeism, and overuse of health care resources. These stress outcomes are the usual focus of medical and mental health intervention, but the larger model of the stress pathway provides primary care clinicians with potent opportunities for comprehensive preventive health care.

STRESS OUTCOMES IN ORGAN SYSTEMS

Each organ system has a unique susceptibility to stress. The following is a brief overview of some of the stress implications in specific systems.

Cardiovascular

Cardiovascular disease is the leading cause of mortality in the United States. Stress contributes to all expressions of heart disease, including coronary artery disease, congestive heart failure, and sudden cardiac death. Since fully a third of sudden cardiac deaths and myocardial infarctions cannot be explained by the severity of the standard cardiac risk factors—family history, hypertension, dyslipidemia, diabetes, or tobacco use—stress may explain some of this variance. Table 29–1 outlines the pathways that may mediate between stress and cardiovascular disease. For example, one of the hemodynamic risk factors, hypertension, is partially the result of mental stress. Changes in vessel caliber contributing to vascular constriction, coupled with surges in cardiac output under conditions of stress, often lead to circadian variation in blood pressure levels. The assessment of these peak levels of blood pressure may be helpful in identifying patients at risk for stress-related cardiovascular disease.

Table 29–1. The cardiovascular consequences of mental stress and intensity.

1. **Hemodynamic**—blood pressure elevations caused by deleterious change in vascular constriction or cardiac output increasing susceptibility to endothelial damage and plaque fracture
2. **Hypertrophic**—the dangerous thickening of the walls of the left ventricle accelerated by catecholamine excesses and hemodynamic overload
3. **Lusitropic**—the stiffening of the left ventricle, reducing cardiac compliance and ease of filling
4. **Arrhythmogenic**—catecholamine-driven increases in heart rate and cardiac electrical instability
5. **Metabolic**—deleterious derangements of cholesterol, insulin, glucose, electrolyte, and hormonal profiles
6. **Coagulative**—accelerated clotting due to enhanced platelet activation and decreased fibrinolytic activity during stress
7. **Cardiotoxic**—catecholamine myocarditis resulting in coagulative myocytolysis with direct nonischemic damage to cardiac muscle cells
8. **Ischemic**—dynamic coronary vascular constriction during stress, leading to ischemic perfusion defects and often chest pain

Immune

Clinical expressions of immune deficiencies are in part the result of stress. They range from the common cold to some forms of cancer. Although research on the relationship between stress and cancer is still inconclusive, there is a suggestion that stress may interact with personality traits, such as a helpless, hopeless way of responding to stressors and a rational, nonemotional response to stressful events, in the etiology of cancer. Other immune-mediated diseases such as rheumatoid arthritis and systemic lupus erythematosus may show a pattern of exacerbation brought on by stress. Another manifestation of immune dysfunction is the effect of psychological stress on the slowing of wound healing.

Neurological

All forms of stroke show a circadian expression in their presentation, with peaks during the early morning hours when catecholamines are highest. Dizziness, vertigo, and other balance disorders often have stress as a causative or contributing factor. One of the most common neurologic expressions of stress in clinical practice is headache. Both tension headache and migraine headache are substantially influenced by patient stressors.

Gastrointestinal

Peptic ulcer disease may have an association with stress. Gastric hyperacidity and excess pepsin production are hallmarks of the sympathetic arousal that occurs during stress. Irritable bowel syndrome (IBS), which is characterized by abdominal pain with altered bowel habits (constipation or diarrhea) in the absence of a definable lesion or structural abnormality, frequently correlates with periods of emotional stress. The human "defense reaction" (fight or flight response) promotes activation of the cardiovascular system along with inhibition of gastric motility.

Musculoskeletal

Some forms of arthritis show stress-related exacerbations. Complex syndromes such as fibromyalgia seem to have a psychosocial trigger. Temporomandibular joint (TMJ) dysfunction and its related pain syndrome are frequently associated with mental stress. Chronic pain tends to show a course that correlates to stress in a person's life.

Pulmonary

Asthma and chronic obstructive pulmonary disease appear to be worsened by stress. Conversely, one of the more powerful self-regulatory stress-control techniques is relaxed abdominal breathing. Asthmatics who participate in stress reduction programs have shown improved physical activity and decreased medical visits.

Reproductive and Genitourinary

The neurohormonal, vascular, and immunologic effects of stress have significant effects on the reproductive and genitourinary systems. Changes in estrogen and testosterone levels can show marked association with environmental and psychological stressors. Amenorrhea frequently occurs during stressful times in the lives of women. Fertility also can be affected by stress. Dysmenorrhea, dyspareunia, endometriosis, and impotence all have substantial stress and strain connections.

Dermatologic

A variety of skin lesions and rashes have been associated with the stress response. Stress-induced vasomotor changes may aggravate inflammatory dermatoses. Vasodilation is seen as responsible for the thermal aggravation often expressed as pruritus. This lowering of the itch threshold by vasodilation may account for the pruritus seen with many dermatologic syndromes. Emotional stress, fear, and pain are all accompanied by substantial drops in skin temperature of the fingers.

DIAGNOSIS

Given the multivariate, multiple-pathway nature of the stress response, clinical diagnosis of stress assumes a multifactorial approach. Traditional medical diagnosis and treatment occurs at the point of illness manifestation in target organ systems. From the broader perspective of stress medicine, however, each of the lenses in the optical model (see Figure 29–1) is a potential focus of diagnosis.

The Medical Interview

The richest source of data concerning stressors, perception, coping, and arousal reduction strategies is the medical interview (see Chapter 1). Having the stress model in mind allows the primary care clinician to inquire about current and recent life stressors and to make note of significant clusterings of stressors that precede illness onset. A careful history should uncover whether life stressors are temporally related to the onset of chronic disease and to periods of disease exacerbation.

During the interview, the clinician can ask patients about their beliefs, expectations, self-perceptions, and needs that influence how stressors are perceived. For example, asking patients how much control they prefer in their lives and how much control they perceive having over specific life events can determine whether there is congruence or incongruence between preferred control and perceived control. Incongruence tends to amplify the effect of stressors. It is also helpful to ask patients how they view their own resources (internal and external) for coping with stressors, since the more the perceived threats exceed the perceived personal resources, the greater the stress involved.

Patients' approaches to coping with stressors should also be probed in the interview. The presence or absence of social supports, as well as patients' ability to access these supports through self-disclosure, are critical data for facilitating stress management. The perceptual and coping styles uncovered in the interview have implications for primary care management of the patient's health, both in prevention and intervention.

It is also important to assess patients' approaches to arousal reduction and to ascertain the balance of health-enhancing and health-degrading strategies. The following questions can be helpful in this regard: "What are the signs to you that you are experiencing stress? " "What are the physical symptoms? " "What happens in your emotional life? " "How do you act differently when you are stressed? " Methods used to mitigate this arousal can then be ascertained: "When you notice these signs of stress, what do you do to reduce the intensity of the physical symptoms? " It is also important to elicit the short- and long-term outcomes of these strategies: "How does this strategy work for you? " "How does it affect the way you feel immediately? several hours later? the next day? " Sometimes it is helpful to ask about specific arousal reduction techniques: "Do you practice a form of meditation or relaxation exercise? " "Do you get regular physical exercise? " When questions about substance use or tobacco use are asked in the interview, it is helpful to ask whether their use is associated with periods of stress.

Self-Report Questionnaire

A multitude of self-report questionnaires and inventories have been developed for research purposes that measure stressors and many of the variables listed in Figure 29–1 related to perception and coping. Given the limitations of patient and support staff time in primary care settings, it is recommended that any questionnaire be simple, brief, and provide data that can be used by the provider in counseling patients in the area of stress management. An example of such an instrument is the Life Stress Inventory developed by one of the authors (JFC) and shown in Appendix 29–A. Borrowing from the life event scaling studies and the critical role that perceived control plays in mediating stress, this inventory asks patients in an open-ended way to list the major events (and expected nonevents), changes, and stressors that have occurred during the previous year. They are asked to check those stressors that are current, ongoing problems. In addition, patients are asked to rate each stressor on a scale of 1 to 10, indicating the extent of perceived control they had over these events. The provider can take the mean of the control ratings and place that number (1 to 10) in the "control score" blank. This instrument provides both qualitative and quantitative data on the nature of patient's stressors, those that are a current source of struggle, and their perceived control over these events. The higher the external control score, the more at risk the patient is for the adverse consequences of stress. Examining with patients those stressors that seem under their control can allow the provider to suggest lifestyle changes in those areas. In some instances, patients can be counseled to adjust their perceptions of no control in the direction of greater control. For example, a patient who perceives no control over her work hours can be helped to see areas in which limits can actually be set. In other cases patients can be led to consider changing their expectations and accepting areas that are truly beyond their control.

Assessing Blood Pressure Responses to Stress

In addition to patient self-reporting in the medical interview and on questionnaires, stress can be assessed in the office setting by direct measurement of physiologic responses. Of all the physiological consequences of mental stress, blood pressure and heart rate may be the most clinically accessible. Blood pressure—both systolic and diastolic—tends to elevate during times of mental stress and fall during periods of calm and relaxation. Heart rate varies in a similar fashion. Both the absolute values of the peak pressures and pulses during stress and the variation from the resting state may have clinical diagnostic and prognostic significance in the analysis of stress and disease in primary care medicine. The "defense reaction," a common response to challenges in everyday life, occurs whenever interesting, irritating, or otherwise challenging mental stimuli are at hand. In the laboratory setting the peak ambulatory blood pressure levels associated with defense reactions have been approximated by standardized stress tests. One such standardized test consists of measuring blood pressure at rest, during mental arithmetic and time-reaction tests (β-adrenergic challenge that increases cardiac output), and during a cold pressor test (α-adrenergic or vasoconstrictive challenge). These blood pressure readings have been found to correlate with ambulatory blood pressure variations obtained in the same subjects during the work day. Blood pressure reactions to the challenge tests have been demonstrated to be predictive of future cardiovascular events.

The mathematics challenge has been shown to induce cardiac ischemia in susceptible patients and cause blood pressure elevations equivalent to those that occur with exposure to environmental stress. The cold pressor test, which has been used in research settings for several decades, has been shown to reliably predict coronary heart disease (CHD). A diastolic blood pressure rise of more than 20 mm Hg was associated in one study with hyperreactors 2.4 times more prone to CHD than their normal-reactor counterparts.

MANAGEMENT: PREVENTION & INTERVENTION

The model of stress shown in Figure 29–1 offers the clinician various foci for illness prevention and intervention, just as it does for diagnosis. The clinician familiar with this model should be able to tailor specific psychological, social, behavioral, and pharmacologic strategies to the unique needs of individual patients. This is preferable to referring the patient for "stress management," since this generic term does not address the multiplicity of stress-related variables and pathways discussed earlier.

Communicating With Patients About Stress

A primary component of stress prevention and treatment involves the way stress is discussed with patients. Avoiding the miscommunication that "it's all in your head" is of great importance. Equally important is avoiding the message that "you are responsible for your illness," which implies greater personal control over somatic processes than is realistic. Here the risk is that of inducing guilt in patients who become ill and who feel they have failed at being a "better person." Avoiding negative emphases, for example, "Your hectic pace is going to kill you," in favor of a positive framing of the health benefits of stress management is more likely to have a positive influence (see Chapter 6). For example, the clinician can express optimism about the patient's ability to influence health as follows: "Fortunately there are many avenues available for examining and changing your habits of thought and ways of responding to life challenges. I'd like to give you an overview of some strategies that we can discuss now and in future appointments." Showing the patient a model such as that in Figure 29–1 can be helpful as part of this discussion.

Another important communication is framing beneficial life-style changes as the patient's choice. Rather than using the stress model to assume more responsibility for patients' lives, the primary care provider can act as a consultant and coach, clearly giving feedback to patients about the patterns of stress revealed by the diagnostic work-up and offering concrete strategies for health promotion along with likely consequences for adherence and nonadherence (see Chapters 16 and 17).

Counseling About Perception & Coping

The perception and coping variables listed in Figure 29–1 represent potential topics for primary care counseling with patients. Depending on the clinician's expertise, inclination, and time, this could be done during a portion of several primary care visits. For example, a parent who is feeling stressed because of a teenager's oppositional behavior could be invited to reflect on how much parental control is needed and coached on ways of setting realistic limits. With an accountant feeling overwhelmed about a recent promotion to senior management, the clinician could elicit his recollections of previous adaptations to challenging life changes in order to help him become cognizant of his own resources.

Referring a parent of a child with recently diagnosed leukemia to a support group of other parents is an example of a coping strategy. Encouraging a widower to confide feelings of sadness to close friends is an example of helping a patient improve his use of social supports. Referring a teacher with a chronically explosive temper for short-term anger management therapy would potentially reduce a cardiac risk factor.

Counseling patients about time management offers a rich opportunity for clinicians to raise questions to patients of their values and missed opportunities for personal renewal. For example, the clinician can ask the patient to reflect on those important but nonurgent activities that can contribute to

Table 29–2. Nonpharmacological interventions related to perception and coping.

1. Improve time management.
2. Improve sense of humor.
3. Pursue personal and vocational activities consistent with life values.
4. Explore the meaning and purpose of life.
5. Cultivate spiritual and transcendent activities.
   a. prayer
   b. communal religious observances
   c. spiritual retreat
   d. seasonal ritual celebrations
6. Increase emotional self disclosure.
7. Pursue short-term psychotherapy.
8. Clarify values.
9. Cultivate social support network.
10. Increase assertiveness.
11. Reduce exposure to unnecessary stressors.
12. Monitor sensory input.
13. Help others.

personal well-being (eg, time spent playing with a child), but which are consistently postponed in favor of more urgent but less important tasks (eg, keeping track of the performance of stocks). A list of potential nonpharmacologic strategies related to perception and coping that can be suggested to patients is shown in Table 29–2.

Nonpharmacological & Pharmacologic Strategies for Improving Physiologic Processes

Once identified in clinical practice, sympathetic hyperreactors may benefit from both nonpharmacological and pharmacological treatment interventions. The nonpharmacological treatment of blood pressure elevations related to stress is outlined in Table 29–3. Included are strategies for exercise, diet, and weight control. Principles for the pharmacologic treatment of blood pressure elevations related to stress are summarized in Table 29–4. Effective outcomes are achieved when the blood pressure reduction is accompanied by concomitant improvement in other cardiovascular and noncardiovascular components of sympathetic excess. Table 29–5 ranks antihypertensive medication according to effectiveness in controlling sympathetic hyperreactivity.

Arousal Reduction Strategies

For patients showing a high degree of autonomic hyperreactivity, the clinician can provide or suggest several arousal reduction strategies that can work syn-

Table 29–3. The nonpharmacological treatment of blood pressure elevations related to stress.

Exercise
1. Pursue daily aerobic exercise.
2. Improve physical fitness and stamina.

Diet and Weight Control
1. Reduce excess body weight and fat.
2. Reduce alcohol intake to less than one ounce per day.
3. Reduce dietary sodium.
4. Increase dietary potassium.
5. Increase dietary calcium.
6. Increase dietary omega-3-rich fish.

ergistically with perception and coping skills, as well as with pharmacological interventions. These strategies are listed in Table 29–6.

Referral for Psychotherapy

The clinician may choose to refer patients for psychotherapy or to educational groups to achieve some of the desired outcomes in the areas of perception, coping, and arousal reduction techniques. These referrals are more effectively targeted to the unique needs of patients if the clinician uses the multifactorial model in Figure 29–1. This model can also aid the primary care clinician in communicating with the psychotherapist about possible foci for treatment. Psychotherapy may be more effective than primary care counseling for altering dysfunctional belief systems (eg, no control of one's life) or coping habits (eg, excessive need for achievement) that amplify stress.

Table 29–4. The pharmacological treatment of blood pressure elevations related to stress.

Cardiovascular Treatment Guidelines
1. Control blood pressure and heart rate at rest.
2. Control blood pressure and heart rate during physical and mental stress for 24 hours.
3. Avoid increases in heart rate (ie, reflex tachycardia).
4. Avoid increases in renin/angiotensin.
5. Avoid sympathetic stimulation and catecholamine release.
6. Optimize renal hemodynamics.
7. Improve the hemodynamics of stress.
8. Enhance target organ perfusion.
9. Strive to reduce sympathetic arousal.
10. Lower the threshold for arrhythmogenesis.
11. Optimize the clotting profile (ie, inhibit platelet aggregation and thrombus formation).
12. Optimize the lipid profile.
13. Control or reverse left ventricular hypertrophy.
14. Control or promote regression of atherosclerosis.
15. Improve coronary blood flow.
16. Improve cardiac compliance and diastolic relaxation.
17. Avoid metabolic consequences (ie, reductions in potassium and magnesium).
18. Improve insulin resistance and glucose tolerance.
19. Enhance exercise motivation and performance.
20. Avoid exacerbations of non-cardiovascular stress-related symptomatology (ie, headache, diarrhea, dyspepsia, fatigue, tachycardia, anxiety, etc).

Noncardiovascular Considerations
1. Evaluate and treat stress-related symptomatology noted in other organ systems (ie, headache, irritable bowel, fatigue, dyspepsia, etc)
2. Consider anxiolytics.
3. Consider antidepressants.
4. Consider hypnotics for sleep enhancement.

Table 29–5. Blood pressure medication and control of sympathetic hyperreactivity: a rank order of efficacy.

1. Nondihydropyridine calcium antagonist—limits heart rate (eg, verapamil)
2. Angiotensin converting enzyme (ACE) inhibitor
3. β-blocker
4. α-blocker
5. Centrally acting alpha agonist
6. Dihydropyridine calcium antagonist—does not limit heart rate (eg, nifedipine)

Table 29–6. Health-enhancing arousal reduction techniques.

1. Meditation
2. Self-hypnosis
3. Relaxation exercises
4. Time in nature
5. Massage
6. Abdominal breathing
7. Singing
8. Tai-chi
9. Listening to soothing music

CASE ILLUSTRATIONS

Case illustration 1:

History: A 46-year-old manager of a computer store presented with concern over palpitations that occurred the previous week at work. He noted "skipped" heart beats intermittently during the previous 2 months, but they intensified during the previous week as work pace accelerated. The patient played racquetball once per week and noticed no chest pains or palpitations during the game. He had no history of hypertension or lipid abnormalities, and denied nausea, shortness of breath, or diaphoresis.

Related History: As the holiday season approached, the patient also noted sleep disturbance, eczema of the hands, heartburn, and unusually loose stools. He also gained 8 lb and noted increased irritability with his children. Screens for depression and anxiety disorder were negative.

Medical Assessment: Physical examination revealed a normal male 20 lb overweight with a resting pulse of 92. No other abnormalities were noted except for an occasional "skipped" beat during manual heart rate monitoring. The resting blood pressure in the sitting position was 141/92 but rose to 166/102 with a mathematics challenge (Serial 7's).

Recommendations: The patient was encouraged to hire extra help for his retail business during the holiday season. He agreed to ask a trusted employee to remind him to leave the store each day by noon for an hour of walking, reflection, and relaxation. The nursing staff provided a brief instruction in diaphragmatic breathing techniques. A sleeping medicine was given to be used as needed.

Disposition: Over the next 2 months the daily hour program of walking and relaxation resulted in a 6-lb weight loss. Heartburn, loose stool, and sleep disturbance improved. The patient's palpitations resolved. Sleeping medication was discontinued. At follow-up his resting blood pressure was 126/84, and after mathematics challenge was 143/90.

Case illustration 2:*

History: A 54-year-old female with a history of chronic migraine headaches, hypertension, hypercholes-

terolemia, mild obesity, and smoking presented to a new primary care physician. She was treated by her previous physician with Tylenol #3, 1 tablet twice a day, for the migraines, and she routinely called in halfway through the month for extra refills. Other medications included propranolol 10 mg bid for blood pressure elevation and migraine prophylaxis, as well as over-the-counter antacids for occasional heartburn.

Patient Interview: The patient appeared angry and complained that the medication was not helping her pain. The new physician listened to her complaints and agreed at the end of the visit to refill her medications, but told her he would not prescribe more than the previous doctor. He asked her to return for her annual Pap smear, at which time he would take a history and do a physical examination.

Social History: At the follow-up appointment the physician took a social history, which revealed that the patient had been smoking a pack of cigarettes every day for the last 35 years but did not use alcohol or street drugs. Although never married, she had been involved in a 10-year relationship with her current boyfriend, who suffered from severe emphysema and was dependent on oxygen. Three years previously this man had assumed responsibility for raising his two granddaughters (ages 8 and 11) because his daughter, the girls' mother, was a drug addict serving time in prison. The patient was not consulted about this custody decision. She accepted the stressor out of love for her partner, who was also dependent on her. The oldest granddaughter was now 14 and had become unruly, rebellious, sexually active, and aggressive. She had asked the patient for help obtaining birth control. Although the patient wanted to leave this demanding social situation, she saw it as her responsibility to care for her partner and the two children. The history correlated these recent life events with increased frequency of migraines and initiation of daily use of Tylenol #3.

Physician Facilitation of Emotional Self-Disclosure: The physician actively listened to the patient's self-disclosure, which was accompanied by crying. At the end of the interview the patient thanked the physician, who noted that she had not complained of migraines during that visit.

Brief Counseling and Referral for Family Therapy: In the follow-up visit the physician counseled the patient to realize that she was not isolated. He validated her efforts to work with the situation, even though she had the real option of leaving. He recommended family therapy, to which the patient agreed. Further medical treatment was deferred until after the

---

*The authors are grateful to Kerry Kuehl, MD, for sharing this case.

family had engaged in therapy. The patient made no mention of pain medication during this visit.

Change of Medication and of Life-Style: Prior to the next visit, which was several months later, there were no further calls for pain medication refills. At that visit the patient stated that the migraines, although still present, were not as disabling. The focus of the visit was on improving management of hypertension, high cholesterol, and migraines. They discussed starting an exercise program, initiating a low-fat diet, weight loss, and quitting smoking. The physician discontinued the propranolol and Tylenol #3 and started the patient on a low-dose calcium channel blocker. They discussed starting hormone replacement therapy to lower the patient's risks of premature cardiovascular disease and osteoporosis. The physician remarked that the patient appeared to be gaining control over the life events involving her family.

Disposition: After several months of family therapy the patient had established a primary care relationship with a pediatrician to help her with the medical and hormonal issues of the grandchildren. Her boyfriend had increased his level of help. She had lost 8 lb over 4 months, started walking 4 days a week for 30 minutes, and began a low-fat diet. She began hormone replacement therapy, and her headaches and blood pressure were well controlled without pain medication. She agreed to start a smoking cessation program within the year. The patient demonstrated a marked change in attitude and treatment of office staff, and the primary care provider developed a changed perception of her and an appreciation of the healing potential in "drug-seeking patients."

CONCLUSION

The relationship between stress and disease is well established, although the specific pathways are complex and multifactorial. Primary care clinicians increasingly are asked to examine the cost-effectiveness of the time spent with their patients with a view to improving outcomes within the constraints of available financial and human resources. Attention to the function of stress in patients' illnesses has potential for improving treatment outcomes and preventing or delaying the onset of costly target organ disease or the exacerbation of chronic illness. Applying a multidimensional stress model that includes patients' perceptions, coping strategies, physiological arousal mechanisms, and arousal reduction strategies offers the primary care provider multiple opportunities for influencing the ecology of disease.

SUGGESTED READINGS

Black PH: Central nervous system-immune system interactions: Psychoneuroendocrinology of stress and its immune consequences. Antimicrob Agents Chemother 1994;38(1):1.

Boone JL: Stress and hypertension. In Boone JL (editor): *Primary Care: Clinics in Office Practice: Hypertension.* Saunders, 1991.

Christensen JF: The assessment of stress: Environmental, intrapersonal, and outcome issues. In McReynolds P (ed), *Advances in Psychological Assessment,* Vol 5, Jossey-Bass, 1981.

Eliot RS: The dynamics of hypertension—An overview: Present practices, new possibilities, and new approaches. Am Heart J 1988;116(2):583.

Eliot RS: Stress and the heart. Postgrad Med 1992;92:237.

Folkow B: Physiological organization of neurohormonal responses to psychosocial stimuli: Implications for health and disease. Ann Behav Med 1993;15(4):236.

Holmes TH, Rahe RH: The Social Readjustment Rating Scale. J Psychosom Res 1967;11:213.

Julius S, Jamerson K, Mejia A, et al: The association of borderline hypertension with target organ changes and higher coronary risk: Tecumseh Blood Pressure Study. JAMA 1990;264(3):354.

Kannel WB: Hypertension and other risk factors in coronary heart disease. Am Heart J 1987;114:918.

Keys A et al: Mortality and coronary heart disease among men studied for twenty-three years. Arch Intern Med 1971;128(2):201.

Kiecolt-Glaser JK et al: Slowing of wound healing by psychological stress. Lancet 1995;4:1194.

Kobasa SC: Stressful life events, personality and health: an inquiry into hardiness. J Pers Soc Psychol 1979;37:1.

Leor J, Poole WK, Kloner RA: Sudden cardiac death triggered by an earthquake. N Engl J Med 1996;334:413.

Morales-Ballejo HM et al: Psychophysiologic stress testing as a predictor of mean daily blood pressure. Am Heart J 1988;116(2):673.

Muller JE, Tofler GH: Circadian variation and cardiovascular disease. N Engl J Med 1991;325(14):1038.

Rahe RH, Arthur RJ: Life change and illness studies: Past history and future directions. J Hum Stress 1978;4:3.

Schnall PL et al: The relationship between "job strain," workplace diastolic blood pressures and left ventricular mass index. JAMA 1990;263(14):1929.

Seyle H: *Stress in Health and Disease.* Butterworth, 1976.

Sobel D: Mind matters, money matters: The cost-effectiveness of clinical behavioral medicine. Ment Med Update 1993;1.

Steptoe A. The links between stress and illness. J Psychosom Res 1991;35:633.

Wilkin JK, Trotter K: Cognitive activity and cutaneous blood flows. Arch Dermatol 1987;123:1503.

Appendix 29–A. Life Stress Inventory.

In the blanks below list the major events, changes, or stressors that have happened to you within the last year. Also list those events that you expected but that failed to occur. In the next column place a check next to those stressors that are current, on-going problems. In the last column opposite each stressor, indicate the degree to which this event has been under your control by writing a number corresponding to the scale at the top.

Life Event or Stressor	Current Problem	Within Your Control	Outside Your Control
		1 2 3 4 5 6 7 8 9 10	

1. _____   _____   _____

2. _____   _____   _____

3. _____   _____   _____

4. _____   _____   _____

5. _____   _____   _____

6. _____   _____   _____

7. _____   _____   _____

8. _____   _____   _____

9. _____   _____   _____

10. _____   _____   _____

Control Score _____

John F. Christensen, PhD

Pain

30

Gregory Smith, PhD, & Douglas Beers, MD

There are among us those who haply please
to think our business is to treat disease.
And all unknowingly lack this lesson still
'tis not the body, but the man is ill

S. Weir Mitchell (cited in Turk, Meichenbaum, and
Genest, 1983).

INTRODUCTION

Pain is commonly a symptom of an underlying disease process or injury. It derives from nociceptive input and is modulated by central nervous system activity, physical movement, psychologic status, and environmental stressors. Pain is not directly measurable, and its significance is therefore not fully understood.

Pain behavior is the verbal and nonverbal expression of pain that describes both the nociceptive input and the modulation or suffering that together comprise the problem of pain (Table 30–1).

This chapter addresses treatment concepts of several differing pain problems, including acute pain; chronic periodic pain; such as migraine headaches, chronic intractable pain; such as chronic low back pain, and chronic progressive pain such as cancer pain. Special attention is given to issues of evaluation and treatment related to cross-cultural differences, workers' compensation, and pain center treatment. Guidelines, tools, and techniques are highlighted to better assist the primary care physician in the treatment of various pain problems.

This chapter examines the evaluation and treatment approaches of various pain problems in a managed care environment. It is assumed that the primary care physician has the responsibility for treatment and use of appropriate referrals, consultations, and treatments. Behavioral management of patient care and use of appropriate referral sources in a timely way is cost-effective as well as being good patient care.

A patient dealing with pain comes to medical attention with a number of possible feelings and goals:

1. The patient may simply want to discover the cause of the pain to allay his or her fears about serious disease.
2. The patient may be interested only in relief from the nociceptive stimulus.
3. The patient may want to regain impaired function to return to normal work or recreational activities.
4. The patient may want medical and social acknowledgment that the pain is preventing normal activities.

The effectiveness of the patient-doctor relationship is defined largely by the physician's ability to acknowledge the patient's problem, address the patient's goals, and establish a collaborative approach on which both the doctor and patient can agree. Because the primary concerns of the doctor and patient are often different, the potential for miscommunication can occur with patients suffering from acute as well as chronic pain. Pain is a symptom not perceivable to the observer. Pain behaviors are the functional medium for observing pain. Moreover, pain behaviors are often embedded in family interactions and dynamics that can lead unintentionally to reinforcing a sick role or to family dysfunction, which can promote increases in the pain behaviors (see Chapter 9). It is therefore important to modify the "three-function model of the medical interview" as an ongoing format for the evaluation and treatment of patients presenting with pain (Table 30–2) (see Chapter 1). In this model, all functions are openly and simultaneously pursued throughout treatment.

The three-function model allows for a streamlined diagnostic evaluation, ongoing relationship building, and early return to function. Patients' anxieties about pain and their use of medical resources often stem from unrealistic expectations of the role of healing. Establishing a diagnosis and an expectation for return to function can help control excess use of both pain medications and diagnostic and consultative services.

Table 30–1. Pain behaviors.

Pain behaviors can be separated into three categories:
1. **Pain complaints:** Verbalizing the presence of pain, complaining, moaning, grimacing.
2. **Impaired functioning:** Such as reduction of activities, avoidance of certain activities, impaired interpersonal and sexual relationships.
3. **Somatic interventions:** Such as taking medications or seeking treatment.

Table 30–3. Pain types.

1. **Acute pain:** usually self-limiting and of less than 6 months' duration (for example postsurgical pain, dental pain, pain accompanying childbirth).
2. **Chronic periodic pain:** acute but intermittent (for example migraine headaches, trigeminal neuralgia).
3. **Chronic, intractable, benign pain:** present most of the time, with intensity varying (for example low back pain).
4. **Chronic, progressive pain:** often associated with malignancies.
5. **Experimentally induced pain:** nociceptive stimulation produced in a laboratory setting (for example electric shock, radiant heat, muscle ischemia).

Identifying pain as an issue and dealing with it in a comprehensive medical and behavioral way must coexist with a diagnostic evaluation of both medical and psychological causes of that pain. This avoids a costly, lengthy, and frustrating cycle of "rule out" diagnoses.

The next section discusses four cases representing common pain types (Table 30–3). In each case the approach to evaluation and treatment uses the three-function model. We suggest specific questions representative of the three functions that can be asked initially and at any time during treatment (Table 30–4).

ACUTE PAIN: CARPAL TUNNEL SYNDROME

Case illustration 1: Ann is a 28-year-old woman with insulin-dependent diabetes mellitus who presented with bilateral hand and wrist pain with radiation to the elbows and shoulders. The pain began 2 months earlier and increased with work (data entry) and in the morning. Pain and tingling in the median nerve distribution was increased with Tinel's and Phelan's maneuvers, consistent with carpal tunnel syndrome. There was no discernible weakness or wasting in the hands.

Wrist splints afforded no relief. Nerve conduction studies confirmed slowing in the median nerve at the carpal tunnel. She had stopped work at the time of the first visit and filed a worker's compensation claim for carpal tunnel syndrome.

She does not want to return to her previous job and would like to use the time to identify an alternative employer. She is not eager to consider surgery at this time.

Table 30–2. Three-function model of the medical interview.

1. **Data gathering:** Elucidate the etiology (physical and psychologic) of the pain. Arrive at a tentative working diagnosis even while considering alternative hypotheses.
2. **Relationship building:** Collaborate on the meaning the pain has in the patient's life and on the understanding of "pain behaviors" and pain dysfunction (both physical and social).
3. **Management:** Explain the role of pain medications, including the duration of their use, the importance of time contingency, and an expectation of the degree of relief.
   a. Plan the use of physical and other therapies designed to improve function.
   b. Acknowledge the roles and limitations of rest.
   c. Establish the value of return to normal work and recreational activity to overcome pain behavior and dysfunction.

Several common pain management traps are evident in this case:

1. The overprescription of rest as a treatment modality.
2. Failure to build into a treatment regimen a restoration of activity level.
3. Positive reinforcement of pain behaviors.

In order to engage this patient in collaborative management of the pain problem, a number of behavioral techniques can be used. Although there is a very close link between nociceptive input and pain behavior in the acute phase of the injury, the doctor should discuss with the patient how pain behaviors can, in the chronic phase, become a more prominent problem. In the acute phase, this patient has been conditioned to believe that the persistence of pain means a continuation of the precipitating factor. As a behavior, pain is readily conditioned. For example, pain behaviors in the subacute condition can become linked to the anticipation of positive consequences (worker's compensation), of avoiding aversive consequences (unpleasant work environment), and excessive guarding (significantly reduced activity level). It is important to note that persistence of the pain does not imply an emotional problem.

Table 30–4. Five questions to ask patients.

1. What does pain keep you from doing that you would otherwise do (work, sex, etc—all can mean something about the effect or etiology of pain behaviors)? Conversely, what do you do in spite of the pain?
2. How has pain affected those around you? When you're hurting what does your spouse (partner) do?
3. What is your goal in seeking help for this pain? What do you hope will be the benefit of coming here today? (Diagnosis, fear reduction, pain relief, return to work, remain out of work, etc).
4. How has this pain affected other health issues? Do you have other physical problems that are now worse since the pain has started? (Exercise program; obesity; unrelated aches and pains; worry; eg, cancer; heart disease; etc).
5. What told you that this pain was one that warranted medical attention? What's different about this pain from other pain problems you've had in the past?

Case illustration 1 (Contd.): Further evaluation reveals that during the weekends or time away from work Ann holds her hands in a somewhat immobilized position, that greatly reduces her pain. She reports that after this period of "rest" she can resume many of her activities around the home. Her husband expresses concern about her pain but is uninvolved in her daily activities. Ann does report maintaining her exercise and diet program throughout, even with the reduced mobility of her hands. She also indicates that she hopes to better control the pain and to locate alternative employment that would not exacerbate her pain. Further inquiry reveals that she feels too much pressure from her boss, sees little chance for advancement, and dislikes her coworkers.

The significance of the pain complaint in the patient's life has become clearer. Although she reports an acute onset of carpal tunnel symptoms, she also reports a method of managing the symptoms that was initially effective. The influence of her injury was largely felt in the work setting rather than at home. Although it may be appropriate for her to consider changing employment, the consequences of doing so while filing for worker's compensation may have the effect of increasing and prolonging the pain behavior.

During the patient's first appointment and evaluation a realistic projection of the duration of the pain should be agreed on, (4–8 weeks) as well as a plan for active physical therapy and a resumption of normal activity. An early elucidation of the expectations of treatment allows the patient the opportunity to focus on work dissatisfaction independent of the pain behavior. Appropriate referral for behavior therapy and vocational rehabilitation may be considered. Addressing all of these issues during the first session also decreases the patient's uncertainty and therefore the need to use further diagnostic and consultative resources.

CHRONIC PERIODIC PAIN: MIGRAINE HEADACHE

Case illustration 2: Lisa is a 39-year-old woman who sought care for her long-standing migraine headaches. These headaches first appeared at age 18, at which time they were characterized by severe left orbital and temporal pain associated with nausea, nasal stuffiness, and photophobia. They were often preceded by a scintillating scotoma in the right temporal visual field. Her work-up included a normal lumbar puncture, several normal EEGs, CT scans, and blood chemistries. She was virtually headache-free for 1 year following a pregnancy in her early twenties. Headaches gradually recurred but remitted again for a year after a hysterectomy for endometriosis in her early thirties. She now reports an increasing frequency, duration, and severity of the headaches over the past 2 years, with more photophobia, nausea, and vomiting.

Treatment modalities have included analgesia (aspirin, acetaminophen, NSAIDs, narcotics), abortive agents (DHE injections, ergotamines [Cafergot], sumatriptan), prophylactic medication (amitriptyline, cyproheptadine, phenytoin, valproic acid, propranolol), and vitamins that have had only transient benefit. Dietary and activity prescriptions have also been of minimal success. Her main source of relief over the past year has been repeated after-hours visits for IM narcotics. She has seen multiple internists, neurologists, allergists, and emergency room physicians.

Long-standing recurrent incapacitating nonmalignant pain provides a number of management traps:

1. Doctor "shopping" or seeking assistance from a series of caregivers without resolution.
2. A clear fluctuation in the frequency and intensity of headache apparently due to physiologic changes, but without an exploration of possible behavioral or social changes associated with these fluctuations.
3. Failure to explore the significance the headache has had in the patient's life.

Case illustration 2 (Contd.): Further history revealed that Lisa's headaches in late adolescence were infrequent (several per year) and were managed conservatively. Her single severe attack resulted in a hospitalization that was a source of embarrassment to her and her husband. During the early years of her marriage, she continued to have infrequent, but more severe headaches. During a period of 6 months of treatment with oral contraceptives, she suffered a transient exacerbation. As her daughter grew older and her job responsibilities increased, the frequency and severity of headaches grew. She further reported that she was best able to control her pain by being alone in a quiet room, reading or listening to quiet music.

The patient is now identifying what may be a clear relationship between marital or social stress and her headache complaint. Whereas the headache can provide "time-out" from the conflicts at hand, it does not interfere with other activities such as listening to music or reading. She further describes that the headaches did not have a significant effect in her early life.

Case illustration 2 (Contd.): The headache pattern remained unchanged until 1 $\frac{1}{2}$ years ago. At that time Lisa and her husband relocated as a result of her husband's work and they moved into a home that required major remodeling, the responsibility of which was largely the patient's. She had difficulty replacing her former employment and considered a new career. Although she reported enthusiasm for the remodeling and the relocation, Lisa also reported a marked increase in the frequency of the headaches. She was unable to work around the house remodeling or participate in stressful family discussions when she had the headache but was otherwise able to prepare meals, do housework, and drive as far as 30 miles one way for social or medical visits. She reported that when she retreats to her room with a headache her husband and children attend to her until she starts to improve. She also indicated that her husband returned home early from work during times of severe headache. She has seen a cascade of physicians in various specialties with a variety of diagnostic tests and specialty work-ups. Her average length of adherence with any one physician was five visits; new referrals were made after several visits. She reported with embarrassment that she had been unable to keep up with her diet and exercise program and was increasingly overweight. She felt otherwise in good health, with no other medical problems.

Although the headache event is likely to have both muscle contraction and vascular components, there appear to be a number of clear situations or conditions that accompany the onset of the headache. Moreover, it is clear that in early adulthood the headache was manageable without medications and with minimal medical attention. The primary behavioral reinforcing events for the headache complaint therefore appear to be (1) avoidance of stressful marital or environmental situations and (2) increased attention from others. A possible secondary reinforcer may be the conditioned use of narcotics in a failed effort to control the headache.

The following treatment course of action was undertaken:

1. It was agreed that the best course of treatment was to use as little narcotic medication as possible. Even though narcotics were found to be useful by the patient, she recognized their addictive potential and agreed to use them only with the direction of the primary care physician. Patient and physician medication management responsibilities were also outlined.
2. It was agreed that the patient would not seek additional medical evaluation or treatment without discussing it with her primary physician first.
3. The primary physician agreed to be available within a 12-hour period of being contacted about a headache to discuss the headache and the possible situation surrounding it. It was agreed that these conversations were to last no longer than 5–10 minutes.
4. An effort was made to encourage active participation: A course of biofeedback training and instruction in neck exercises was arranged to place a share of control with the patient.
5. A family conference affirmed to all that the headaches were to be treated as both symptoms of stress and as problems in themselves.
6. If this plan did not show significant benefit in a specified time, referral to a pain center would be made.
7. Finally, the physician would be available for treatment of other medical complaints.

In this way, the primary care physician redefined the headache complaint: It does not need immediate or intensive medical care, it does not need further diagnostic evaluation, and it does not need different medication trials. By establishing a meaningful relationship with the patient, acknowledging the severity of her complaint, setting clear expectations for how to respond to symptoms, and securing the patient's commitment to work within these limitations, a framework for pain management was agreed on. Appropriate referral for pain management to a pain control program or a psychologist for psychotherapy should be the next contingency plan.

CHRONIC INTRACTABLE PAIN: CHRONIC LOW BACK PAIN

Case illustration 3: Michael is a 45-year-old man with known controlled hypertension, who presented with low back pain. He reported that while working on a farm a year ago, he experienced a motor vehicle accident, resulting in a herniated disc in his lumbar spine. A lumbar laminectomy and discectomy followed with some recovery for approximately 3 months. Since that time he had been seen twice a week for 6 weeks for passive physical therapy (hot packs, ultrasound massage, gentle stretching) and provided additional pain medication, including oral narcotics and anti-inflammatories by his surgeon. He had not returned to work since the day of injury and was currently involved in vocational rehabilitation.

On physical examination the patient was tender to palpation across his low back bilaterally. Passive straight leg raising was normal. Sharp, dull, and light touch sensation were intact throughout, with symmetric reflexes in both lower extremities.

Imaging studies revealed old surgical repair of a herniated disc without other abnormalities. Recent nerve conduction studies were unremarkable for nerve slowing. The patient's surgeon, who had "nothing more to offer," referred him back to his primary care physician for continued treatment.

Chronic low back pain commonly displays the characteristics seen here:

1. Subjective complaint of pain without substantial objective findings.
2. Prominent pain behaviors (eg, avoidance of work).
3. Use of "passive" instead of "active" physical therapy.
4. Continued use of narcotic medication to manage the pain.

Case illustration 3 (Contd.): The patient went on to report that he spends much of the day sitting in his reclining chair in front of the television set either watching television or reading. He moves from the chair two or three times each day, primarily for meals. He frequently naps during the day and reports disrupted sleep at night, averaging 5–6 hours. He feels depressed, hopeless about his recovery, and believes that unless his pain is relieved he will be unable to return to work. He acknowledges that his spouse and children are angry with him and his inability to return to work.

On further questioning it is discovered that the social "cost" of the pain behavior is high. Michael's daily activities are greatly impaired, his self-esteem and affect have plummeted, and he is further emotionally isolated from his family by his pain. In such a circumstance where a patient's pain behaviors are well entrenched the doctor must accurately establish the expectations for recovery and the outcome of treatment. Because the patient is probably still focused on the pain as a continuation of the original precipitating event, it becomes necessary to identify and deal more with the patient's pain behaviors.

Although Michael reported feelings of depression, it is inaccurate to say that the pain is caused by the depression. It has been shown, however, that the intensity of pain often diminishes with a trial of an antidepressant medication.

The treatment for chronic low back pain is primarily focused on improving patients' activity level, diminishing their reliance on medications, and reducing pain behaviors (eg, changing the focus of treatment from decreasing pain-limiting activities to increasing activity level for meaningful tasks). In this way the doctor assists in "managing" the pain behavior.

After a careful explanation by the doctor of the anatomy, physiology, and probable cause of Michael's low back pain, a collaborative discussion followed, leading to an agreement on the following treatment plan:

1. A course of physical therapy using primarily active exercises (eg, aerobic, walking, strengthening, and stretching), would be started. In addition, the patient agreed to take progressively longer walks each day. It was expected that with increased activity there would be an initial increase in pain. For that reason, it was agreed that the patient could continue to use his analgesic medication for a short time.
2. Analgesic oral medication was placed on a time-contingent basis, extending the number of hours between pills without increasing the dose. This regimen avoided linking the patient's pain behavior with the timing and amount of dosing. This was managed through weekly dispensing of the medications through the pharmacy. It was agreed that any request for change in his medication regimen would be directed only to the doctor, not emergency rooms or other physicians.
3. The patient would be seen once monthly by the doctor. It was agreed that after the first 4 weeks of physical therapy, a medication taper would begin, reducing the number of pills taken over a 3-week period to zero. A primary focus of future visits would be discussion about daily activities or return to work goals rather than the pain.
4. If, by the end of the second month, functional activity levels were not substantially greater,

progress toward return to work was not made, or he was not yet off narcotic medication, then referral to a pain management facility would be made.

The doctor has now, in collaboration with the patient, established the parameters of treatment, clarified the expected outcomes in terms of function, discontinued the use of narcotic medications, and progressed toward meaningful employment goals. These steps define the treatment effort to reducing pain behaviors. In this way the doctor becomes a "change agent." Patients who respond favorably to treatment of pain behavior usually report either that the pain is significantly reduced or that it does not bother them as much as it used to. When pain behavior is more entrenched (the patient is unresponsive to treatment) early referral to a comprehensive pain management facility is indicated. Treatment in a pain management facility is typically intensive and primarily involves the reduction in pain behaviors and increase in functional activities. The variety of techniques used to increase functional activity include active physical therapy, improved physical tolerances often through occupational therapy, biofeedback, cognitive behavior therapy, management of medications, stress management techniques, relaxation counseling, hypnotherapy, transcutaneous nerve stimulation, vocational counseling, and coping skills training. Treatment is typically offered 6–8 hours/day, 5 days/week, for 3–4 weeks with active follow-up. At the end of treatment patients are usually referred back to their primary care provider with specific recommendations for future treatment or management.

Use of counseling for treatment of depression, marital therapy for treatment of marital difficulties, and nutritional counseling for dieting in addition to behavioral treatments for pain (Table 30–5) are useful adjunctive therapies that can be added to the treatment regimen.

Table 30–5. Behavioral treatment methods for pain.

- **Biofeedback:** Computer-assisted measurement of physiologic changes previously thought to be involuntary, for the purposes of training the patient to bring them into voluntary control. Measurements often include surface electromyelography, temperature, galvanic skin response, respiration, pulse transit time, and distal plesmography.
- **Autogenic training:** A series of mental exercises designed to produce relaxation imagery that may be guided by a practitioner through suggestion or can be coupled with relaxation and exercises.
- **Progressive muscle relaxation:** A systematic approach to relaxation exercises involving the tensing and relaxing of muscle groups from head to foot.
- **Hypnosis:** A state of enhanced focus or awareness that can lead to increased levels of suggestibility. This can be helpful in the blocking of painful sensation. (hypnoanalgesia).
- **Cognitive behavioral therapy:** The approach often involves the monitoring of automatic thoughts that are negative; recognizing the connections between thoughts, affect, and behavior; and altering and replacing dysfunctional thoughts with more reality oriented interpretations.

CHRONIC PROGRESSIVE PAIN: PAIN IN CANCER PATIENTS

> *Case illustration 4:* Jorge is a 58-year-old Hispanic man who was diagnosed with colon cancer, Dukes stage C, 18 months before presenting with progressive weight loss and right upper quadrant pain. Chemistries and imaging studies confirmed multiple metastases in his liver. He was increasingly fatigued and was forced to leave his job as an electronics technician. He now reported his pain to be expanding to include the entire abdomen, present constantly, but worse in the evening and with any activities. He was married with five children, and his spouse was employed. They arranged a schedule to allow at least one of his children to be present to help him and his wife each day. Despite this help, he was becoming increasingly incapacitated and complained of pain with minor tasks. His family was concerned that he was "always in pain and losing the will to live."

Cancer pain represents another physical and psychological challenge to primary care providers and patients alike. Often pain is an outgrowth of simple tissue destruction by advancing tumor mass. Accompanying this, however, is the progressive loss of "hardiness" (strength, independence, and social identity) that accompanies the cancer. Patients often believe that cancer is a painful condition; for example, it has been shown that sciatic pain hurts more by verbal report and requires more analgesia after a malignant diagnosis is made. In addition, the patient suffers changes in a number of key roles in the face of the disease. As Jorge gives up the roles of parent, spouse, and worker, his pain behavior increases to match his new dependency. Finally, anxiety about both deteriorating health and family responses increases the pain.

> *Case Illustration 4 (Contd.):* A meeting with the patient and family was scheduled specifically to address the issue of pain. A careful and complete examination to evaluate all pain complaints was performed. The family's concerns were also solicited. Finally, the concepts of cancer pain treatment were reviewed, with an explanation of the importance of identifying and dealing with biological, social, and psychological issues that affect the pain. At the time of this examination, only abdominal pain with radiation to the back was identified as a limiting pain.

Although cancer has a devastating and lasting effect on family function, involving the family in treatment decisions and planning is crucial. In many families, including many Hispanic families, it is particularly important to identify the head of the household as well as primary caregiver. In this case, although Jorge is the head of the household, it is customary that once he becomes sick he be cared for by the family and that he take on a sick role. It becomes important, therefore, to involve his spouse, who is the primary person in charge of caregiving, in discussions involving treatment decisions and planning.

An early discussion of the effect of the pain on the patient and his family is key to the collaborative treatment of pain. If they do not understand how the physician needs to integrate treatment as an aspect of daily life, the patient and family often feel that reports of pain are being discounted or diminished. Similarly, soliciting and supporting the use of home and cultural remedies can further this communication and collaboration (see Chapter 13). Medications to control cancer pain must be used effectively, regularly, and in adequate doses. Narcotics should be used around the clock in long-acting form rather than on a PRN basis. PRN medications encourage both patient and family to gauge the pain, thus providing an unnecessary focus on the pain. The use of inadequate pain medication also sets up a distrustful resentment between patient and physician. Specific adjunctive medication can be used to afford more relief with less sedation (NSAIDs for bone pain, steroids for pain associated with local inflammation and edema, baclofen (Lioresal) for muscle spasm, sedatives for insomnia).

Cognitive-behavioral interventions can be tailored to the specific family and cultural circumstances of the patient. In the case of Jorge, his family expects him to yield his roles and need help as his disease and pain behavior increase. Therapy can thus be directed to both patient and family with the goal of increasing the patient's independence and decreasing the family's tendency to respond to all of his pain behaviors with fear. In addition, Jorge believes that cancer is painful and disabling, neither of which is to be tolerated. This attitude engenders helplessness and suffering. Behavior therapy could address this belief with techniques to provide control over his pain, such as a single-symptom autogenic training, relaxation, hypnosis, or cognitive behavioral therapy. For example, the patient can be trained to interpret sensations as routine rather than threatening. In this way, he and his family can learn to accept rather than potentially distort his disease and pain.

SUMMARY

In this chapter we presented an approach to the treatment of persons suffering various types of pain that emphasizes the evaluation and treatment of not only the biologic, but also the psychologic and social implications of the problem.

The primary care physician is encouraged to make good use of the three-function model for interviewing and ongoing communications with his or her patient. Key factors to attend to in the treatment of pain are:

- **Identifying pain as an issue:** Deal with it in a comprehensive medical and psychologic way at onset, instead of when it becomes a problem.

■ **Pain behaviors:** Whereas the patient may be quick to understand the pain largely as derived from the precipitating event or factors, the treating physician must always attend to the social consequences of the pain and its implications in the life of the patient at work, at home, and in play.

■ **Meaning of the pain:** Cultural influences may dictate differing attitudes and roles in the expression of the pain.

■ **Doctor as "change agent":** In addition to providing direct treatment and advice, the doctor, through the patient-doctor relationship, can improve adherence to treatment.

■ **Function-, not dysfunction-oriented:** The interests and attention of the doctor influence greatly the thoughts and behaviors of the patient. By commenting on improved functioning as an indicator of healing, the doctor can redirect the patient's attention away from pain and toward increased functioning.

SUGGESTED READING

Bonica T (editor): *The Management of Pain.* Vols. 1 and 2, 2nd ed. Lea & Febiger, 1990.

Cutler R et al: Does nonsurgical pain center treatment of chronic pain return patients to work? Spine 1994; 19(6):643.

Fields H, Liebeskind, J (editors): *Pharmacological Approaches to the Treatment of Chronic Pain: Concepts and Critical Issues.* IASP Press, 1994.

Fishbain DA et al: Types of pain treatment facilities and referral selection criteria. Arch Family Med 1995;4:58.

Fishman B, Luscalzo M: Cognitive-behavioral intervention in management of cancer pain: Principles and applications. Med Clin North Am 1987;71(2):271.

Fordyce WE (editor): *Behavioral Methods in Chronic Pain and Illness.* Mosby, 1976.

Jacox A et al: *Management of Cancer Pain,* No. 9. AHCPR Publication. 94-0592. Rockville, MD. Agency for Health Care Policy and Research, US Department of Health and Human Services, Public Health Service, March 1994.

Kobasa SC: Stressful life events, personality, and health: An inquiry into hardiness. J Pers Soc Psychol 1979;37:1.

Maddi SR, Kobasa SC (editors): *The Hardy Executive: Health Under Stress.* Dow-Jones-Irwin, 1984.

Merskey H, Bogduk N (editors): *Classification of Chronic Pain. Description of Chronic Pain Syndrome and Definitions of Pain Terms,* 2nd ed. IASP Press, 1994.

Sullivan MD et al: Chronic pain in primary care. J Family Prac 1991;32(2)193.

Turk D, Meichenbaum D, Genest M (editors): *Pain and Behavioral Medicine: A Cognitive Behavioral Perspective.* Guilford Press, 1983.

31

HIV/AIDS

Jeffrey H. Burack, MD, MPP, BPhil, Mitchell D. Feldman, MD, MPhil, & Thomas J. Coates, PhD

INTRODUCTION

Infection with the human immunodeficiency virus (HIV) is associated with a daunting range of social, emotional, and neuropsychiatric complications. Despite encouraging developments in the treatment of HIV infection and its sequelae, progression to the acquired immunodeficiency syndrome (AIDS) and to premature death are generally viewed as inevitable. Persons at highest risk for HIV/AIDS (we use the term HIV/AIDS to designate the entire spectrum of clinical manifestations of HIV disease, from asymptomatic infection through advanced AIDS) are disproportionately likely to suffer behavioral and mood disorders and to be socially disenfranchised and economically disadvantaged. Once infected, they must contend with a widely feared and stigmatized, contagious, and often progressively debilitating medical condition; the loss of capabilities and bodily integrity; multiple bereavements and stressors; and their own suffering and mortality. Finally, HIV may cause organic neuropsychiatric disease in a variety of ways: by directly infecting the central nervous system (CNS); by disabling the immune system, thereby opening the door to opportunistic infections and neoplasms that may in turn involve or affect the CNS; and as a result of the medications and therapies used in treatment of the virus and its complications.

EPIDEMIOLOGY

It is estimated that 700,000–900,000 US residents (around 0.3% of the population) are currently infected with HIV, and about 60,000 persons are infected annually in the United States. Half of these new infections occur in persons younger than 25, one

fourth in persons younger than 22, and 1 out of 92 young Americans between the ages of 27 and 39 is infected with HIV. Each year, around 60,000 Americans are diagnosed with an AIDS-related opportunistic infection, and through 1996, more than 350,000 persons residing in the United States who were diagnosed with AIDS had died. AIDS is the leading cause of death among all Americans aged 25 to 44, irrespective of race or gender, and in fact, heterosexual transmission of HIV infection, especially to women, is rising exponentially. Women have been increasingly affected by AIDS in recent years; there are now more AIDS cases among women secondary to heterosexual exposure than as a result of injection drug use. Although AIDS in the United States affects primarily young, urban adults, every state has reported at least one case, and 10% of cases have been reported in adults 55 years and older. Among men, two thirds of cases are in homosexual and bisexual men, with less than 5% reporting heterosexual exposure as their sole risk factor.

Some groups in the United States have borne a disproportionate share of the burden of HIV infection, and the gap between those most affected and the rest of the US population continues to widen. For example, HIV/AIDS disproportionately affects Hispanics and African-Americans, and fully half of the 60,000 new annual infections occurring in the United States are the result of drug users sharing injection equipment. One quarter of new infections occur as a result of heterosexual transmission from injection drug users to their sexual partners. Although some success has occurred through education, as demonstrated with the reduction in homosexual transmission among white men over age 30, HIV incidence continues at unacceptably high rates among young gay men, gay men of color, and men who inject drugs. Hemophiliacs have a high seroprevalence rate, but they make up only about 1% of the total cases reported to date.

Clearly, HIV infection is a major public health problem in the United States, one that all primary care practitioners must become competent in treating.

THE PSYCHOSOCIAL EFFECTS OF HIV/AIDS

OVERVIEW

Although the course of HIV/AIDS is different for every patient, certain clinical and life events may be reliably anticipated to provoke negative psychological consequences, ranging from mild anxiety and discouragement to devastation and suicide. Bereavement may occur at any time in the course of illness, and particularly for members of high-prevalence communities, losses of friends and loved ones may be repeated and frequent, allowing little time for emotional recovery between episodes of grieving. Rejection and ostracism by family and community may occur when they learn of one's HIV infection. Persons with HIV/AIDS may also suffer discrimination in employment, education, housing, and health care. Later in the course of illness, one may have to deal with the loss of employment or a reduction in responsibilities, consequent financial hardships compounded by heavy medical expenses, and dislocation or alienation from established social networks. Fatigue, pain, and other symptoms may diminish quality of life. Weight loss and disfiguring skin lesions may lead to loss of pride, self-image, and bodily integrity. Increasing disability may require a loss of independence and even a move to a residential facility.

The stress of these life events is superimposed on a predictably distressing series of clinical milestones in the progression of HIV infection. These include serologic diagnosis, threshold changes in surrogate markers, the onset of symptoms, diagnosis of serious complications, and approaching death. Any one of these milestones may precipitate a crisis of fear or despair. At each, the physician must proactively explore the patient's understanding of and emotional response to the change in status, and be prepared to intervene with counseling or other therapy aimed at reducing depression or anxiety. The very decision to seek serologic testing may result from anxiety, for example over being informed that a former sexual partner is infected, or from worrisome symptoms, or may instead reflect a positive decision to take control over one's health. It may in any case be followed closely by the devastating discovery that one has been infected with the virus oneself, or is HIV-positive. Even those who test negative may not be spared adverse emotional consequences: many, for example, suffer survivor guilt, particularly if a spouse, partner, or other loved one has tested positive.

COUNSELING PATIENTS WHO TEST POSITIVE FOR HIV

HIV infection is generally diagnosed when an enzyme-linked immunosorbent assay (ELISA) is reactive and confirmed by a Western blot test positive for the presence of HIV antibody. Patients tested in the potential "window period" of 6 months after possible exposure should be offered repeat testing if they are seronegative. By 6 months after exposure, 95% of infected patients should test positive; measurement of viral load allows for earlier diagnosis.

Patients who test positive for the presence of HIV may experience and express a variety of emotional responses (see Chapter 3). In general, the primary care provider should allow the patient to express his or her feelings, and should actively listen to the expressed emotions in a nonjudgmental manner. Effective use of empathic statements such as: "I can understand how difficult this must be for you" and "We can work on this together" can help the patient to feel a little less overwhelmed and helpless when presented with a positive test result.

The range of emotions expressed by patients are as varied as the patients themselves. Therefore, clinicians should be alert to the potential range of emotional responses expressed by patients and then check their understanding with a reflective statement such as "You seem sort of frightened by this news." Often, the emotion that unexpectedly wells up in the physician (eg, sadness, anger, panic) is indicative of what the patient is also feeling. The physician should use these personal emotions as diagnostic information to help gain insight into the patient's feelings.

Paradoxically, although many persons seek testing to resolve the uncertainty of not knowing their status, testing positive can create additional uncertainty. This can be quite unsettling for patients, especially those for whom maintaining tight control over their lives has been highly valued. Suddenly they are confronted with not knowing how long they will remain well, who will care for them if they become ill or debilitated, how they will support themselves, and many other unknowns. The physician can help the patient cope with this sudden uncertainty by providing both information and emotional support. It may be helpful to say: "Many people who test positive are concerned because they do not know what to expect—is this true for you?" Some patients are comforted by the physician's acknowledgment that they are the same persons they were before the test, but now they have information that can be addressed. For example, the clinician can say: "You are the same person today as you were yesterday, only now you *know* that you are HIV-positive. It is important that you have this information so that we can now work on keeping you healthy for as long as possible." Patients should be given up-to-date information about treatment, prognosis, and other medical data, especially if they request it. It has been shown that distress can be decreased if patients are informed about their disease and the treatment options.

Physicians should also remember that informing patients of their HIV status is different from informing them of other medical illnesses because of the stigma still associated with AIDS. This may be especially true for gay men who also have to deal with the social and personal consequence of being gay, such as discrimination, homophobia, and feelings of shame and isolation. It may be important to address these issues of social stigma and shame to help patients cope with their seropositive status. Referral for individual counseling is often helpful.

Other emotions that the seropositive patient may express include anger, fear, denial, and depression. Patients may feel angry for many reasons: about having an incurable illness, about perceived loss of control, about current or future discrimination. Allow patients to express their anger and frustration; often the anger dissipates with empathic listening alone.

Fear is often a less evident emotion and may need to be elicited with questions such as: "What are your major fears about HIV?" and "From your experience with other people with HIV, what kinds of things are most frightening for you?" Seropositive persons may fear loss of job, friends, or health insurance or have more global fears of declining health, increasing pain, or becoming a burden on family or friends.

These fears should be acknowledged as legitimate, and when possible, the physician can help the patient to deal concretely with those problems that can be anticipated and ameliorated. It may be helpful to have the patient make two lists: one with all of the current or anticipated problems that are to some extent controllable and another list of those that are basically uncontrollable. The controllable problems can be addressed through specific **problem-solving** strategies, but the clinician should focus on **emotion-handling skills** for the basically uncontrollable problems and emotions that arise (see Chapters 1 and 2).

Denial is a common response to the news of a positive HIV test. For some patients this may initially be a healthy way of not allowing themselves to be overwhelmed by potentially devastating information. In fact, most people need several months to a year just to come to terms with the diagnosis. If, however, denial leads patients to harm themselves (for example, by refusing potentially life-enhancing or life-extending treatment) or to harm others by exposing them to HIV, the physician needs to challenge the denial. This can be done gently, for example, by saying "I wish that you were not infected," but such statements may need to be repeated at subsequent visits until the patient is ready to accept the fact and consequences of seropositive status.

Depression and anxiety are also common responses in persons who test positive for HIV. The clinician should assess the severity and duration of these symptoms to determine the appropriate treatment. Some studies have found that the risk of suicide is substantially increased in the 3–6 months following a serologic diagnosis, so all patients should be screened for suicidal ideation. It is best to use direct, nonjudgmental questions: "Do you find yourself thinking about dying or death?" "Do you think about taking your own life?"

In the weeks and months following a positive test, the provider can assist patients in coping more effectively by assessing the inpatient's social support system and helping them to reset goals. Providers should assess their patients' support system very early in the disease process. This can be done simply by asking: "If you were to get sick, who could you rely on to help?" "Who can you talk to about your concerns and issues?" If patients are isolated, provide them with phone numbers of local AIDS service organizations. Family members can also provide valuable support, but often HIV-infected people avoid seeking their help, or the family has previously rejected them because of their lifestyle.

Resetting of goals can be a valuable coping strategy for the seropositive person. The physician can play a crucial role in helping people to understand that although their disease may limit their experience, they can continue to have a life worth living. Long-term survivors who adjust to their disease and develop goals and patterns that are achievable report a higher quality of life than those long-term survivors who are unable to adjust. As the patient's HIV disease progresses, the provider can continue to ask: "What is it that gives you satisfaction now?" Helping patients to focus on things that are pleasurable helps them to redirect attention to these activities and maintain a satisfactory quality of life.

WORKING WITH ASYMPTOMATIC & SYMPTOMATIC PATIENTS

Most persons remain asymptomatic for 5–10 years after infection with HIV. During this stage, regular preventive medical care generally includes periodic testing of surrogate markers of disease progression, particularly CD4 lymphocyte, or T-cell, counts, and increasingly RNA or DNA measures of circulating viral burden. Waiting for and receiving the results of a T-cell count can be intensely stressful. Physicians must be careful to counsel patients prior to testing about the day-to-day, even hour-to-hour variability in the test, about the limited clinical significance of a one-time change in counts, and about plans for repeat testing or otherwise following up in the event of specific results. Nevertheless, the clinician must anticipate that, despite reassurances, any decline in CD4 count may be deeply discouraging and viewed as ominous. This is particularly true when the CD4 count drops below one of the thresholds, which, although perhaps serving only as rules of thumb to experienced physicians, within our current understanding still represent momentous clinical benchmarks in the course of HIV/AIDS and are understood to do so by many patients. These include a CD4 count of 500/mm³, at which many experts recommend initiating antiretroviral therapy and below which symptoms are much more likely; 200/mm³, which presently confers an automatic diagnosis of AIDS and below which the risk of opportunistic infections increases dramatically; and 50/mm³, below which expected survival is measured in months and the risks are high of severe complications and disability.

The initial onset of HIV-related symptoms, although perhaps expected by and of little prognostic importance to the physician, may be extremely upsetting to the person with HIV. The first experience of oral thrush or hairy leukoplakia, night sweats, or diarrhea, or the appearance of lesions of Kaposi's sarcoma, may require recognition for the first time of being sick. Prior to this moment, HIV may have been an abstraction, a risk factor, a concern for the future; now it has suddenly become a "condition," an essential and life-threatening feature of the person. Fear, anxiety, sadness, depression, rage, and denial may all be appropriate responses, and the physician must be prepared to intervene. Crisis counseling provides a useful model. It asserts that it is important for patients to experience, express, and receive empathy for emotions and also to make specific plans for coping. Making specific and detailed plans helps sustain a sense of control over one's illness and one's life. The physician should be prepared to refer the patient to available community support and self-help services.

The diagnosis of AIDS, based on a low CD4 count or the occurrence of any of a number of serious opportunistic complications of immunosuppression, may be another such time of crisis. Patients can no longer take comfort in having HIV but not AIDS; society classifies and treats them differently, and indeed the mortality statistics begin to look grim and menacing. Patients at this stage are likely to be taking multiple medications, which may have neuropsychological toxicities or disturbing or uncomfortable side-effects. Particularly important are efforts to maintain hope, energy, and dignity in the face of inexorably progressive illness, which the physician must support, all the while balancing these efforts against the obligations to give accurate and relevant clinical information and to intervene speedily to detect and treat new problems. It is therefore often around this point that not only the patient but also the physician can benefit from increased social support. Developing a multidisciplinary management team not only permits appropriate expertise to be brought to bear on the patient's various medical, personal, and social problems, but also allows team members to share ideas and emotions, to validate and support one another, and to offer mutual aid and relief when issues become overwhelming (see Chapter 8).

Persons with advanced AIDS are often battling multiple chronic infections and may suffer from HIV-associated dementia or wasting syndrome. They may be contending simultaneously with a multitude of physical, emotional, and spiritual ailments, not least of them the dying process and the approach of death itself. Specific issues related to the care of dying persons are covered in Chapter 35. This is often a period of reconciliation with significant persons and of arranging one's material and spiritual affairs. Ensuring access to palliative and pastoral care, as well as to appropriate legal, financial, and social services, becomes essential to routine management. It is well established both that physicians often provide inadequate pain relief to their dying patients, but also that suffering as death approaches is complex, metaphysical, and not limited exclusively or even primarily to physical pain. Physicians caring for patients with advanced HIV/AIDS must become expert in the exploration and relief of suffering. Patients commonly request assistance with suicide, or even active euthanasia. Above all, however, dying persons fear abandonment; this is particularly true for those dying of a socially stigmatized disease, who have often been shunned by the broader society and bereaved of or abandoned by loved ones. As the goals of medical care evolve away from curing illness and toward easing death, physicians must diligently and explicitly reinforce their commitment to caring for their patients to the end, come what may, and reassure them that there is much that can be done to assist in the relief of suffering (see Chapter 35).

Case illustration: Ernesto is a 39-year-old gay Salvadoran-American architect with HIV infection and a CD4 count of 140/mm³. He has a history of oral thrush and takes a protease inhibitor, zidovudine, trimethoprim-sulfamethoxazole, and fluconazole. He has used methamphetamine in the past. One year ago, his partner of 12 years died of AIDS after a protracted struggle with HIV-associated dementia which left him bed-bound, mute, and diapered. Over the last several months, Ernesto has noticed difficulty concentrating at work, has been more irritable and withdrawn, and has lost weight. Several coworkers have mentioned that he seems "not himself," and one suggested that his comments at an important meeting had been "off the wall" and had caused the loss of a major client. Twice in the past month Ernesto has found himself standing on a street corner, not knowing how he got there. Fearing that he was becoming demented and would lose his job if the truth were known, he did not seek medical care, but instead doubled his zidovudine dose and stopped taking his other medications.

Five days ago Ernesto staggered and fell at home, striking his head on a table. In the emergency room, where he went to have his laceration sutured, he was diagnosed with dehydration and depression, and given a prescription for fluoxetine. Today, he has come to see his primary care physician to have his sutures removed. He complains of a headache and a cough. The physician notes a temperature of 39 °C, rapid respirations, weight loss of 10 kg over the past 3 months, cervical lymphadenopathy, oral thrush, and pulmonary rales. The patient is slow to respond to questions and shows poor concentration on the mini-mental status examination. The chest roentgenogram is suggestive of *Pneumocystis carinii* pneumonia. Arterial blood gas shows a pO_2 of 72 mm Hg. His physician sends him home with prescriptions for trimethoprim-sulfamethoxazole and prednisone.

Two days later, he is brought back to the emergency room by the police, who found him standing on the street in soiled clothing, yelling incoherently and threateningly at passersby. The emergency room physician notes a temperature of 38.7 °C, an unsteady gait, a hemoglobin of 8 g/dL, and a serum sodium of 122 mEq/L. Ernesto appears delirious and disoriented. Computed tomography of the head with contrast reveals diffuse meningeal enhancement and mild hydrocephalus. Because the patient cannot give consent, he is restrained so that a lumbar puncture can be performed. Analysis of the cerebrospinal fluid reveals elevated protein, decreased glucose, and a lymphocytic pleocytosis with 167 cells/mm³. Cryptococcal antigen and India ink preparation are negative, as are treponemal tests and Gram's and acid fast stains. Ernesto is admitted, and empiric therapy is begun for tuberculous meningitis. Fiberoptic bronchoscopy is performed the next day and reveals both *Pneumocystis* and *Mycobacterium tuberculosis.* His delirium, headache, and hyponatremia resolve rapidly, and he is discharged 2 weeks later.

Ernesto is seen by his physician in follow-up 3 weeks after discharge. He continues to take three antituberculous drugs—isoniazid, rifampin, and pyrazinamide—in addition to his regular medications. His neurologic and mental status examinations are normal, and his respiratory symptoms have resolved. He continues to report difficulty concentrating and solving complex problems, however. He has had to stop working, has trouble sleeping, has little interest in socializing, and is preoccupied by thoughts of his deceased partner. He feels hopeless and discouraged. The physician considers stopping his isoniazid but is concerned that his tuberculosis might relapse. Instead, he initiates treatment for depression with nortriptyline. Two months later, his depression has resolved, though he is still unemployed and feels his mental acuity has never returned to normal.

Ernesto's case illustrates several important principles in the evaluation and management of psychological, behavioral, and cognitive abnormalities in persons with HIV/AIDS:

1. Always consider and exclude **secondary CNS pathology** and, particularly, treatable conditions.
2. Always consider **drug effects** and interactions.
3. Be aware of the clinical presentation, diagnosis, and management of **primary HIV disease** of the CNS.
4. Psychiatric and behavioral problems are often **multifactorial:** just because CNS disease is

present, for example, doesn't mean that depression is not present as well.
5. Treatment for psychiatric and behavioral problems is generally undertaken with the **same interventions** and pharmacological agents and is guided by the same principles as are standard for non-HIV-infected persons, with the few exceptions to be described later on based primarily on drug toxicity.
6. Be aware of the **complex psychosocial context** in which any HIV-related pathology arises.

MANAGEMENT OF NEUROPSYCHIATRIC COMPLICATIONS OF HIV/AIDS

SECONDARY CNS PATHOLOGY

Many AIDS-associated infections or neoplasms of the CNS may first present with neuropsychiatric manifestations. Earlier in the course of HIV/AIDS, patients are at risk for primary HIV meningitis, neurovascular syphilis, and meningitides due to *Mycobacterium tuberculosis, Streptococcus pneumoniae,* and other pathogenic bacteria. As immunosuppression advances, and particularly as the CD4 count falls below approximately 200/mm³, the risk of opportunistic complications increases, most notably meningitis caused by *Cryptococcus neoformans,* encephalitis due to *Toxoplasma gondii,* cytomegalovirus and other herpesviruses, primary CNS lymphoma, brain abscesses due to disseminated bacterial or fungal infection, and progressive multifocal leukoencephalopathy (PML), believed to be caused by a papovavirus. Presentation of any of these conditions may be subtle. Most often, but not always, other suggestive signs or symptoms are present, such as headache, meningismus, or fever in meningitis; focal neurologic deficits associated with space-occupying CNS lesions; or other organ system manifestations of infection. The first questions the physician ought to ask, then, when confronted with a significant change in level of consciousness, behavior, cognition, or even mood are: What secondary CNS complications of HIV/AIDS could possibly be present, and what must be done to identify or exclude them?

DRUG EFFECTS

Many of the innumerable medications used to treat HIV/AIDS and its complications have common neuropsychiatric side effects. Some are new drugs for which toxicity profiles are not yet fully understood. Patients, particularly with advanced AIDS, often take many medications simultaneously, some of which may interact and exacerbate one another's toxicities. Toxicities may be related to cumulative dose or to circulating levels but alternatively can be unpredictable and idiosyncratic. Furthermore, the homeostatic mechanisms responsible for maintaining therapeutic drug levels, may be disrupted by end organ involvement, such as decreased renal excretion, hepatic metabolism, or cardiac output; diminished body fat; immunologic dysregulation; and a predisposition toward dehydration. Patients are therefore more susceptible even to the side effects of more commonly used medications. The rule of thumb for prescribing ought to be "say no, start low, and go slow": avoid unnecessary medications, use reduced dosages of those that are necessary, and increase doses slowly and cautiously.

Drug effects and toxicities must always be considered in the initial differential diagnosis of any neuropsychiatric abnormality. Table 31–1 describes the adverse reactions associated with some drugs commonly used in the treatment of HIV/AIDS. A few general principles ought to be borne in mind. First, alternative agents should be selected or dosages adjusted in cases of known renal, hepatic, or cardiac dysfunction. For example, patients on renal dialysis usually require smaller doses, and dosing must be timed carefully around dialysis if it is essential to maintain consistent circulating drug levels. Second, caution must be used in the coadministration of medications with similar side effect profiles or those that significantly affect one another's pharmacodynamics. An example of the first situation is the simultaneous use of any combination of antidepressants, antihistamines, neuroleptics, or antimotility agents, all of which have substantial anticholinergic effects. The second concern arises in the use of agents such as rifampin, which induces the hepatic cytochrome P450 enzyme system and thereby accelerates metabolism of many other drugs. Third, adherence to complex medication regimens may be difficult and distasteful. Incorrect dosing may result in undertreatment for some conditions, but confusion may also result in inadvertent overdosing. Every effort must be made to simplify the regimen and to use the lowest doses of the fewest drugs likely to be effective. The assistance of a pharmacist is invaluable in sorting out these concerns. If possible, the regimens of patients with advanced HIV/AIDS should be periodically reviewed by a pharmacist for possible interactions and toxicities, redundancy, and appropriateness of dosing.

Establishing a drug as the cause of a neuropsychiatric abnormality can be difficult, as there is most often no definitive test available to do so. The physician must be attuned to the temporal relationship between the onset or exacerbation of symptoms on the one hand, and any new medications or dosage increases on the other. In cases in which the temporal relationship suggests causation and the symptom is a known common effect of the drug, the drug can be discontinued or reduced in dose. In less well defined circumstances, the physician's initial strategy might include stopping all nonessential drugs. Most drug-induced neuropsychiatric side effects resolve within several days of stopping the agent. If necessary, medications can be added back one by one. Recurrence of symptoms after rechallenge strongly suggests a causal relationship. Consultation with a pharmacist or psychiatrist might be helpful in more perplexing cases.

Finally, there may be other pharmacological causes of neuropsychiatric disturbances, including alternative or nontraditional medical therapies and use of alcohol or illicit substances. The toxicities of most nontraditional therapies have not been well studied, but it is likely, for example, that plant alkaloids present in many herbal or "natural" remedies have psychoactive properties. The physician must be prepared to explore the use of such therapies in a nonthreatening manner. Persons with HIV/AIDS on average have higher levels of substance abuse, in part because of the association between preexisting drug use and the risk of acquiring HIV, and perhaps because of self-medication for depression or anxiety. Stimulant drugs such as cocaine or amphetamines can cause agitation, psychosis, or delirium, as can withdrawal from sedating drugs such as benzodiazepines and alcohol. Sedatives and narcotics can of course cause somnolence, confusion, and psychomotor slowing but can also cause paradoxical reactions, including agitation, paranoia, and rage. This may be especially true of the short-acting benzodiazepines, including triazolam (Halcion) and alprazolam (Xanax).

PSYCHIATRIC COMPLICATIONS

Depression

Major depression is the most common psychiatric diagnosis for persons with HIV/AIDS. The lifetime incidence is unknown but rises dramatically as the disease progresses. As with non-HIV-infected depressed patients, the cardinal symptoms include depressed mood, anhedonia, feelings of worthlessness and hopelessness, disturbances in sleep and appetite, weight loss or gain, fatigue, psychomotor slowing, agitation, and preoccupation with morbid thoughts. A family history of an affective disorder or alcoholism may be present. Depression may be more difficult to diagnose in the presence of HIV/AIDS, however, for several reasons. First, its manifestations, and particularly the vegetative symptoms of fatigue, weakness, weight loss, and loss of libido, overlap with the constitutional symptoms commonly attributable to HIV infection or its supervening complications. Second, the multiple losses that many persons with HIV/AIDS endure may result in a chronic grieving state that shares many of

Table 31–1. Psychiatric side effects of drugs used to treat HIV infection

Drugs	Adverse Reaction	Comment
Antiretrovirals		
Zidovudine (AZT)	Mania, anxiety, auditory hallucinations, confusion	Idiosyncratic reaction; resolves within 24 h after stopping drug
Didanosine (ddl)	Anxiety, irritability,	Idiosyncratic reaction; self-limiting, does not require drug
Zalcitabine	insomnia	discontinuation
Antivirals		
Acyclovir	Lethargy, delirium, hallucinations,	Dose-related reaction, more common after high-dose oral or
Ganciclovir (DHPG)	agitation, paranoia	parenteral therapy, or in patients with renal impairment. Uncommon with DHPG
Foscarnet	Hallucinations, confusion	Association uncertain. Alterations in calcium and magnesium levels are contributory.
Antimicrobials		
Amphotericin B	Delirium, confusion	Rare reports; might be related to hyperthermia and irreversible leukoencephalopathy
β-lactam antibiotics	Confusion, paranoia, hallucinations, mania, coma	Dose-related; high doses in patients with renal dysfunction; increased risk with procaine penicillin
Quinolones	Psychosis, delirium, seizures, anxiety, insomnia, depression	Dose-related, high doses in patients with renal dysfunction
Sulfonamides	Psychosis, delirium, confusion, depression, hallucinations	Dose-related; high doses in patients with renal dysfunction and the elderly. Direct neurotoxic effect
Isoniazid (INH)	Paranoia, confusion, anxiety, hallucinations	Doses exceeding 17 mg/kg/day. IV pyridoxine recommended
Dapsone	Mania, psychosis, anxiety	Several reports in patients with overdosages; resolves within 24 h after discontinuation
Anabolic steroids	Mania, psychosis, depression, aggressiveness	Anecdotal reports in patients receiving 10–100 times the recommended doses; abrupt withdrawal after prolonged usage
Dronabinol (Marinol)	Anxiety, confusion, psychosis, mania, depression, hallucinations	Dose-related; self-limited, usually resolves within 12 h after acute usage; abrupt withdrawal produces similar symptoms
Opiates	Delirium, psychosis, depression, nightmares, hallucinations	Dose-related; might be more frequent with tincture of opium and long-acting narcotics; responds to dose reduction
Corticosteroids	Mania, "steroid psychosis," depression, euphoria	Dose-related > 40 mg/daily of prednisone; resolves with dosage reduction
Tricyclic antidepressants, neuroleptics, and other anticholinergics	Confusion, hallucinations, delirium, psychosis, mania, anxiety	Dose-related; resolves within 24–72 h after stopping the drug. Physostigmine 1–2 mg IM/IV can reverse toxicity.
Fluoxetine	Anxiety, insomnia, mania	Administer in morning; can inhibit metabolism of TCAs and phenytoin and increase their toxicity
Benzodiazepines	Confusion, disorientation, paradoxical agitation, paranoia and rage; rebound anxiety and insomnia	Related to abuse and abrupt withdrawal after prolonged therapy. Increased risk with short-acting agents

the affective aspects of depression. Third, thoughts of death and suicide may be viewed as appropriate or rational as disease progresses. Fourth, organic impairment due to the HIV-associated dementia complex may have affective manifestations. Finally, medication use, and the use of or withdrawal from other psychoactive substances, can have mood-altering effects as described previously. Nevertheless, it must be emphasized that major depression is diagnosed by the same criteria for HIV-infected as for non-HIV-infected persons and should never be treated as a normal finding. Persons with symptoms consistent with major depression should be presumed to have the disorder until proven otherwise (see Chapter 22).

The physician should screen for depression frequently with open-ended questions such as "How have things been going for you lately? " or "How are you coping with all of this? " Certain clues may help to distinguish depressive from constitutional symptomatology. For example, progressive fatigue that worsens with exertion and over the course of the day is characteristic of somatic disease, whereas an inability to get going in the morning that improves with activity may suggest depression. Similarly, nondepressed patients may report that nausea or dysgeusia (an abnormal sense of taste) interfere with their appetite, whereas depressed patients often report simply no interest in eating. Nondepressed patients often report their symptoms and limitations with frustration and concern, whereas apathy and resignation are more characteristic of major depression. Anhedonia and a sense of worthlessness are never symptoms of a somatic condition, and should therefore be directly investigated as specific indicators of depression. Screen for anhedonia by asking patients if they still engage in pleasurable activities.

The treatment of depression in HIV/AIDS is essentially the same as in the non-HIV-infected population. Regular, empathic listening and short-term psychotherapeutic techniques may be very effective. Explicit recognition and validation of the patient's losses and fears help to establish a trusting therapeutic relationship and may permit jointly developing strategies to cope with them. Normalizing depression as a common ailment, particularly frequent in the setting of HIV/AIDS, and amenable to treatment, is important. The use of antidepressant medication remains central but ought to be undertaken with particular caution because of the increased risk of adverse effects. As with other patients, choosing among the many available agents, all of which are essentially equally efficacious, should be largely a matter of selecting the most desirable or tolerable side effect profile.

The clinician must be alert to how the activity and toxicity profile of particular agents may actually help in simultaneously addressing other concerns of the patient. For example, sedating agents like trazodone may be effective in patients who suffer insomnia, and doxepin may also relieve pruritus. A tricyclic antidepressant such as nortriptyline is an ideal choice in a patient with neuropathic pain, who may also benefit from the drug's synergy with other analgesics. Drugs like nortriptyline and desipramine, for which blood levels can be monitored, may be selected in patients with impaired renal or hepatic function. The risk of cardiac arrhythmias associated with tricyclic drugs may be increased in persons taking imidazole antifungal agents (such as fluconazole or itraconazole), whereas the selective serotonin reuptake inhibitors may exacerbate sexual dysfunction or agitation.

Tearfulness, anhedonia, preoccupation, agitation, and insomnia may characterize an acute grief reaction, which can be expected in the wake of bereavement or at any of the life transition points or disease progression benchmarks mentioned previously. Grieving persons often need emotional and social support and spiritual counseling, and group or individual psychotherapy may be effective in encouraging adaptation. It is appropriate to treat short-term insomnia or agitation with limited courses of medium-acting benzodiazepines such as lorazepam (Ativan) or temazepam (Restoril). If vegetative symptoms persist or normal social functioning remains significantly impaired beyond 2–4 weeks after the acute loss, treatment for major depression is often appropriate.

Studies have demonstrated that persons with HIV/AIDS commit suicide at rates several times the population norm, and the true incidence may be much greater, since many suicides are reported as unexplained deaths or attributed to HIV or its complications. Major depression dramatically increases the risk of suicide, which ought to be viewed no more as the result of a "rational" choice in persons with HIV than it would be in the depressed non–HIV-infected population. Attempting suicide is correlated with a history of psychiatric treatment, substance abuse, persistently high levels of psychological distress, HIV-related interpersonal and occupational problems, poor perceived social support, and recent evidence of disease progression. Physicians should be prepared to intervene under such circumstances with crisis counseling, social support, and even psychiatric hospitalization.

Nevertheless, as disability, suffering, and loss of dignity progress, suicide may indeed appear for many to be an attractive and rational alternative to continued deterioration. Perhaps most importantly, the idea that suicide is eventually an option is a comfort to many persons with HIV/AIDS and other chronic degenerative diseases, for whom it represents ultimate control over their condition, and a hedge against the fear of complete dependence and debilitation. Physicians must walk a fine line, detecting and intervening to prevent depression-associated suicide, but remaining careful not to take away the comfort and hope that ultimate control over one's fate confers. Regardless of the physicians' own ethical or religious position on suicide, they must be willing to openly and honestly probe and discuss the patient's suicidal thoughts and, most importantly, the fears and concerns that have led to them. As with requests for assistance in suicide, a discussion of suicide with one's physician is often a disguised cry for help. It may reflect exasperation or exhaustion over symptoms inadequately treated, fear of uncontrollable future pain or suffering, anxiety over burdening caregivers, or the desperate need to be reassured that one will not be abandoned by care providers in one's time of greatest need. What begins as a discussion about suicidal thoughts often ends in the discovery of previously unsuspected or unarticulated fears and needs, a situation that permits physician and patient to work together to chart a clear, practical course to address them (see Chapter 35).

Anxiety

As with some of the symptoms of depression, anxiety may be a normal response to many of the stressors associated with living with HIV. Symptoms of anxiety may include poor concentration, motor restlessness, preoccupation or intrusive thoughts, insomnia (particularly trouble falling asleep), and fatigue. Persons with poor coping skills may be particularly prone to periods of uncontrollable anxiety. Withdrawal from nicotine, alcohol, or illicit drugs, or overuse of caffeine may cause symptoms of anxiety. Some medications used in HIV/AIDS, particularly corticosteroids, decongestants, and nucleoside analogue antiretrovirals, can produce anxiety or agitation, and, rarely, anxiety may be the presenting manifestation of underlying secondary CNS disease.

Treatment is indicated if anxiety impairs social or occupational functioning, or is persistently uncomfortable. In general, regular emotional and social support should be offered. Pharmacotherapy generally involves the use of benzodiazepines, which is complicated by their addictive potential and possible untoward side effects. Psychiatric consultation is indicated when a physician considers prescribing these drugs for longer than a limited period of 2–4 weeks. For episodic and unpredictable bouts of anxiety, shorter- to medium-acting benzodiazepines, such as lorazepam (Ativan) or alprazolam (Xanax), are generally more effective, due to their more rapid onset of action, and are safer because they have fewer active metabolites. The physician should carefully monitor the frequency of prescriptions for short-acting anxiolytics: a pattern of escalating use may suggest that a longer-acting agent or antidepressant therapy is preferable. For chronic disabling anxiety, longer-acting benzodiazepines such as clonazepam (Klonopin), which maintain more stable blood levels, may be more effective. Buspirone (BuSpar), a nonaddicting, nonsedating anxiolytic, is also useful in the long-term treatment of chronic anxiety.

Patients with a chronic disease such as HIV also may be at greater risk for panic disorder than the general population. Panic attacks are characterized by intense, unexpected episodic anxiety associated with physical symptoms, such as chest pain, palpitations, shortness of breath, perioral and digital paresthesias, and a sense of impending doom. These episodes are generally terrifying. Treatment for panic in patients with HIV is similar to that for other patients and generally involves antidepressant medications, although anxiolytics also may provide very effective adjunctive therapy (see Chapter 23).

Insomnia may complicate depression or anxiety disorders; may be a side effect of medications, including antiretrovirals; or may indicate excessive caffeine or stimulant use. Decreasing levels of daytime activity, due to fatigue, disability, or unemployment may cause nocturnal insomnia, particularly if the patient also takes daytime naps, as may the disruption of routine that accompanies hospitalization or a change in living circumstances. Sleeplessness may result from the inability to get comfortable, due to pain or dyspnea, or from fears of fecal incontinence during bouts of diarrhea. The physician should carefully investigate the precise nature of the sleep disorder and identify and address possible causes. Nonpharmacological approaches should be tried, including limiting evening caffeine, alcohol, and fluid intake; creating a conducive sleeping environment; and learning relaxation techniques. As noted earlier, a sedating antidepressant given at bedtime may be an ideal therapeutic choice for the patient with depression, agitation, and increased sleep latency. For many nondepressed patients, and particularly for those with cognitive impairment who are at risk for adverse reactions to benzodiazepines, moderate bedtime doses of chloral hydrate (500–1000 mg) are safe and effective. Diphenhydramine (Benadryl) may also be effective but often causes anticholinergic side effects in the doses necessary to treat insomnia.

Delirium

Delirium is an acute confusional state that includes disorientation and an altered sensorium. It is *never* simply a manifestation of HIV/AIDS and should always be considered to reflect a potentially life-threatening metabolic disruption that has affected the CNS. Patients with cognitive impairment due to the HIV-associated dementia complex or other underlying brain pathology are at particular risk for having delirium precipitated by a metabolic insult, but the dementia itself is never the sole cause of delirium. The list of possible complications of HIV/AIDS that may cause delirium is long and includes disorders of perfusion and gas exchange (hypotension, hypoxia, hypercapnia); fluid and electrolyte abnormalities (dehydration, hyponatremia, hypoglycemia, hyperkalemia, hypercalcemia, uremia); endocrine disorders (adrenal insufficiency, exogenous corticosteroids); CNS injury, infection, or neoplasm; sepsis and other systemic infections; medication side effects (anticholinergics, sedatives, some antimicrobial and antineoplastic agents); and alcohol or drug intoxication or withdrawal. Delirium is generally of abrupt onset and is marked by fluctuating consciousness, poor attention, disorganized thought and speech, and perceptual abnormalities such as visual or auditory hallucinations. It may also be accompanied by either extreme agitation or apathetic withdrawal.

The search for and correction of the underlying abnormalities must be undertaken emergently, in a closely supervised setting such as an intensive care unit. Depending on patients' level of consciousness, frequent attempts may be made to keep them oriented, with careful attention paid to lighting and noise so that sensory stimulation is adequate but not overwhelming. Mechanical restraints should be avoided if possible but might be necessary to prevent patients from injuring themselves or from pulling out lines and catheters. Agitation commonly complicates delirium and can be managed with escalating doses of medium-potency neuroleptics and, if necessary, with short-acting parenteral anxiolytics.

Mania

Mania can be a terrifying and dangerous complication of HIV/AIDS. As in non–HIV-infected persons, mania is characterized by hyperactivity and psychomotor restlessness, euphoric or irritable mood, insomnia and perceived decreased need for sleep, pressured or rapid speech, grandiosity or paranoia, racing thoughts, distractibility, hypersexuality, and reckless or disinhibited hedonistic behavior. Mania in HIV/AIDS is considered an organic rather than a functional disorder because it almost never occurs without either significant underlying brain disease, use of known precipitant drugs, or both. Mania is rarely observed except in patients with underlying HIV-associated dementia complex (see next section), but it may be the first manifestation of that disorder. Medications reported to cause mania include high-dose corticosteroids, antidepressants, and, rarely, zidovudine, and stimulant drugs such as cocaine and amphetamine derivatives. Extreme stressors associated with HIV may precipitate manic episodes in patients predisposed to but previously undiagnosed with bipolar disorder; many of these patients have a family history of bipolar disorder or major depression. Most uncommonly, intense anxiety and distress may produce mania in a patient with no evident predisposition.

Treatment involves first discontinuing any potential pharmacological precipitant and ensuring a safe social environment. Pharmacotherapeutic agents effective in treatment of non–HIV-infected patients are also useful here, but their relative usefulness is changed by potential toxicities. In particular, lithium, the mainstay of treatment for other manias, is risky in patients with advanced HIV/AIDS, in whom levels appear to fluctuate unpredictably. Dehydration, due to diarrhea, vomiting, fever, or poor intake, can quickly result in toxic lithium levels, further complicating management, and patients with HIV/AIDS seem to be more susceptible to toxic side effects even within the therapeutic range. Carbamazepine (Tegretol) is relatively contraindicated in patients with advanced disease because of potential myelosuppression, and it must be used with caution, particularly in conjunction with other myelotoxic drugs such as zidovudine or ganciclovir. Valproate (Depakote) is therefore the agent of choice for mania associated with HIV/AIDS, although patients must be monitored carefully for evidence of hepatotoxicity or thrombocytopenia. Neuroleptics, benzodiazepines, and calcium channel blockers, particularly verapamil, may be useful in preventing recurrences of mania.

Psychosis

As with mania, frank psychosis occurring in persons with HIV/AIDS and without an obvious pharmacological cause generally indicates underlying HIV-associated dementia. Psychotic symptoms include hallucinations, typically auditory rather than visual; delusions, which tend to be paranoid in content; looseness of association; and flight of ideas. Personal care and hygiene may be neglected, and the risk of violence to self or others is increased. Use of or withdrawal from many illicit drugs, including amphetamines, phencyclidine, cocaine, alcohol, marijuana, and opiates, may cause a transient psychosis, and psy-

chosis caused by methamphetamine in particular may last for days or weeks. Psychosis may complicate administration of the anticytomegalovirus drugs ganciclovir and foscarnet, anabolic or corticosteroids, zidovudine, opiates, other psychoactive pharmaceuticals including sedatives and antidepressants, and, very rarely, a host of ordinary antimicrobial agents (Table 31–1). Psychosis is also an infrequent but not-unheard-of first manifestation of underlying secondary CNS infection or neoplasm.

Treatment of HIV/AIDS-associated psychosis involves identification and removal of precipitating drugs and treatment as appropriate of underlying disease. Psychiatric consultation is essential to confirm the diagnosis, identify possible secondary causes, and optimize management. Neuroleptic antipsychotic agents are as effective as in other clinical situations, but the choice of agent should be guided by the increased susceptibility of persons with advanced HIV/AIDS to side effects and toxicity, including the neuroleptic malignant syndrome. High-potency agents like haloperidol (Haldol) are more likely to cause extrapyramidal effects, and low-potency agents such as thioridazine (Mellaril) may cause unacceptable sedation and anticholinergic manifestations. Midpotency agents are typically recommended, including perphenazine (Trilafon) and molindone (Moban).

Primary CNS Disease—The HIV-Associated Dementia Complex

HIV-associated dementia, commonly known as AIDS dementia, is perhaps the most dreaded complication of HIV/AIDS. To the typical young person afflicted with HIV/AIDS, there is nothing more terrifying than the prospect of the loss of dignity and of meaningful human interaction, compounding all the other burdens of the disease. Many patients have watched others deteriorate to a demented and dependent condition. Besides the fear of ending up in such a state, they may wish not to impose on loved ones the responsibilities of caring for them. The threat of dementia, or the appearance of symptoms that may suggest it, are among the factors most likely to drive persons with HIV to consider suicide. Yet only one of every eight people with advanced AIDS develops clinical evidence of HIV-associated dementia. Of those who do, antiretroviral drugs may significantly ameliorate the condition of many, and psychopharmacological agents and environmental manipulation can mitigate its consequences. HIV-associated dementia lies at the severe end of a continuum of impairment called the **HIV-associated dementia complex,** of which most cases involve only mild abnormalities. The primary care provider must be able to counsel patients about the prevalence, signs, and symptoms of cognitive impairment; must be alert to the criteria for and use of testing in the diagnosis of the HIV-associated dementia complex; and must be aware of appropriate management strategies.

Clinical Features: The HIV-associated dementia complex is a subcortical dementia resulting from direct infection of the brain by HIV and is accompanied by demyelination of cerebral white matter. Although it is always a diagnosis of exclusion, HIV-associated dementia is rarely evident when the CD4 count is above 200/mm³; suggestive symptoms or signs in patients with higher counts should prompt the search for another cause. The complex includes not only cognitive but also motor and behavioral disturbances. These may be of different degrees of severity, so that some patients may have disabling cognitive impairment without detectable motor deficits; and for some, behavioral manifestations may be the most troubling. The American Academy of Neurology AIDS Task Force (AANATF) developed diagnostic criteria to distinguish **HIV-associated minor cognitive motor disorder** (HMCMD), in which only mild impairment is evident in attempting complex tasks, from **HIV-associated dementia,** in which there must be significant impairment of activities of daily living. Diagnostic criteria are displayed in Table 31–2. Early and accurate detection may permit treatment at a stage when it is more likely to be effective at restoring or preserving function. It may also permit planning for the time when the patient may no longer be capable of competent decision making, for example regarding medical treatment and end-of-life care, or the management of financial affairs.

Typically, patients with early HMCMD may notice some deficit in attention, concentration, or memory; or in motor coordination or balance. They may be more emotionally labile or irritable in stressful situations, particularly in the workplace. In more familiar settings, no abnormalities may be apparent. In moderately advanced HIV-associated dementia, there are more obvious difficulties with memory, concentration, or comprehension of complex information. Speech and thought may appear slowed and impoverished, and affect may seem "flat." Some disinhibition and socially inappropriate behavior may be apparent. Gross motor abnormalities are not yet evident, but careful neurological testing may reveal a new tremor or an impairment of balance, gait, or coordination. As impairment progresses to full-blown HIV-associated dementia, all activities of daily living are compromised. Attention deficits may make reading or participating in conversation impossible. Short-term memory is severely impaired, and frank disorientation may ensue. Speech may be slowed and impoverished to the point of muteness, accompanied by utter lack of emotional expression. Motor deficits may progress to include generalized weakness and uncoordination or ataxia, requiring assistance in ambulation and eventually confinement to bed or wheelchair, and in some patients, bowel and bladder incontinence may ensue.

Diagnosis: Diagnostic evaluation begins with a careful and sensitive history, including, if possible, soliciting the observations of loved ones, friends, or colleagues. Areas of particular interest include the performance of complex cognitive or motor tasks, problems with memory, activities requiring concentration, and changes in or lability of emotional responses. Thorough neurological and mental status examinations are essential. Once a constellation of cognitive, behavioral, and motor findings is established, laboratory and imaging studies are essential to exclude other etiologies, and in particular, treatable infections or neoplasms. Blood chemistries, serologies, and cultures can help rule out endocrine and other metabolic causes of dementia, as well as cryptococcal infection and neurosyphilis. Likewise, although cerebrospinal fluid (CSF) examination may show elevated protein and pleocytosis, there are no findings pathognomonic for HIV-associated dementia, and lumbar puncture is performed to exclude fungal, bacterial, mycobacterial, treponemal, herpesvirus, and neoplastic meningitides. Computed tomography or magnetic resonance imaging commonly show diffuse white matter degeneration and generalized atrophy, but these studies may be normal in many patients and are helpful primarily to exclude lymphoma, toxoplasmosis, and progressive multifocal leukoencephalopathy.

The most difficult challenge, when the rest of the work-up is unrevealing, lies in distinguishing the manifestations of HMCMD from depression. Neuropsychological testing uses a battery of standardized tests to assess the behavioral, emotional, and cognitive components of cerebral dysfunction and is therefore particularly useful in the evaluation of patients with subtle abnormalities or who do not have characteristic motor involvement. Formal testing of specific cognitive and motor skills may help to distinguish HIV-associated dementia from other diagnoses, and in particular from the pseudodementia common in depression. It may also be useful in uncovering significant compromise in a well-compensated patient, quantitatively assessing the severity of disease and establishing baseline functioning so as to better tailor interventions and assess response to therapy (see Chapter 26).

Management and Treatment: The mainstays of management for the HIV-associated dementia complex, as for other progressive dementias, are environmental adaptations and behavioral interventions designed to reduce the condition's impact on the patient's functioning, dignity, and quality of life. A multidisciplinary team approach is essential for problem recognition and problem solving and should include professionals in medicine, nursing, mental health, social services, physical and occupational therapy, and direct patient assistance, as well as loved ones and caretakers. The physician can suggest small practical interventions, such as the use of appointment or reminder books, "medi-set" pill organizers, and prominently displayed clocks and calendars, which may assist patients with diminishing function. As de-

Table 31–2. Criteria for clinical diagnosis of HIV-1–associated dementia complex.

HIV-1–associated cognitive/motor complex

All of the following diagnoses require laboratory evidence for systemic HIV-1 infection (ELISA test confirmed by Western blot, polymerase chain reaction, or culture):

I. Sufficient for diagnosis of AIDS

   A. HIV-1–associated dementia complex

   Probable (must have *each* of the following):

      1. Acquired abnormality in at least two of the following cognitive abilities (present for at least 1 month): attention/concentration, speed of processing of information, abstraction/reasoning, visuospatial skills, memory/learning, and speech/language. The decline should be verified by reliable history and mental status examination. In all cases, when possible, history should be obtained from an informant, and examination should be supplemented by neuropsychologic testing. Cognitive dysfunction causing impairment of work or activities of daily living (objectively verifiable or by report of a key informant) This impairment, should not be attributable solely to severe systemic illness.

      2. At least *one* of the following:

        a. Acquired abnormality in motor function or performance verified by clinical examination (eq, slowed rapid movements, abnormal gait, limb incoordination, hyperreflexia, hypertonia, or weakness), neuropsychologic tests (eg, fine motor speed, manual dexterity, perceptual motor skills), or both.

        b. Decline in motivation or emotional control or change in social behavior. This may be characterized by any of the following: change in personality with apathy, inertia, irritability, emotional liability, or new onset of impaired judgment characterized by socially inappropriate behavior or disinhibition.

      3. Absence of clouding of consciousness during a period long enough to establish the presence of #1.

      4. Evidence of another etiology, including active CNS opportunistic infection or malignancy, psychiatric disorders (eg, depressive disorder), active alcohol or substance use, or acute or chronic substance withdrawal, must be sought from history, physical and psychiatric examination, and appropriate laboratory and radiologic investigation (eg, lumbar puncture, neuroimaging). If another potential etiology (eg, major depression) is present, it is not the cause of the above cognitive, motor, or behavioral symptoms and signs.

   Possible (must have *one* of the following):

      1. Other potential etiology present (must have each of the following):

        a. As above (see *Probable*) #1, 2, and 3.

        b. Other potential etiology is present but the cause of #1 above is uncertain.

      2. Incomplete clinical evaluation (must have *each* of the following):

        a. As above (see *Probable*) #1, 2, 3.

        b. Etiology cannot be determined (appropriate laboratory or radiologic investigation not performed).

II. Not sufficient for diagnosis of AIDS

   B. HIV-1–associated minor cognitive/motor disorder

   Probable (must have *each* of the following):

      1. Cognitive/motor/behavioral abnormalities (must have *each* of the following):

        a. At least two of the following acquired cognitive, motor, or behavioral symptoms (present for at least 1 month) verified by reliable history (when possible, from an informant):

          1) Impaired attention or concentration

          2) Mental slowing

          3) Impaired memory

          4) Slowed movements

          5) Incoordination

          6) Personality change, irritability, or emotional liability

        b. Acquired cognitive/motor abnormality verified by clinical neurological examination or neuropsychological testing (eg, fine motor speed, manual dexterity, perceptual motor skills, attention/concentration, speed of processing of information, abstraction/reasoning, visuospatial skills, memory/learning, or speech/language).

      2. Disturbance from cognitive/motor/behavioral abnormalities (see #1) causes mild impairment of work or activities of daily living (objectively verifiable or by report of a key informant).

      3. Does not meet criteria for HIV-1–associated myelopathy.

      4. No evidence of another etiology, including active CNS opportunistic infection or malignancy, or severe systemic illness determined by appropriate history, physical examination, and laboratory and radiologic investigation (eg, lumbar puncture, neuroimaging). The above features should not be attributable solely to the effects of active alcohol or substance use, acute or chronic substance withdrawal, adjustment disorder, or other psychiatric disorders.

   Possible (must have *one* of the following):

      1. Other potential etiology present (must have *each* of the following):

        a. As above (see *Probable*) #1, 2, and 3.

        b. Other potential etiology is present and the cause of the cognitive/motor/behavioral abnormalities is uncertain.

      2. Incomplete clinical evaluation (must have *each* of the following):

        a. As above (see *Probable*) #1, 2, and 3.

        b. Etiology cannot be determined (appropriate laboratory or radiologic investigations not performed).

mentia progresses, efforts must be directed at creating a safe, familiar, and simplified environment, in which disorienting, excessive, or inadequate sensory stimulation are avoided. Patients must be frequently and actively oriented and distracted or redirected from inappropriate or problematic behavior.

Antiretroviral therapy may be of limited overall benefit. High doses of zidovudine (AZT)—generally

800–1200 mg/day—have been shown to be of benefit to patients with HIV-associated dementia, producing improvement in neuropsychological test scores and in subjective functioning. The higher doses, which are required because of relatively poor penetration of the blood-brain barrier, may result in greater systemic toxicity, particularly since the typical patient with HIV-associated dementia has advanced AIDS, with multiple comorbidities and many potentially interacting medications. For other antiretroviral drugs, including the other nucleoside analogue reverse transcriptase inhibitors and the newly licensed protease inhibitors, levels attainable in the CSF are even lower, and efficacy in treating CNS disease has not been established. Even the clinical benefits obtained with AZT tend to be modest and should not be held out as a cure for dementia, nor even as likely to prevent progression.

Pharmacotherapy plays an important role in the management of specific behavioral manifestations that may complicate HIV-associated dementia. The cornerstone of drug choice is careful attention to potential adverse effects, and psychiatric consultation should be sought to assist with therapeutic decision making and treatment oversight. Agitation or even frank psychosis is not uncommon as dementia advances. As noted earlier, because of the increased susceptibility of persons with advanced HIV/AIDS to toxicity, midpotency neuroleptic antipsychotic agents are to be preferred. Benzodiazepines should generally be avoided, particularly long-acting agents like diazepam (Valium), which tend to exacerbate cognitive dysfunction and may cause excessive sedation or behavioral disinhibition. Frank mania may occur in 16–20% of persons with HIV-associated dementia and may occur also in earlier stage HMCMD. As noted previously, valproate (Depakote) may often be the safest agent for management of acute HIV/AIDS-associated mania.

Psychostimulant treatment is occasionally recommended for severe psychomotor slowing and depression, particularly for patients who stop eating, communicating, or moving because of profound apathy. Low doses of methylphenidate (Ritalin) or dextroamphetamine (Dexedrine) have been used with some success. If these agents are to be effective, improvement in activity level and mood are usually evident within hours to days of beginning treatment. The temptation to use psychostimulants ought never to obscure the consideration and appropriate treatment of depression, particularly in earlier stages of the HIV-associated dementia complex, when grief and withdrawal are common responses to awareness of impairment. At the other end of the disease spectrum, treatment with stimulants in very advanced HIV-associated dementia may reflect magical or wishful thinking on the part of medical providers or caregivers, whose subtle but vain hope may be to pharmacologically restore the vanishing personality for whom they grieve. The suggestion that psychostimulants be tried should therefore always prompt a serious reevaluation of the patient's overall condition and assessment of whether treatment is truly likely to benefit the *patient* by improving her or his quality of life. In many circumstances, more aggressive palliative measures may be indicated to reduce the patient's suffering.

HIV PREVENTION IN CLINICAL PRACTICE

Each new HIV infection requires transmission from an infected to an uninfected person. Despite this simple but powerful fact, prevention is underemphasized in clinical practice. In part, this has been in an attempt to minimize discrimination against and stigmatization of infected individuals. Clinicians can and should encourage personal responsibility, however, so that infected individuals do not spread HIV beyond themselves.

Physicians should encourage antibody testing among uninfected patients who in the past were or who are currently placing themselves at risk for HIV infection. Screening need not be laborious or intensive. The primary care practitioner should focus on those patients who are at high risk and concentrate prevention efforts on them. A simple set of screening questions (Table 31–3) can help to identify most individuals who need screening and more intensive HIV education.

HIV antibody testing should be encouraged for anyone who might be at risk for HIV infection and also for women who are pregnant or contemplating pregnancy. Use of antiretrovirals to decrease vertical transmission is highly efficacious and is a choice that can be offered to HIV-positive pregnant women. Whereas 90% of Australian gay men know their antibody status, US estimates place the percentage at 65% for gay men, 50% for injection drug users, and 30% for heterosexuals with multiple partners. Individuals can be encouraged to use anonymous testing centers, and physicians can provide testing with counseling in their medical practices. In addition, home HIV testing, still in the regulatory phase, may allow for complete anonymity.

Table 31–3. Screening questions to determine HIV risk.

For all patients:
- Did you receive a transfusion of blood or blood products between 1978 and 1985?
- Have you ever used any kind of injected drug?
- Have you ever had sex with someone who has used, or might have used, injected drugs?
- Do you have any reason to suspect that you might be at risk for HIV infection or AIDS?

For men
- Have you ever had sex with a man?
- Have you ever had sex with a prostitute?

Physicians should be alert to the possibility of primary infection—the period after which individuals have been infected but before they develop antibodies. Infectivity in the primary infection period is estimated to be 50–2000 times greater than in the subsequent asymptomatic period. Thus, primary infection may play a significant role in the further transmission of HIV. Individuals reporting symptoms of initial HIV infection and also recent risky behavior might be offered direct testing of the virus (HIV antigen or viral burden), and counseled to motivate them to safer practices.

Physicians need to assist patients in maintaining safer practices. Many individuals at highest risk for HIV (eg, gay men, injection drug users) have stopped practicing unprotected anal intercourse or sharing of injection equipment. And it is the rare HIV-infected individual who deliberately infects others. Occasional lapses are more common, however, and the physician needs to be open to discussing these lapses with patients in a nonjudgmental manner. Failure to maintain safe practices should not be a surprise, but rather should be expected and planned for in clinical practice. Of course, failure to maintain safe practices, especially in high prevalence areas, can be extremely dangerous. Especially prone to lapses are younger gay men, gay men of color, and men who use or abuse mind-altering substances. In addition, many gay men continue to engage in oral sex based on the fact that the risk of transmission of HIV is considerably less for this practice than for anal intercourse. These gay men are those who are likely to seek repeat testing to ensure that their behavior has not caused them to become infected. Finally, although many injection drug users have changed injection practices, they have not adopted safer sexual practices in great numbers, and, as a result, considerable heterosexual transmission continues to occur between injection drug users and their sexual partners.

Knowledge alone is rarely sufficient to motivate behavior change. Similarly, fear is not likely to be a motivator for individuals who persistently or even occasionally practice high-risk behaviors. Individuals who persist in high-risk behavior may do so for a variety of reasons, and it is important to discover these reasons in order to determine the right prescription for change. The physician should attempt to understand why risky behaviors may be continuing in order to provide the best advice. Recent data have revealed, for example, that substance use is often involved in many new HIV transmissions. Younger gay men are most likely to engage in high-risk practices with steady partners or boyfriends, suggesting that the de-

sire for intimacy may override concerns about transmission. Individuals who have been sexually abused in childhood are at higher risk for HIV as well.

One way to discover why a person may be engaging in unsafe practices is to ask them about the circumstances surrounding their most recent risky acts. The major reasons are most likely to be inebriation, lack of availability of condoms or clean needles, lack of concern for safety, and coercion or lack of power in the relationship. Referral to agencies for help with these concerns can go a long way toward helping people overcome barriers to safety.

A variety of motivational strategies can be used in clinical practice to assist patients in reducing high-risk behaviors. These include appealing to altruism, ascertaining that individuals have appropriate communication skills to insist on condom use, ensuring that individuals know where to obtain clean needles and syringes, and also maintaining lists of service agencies so that appropriate referrals can be made.

Treatment of HIV infection may also be highly efficacious in reducing transmission. If drug regimens are effective in reducing virus circulating in blood or available in vaginal secretions or semen, maintaining individuals on effective regimens can be important in reducing new infections.

Physicians and other health care providers should remember that HIV prevention is one of the success stories of the decade. Although there are still 40,000 new infections in the US every year, successful strategies have been identified and put in place that actually work. Table 31–4 outlines some of the steps clinicians can take to promote HIV prevention. The goal is not to demand perfection but rather to move individuals toward safer practices. Physicians should work in their clinical settings and through their medical societies to help prevent the spread of this dread disease.

Table 31–4. What clinicians can do to prevent HIV transmission.

- Conduct risk assessment with all patients.
- Encourage all at-risk patients to consent to HIV antibody testing.
- Encourage all women who are pregnant or who want to get pregnant to consent to HIV antibody testing.
- Urge all high-risk or infected patients to practice safer sex all the time.
- Refer patients to HIV prevention, education and support services.
- Remind every HIV-positive patient at every visit that adherence to therapy is of utmost importance.
- Serve as a community advocate for sound HIV prevention policies.

SUGGESTED READINGS

American Academy of Neurology AIDS Task Force: Nomenclature and research case definitions for neurologic manifestations of human immunodeficiency virus type 1 (HIV-1) infection. Neurology 1991;41:778.

Boccellari A, Zeifert P: Management of neurobehavioral impairment in HIV-1 infection. Psychiatr Clin North Am 1994;17:183.

Coates T, Lo B: Counseling patients seropositive for human immunodeficiency virus: An approach for medical practice. West J Med 1990;153(6):629.

Capaldini L: HIV Disease: Psychosocial issues and psychiatric complications, In: Sande M, Volberding PA (editors): *The Medical Management of AIDS,* 4th ed. Saunders, 1995.

Perry SW: Organic mental disorders caused by HIV: Update on early diagnosis and treatment. Am J Psychiatry 1990;147(6):696.

Sidtis JJ, Price RW: Early HIV-1 infection and the AIDS dementia complex. Neurology 1990;40:323.

Mistakes in Medical Practice

32

Albert W. Wu, MD, Stephen J. McPhee, MD, & John F. Christensen, PhD

INTRODUCTION

Mistakes are inevitable in the practice of medicine. They result, in part, from the complexity of medical knowledge, the uncertainty of clinical predictions, the pressures of time, and the need to make treatment decisions despite limited or uncertain knowledge. Although much attention has been focused on the effects of errors on patients, it must be understood that medical mistakes are correspondingly distressing for physicians, evoking intense emotions of shock, remorse, guilt, anger, and fear.

If dealt with effectively, mistakes can also provide powerful learning experiences for physicians; however, difficulty in dealing with them may impede both learning and efforts to prevent future errors. Professional norms that assume infallibility and treat mistakes as anomalies pose significant barriers to learning from them. Judgmental institutional responses and fear of litigation are further disincentives to the open discussion of mistakes. Although some individuals may learn from their own mistakes and make subsequent changes in practice, others are less likely to benefit from these lessons.

Definition

A medical mistake can be defined as an act of commission or omission that has serious, or potentially serious, consequences for the patient, and which would be judged wrong by knowledgeable peers at the time it occurs. The usual definition excludes unavoidable bad outcomes and foreseeable complications of disease or correctly performed procedures. Mistakes differ from negligence or malpractice in that a mistake is not necessarily the proximate cause of harm to a patient. It is clear that not all judgments that precede bad outcomes are necessarily wrong. Several factors, such as the severity of the outcome and the perceptions of colleagues and others—including the patient and family—may cause an event to be considered as a mistake.

Prevalence

Most of the relatively few studies of mistakes have focused on the hospital setting and have examined injuries rather than errors. Although the overall prevalence of medical mistakes is difficult to ascertain, it appears that they are common. Iatrogenic events occurred in the care of 36% of patients hospitalized on a general medical service in a teaching hospital. A large study of patients hospitalized in New York State in 1984 found that injuries occurred in nearly 4% percent of hospitalizations, with a quarter of these events judged to have been due to negligence. In a survey of 254 medical residents, 114 responded (45%) and reported a significant mistake made during the prior year. On an academic medicine service, preventable adverse events occurred in 4% percent of more than 3146 admissions. Autopsy studies show that medical diagnoses are often found to have been mistaken. Other studies document that medical errors are common in hospitalized patients, although most mistakes do not produce adverse outcomes. The prevalence of mistakes in outpatient practice has not been studied.

Types

Mistakes occur in every aspect of medical practice—in diagnosis, in decision-making, in ignorance of facts, in the pace of evaluation or its timing, in prescribing medications, or in performing procedures. Mistakes can be classified along a number of dimensions, including cause, outcome (whether the patient was injured, and, if so, how severely), quality of care (whether the care was standard or substandard), and locus (where in the process of medical care the error occurred). Mistakes can also be classified as errors of commission and errors of omission. Table 32–1 shows one classification of the types of medical mistakes.

The Harvard Medical Practice Study found that among 1133 patients with disabling injuries caused by medical treatment, 28% were judged to be due to negligence. The most common adverse event involved performance or follow-up of a procedure or operation

Table 32–1. Types of medical mistakes.

Error	Example
Diagnosis or evaluation	Missed diagnosis
Medical decision-making	Inappropriate or premature discharge
Treatment	Waiting when treatment is indicated
Medication	Incorrect dosage
Procedural complications	Faulty technique
Faulty communication	Failure to convey information during sign-out
Inadequate supervision	Failure to review treatment plan

Source: Adapted, with permission, from Wu AW et al: Do house officers learn from their mistakes? JAMA 1991;265:2089. © Copyright 1991, American Medical Association.

(35%). Failure to take preventive measures (eg, failure to guard against accidental injury) were the next most common (22%), followed by diagnostic errors (eg, failure to use indicated tests, act on test results, or avoid delays in response) (14%), errors involving drug treatment (9%), and system errors (2%).

A review of New Jersey malpractice claims from 1977 to 1989, for which payment was made or negligence determined, found that errors in patient management (eg, diagnostic errors, decision errors, improper management, medication errors, unnecessary treatment, or problems in communication), were more common than were errors in technical performance or medical and nursing staff coordination.

Causes

Physicians report a variety of reasons for their mistakes and frequently attribute the mistakes to more than one cause. In one study, house officers most often reported that mistakes were caused in part because they did not possess specific essential knowledge (eg, being unaware of the significance of a prolonged episode of ventricular tachycardia). Almost as often, they cited "too many tasks" (one resident neglected to continue a required medication because he was "too busy with other sick patients, and supervising interns and students."). Fatigue was a significant factor (after inadvertently ordering potassium replacement as a bolus, one resident commented, "It was 3:00 AM, and I'm not sure I was completely awake"). A study of an inpatient medical service, found cross-coverage to be a significant predictor of preventable adverse events. Table 32–2 summarizes common causes of medical mistakes.

The pressures of practicing medicine in a managed care setting, especially in capitated systems with higher demands for productivity, may increase the risk that a hurried physician will overlook important diagnostic information or make a prescription error.

Table 32–2. Common causes of medical mistakes.

- Ignorance
- Inexperience
- Faulty judgment
- Hesitation
- Fatigue
- Job overload
- Breaks in concentration
- Faulty communication
- Failure to monitor closely
- System flaws

Similarly, the incentives offered by third-party payers to order fewer diagnostic tests and to limit the number of referrals to subspecialists can lead to errors of omission.

Circumstances

Mistakes seem to occur more frequently during residency training, possibly because interns and residents are learning new skills, honing their clinical judgment, and accepting new responsibilities. Although first-year residents in one study made the highest proportion of prescription errors (4.25 per 1000 orders), more experienced physicians have also reported making serious medical mistakes.

Many mistakes happen in the inpatient or emergency room setting. Severely ill patients, with unstable conditions such as those in intensive care or emergency departments, require rapid assessment of a complex clinical picture and multiple procedures, evaluations, and decisions, thus presenting many opportunities for mistakes to occur. In the Harvard Medical Practice Study, reviewers found that about 73% of negligent adverse events occurred in the hospital, 8% in the emergency room, and 8% in the physician's office.

Patient characteristics can also increase the risk of mistakes. The risk of iatrogenic events increases with age, the length of the hospital stay, and the number of drugs prescribed. Older patients, for example, are likely to have advanced disease and comorbid conditions and to be taking numerous medications. These factors increase both the risk of errors and the likelihood that complications of treatment will make these errors consequential.

Serious medical mistakes certainly occur in office practice. Some practicing physicians contend that the probability of making a serious error increases with the number of years in practice, particularly with the current pressures to increase productivity (see Chapter 7).

THE OUTCOMES OF MEDICAL MISTAKES

Consequences for Patient & Family

Minor errors may produce no serious consequences. Sometimes more serious errors, if recognized and corrected, may have no major consequences. In such cases, there may be no judgment that a mistake has occurred, or it may be disregarded as a minor occurrence. Serious errors, however, often have significant and multiple consequences for the patients involved, such as physical discomfort, emotional distress, additional therapy or procedures, prolonged hospital stay, worsening of disease, or death. Mistakes can also cause distress for family members, including worry, anger, and guilt, particularly if they were involved in making treatment decisions.

Consequences for Physicians & Colleagues

Physicians also experience emotional distress in reaction to a medical mistake. After a fatal mistake involving a young patient, one house officer wrote, "This event has been the greatest challenge to me in my training." Clinicians report a variety of emotional responses from remorse, anger, guilt, and feelings of inadequacy to fear—particularly the fear of negative repercussions, such as malpractice suits.

Physicians occasionally report persistent negative psychological effects from mistakes. After a mistake caused the death of a patient, one house officer commented, "This case has made me very nervous about clinical medicine. I worry now about all febrile patients, since they may be on the verge of sepsis." For another house officer, a missed diagnosis made him reject a career in subspecialties that would involve "a lot of data collection and uncertainty."

Consequences for the Physician-Patient Relationship

In some cases, depending on the severity of the outcome for the patient and the quality of communication between physician and patient, the physician-patient relationship may be harmed by a mistake. For the physician, feelings of guilt, shame, or shaken confidence may lead to avoidance of the patient or to a diminution of open and frank discussion. One physician, for example, reported that his guilt from the death of a patient led him to act like an indentured servant to the patient's family, attempting to expiate his "crime" over a prolonged period of time by spending more time with the family and reducing his fees.

For the patient, learning about a mistake may cause alarm and anxiety, destroying the patient's faith and confidence in the physician's ability to help. There may be anger, an erosion of trust, decreased respect, or feelings of betrayal that diminish openness. Patients may become disillusioned with the medical profession in general, causing them to decline or reduce their adherence to beneficial treatments or habits.

To the extent that doctor and patient can discuss their emotions directly and with mutual acceptance, the relationship is likely to endure; it may even deepen with time. The negative effect of a mistake on the doctor-patient relationship may also be mitigated if there is a history of shared decision-making, which diffuses the responsibility of the physician, especially when there has been uncertainty about treatment.

It should be noted also that mistakes that are nationally—or even locally—reported in the press can damage public trust in the medical profession. Any loss of credibility can be harmful to the public health by creating cynicism about medical care and research findings and discouraging individuals from seeking care or adopting healthful behaviors.

RESPONDING TO MEDICAL MISTAKES

The way in which physicians respond to mistakes can turn these experiences into powerful opportunities for learning and for personal growth.

Individual Responses

Coping with Mistakes: Two major modes of coping are **problem-focused,** in which coping is directed at the problem causing the distress; and **emotion-focused,** in which coping is directed at managing the emotional distress caused by the problem. Effective coping can prevent such unhealthy responses as denial, cynicism, and excessive concern. The use of effective coping strategies can also play a role in modulating physician stress and increasing physician work satisfaction.

Table 32–3 briefly summarizes some of the many possible strategies for coping with medical mistakes. Among these, accepting responsibility and problem-

Table 32–3. Potential strategies for coping with medical mistakes.

Approach	Strategy
Problem-focused	Acceptance of responsibility Consultation to understand nature of mistake Consultation to correct mistake Planned problem-solving (eg, obtaining extra training)
Emotion-focused	Pursuance of social support Disclosure to colleague, friend, or spouse Disclosure to patient Emotional self-control (eg, repressing one's emotional response) Escape-avoidance Distancing Reframing of mistake (eg, recognizing it as inherent in practicing medicine)

Source: Adapted, with permission, from Wu AW et al: How house officers cope with their mistakes. West J Med 1993;159:565; and Christensen JF et al: The heart of darkness: The impact of perceived mistakes on physicians. J Gen Intern Med 1992;7:424.

solving techniques may be those most often used. As an example, "accepting responsibility" would include such statements as: "I made a promise to myself that things would be different next time"; "I criticized or lectured myself"; and "I apologized or did something to make up." Seeking social support and controlling emotions may be somewhat less frequently employed, and escape-avoidance and distancing are used even more rarely.

Accepting responsibility is a prerequisite to learning from a mistake, and physicians who cope by accepting responsibility for their mistakes seem to be more likely to make constructive changes in practice. They may also be more likely to experience emotional distress, however, as in the case of the resident who described persistent feelings of guilt and shame after realizing that inappropriate management of a diabetic patient's foot ulcer led to an amputation.

Disclosure to Patients and Families: It is difficult to disclose mistakes to patients or their families, and several reports suggest that physicians are reluctant to tell patients about mistakes. In one study, such disclosure was reported by less than one quarter of house officers, yet legal and ethical experts suggest that those involved should generally be told about errors. Disclosure of a mistake also fosters learning by compelling the physician to acknowledge it truthfully. In addition, disclosing a mistake to the patient may be the only way for the physician to achieve a sense of absolution.

Telling patients about mistakes is made more difficult by the lack of guidelines about how to do so, and all physicians must develop their own approach to each case. Disclosure and discussion of an error with the patient or family can be made easier by several techniques. Physicians should first try to acknowledge their own emotions. Before approaching the patient or family, it may be helpful to perform a simple relaxation exercise and to remind oneself that the event and present feelings do not define the physician as either a healer or a person. Rehearsing a few simple, direct statements ahead of time can provide a road map for the physician in this awkward moment. When meeting the patient or family, the physician should make a brief, direct statement, accompanied by a genuine apology. Such directness may help avoid the kind of long and rambling discussion that often increases anxiety for both physician and patient.

The physician who has mistakenly prescribed a medication without checking the patient's allergies, for example, might tell the patient: "Mr. Jones, I've discovered what made you sick last week. I regret to say that I failed to check whether you were allergic to the antibiotic before I prescribed it. You are allergic to it, and that information is clearly written in your chart. I feel awful that my not checking has caused you so much distress. I am truly sorry." It would then be appropriate to pause and allow the patient to respond.

Reflecting and accepting the patient's feelings can help to begin to heal the relationship more effectively than overwhelming the patient with information and explanations. The doctor-patient relationship can be enhanced by honesty in this most difficult and sensitive moment (see Chapter 3).

Disclosure to Colleagues: Physicians also seem to be reluctant to tell their colleagues about mistakes. Some physicians report that they find this kind of discussion both threatening, because of the fear of judgment by colleagues, and unhelpful, because of the tendency of colleagues to minimize the mistake. Most often, discussing mistakes with colleagues serves the purpose of problem-focused coping: correcting a mistake. Sharing mistakes with colleagues can also prevent isolation and start the necessary process of remorse and learning.

Changes in Practice: Table 32–4 summarizes changes in practice that often follow medical mistakes. These changes can be constructive, or they can be defensive—and maladaptive—in nature. Constructive changes cited by physicians include paying more attention to detail, confirming clinical data personally, changing protocols for diagnosis and treatment, increasing self-care, changing methods of communication with staff, and being willing to seek advice.

Physicians also report making defensive changes, however. These include an unwillingness to discuss the mistake, avoidance of similar patients, and—in some circumstances—ordering additional tests. Defensive changes in practice are more likely to occur if the institutional response to a mistake is punitive or judgmental.

Learning from Mistakes: Several factors may determine the extent to which physicians learn from mistakes. When negative emotions such as shame,

Table 32–4. Common changes in practice following mistakes.

Constructive Changes	Defensive Changes
Increasing information-seeking	Being unwilling to discuss the error
■ Asking advice	Avoiding patients with similar problems
■ Reading	Ordering additional but unnecessary tests
Increasing vigilance	
■ Paying more attention to detail	
■ Confirming data personally	
■ Changing data organization	
■ Ordering additional tests as appropriate	
■ Improving screening for disease	
■ Improving communication with patients	
Improving self-pacing	
Improving communication with staff	
Supervising others more closely	

guilt, or humiliation follow from the mistake, the physician's energy may focus on the emotional aspects of coping. Addressing these negative emotions directly can enhance the physician's ability to learn new information or new approaches to the problem. The cause to which the physician attributes the mistake can also affect learning. Physicians in one study were more likely to report constructive changes if the mistake was caused by inexperience or faulty judgment in a complex case; they were less likely to do so if they believed that the mistake was caused by overload. Physicians who responded to the mistake with greater acceptance of responsibility and more discussion were also more likely to report constructive changes.

Responding to Colleagues Who Make Mistakes: There are several important considerations when responding to a colleague who discloses a mistake. It is important to try to elicit or accept the colleague's self-assessment and to not minimize the importance of the mistake. At this point, a selective and discreet disclosure of one's own mistakes can reduce the colleague's sense of isolation and legitimize the discussion. It is then appropriate to inquire about the emotional effect of the mistake and how the colleague is coping with it. An important consideration here is that negative emotions are not necessarily problems to be solved, and they can often be mitigated by acknowledging them. The clinician should return to the content of the mistake and help the colleague to correct it with problem-solving techniques, making the necessary changes in practice, and incorporating the new lessons that have been learned.

Witnessing Mistakes by Others: When a physician sees a mistake made by another physician, the observer has several options: passively waiting for the physician to disclose the mistake, telling the patient directly oneself, advising the physician to disclose the mistake, or arranging a joint meeting to discuss the mistake. Although some physicians may feel an obligation to report mistakes they have seen, most are reluctant to say anything.

The simplest option, of course, is to wait for the physician who made the mistake to report it. There is no assurance, however, that the patient will actually be informed. Telling the patient directly may be awkward, particularly if the observing physician does not know the patient, and may interfere with the existing doctor-patient relationship. Advising the physician who made the error to tell the patient may fulfill the observing physician's responsibility for disclosure, but the patient may still not be informed. Simultaneously advising the physician and the hospital or clinic quality-assurance or risk-management personnel would increase the likelihood that the patient would be told. Arranging a joint conference would satisfy the observer that appropriate disclosure was made while preserving the primacy of the relationship between the patient and the treating physician (Figure 32–1).

Institutional Responses

Hospitals: Physicians sometimes feel that the hospital atmosphere inhibits them from talking about their mistakes and that the administration is judgmental about mistakes. Some institutions have formal settings for discussing mistakes, such as morbidity and mortality conferences. Such important issues as a discussion of the physician's feelings about the mistake and disclosure by colleagues of how they coped with their own mistakes, however, are commonly avoided in these conferences. The risk-management departments of hospitals could take a leading role in this area—promoting comprehensive, supportive forums for discussing mistakes, using emotion-focused coping to maximize problem-focused learning and minimize future errors.

Graduate Medical Education: Although some physicians feel that public disclosure of mistakes is counterproductive, others assert that physician fallibility and methods of dealing with medical errors are appropriate topics for medical school and subsequent training. Although they may initially be reluctant, physicians sometimes find discussing a mistake to be a positive experience: "Presenting this case at interns' report was difficult—I felt under a lot of scrutiny from my peers. In the end, I felt as though I had gotten more respect from presenting this kind of case rather than one where I had made a great diagnosis."

Mistakes can be discussed in attending rounds, at morning report, or at morbidity and mortality conferences. When mistakes are discussed in these conferences, it is important to address issues such as overwork, shared responsibility with other physicians (eg, consultants, attending physicians), and appropriate protocols for communicating with staff. In addition, while ensuring that everyone involved learns from the mistake, care should be taken that errors are seen as an unfortunate inevitability in the practice of medicine and that there are appropriate ways of coping with them and of responding to colleagues who make them.

Primary Care Practice Groups: As group practice becomes the norm in managed care settings, it is important that such groups implement procedures for responding to mistakes. Collegial support should be an explicit rule, providing a safe and confidential setting for discussion of the mistake (see the guidelines discussed earlier, for responding to a colleague's mistake). It would also be wise for the practice group to formalize—and thus legitimize—periodic discussions about mistakes; these could broaden the scope of the emotion-focused support, allow members to learn from colleagues' mistakes, and address system flaws that contribute to the mistakes. A bonus of this approach is in the gain in personal well-being of the group members—a nonspecific, yet significant, contribution to the practice climate.

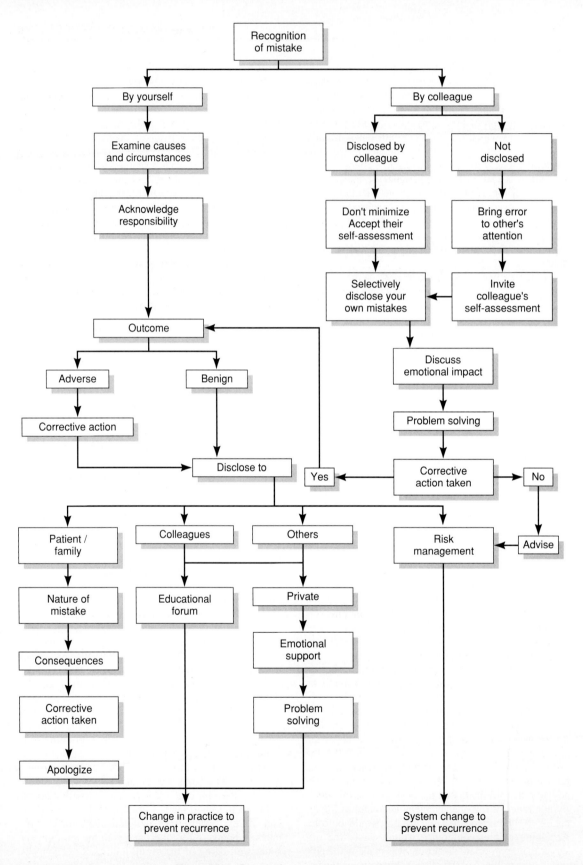

Figure 32–1. Process for responding to a mistake.

PREVENTING MISTAKES

Reducing the frequency and severity of mistakes is of the highest priority. There are several ways to help physicians learn from their mistakes and to make constructive changes in practice.

Physician Responsibility

As noted earlier, physicians should be encouraged to accept responsibility for their mistakes. Although those who do so seem more likely than those who do not to make constructive changes in practice, accepting responsibility for mistakes can engender emotional distress. It is therefore important for colleagues and supervising physicians to respond with sensitivity to the distress of practitioners acknowledging their mistakes. The probability of future mistakes can be reduced if the current error can be reviewed in a way that decreases emotional distress, invites disclosure of uncertainty in diagnosis and management, and leads to a discussion of appropriate changes in practice.

Administration & Supervision

Efforts to forestall errors must also take place at administrative levels. More active supervision may prevent some mistakes or mitigate their adverse effects. Senior physicians should be more available to their less-experienced colleagues for making critical decisions about patient care, especially in complex cases that require more mature clinical judgment. Group practice administrators and training-program directors should correct problems in staffing, scheduling, and the nature of work—which may all contribute to mistakes. Serious attention must be paid to the workload. Sleep deprivation during training may be a source of errors; job overload, fatigue, and being expected to perform too many tasks can also lead to mistakes. Working under these conditions may teach house officers to tolerate and rationalize errors; in addition, it may make them less likely to seek the corrective information that could help prevent future mistakes.

Identifying & Reporting Errors

Delineating the cause of a mistake often suggests specific strategies for preventing future mistakes. Routine mechanisms to identify adverse events, such as anonymous reporting by physicians and nurses, or computerized feedback about adverse drug reactions, are necessary to provide information about the ubiquity, frequency and nature of mistakes. Developing routine methods of conveying information, such as computerized forms that standardize the type and amount of information exchanged between covering physicians, can also reduce errors.

Fail-safe mechanisms, such as the computerized systems now used by some pharmacies, should be put into place to prevent medication errors, including overdoses, incorrect routes of administration, drug interactions, and allergies. Computerized ordering systems should facilitate implementation of such programs and allow the use of checklists and guidelines to promote and improve standards of practice.

Managed Care

The demands of practicing in a managed care setting may increase a busy physician's susceptibility to making mistakes. Fatigue, information overload, and increased pressures to be a more productive member of the practice by seeing more patients for shorter visits can lead the physician to overlook important information. In addition, the role of the physician as the gatekeeper of referrals to specialists in most managed care plans, along with financial incentives for holding down the number of referrals, tests, hospital admissions, and hospital days, has the potential for increasing errors of omission. Ironically, the risk of malpractice litigation may counter this tendency by inducing physicians to practice defensively by ordering more tests. Within the extremes of these incentives and disincentives, there is a need for continuing education of physicians on standards of practice with regard to tests, referrals, and further treatment.

Both physicians and institutions should make whatever changes in practice are warranted to prevent new mistakes or the recurrence of similar events. Recognizing and dealing with mistakes honestly and directly can improve the quality of patient care and lead to a more rewarding practice.

SUGGESTED READINGS

AMA Principals of Medical Ethics 1957; 4.

Anderson RE, Hill RB, Key CR: The sensitivity and specificity of clinical diagnostics during five decades: Toward an understanding of necessary fallibility. JAMA 1989;261:1610.

Applegate WB: Physician management of patients with adverse outcomes. Arch Intern Med 1986;146:2249.

Bosk CL: *Forgive and Remember: Managing Medical Failure.* University of Chicago Press, 1979.

Brennan TA et al: Incidence of adverse events and negligence in hospitalized patients: Results of the Harvard Medical Practice Study I. N Engl J Med 1991;324:370.

Burnhaum JF: Sounding Board: Secrets about patients. N Engl J Med 1991;324:1130.

Calnan M: Clinical uncertainty: Is it a problem in the doctor-patient relationship? Sociol Health Illness 1984;6:74.

Carmichael DH: Learning medical fallibility. South Med J 1985;78:1.

Christensen JF, Levinson W, Dunn PM: The heart of darkness: The impact of perceived mistakes on physicians. J Gen Intern Med 1992;7:424.

Classen DC et al: Computerized surveillance of adverse drug events in hospital patients. JAMA 1991;266:2847.

Colford JM, McPhee SJ: The raveled sleeve of care: Managing the stresses of residency training. JAMA 1989;261:889.

Dearden CH, Rutherford WH: The resuscitation of the severely injured in the accident and emergency department: A medical audit. Injury 1985;16:249.

Dubovsky SL, Schrier RW: The mystique of medical training: Is teaching perfection in medical house-staff training a reasonable goal or a precursor of low self-esteem? JAMA 1983;250:3057.

Folkman S, Lazarus RS: *The Ways of Coping.* Consulting Psychologist Press, 1988.

Gillon R: Doctors and patients. Br Med J 1986;292:466.

Hilfiker D: Facing our mistakes. N Engl J Med 1984;310:118.

Kravitz RL, Rolph JE, McGuigan K: Malpractice claims data as a quality improvement tool, 1. Epidemiology of error in four specialties. JAMA 1991;266:2087.

Laine C et al: The impact of regulation restricting medical house staff working hours on the quality of patient care. JAMA 1993;269:374.

Leape LL et al: The nature of adverse events in hospitalized patients: Results of Harvard Medical Practice Study II. N Engl J Med 1991;324:377.

Leape LL: Error in medicine. JAMA 1994;272:1851.

Lesar TS et al: Medication prescribing errors in a teaching hospital. JAMA 1990;263:2329.

Levinson W, Dunn PM: Coping with fallibility. JAMA 1989;261:2252.

Lo B: Disclosing mistakes. In: Lo B (editor): *Problems in Ethics.* Williams & Wilkins, 1994.

Meyer BA: A student teaching module: Physician errors. Fam Med 1989;21:299.

Millman M: Overlooking medical mistakes. In: *The Unkindest Cut: Life in the Backrooms of Medicine.* Morrow, 1977.

Mizrahi T: Managing medical mistakes: Ideology, insularity and accountability among internists-in-training. Soc Sci Med 1984;196:135.

O'Neil AC et al: Physician reporting compared with medical-record review to identify adverse medical events. Ann Intern Med 1993;119:370.

Paget MA: *The Unity of Mistakes: A Phenomenological Interpretation of Medical Work.* Temple University Press, 1988.

Petersen LA et al: Does housestaff discontinuity of care increase the risk of preventable adverse events? Ann Intern Med 1994;121:866.

Petersen LA et al: Housestaff-based intervention increases continuity of inpatient care and prevents medical injuries [Abstract]. J Gen Intern Med 1994;9(Suppl 2):63.

Quill TE, Williamson PR: Healthy approaches to physician stress. Arch Intern Med 1990;150:1857.

Sorensen JR: Biomedical innovation, uncertainty, and the doctor-patient interaction. J Health Soc Behav 1974;15:366.

Steel K et al: Iatrogenic illness on a general medical service at a university hospital. New Engl J Med 1981;304:638.

Vincent CA: Research into medical accidents: A case of negligence? Br Med J 1989;299:1150.

Vogel J, Delgado R: To tell the truth: Physicians' duty to disclose medical mistakes. UCLA Law Review 1980;28:521.

Warner E. Telling patients about medical negligence. Can Med Assoc J 1983;129:366.

Wu AW et al: Do house officers learn from their mistakes? JAMA 1991;265:2089.

Wu AW et al: How house officers cope with their mistakes: Doing better but feeling worse? West J Med 1993;159:565.

Domestic Violence

33

Mitchell D. Feldman, MD, MPhil

INTRODUCTION

Domestic violence is defined as any intentional, controlling behavior consisting of physical, sexual, or psychological assaults in the context of an intimate relationship. The data on domestic violence underscores the magnitude of the problem. In a landmark study, 28% of a random nationwide sample of couples reported violence at some point in their history; almost 4% of the women reported severe violence. If these figures are extrapolated to the general population, it is estimated that 4–8 million women are subject to battering each year.

Studies of emergency departments and outpatient medical settings suggest that battered women are high users of medical services. Up to 23% of women using emergency services are there for complaints directly attributable to domestic violence. Because their complaints are frequently misdiagnosed, they may return time and time again, often with increasingly severe trauma.

Despite its magnitude in society and in medical settings, domestic violence could be, until recently, accurately labeled a "silent epidemic." Considered a private, family problem by the government, and a social problem by the medical establishment, victims of domestic violence often had nowhere to turn. This predicament has gradually improved. Domestic violence is now acknowledged to be an important public health problem, and the American Medical Association has released diagnostic and treatment guidelines for practicing physicians. All primary care practitioners must be knowledgeable about and comfortable with the evaluation and care of patients who are subjected to domestic violence.

EPIDEMIOLOGY

Research conducted in a variety of medical settings has reported on the prevalence of domestic violence.

Cross-sectional studies from outpatient primary care clinics and emergency department settings have found the prevalence of domestic violence among women to be from 5.5% to 23%; lifetime prevalence rates up to 54% have been reported. Similar rates have been uncovered by well-done studies from obstetric/gynecologic outpatient clinics.

Unfortunately, all of the major studies to date ask about violence exclusively in the context of heterosexual relationships. Although few rigorous studies have been conducted, it would appear that a similar prevalence of domestic violence exists in gay and lesbian relationships, often with the same physical and emotional consequences. Primary care providers should be aware that because of homophobia, it is often more difficult for gay and lesbian patients to disclose that they are in abusive relationships. In addition, the commonly held bias that violence does not occur in these relationships ("women can't hurt women") further lowers detection rates.

Men report being physically abused by their female partners at rates just below those reported by women. The injuries inflicted by women on men, however, are insignificant when compared with same sex or male-on-female violence, so should not be considered a significant public health or medical problem.

DIAGNOSIS

Many battered women seek medical care both for the direct and indirect sequelae of their battering. Yet only a small percentage of them are diagnosed and treated appropriately. The following case is illustrative of the type of patient commonly seen in the primary care setting.

Case illustration: A 40-year-old nurse presents to the general medical clinic with a chief complaint of a headache. She reports having been in a motor vehicle accident 3 days earlier and striking her head on the dashboard. She says that her friends encouraged her to come in, and she is accompanied to the clinic (but not the office) by her partner. On physical examination she appears tense and sad, with bilateral periorbital ecchymoses.

History

A thorough history is the cornerstone of the diagnosis of domestic violence. Because the presentation is often subtle, with few dramatic injuries, detection requires a high index of suspicion. There are many clues in the medical history, as shown by the case illustration, that should prompt the physician to evaluate the patient for domestic violence (Table 33–1). Clues that should prompt further inquiry include:

- Delay in seeking care
- Illogical explanation of injury
- Multiple somatic complaints
- Depression, anxiety, and other mental disorders
- Pregnancy
- Substance use
- Recent diagnosis of HIV
- Family history of domestic violence
- Overbearing partner

Delay in Seeking Care: Patients who have been assaulted often delay seeking medical attention for 2 or more days, in contrast to accident victims who generally seek out medical attention immediately.

Illogical Explanation of Injury: Injuries that are attributed to a mechanism that seems illogical should always raise concern. For example, periorbital ecchymoses ("black eyes") are generally not caused by a motor vehicle accident, or by anything other than a fist.

Multiple Somatic Complaints: Some women may present with vague somatic complaints as their only symptom of domestic violence. Fatigue, sleep disturbances, headache, gastrointestinal complaints, abdominal and pelvic pain, genitourinary problems such as frequent urinary tract and genital infections, chest pain, palpitations, and dizziness are just some of the complaints with which women present. Domestic violence should be ruled out as a sole or contributing cause of these problems.

Depression, Anxiety, and Other Mental Disorders: Depression, eating disorders, and anxiety disorders such as chronic posttraumatic stress dis-

Table 33–1. When to screen for domestic violence.

Delay in seeking care
Illogical explanation of injury
Multiple somatic complaints
Depression, anxiety, and other mental disorders
Pregnancy
Substance use
Recent diagnosis of HIV
Family history of domestic violence
Overbearing partner

order and panic disorder are more common among victims of domestic violence than occurs in the general population. If present, the primary care provider should always screen for the presence of domestic violence. These emotional disturbances should be thought of as a consequence, not a cause, of the domestic violence. Some patients may feel hopeless and turn toward suicide as a way out. In fact, 1 of every 10 battered women attempts suicide. Of those, 50% try more than once.

Pregnancy: Many studies have demonstrated that women are at increased risk of physical and sexual abuse during pregnancy. Clues to be alert for include delay in seeking prenatal care, depressed or anxious mood, injuries to breasts or abdomen, frequent spontaneous abortions, and preterm labor. In addition to the physical and emotional trauma to the pregnant woman, these assaults can result in placental separation, fetal fractures, and fetal demise.

Substance Abuse: Although violence and substance abuse often coexist, it is inaccurate and generally not helpful to frame domestic violence as secondary to the substance abuse. Although the perpetrator, and at times the woman herself, often asserts that the violence was a consequence of altered behavior from drugs or alcohol, in fact, the violent behavior must be addressed as a separate issue and is unlikely to end even if the substance abuse does.

Conversely, some studies have also found an increased rate of substance use in victims of domestic violence. At times, this may take the form of increased use of pain medications or anxiolytics in an effort to cope with the assaults. It is even more imperative in this instance that physicians not attribute the domestic violence to the substance use; it is precisely this mentality of "blaming the victim" that has often prevented the appropriate evaluation and treatment of domestic violence in all medical settings.

Recent Diagnosis of HIV: Women are the fastest growing group of persons with HIV in the United States. Some women have reported an initiation or escalation of domestic violence when they have informed their partner of their seropositive status. Although it is an accepted ethical principle that sexual partners be notified of HIV-positive results, physicians should assess their patient's risk of violence while discussing the issues surrounding notification. If there is any suspicion of a risk of violence, a safety plan should always be part of post-test counseling.

Family History of Domestic Violence: Patients who report a family history of domestic violence, particularly those who witnessed parental violence as a child or adolescent, are at increased risk themselves even if they are not presently in an abusive relationship. Such women should therefore be educated and screened more carefully.

Overbearing Partner: An overbearing partner who, for example, insists on accompanying the patient into the examining room, acts overly solicitous or concerned (sometimes to the point of knocking on the examining room door to inquire about her well-being), or is hostile to the health care team may be a clue to the presence of domestic violence. Never probe about domestic violence if the perpetrator is in the examining room as this may serve to escalate the violence and put the patient in extreme danger.

***Not* Socioeconomic or Ethnic Status:** Many health care providers mistakenly believe that domestic violence disproportionately affects persons in particular ethnic or socioeconomic groups; in fact, it cuts across all ethnic groups and all economic strata. Although some studies have found that women who are uninsured or on medical assistance are at increased risk of domestic violence, this is most likely due to selection bias in the studies. Women from lower socioeconomic status (SES) groups may be overrepresented in some statistics because those from higher SES groups have more resources available to them and the abuse is therefore more likely to remain hidden. Women with fewer resources are forced to take refuge in shelters or county hospital emergency departments, for example, whereas their middle-class counterparts may flee to a hotel or their offices and are therefore missed by many of the surveys.

Physical Examination

The physical examination may provide the first clues of the presence of domestic violence (Table 33–2), including:

- Inappropriate behavior
- Multiple injuries
- Central pattern of injury
- Injuries at different stages of healing

Inappropriate Behavior: Behavior that appears to be inappropriate at the time of the physical examination may be a sign of domestic violence. Fright, inappropriate embarrassment or laughter, anxiety, passivity, shyness, and avoidance of eye contact may all be clues that the patient has been battered.

Multiple Injuries: Battered women are more likely to have multiple injuries than are ordinary accident victims. Victims of domestic violence, for example, typically have injuries to the head, neck, abdomen, and chest, whereas accident victims often are able to protect themselves, at least in part, and present with less widespread trauma. The common emotional

reactions to assault of denial, confusion, and withdrawal may also lead to more extensive injuries.

Central Pattern of Injury: Victims of domestic violence often experience injuries such as bruises, lacerations, burns, bites, and more severe injuries secondary to assaults with a deadly weapon or repeated beatings that cause massive internal injuries and fractures. Injuries are most commonly seen in the central areas of the body—the head, neck, chest, abdomen, breasts and occasionally upper arms from fending off blows.

Injuries at Different Stages of Healing: As with child abuse, multiple injuries at different stages of healing should always prompt an inquiry about domestic violence.

In summary, primary care providers must be alert to the signs and symptoms of domestic violence. It is important to remember that most domestic violence victims do not present with injuries that require emergency treatment or lead to hospitalization. In fact, for many patients, even in emergency departments, the presenting complaint is often medical or psychological, rather than an actual physical injury. For this reason, domestic violence will only be detected if the physician frequently includes it on the differential diagnosis and actively screens for it during the medical encounter.

Screening for Domestic Violence

Questions about domestic violence should be a routine part of the history and physical examination for all female patients. This can be done by including questions about abuse on the medical history questionnaire, verbally as a part of the social or past medical history, or (preferably) both. It may help some women to answer honestly by screening with the following sorts of questions: "We all fight at home. What happens when you or your partner fight or disagree? " or "Because abuse and violence are so common in women's lives, I've begun to ask about it routinely. At any time, has a partner hit or otherwise hurt or threatened you? " (see Table 33–3 for suggested screening questions). If the answer is vague or evasive, more direct questions must be asked to determine if abuse is taking place. If this is done in a supportive, nonjudgmental manner, the vast majority of patients feel comfortable and respond honestly.

Table 33–2. Physical examination clues to the presence of domestic violence.

Inappropriate behavior
Multiple injuries
Central pattern of injury
Injuries at different stages of healing

Table 33–3. Screening questions.

- We all fight at home sometimes. What happens when you or your partner fight or disagree?
- Do you feel safe in your home and in your relationship?
- Do you ever feel afraid of your partner?
- Because abuse and violence are so common in women's lives, I've begun to ask about it routinely. At any time, has a partner hit or otherwise hurt or threatened you?
- Does your partner ever force you to engage in sex that makes you feel uncomfortable?
- Does your partner threaten, hit, or abuse your children?

TREATMENT

When domestic violence is detected, five basic tasks must be accomplished (Table 33–4). First, the physician must validate the problem by making a clear statement to the patient that violent behavior is unacceptable, illegal, and that nobody has the right to abuse her. The physician's acknowledgment of the domestic violence as a real issue may be the first step in helping to free her from the relationship. Under all circumstances, avoid language that could be interpreted as blaming the victim for the violence.

Since the majority of women are not ready to leave the relationship when the violence is detected, a main task for the primary care provider is to build the relationship with the patient. Statements that express empathy can be an effective way to accomplish this task, for example: "I really respect the way you have been dealing with this" and "we can work on this problem together." It is important to help the patient set realistic goals (eg, obtain the skills required for a particular job) so that she is not set up for disappointment when she is unable (or unwilling) to leave the relationship. Above all, the physician should avoid recapitulating the power and control dynamics that so often characterizes the patient's abusive relationship. Never insist that she leave the relationship and always allow her the autonomy to make her own decisions.

Second, it is essential to assess the patient's safety thoroughly. Is it safe for her to go home? Other potential options (such as friends, shelters, etc) should be explored and an emergency escape plan reviewed if she chooses to return home. For women not returning home, advising them to inform one or two coworkers about the situation is prudent as the perpetrator may attempt to hurt them at work. Are there weapons in the home, and are there children who are potentially at risk? Assess risk factors for escalating violence, such as an increase in the frequency and severity of assaults, an escalation in threats, and the availability of a firearm.

Third, it is imperative that physicians and other health care providers document clearly and completely when they encounter domestic violence. The medical record should include a complete description of the assault with quotes, if possible, from the patient's own account. Include relevant details in the past medical history and social history. Be sure to write legibly; successful prosecution should never be compromised by sloppy record keeping. Injuries should be described and visually documented, either with a body chart or with photographs, if the patient consents (include the patient's face in at least one photograph). If the police are called, always include the name and any actions taken by the investigating police officer.

Fourth, the patient must be provided with information and appropriate referral. Primary care providers should become familiar with the social and legal services available for battered women in their area. Information about shelters should be provided, if it would not compromise the patient's safety, even if she intends to return home. All patients should be assessed for the presence of psychiatric or substance abuse problems that would benefit from treatment or referral. Physicians should have a basic understanding of legal options, such as restraining orders, so that they can help advise women who wish to take immediate action.

Finally, physicians must be aware of their state's reporting requirements. Although few states currently have statutory provisions specific to domestic violence, more comprehensive laws are being considered by state legislatures around the country. For example, in California, a new law took effect in January 1994 that requires health practitioners to report all incidents of domestic violence to the police that involve an injury. The usual doctor-patient privileged communication is explicitly preempted by this law. It remains to be seen if mandatory reporting laws have the unintended effect of making it more difficult for battered women to discuss domestic violence with their physician and, as a result, further decrease the detection rate.

What to Avoid

Do not insist that the battered woman terminate the relationship, even if you believe that this is the appropriate action. Only she can make that decision. Trying to control her behavior, albeit subtly, recapitulates the same negative dynamic that is taking place in the battering relationship.

Do not recommend couple counseling. This is only appropriate when the male partner acknowledges the problem and wants to change his behavior, and both partners want to preserve the relationship.

Do not use the word *alleged* in the medical record. It implies that you do not believe the woman's story, and you may inadvertently impede her ability to bring her case to court.

Do not ask what the victim did to bring on the violence.

Table 33–4. After detection: five tasks to accomplish

1. Validate the problem.
2. Assess the patient's safety, and review an emergency escape plan.
3. Document clearly and completely.
4. Provide information and appropriate referral.
5. Be aware of reporting and other legal requirements.

BARRIERS

Physician Barriers to Detection

Many studies have revealed that physicians and other health care providers do a poor job of detecting domestic violence, with detection rates rarely exceeding 10%. Several factors are responsible for this dismal record. First, most providers simply lack the appropriate knowledge and training to effectively detect and treat victims of domestic violence. The first step in improving their ability to do so is to disseminate information more widely about its prevalence and consequences. Domestic violence has been little addressed in medical schools, residency training, or continuing medical education. This will change as state and perhaps federal legislation increasingly requires that domestic violence be added to physicians' and other health professionals' education.

Lack of institutional support is another important barrier. Despite the enormity of the problem and the increasing requirements on institutions to have protocols in place, most hospitals and clinics have few, if any, adequately trained support staff, accessible guidelines for practitioners, or information for patients. In addition, with the growth of managed care, there is growing pressure on providers to see more patients and use fewer resources, and this may make it increasingly difficult for issues such as domestic violence to be addressed. Many of the physicians interviewed in one study identified time constraints as the major deterrent to opening the Pandora's box of domestic violence.

It should be noted, however, that the total annual health care costs from domestic violence exceed $44 million, plus the indirect costs of 175,500 lost days from paid work. In addition, the diagnostic and treatment strategies outlined here are not particularly time-intensive. Screening for domestic violence adds less than 1 minute to the typical new patient evaluation; if widely employed, it likely would yield enormous savings through prevention of injury and decreased health care usage.

The third barrier to detection of domestic violence arises from provider discomfort. Many health care providers feel uncomfortable addressing issues other than those that fit neatly into the traditional medical model. Numerous studies have shown that most do a poor job discussing issues with their patients having to do with sex, violence, and substance abuse. Physicians are trained to feel more comfortable dealing with problems that seem to have a clear pathophysiology and treatment. Delving into the cause of a suspicious injury makes them uneasy: it is messy, often not amenable to a straightforward solution, and may raise embarrassing or uncomfortable feelings. We must come to terms with the feelings that domestic violence raises in us, however, if we are to be effective in caring for our patients.

Patient Barriers to Terminating an Abusive Relationship

Primary care providers often have difficulty understanding why more battered women do not terminate their abusive relationship. Why some women remain in these relationships is complex. Some of the reasons include:

1. Fear—for their own safety or for their children. One third of women are not at home when the assault takes place, so it is clear that leaving is no guarantee of safety.
2. Economic—many battered women lack employment skills or experience and would find it very difficult to support themselves and their children. Battering may be the price they decide to pay for economic viability.
3. Psychological—some may find it difficult to leave because of the "psychological dependence" the years of repetitive abuse has created. Battered women are told overtly and covertly that they are worthless; they eventually internalize this and come to believe that they are incapable of surviving on their own, and that they must deserve the beating.
4. Social support—or the lack thereof. Women are often encouraged by well-meaning friends and family members to "try to work things out," or they are advised to stay "for the children's sake."
5. Lack of other options—shelters are often full, friends and family unavailable, legal counsel not accessible.
6. Not all women want the relationship to end, just the battering.

CONCLUSION

Along with the criminal justice system, primary care physicians and other health care providers are most likely to come into contact with victims of domestic violence. They have a professional and ethical obligation to recognize domestic violence and intervene appropriately as well as to exert their influence on a broader level. This may be to push for funding of more shelters (there are only 1300 shelters in the United States, so that three of four women are turned away) or to make sure that teaching about domestic violence is included in all levels of medical education. Screening for and treating domestic violence should become a routine part of the practice and training of medicine. It is time that we confront the epidemic of domestic violence and strive to lessen its impact as one of the most important public health issues of our time.

SUGGESTED READINGS

Alpert EJ: Violence in intimate relationships and the practicing internist: New "disease" or new agenda? Ann Intern Med 1995;123(10):774.

American Medical Association: *Diagnostic and Treatment Guidelines on Domestic Violence.* American Medical Association, 1992.

Flitcraft A: Physicians and domestic violence: Challenges for prevention. Health Aff 1993;Winter:154.

McCauley J et al: The "Battering Syndrome": Prevalence and clinical characteristics of domestic violence in primary care internal medicine practices. Ann Intern Med 1995;123(10):737.

Strauss M, Gelles R, Steinmetz SK: *Behind Closed Doors: A Survey of Family Violence in America.* Doubleday, 1980.

Sugg N, Inui T: Primary care physician's response to domestic violence: Opening Pandora's box. JAMA 1992;267:3157.

Walker LE: *The Battered Woman Syndrome.* Springer, 1984.

Chronic Illness

34

Gail F. Brenner, PhD

INTRODUCTION

The incidence of chronic disease in primary care practice is on the rise. Although chronic diseases comprise a diverse group of pathologic processes, they share in common long-term and frequent medical intervention with little hope for a cure. Moreover, they can tremendously affect people's lives, often requiring significant life changes and reevaluation of priorities. Chronic diseases include the following when their presentation is significant enough to cause impairment: rheumatoid arthritis, lupus, and other rheumatic diseases; neuromuscular diseases such as multiple sclerosis and cerebral palsy; Parkinson's disease; heart disease; stroke; asthma; emphysema; diabetes; and AIDS.

By definition, the management of chronic disease implies longevity in the physician-patient relationship—a relationship that may intensify during exacerbations of the disease. Because the physician-patient relationship needs to be a strong one in cases of chronic disease, communication and interpersonal skills become important in treating these patients. Physicians have the opportunity to provide a supportive environment in which their patients can confront the challenges presented by their illness. This chapter identifies those challenges and provides guidelines to the primary care practitioner for effective intervention, with the ultimate goal of helping people find a way to live meaningfully despite the limitations imposed by their illness. Given the all-encompassing effects of chronic disease, the path to this goal involves instilling in people a sense of control, that is, encouraging them to develop skills and attitudes that will help them to self-manage the multiple manifestations of their disease.

THEORETICAL MODEL OF STRESS & COPING

Stress

A well-known theoretical model of stress and coping provides a useful framework for explaining people's responses to chronic disease and suggests ways in which the physician might intervene. According to this model, stress is experienced when the perceived demands of the environment exceed the available resources for coping with them. Once an event is perceived as stressful, the options and available resources for coping are assessed.

Consider a 29-year-old attorney who has just been diagnosed with insulin-dependent diabetes. Given that he has no prior experience coping with this or similar situations, he defines this event as stressful. He begins to worry about his current and future health status and feels distressed when he considers how the illness will affect his work, his family life, and his daily activities. These thoughts and feelings eventually prompt him to think about how he can cope in a way that will make the experience seem more manageable.

Coping

The goal of coping is to respond cognitively or behaviorally to manage, tolerate, or reduce the effect of a stressful event. The two major methods of coping are problem-focused and emotion-focused. Problem-focused coping consists of active efforts to change something about oneself or the environment. Emotion-focused coping involves efforts to regulate emotional distress. Most often, people tend to take action to solve problems, but when a stressful experience is uncontrollable, that is, nothing can be done to change it, problem-focused coping can be counterproductive. It may even result in chronic distress, whereas efforts at emotional regulation may more successfully provide relief.

In the case of the attorney recently diagnosed with diabetes, with appropriate education he will learn that much of his disease is controllable. He can engage in problem-focused coping responses that will control his blood sugar levels, such as frequent blood sugar testing, taking insulin as needed, and complying with diet and exercise recommendations. He may at times, however, feel afraid about the possibility of future complications and experience frustration about the extent to which his diabetes intrudes on his daily functioning. He may decide to cope with these feelings by distracting himself with an activity he enjoys, by seeking out someone to talk with about his feelings, or by focusing on the present situation and the things he can control. These emotion-focused responses are intended to minimize his emotional distress.

The problem-focused/emotion-focused distinction in coping is useful, not only in understanding people's coping efforts, but in providing guidelines to primary care practitioners about how to facilitate adaptation to chronic disease. It is likely that providers perceive patient reactions such as noncompliance, frustration with medical care, or expressed fear about future disability as requiring a response. The physician asks, "What can I do to help this patient? " This framework conceives of chronic disease as a series of challenges that face both patients and their providers. The remainder of this chapter describes the situations that people with chronic disease often encounter and experience as stressful. It explores how these stressful reactions appear in the provider-patient relationship, and offers suggestions to the primary care practitioner for problem-focused and emotion-focused coping responses.

THE CYCLE OF CHRONIC DISEASE

The experience of living with many chronic illnesses has been described as the interconnection among depression, stress, pain, and the disease process or increased disability (Figure 34–1). Increasing stress in an individual's life, for example, greater work demands, might lead to an increase in activity level, greater fatigue, muscle tension, and the

psychological experience of feeling stressed and overwhelmed. These may contribute to high levels of pain, which in turn can lead to a decline in daily functioning, immobility, and heightened disease activity. This brings to awareness the debilitating aspects of the chronic illness and may negatively affect self-esteem, contributing to depression. Ongoing problems add to this cycle, characterized by poor coping and inability to adapt.

The components of this cycle are addressed in the following sections, with suggestions for problem-focused and emotion-focused coping responses that target patients' thoughts, attitudes, emotions, and behavior. To the extent that these coping responses can be considered and put to use, the cycle of chronic disease can be interrupted, decreasing stress and pain, increasing psychological well-being, and slowing the disease process.

DIAGNOSIS OF CHRONIC DISEASE

At the Time of Diagnosis

Description: It may take years until the correct diagnosis of a chronic illness becomes evident. From the patient's point of view, knowing a problem exists but being unable to define its boundaries, is often frightening and frustrating. Physicians may likewise experience frustration and fear about possibly having missed an important piece of information that would lead to the correct diagnosis. Successful management of this situation can be enhanced by emotion-focused and problem-focused techniques (Table 34–1).

Intervention: Patients often worry that their symptoms may not be taken seriously. Providers can

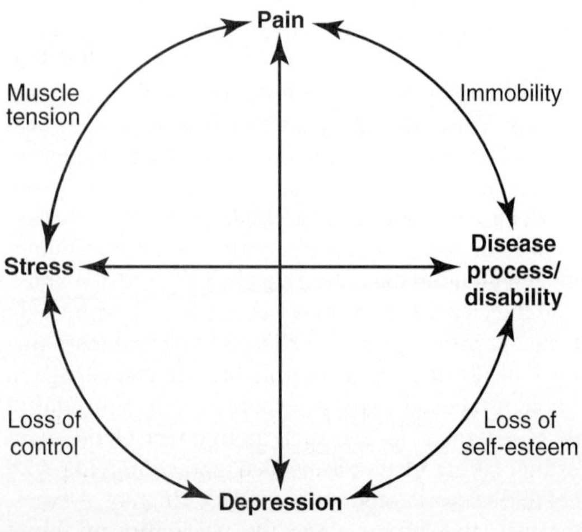

Figure 34–1. The cycle of chronic disease.

Table 34–1. Physician interventions before diagnosis and at the time of diagnosis.

Before Diagnosis
Emotion-focused interventions
1. Ask about and listen to patient's emotional responses.
2. Acknowledge uncertainty.
Problem-focused interventions
1. Suggest palliative measures for symptom relief.
2. Provide patient education about the chronic disease cycle.

At the Time of Diagnosis
Emotion-focused interventions
1. Expect variability in emotional responses.
2. Inquire about the patient's feelings.
3. Reflect back expressed feelings to communicate understanding.
4. Fully attend to the patient, discussing concerns in an unhurried manner.
Problem-focused interventions
1. Schedule a second appointment soon after delivering the diagnosis.
2. Assess patient's preference for information.
3. Discuss the structure of the physician-patient relationship.

provide emotion-focused support by listening to and reflecting back the patient's concerns and by acknowledging that fear and uncertainty are natural at this time. They can also be reassuring about their commitment to their patient's care. Finally, it might be useful for providers to reflect on their own feelings of frustration or concern and acknowledge that these may well be appropriate to the situation.

Problem-focused responses such as palliative measures, including medication, physical therapy, occupational therapy, splints, orthotics, and adaptive devices, are likely to be helpful. In addition, patients can be educated about the cycle of chronic disease and pain control techniques so they can better understand and adapt to their condition.

Communicating About the Diagnosis: Once the diagnosis is clarified, patients are faced with the challenge of adapting to their illness. They may react to the news with shock or disbelief and be unable to absorb information provided at that time. The provider should schedule a second appointment soon after the news is delivered to enable patients to ask questions about the disease and its effect on their life (see Chapter 3).

Some patients are information seekers, who need detailed information to reduce uncertainty; others tend to avoid information and cope by distracting themselves from the stressful experience. Providers should ask about the amount of information the patient prefers, keeping in mind that preferences may change over time. Physicians should discuss the cause of the disease, treatment options, expected course, and possible complications using nontechnical language. Patients' understanding of the information should be checked by asking them to repeat what the doctor has told them.

Patients may also benefit from a brief discussion of the structure of the provider-patient relationship. The provider might state the length of time of the usual appointment and suggest ways to make the best use of that time, for example, that the patient arrive with a list of questions or concerns. Patients may be concerned about physician availability, especially in the event of an acute or urgent medical situation. They are likely to be reassured by having discussed a plan in advance to deal with these situations.

Emotional Responses: Many people with a new chronic illness appear to move through a series of stages as they begin to accept their situation. These stages occur as a function of the many losses inherent in adapting to a chronic condition and may include denial, anger, bargaining, depression, and, finally, acceptance. It is important to remember that responses to learning about a diagnosis vary greatly. The responses might not occur in any particular order and are unlikely to adhere to an expected timetable. Moreover, recent evidence suggests that not all people experience grief and depression in response to significant losses; some appear to adapt without substantial emotional distress.

The primary care provider should remember that patients with a new diagnosis may manifest a number of responses, including shock, denial, acceptance, helplessness, anger, or sadness. They are likely to feel relieved and supported by the physician's willingness to inquire about and show empathy for their experiences. The physician might ask, "How are you feeling about the news I've given you? " or "What's it like for you to learn about your diagnosis? " and respond by showing understanding with a statement like "It must be hard for you to think about how this will affect your life." Touching may help communicate caring and concern. Conversations of this type need to take place in an unhurried manner with the physician fully attending to the patient. Once the patient understands that not only medical, but other personal concerns may be discussed, an effective working alliance begins to form between the physician and the patient.

Cultural Issues: Primary care providers should be aware of culturally based explanations of health and illness. They need to recognize that their perspective may differ from that of their patients and they should attempt to understand the effect of the disease from their patients' points of view.

EFFECT OF CHRONIC DISEASE

Patients with a chronic illness encounter a range of coping challenges that involve nearly every aspect of their lives. The following section details these challenges, discusses variations in the ways people may respond, and suggests effective interventions (Table 34–2).

Case illustration: Jane is a 34-year-old married woman and mother of two young children, who recently experienced a severe flare-up of her rheumatoid arthritis (RA). When her arthritis was in remission, she worked full-time, volunteered at her children's school, and was active on the board of a community organization. She considered herself fortunate to be so functional and was pleased with these multiple roles. With the flare-up, however, she needed to take sick leave from work and, with continued deterioration in her condition, she decided to resign from her volunteer positions. Because of pain and fatigue, she became less able to drive her children to different activities, managing only to do the most essential household chores. She found herself relying more on her husband and close friends for assistance and emotional support. Moreover, her arthritis became more apparent to others, as it affected her gait and the appearance of her hands. As her functional abilities became impaired, she began to feel that she was no longer able to contribute to her relationships and her community, and her self-esteem diminished. In addition, she felt less attractive due to changes in her appearance, and she felt disconnected from her body, as it reacted in unfamiliar and unpleasant ways. She became increasingly depressed and isolated from others.

Table 34–2. Physician intervention in areas affected by chronic disease.

Activity Level
Emotion-focused interventions
1. Elicit the patient's reactions to necessary reductions in activity level.
2. Listen to and reflect feelings expressed by the patient.
Problem-focused interventions
1. Suggest planning the day's activities in advance, leaving time for rest and enjoyment.
2. Encourage flexibility about adapting to change.
3. Positively frame changes in activity level.

Activity Choice
Emotion-focused interventions
1. Use active listening and reflection of feelings.
2. Provide hope by encouraging an active approach to the disability.
Problem-focused interventions
1. Suggest connecting with others through disease-specific organizations or by reading about others' experiences with chronic disease.
2. Prescribe physical and occupational therapy as needed.
3. Encourage use of adaptive living devices.
4. Reinforce patients' progress in adapting to their disease.

Sexuality
Emotion-focused interventions
1. Raise the topic of sexuality with all chronic disease patients.
2. Normalize and validate the patient's experiences.
Problem-focused interventions
1. Ask questions to pinpoint the problem.
2. Encourage communication with the partner.
3. Suggest planning sex when fatigue and pain are reduced, after use of pain medication, and consider alternative sexual practices.
4. Refer for counseling as needed.

Emotional Response
Emotion-focused interventions
1. Reflect on one's own degree of comfort with experiencing and expressing feelings.
2. Remember that listening, reflecting, and being silent are effective.
3. If the patient's feelings are intrusive, suggest distraction by engaging in enjoyable activities.
4. At appropriate times, suggest focusing on positive or controllable aspects of the situation, using humor, and noticing how the present situation has helped one develop desired characteristics.
Problem-focused interventions
1. Refer for mental health treatment as necessary.
2. Encourage active self-management of the disease.
3. Include patients in decision-making about their medical care.

Relationships
Emotion-focused interventions
1. Ask about the effect of the chronic disease on relationships.
2. Validate the difficulty in relationship transitions.
3. Discuss the effectiveness of the physician-patient relationship.
Problem-focused interventions
1. Encourage communication in relationships using effective communication skills.
2. Encourage patients to maintain their usual level of control and decision-making power in their relationships.
3. Refer for individual, couple, or family counseling, as appropriate.

Effect on Activity Level

Description: As a result of pain, fatigue, or physical disability, most people with a chronic disease eventually find that they are unable to maintain their usual level of activity. A common response is to try against all odds to maintain as "normal" a life as possible, sometimes overdoing it. This can result in an increase in disease activity. Others may simply give up and not try to adapt to their new situation. They may feel victimized and controlled by their disease, which leads them to lose their sense of power and become dependent on others. The resulting reduction in activity can be detrimental to their physical condition as well.

Case illustration (Contd.): Jane returned to her busy schedule once her RA was stabilized. She tried desperately to maintain her usual activity despite pain and overwhelming fatigue. She dropped into bed each night exhausted, waking at 5:00 AM to give her joints time to lose their stiffness. Within a month, she was back in her physician's office, complaining of pain, redness, and swelling in her hands and feet, and asking for a change in medication to enable her to keep going. When her physician commented that she seemed more stressed than usual, she began to cry.

Intervention: Provider interventions regarding their patients' activity level can help people adapt to their illness. These interventions are useful both for patients who overdo it and those who give up. The goal is to achieve a state of maximum functionality within the limitations imposed by the disease. Before providing problem-focused assistance, it is useful for the provider to discuss the patient's feelings about the losses incurred by giving up valued activities. Ask open-ended questions such as, "What do you think about (or feel) when you realize that you can't do it all anymore? " and respond by simply listening or labeling the emotion expressed with a statement like, "It seems like you're feeling very sad about your losses."

Using empathic reflection may feel to the provider as though nothing is being accomplished, but such communication skills can be highly effective. When patients feel heard and understood, they are more open to discussing problem-focused strategies for addressing their problems. The provider's input can be helpful as people move through the difficult process of considering which of their activities to reduce or eliminate. In addition, people with chronic disease are likely to benefit from planning each day in advance, making sure to include enjoyable activities and leaving time for a rest or a nap.

Flexibility is essential to successfully adapting to these changes. For example, patients should be encouraged to reevaluate their schedule on a day when they wake up feeling poorly. Framing these shifts in activity level in a positive way helps facilitate patients' acceptance of them. Explaining how rest and relaxation can retard the progression of the disease and contribute to life satisfaction can also be helpful. The changes can be viewed, for example, as an opportunity to have more quality time to spend with one's children.

Effect on Activity Choice
Description: Most people with a chronic disease eventually need to make changes in the kinds of activities in which they participate. These changes can range from giving up a valued hobby or satisfying job to adapting to one's inability to turn a doorknob or climb a flight of stairs. These challenges are significant because they are a constant reminder of their illness and its effects.

Case illustration (Contd.): As Jane's RA progressed, she began having difficulty carrying out her daily activities around the house. She found cooking especially problematic because she could not hold utensils or heavy pots. These problems were caused by her decreased range of motion and flexibility, loss of strength, and pain. She wondered how she could make changes that would enable her to continue to be able to cook for her family.

Intervention: As indicated earlier, physicians should be sensitive to patients' feelings, using active listening and reflection to communicate understanding. Since there are many problem-focused strategies for coping with these activity changes, pa-

tients should be encouraged to adopt an attitude of active self-management and control. The physician can act as a coach, suggesting various coping strategies. Patients might benefit, for example, from connecting with others with similar problems. Local chapters of organizations of people with specific diseases, such as the Arthritis Foundation, are good resources for literature, classes on disease self-management, and support groups.

Patients might also be helped by reading books authored by people with a chronic disease (eg, Pitzele, 1986). Adjunctive treatments such as occupational or physical therapy, as well as use of adaptive living devices, may be helpful. The range of possibilities for adaptive change is unlimited, and people with chronic illness can be encouraged by becoming aware of the options. S. K. Pitzele, for example, offers hundreds of suggestions for modifying activities in every room of the house. It is also helpful to commend patients for their efforts to actively adapt to their condition.

Sexuality
Description: Sexuality is affected by many chronic illnesses. Interest in sex and the physical ability to engage in sexual activity are reduced as a result of fatigue, pain, loss of strength, altered sense of body image, decreased self-esteem, and relationship stress. Patients concerned about sex may raise the topic with their physicians; others may feel burdened by these concerns but reluctant to discuss them.

Case illustration (Contd.): As Jane's arthritis worsened, she and her husband, Ken, began having sex much less frequently. She was usually exhausted and in pain, and the visible changes in her joints made her feel unattractive. In addition, she was afraid of the pain she would experience with sex. She was also aware, however, of the loss of intimacy and the growing rift with Ken. Ken was also feeling the lack of closeness as well as missing the enjoyment of a previously satisfying sex life. Yet he was reluctant to burden her further by bringing up a difficult topic.

Intervention: Primary care providers should try to discuss sexuality with all patients who have a chronic illness. The provider might say "Sometimes people with RA have concerns about sex. Has this been something you've thought about or worried about? " If patients choose to not discuss it, the provider should make known his or her availability to talk and follow up on the issue at a future appointment. If patients do raise concerns, try to pinpoint the source of the problem, such as "What do you think interferes with your having satisfying sex? " An appropriate emotion-focused response is to listen to patients' concerns and validate their experiences by saying, for example, "It's not unusual for people with RA to have that experience." Suggest that patients communicate with their partner about their concerns, possibly by including the partner in a future appointment. Often couples can work together toward solutions once the problem has been identified and discussed.

Practical problem-focused strategies for helping with sexual difficulties include planning sex at a time when the patient is less tired and experiencing less pain, timing medication so the maximal effect occurs when sex is planned, taking a warm bath prior to sex, and using alternative sexual techniques. Referral to a sex or couple therapist might be useful, particularly when the couple has serious communication problems or obvious sexual dysfunction. This might facilitate communication and help the couple discuss options for sex (see Chapter 28).

Emotional Responses to Chronic Disease

In this section, common emotional responses to chronic disease are described followed by a discussion of emotion-focused and problem-focused coping. The goal is to help primary care providers better understand their patients' internal experiences and outward expression of their emotions and to intervene in ways that promote adaptive coping. Adaptive coping means having available a repertoire of responses that can be used to deal with and modulate the ebb and flow of experience.

Keeping in mind the "chronic" in chronic disease, that is, the longevity of the coping process, no set sequence or intensity of emotions should be expected. For example, the grieving that took place with the initial diagnosis may recur years later with a clear increase in physical disability. In addition, people vary greatly in how they react to their experiences—some may feel their emotions intensely, and others may be more modulated or less aware; some may need time to process their feelings, and others feel resolved more quickly. Thus, physicians should be attuned to the feelings their patients are experiencing without expecting them to react in a set way.

Sadness/Grief: One of the common emotions experienced by people with a chronic disease is a sense of sadness and loss accompanied by grieving for the loss. Losses are experienced in many areas: health and well-being, body image, the ability to engage in desired activities including work, the core sense of self, independence, important relationships, and future plans. Although grieving is not always necessary to resolve a loss, many patients benefit from an opportunity to discuss it with their physicians. If they do not, providers may want to ask about how they are feeling and coping. Some patients may see their provider's office as a place where they can talk more openly about their feelings, whereas others may be less willing to show their vulnerability and assert that nothing is wrong. It is often helpful to suggest that discussing feelings is acceptable and often beneficial.

Anger: Patients may feel angry as they process their feelings about their disease. Although a difficult and uncomfortable emotion for many, anger is a normal part of the grieving process. Anger may be expressed overtly but is often suppressed or displaced. This can lead to increased irritability and conflict in relationships. A patient's irritation at her physician's inability to control her symptoms or at her husband's inefficiency in managing household chores that were once her responsibility may reflect her own underlying anger about the effects of the disease. Repressed anger can show itself in behaviors such as noncompliance or missed appointments. Anger may also be expressed in terms of unfairness, as in the patient asking, "Why me?" This question represents a desire to understand events and attribute responsibility for them. People struggle to understand why they developed the disease, wondering whether to blame themselves or others. Eventual acceptance of the disease is facilitated by letting go of the urge to assign blame and focusing attention on the current realities of the disease, including action-oriented coping strategies targeted to aspects of the disease that can be controlled. Patients benefit from acknowledging their anger, understanding that it is to be expected, and communicating it to others in as constructive a way as possible.

Loss of Control: People with chronic disease often experience a sense of loss of control and uncertainty about the future accompanied by anxiety, worry, and fear. Patients worry about future disability, adequacy of financial resources, and ability to maintain significant relationships. As they understand the extent of their loss, they realize that they have no blueprint for the future. A chronic disease imposes on people the need to change without their choosing to do so. They are faced with fear and uncertainty about daily activities that were once taken for granted as well as other issues such as plans for retirement. This uncertainty may manifest itself as anxiety about their medical care.

> *Case illustration (Contd.):* When Jane's physician entered the examining room, she uncharacteristically began by pointing out that he was 10 minutes late. She pulled a list of complaints from her pocket and stated that she was disturbed about the side effects of her medication and the lack of control over her pain. Rather than responding directly to her complaints, her physician reflected that she seemed upset. When she agreed, her physician invited her to talk about it. She talked about the constant pain and discomfort, her recent need to reduce her work hours, and her concern that she could end up in a wheelchair. "I just don't feel like I can count on anything anymore," she asserted. Her physician suggested, "It seems like you feel that your whole world is unstable." "It is," she said sadly, "and sometimes I just don't want to deal with it anymore."

Intervention: To help patients deal with their feelings about their chronic disease, it is useful for providers to reflect on their own styles of experiencing and expressing feelings. To the extent that practitioners can understand and accept their own feelings, they are likely to be more open to those of their patients. Often, the anxiety providers experience with patients with a chronic disease has to do with the feeling that they cannot really do anything to help. In this sense, it is useful to remember that patients may benefit from emotion-focused responses, that is, allowing them to talk about what they are experiencing so that they feel listened to and understood. Once expressed, feelings are no longer carried around only internally, and the patient is less likely to feel burdened by them. Specific responses the physician might make include reflecting the emotion being expressed ("Sounds like you're angry.") and restating the patient's comment ("So what you're saying is that you're disappointed about not being able to enjoy your retirement the way you had planned."). Simply giving the patient time to talk and feel is often helpful (see Chapters 1 and 2).

Another useful method for helping patients deal with their feelings is to alter either their focus of attention or the meaning derived from their current experiences. For example, patients can be distracted from their feelings by refocusing their attention on other thoughts or activities, focusing on the positive aspects of the experience, finding humor in the situation, and reflecting on how the situation has helped them to grow as a person (as in developing patience and greater tolerance). Moving into problem-focused coping by taking active steps to self-manage the problem at hand, as discussed in previous sections, is also appropriate.

Practitioners should acknowledge the uncertainty and provide information to respond to the patient's fears about loss of control. But with some patients, no amount of information can allay all their concerns. Gentle limit-setting with regard to frequency of phone calls and number and length of appointments may be necessary. Patients can be helped by acknowledging their fear and anxiety and by distinguishing between controllable and uncontrollable concerns. When they focus on uncontrollable issues, worry and anxiety increase; recognizing what can be controlled can lead to specific problem-focused coping behaviors that help manage anxiety and decrease a patient's sense of powerlessness.

Physicians can help to foster control by engaging patients as partners in their medical care. If appropriate, give patients a choice of treatment options, allowing them to evaluate the pros and cons of each. Some will seek out information about their illness and potential treatments from a variety of other sources. Acknowledge that they are attempting to restore a sense of control and seriously consider their proposed remedies.

Effect on Relationships

Description: The toll that a chronic illness can take on close relationships should not be underestimated. Given increasing disability, fatigue, and other changes, roles change and people realize that they cannot be quite the same parent, partner, friend, or coworker. The experience of loss can be significant. As the role of one person in the relationship changes, the roles of others change as well. The concerns of partners, children, other family members, friends, and other caregivers should not be overlooked. The patient may fear abandonment, especially at times of greatest need. The provider-patient relationship is also at risk in the context of the patient's impending and eventual debilitation.

Case illustration (Contd.): As Jane's level of disability increased, she noticed differences in how her two children related to her. Her younger daughter, Molly, age 7, seemed committed to not further burdening her mother. Her room was always clean, and she always helped her mother prepare dinner. When Jane encouraged Molly to spend time with friends in the neighborhood, she declined, saying she preferred to stay home in case she was needed. Jane's other daughter, Lauren, age 11, reacted quite differently. Lauren stopped having conversations with her mother about the events of the day and spent most of her time in her room listening to music. She often became angry when Jane said she was too tired to drive her to a friend's house. Jane felt guilty and assumed that her children's reactions were due to her illness, but she did not know how to talk with them about so sensitive a topic.

Intervention: Since relationships are often stressed in persons with chronic disease, the primary care provider should inquire about how things are going at home and acknowledge that transitions in relationships as a result of chronic disease can be difficult. Communication is the key to successfully navigating these transitions. Successful communication requires two components: (1) a structure within which people can openly talk about their feelings, for example, a family meeting at home, a session in the physician's office, or counseling with a mental health professional; and (2) use of effective communication skills.

One important issue that often needs to be discussed is the providing or receiving of help. Problems in this area derive from a mismatch in behaviors that are perceived as helpful by the people in the relationship as well as a discrepancy in the perceived level of need for help. For example, the wife of a man with multiple sclerosis may encourage him to rest with the intention of helping him feel less fatigued, but he may perceive her efforts as further attempts to control his daily activities. People with chronic disease need to maintain as much control as possible in their relationships. This means, at least in part, continuing to make decisions for themselves. Physicians can be helpful to their patients by listening to their concerns about relationships and suggesting possible interventions. Referral to a mental health professional is appropriate, especially prior to the escalation of a problem to a crisis.

Communication is also important in the physician-patient relationship. The relationship can be supported by periodic assessments of its efficacy ("How is our way of relating working for you? ") and the understanding that issues can be discussed as needed.

PROBLEMS WITH ADHERENCE

Patients with chronic disease participate actively in their medical care to varying degrees. Of concern to the provider are those who do not comply with follow-up appointments or medication regimens. Explanations for nonadherence may include financial problems, denial or lack of information about illness severity, cultural beliefs, complexity of dosing schedules, use of multiple medications, adverse side effects, inaccurate expectations about the positive effects of the medication, and the inconvenience of ongoing care. Physicians should try to understand the reasons for poor adherence in a nonjudgmental manner (Table 34–3). In addition, simpler regimens are likely to result in greater adherence. Ultimately, however, it is the patient's responsibility to engage in medical care. Physicians may feel unappreciated if the patient chooses to resist treatment, but they should not view themselves as having failed (see Chapter 17).

Table 34–3. Physician interventions for adherence problems.

1. Assess reasons for nonadherence, including financial concerns and cultural beliefs.
2. Reduce the complexity of medication regimens and dosing frequency.
3. Alter the medication regimen to fit the patient's lifestyle.
4. Provide patient education about the expected effects of the medication.
5. Suggest using a calendar, daily pill box, or diary to keep track of medications.

INDICATIONS FOR REFERRAL

People with a chronic disease can often benefit from a variety of services, including physical and occupational therapy, counseling, pain management programs, social work, nutrition, and employment rehabilitation. Patients should be encouraged to use these services in any way that would be helpful to them. Constraints imposed by managed care, however, may at times limit access to these services. Patients may be helped by referral to community-based resources or by connecting with resources offered by local chapters of national disease-specific organizations.

Referral for mental health services should be offered in the following situations: symptoms of clinical depression or other psychiatric disorder, illness-related concerns that are obstacles to adaptive coping, persistent problems with adherence to medication regimens, and communication problems in close and important relationships. Individual, couple, or family therapy may be appropriate depending on the situation. Cognitive-behavioral therapy may facilitate acceptance of the disease, teach appropriate coping skills, and help the patient to regain a sense of control.

SUMMARY

The effects of chronic disease are broad and severe, affecting physical and psychological well-being, activity level, body image, self-esteem, and important relationships. Primary care providers have a unique opportunity to offer a supportive and affirming environment in which patients can constructively deal with these issues. Intervention strategies are either emotion-focused (aiding in the expression or regulation of emotion) or problem-focused (suggesting concrete ways to take action to affect the multiple manifestations of the disease). The ultimate goal is for patients to find ways to live full, meaningful, and satisfying lives despite the limitations imposed by their disease.

SUGGESTED READINGS

Burkett GL: Culture, illness and the biopsychosocial model. Family Med 1991;23:287.
Delbanco TL: Enriching the doctor-patient relationship by inviting the patient's perspective. Ann Intern Med 1992;116:414.
DiMatteo MR: Enhancing patient adherence to medical recommendations. JAMA 1994;271:79.
Kaplan SH, Greenfield S, Ware JE, Jr: Assessing the effects of physician-patient interactions on the outcomes of chronic disease. Med Care 1989;27(Suppl):S110.
Lazarus RS, Folkman S: Stress, Appraisal, and Coping. Springer, 1984.
Novack, DH: Therapeutic aspects of the clinical encounter. J Gen Int Med 1987; 2:346.

Pitzele SK: We Are Not Alone: Learning to Live with Chronic Illness. Workman Publishing, 1986.
Taylor SE, Aspinwall LG: Coping with chronic illness. In: Goldberger L, Breznitz S (editors): Handbook of Stress: Theoretical and Clinical Aspects, 2nd ed. Free Press, 1993.
Walbroehl GS: Sexual concerns of the patient with pulmonary disease. Postgrad Med 1992;91:455.
Wasner, CK: The art of unproven remedies. Rheum Dis Clin North Am 1991;17:197.
Wortman CB, Silver RC: The myths of coping with loss. In: Monat L, Lazarus, RS (editors): Stress and Coping: An Anthology, 3rd ed. Columbia University Press, 1991.

Death & Dying

35

Michael Eisman, MD, & Timothy Quill, MD

INTRODUCTION

As clinicians, we need to ask ourselves how we want to be treated when we are dying. Answering this question helps us discover and clarify our own beliefs and values concerning the care of dying patients. Although medical practice is usually based on the concepts of healing, cure, and restoration of function, these ideas are called into question when patients are dying. Is death something to be fought at all costs, or is it our responsibility to ease the dying process? Despite the fact that about 2 million people die every year in the United States, death's mystery and finality continue to fascinate and terrify us. Death is not a disease, and dying is not an illness that can be cured. Palliation, not cure, and relief of suffering, not restoration of function, are medicine's primary goals in caring for the dying patient.

> *Case illustration 1:* Ella, a 71-year-old woman, has had pains in her lower chest and upper abdomen for a month before visiting her personal physician. When a chest film shows several nodular masses suggestive of widespread lung cancer, the physician phones Ella and tells her there is a problem, making an office appointment for the next day. At this visit, the doctor discusses the results of the chest film with the patient and her son. Ella, having long suspected she might get cancer from smoking heavily, weeps openly. As the diagnosis is not yet certain, bronchoscopy is recommended, and she is referred to a pulmonologist. The bronchoscopy biopsies show a small-cell lung cancer. The pulmonologist refers Ella to an oncologist who recommends chemotherapy and tells the patient that if she doesn't respond to chemotherapy she will have less than a year to live.
>
> The patient and her son return to her primary care doctor to discuss her options. Ella says she would like to proceed with chemotherapy but wants to stop it if she becomes too ill from the treatments. A Roman Catholic, she has discussed with her priest the morality of refusing extraordinary care, including feeding tubes, if she were to have a terminal condition. She has appointed her son her health-care proxy and discussed with him her desire

not to undergo cardiopulmonary resuscitation. The physician gives Ella a living will; she and her son complete it together. Ella undergoes chemotherapy for several months but grows thinner and weaker.

> Ella lives alone and does not want to die in her apartment. Neither does she want her son to have to provide home care for her when she becomes too dependent to live alone. She also wants to know whether she could die in the hospital or a nursing home. Her doctor agrees to hospitalize her and find other placement when the need arises.
>
> When she becomes confused and is hospitalized, a brain CT scan shows cerebral metastasis. As Ella loses the capacity to make decisions, her son and her physician decide that, based on her previous wishes, she would not want to live under the current conditions. She is moved to a nursing home, with comfort-care orders guiding treatment, and dies 6 months after the initial diagnosis.

The step from a seemingly endless life to one in which death appears clearly on the horizon is a momentous one. We usually live in denial about our own mortality. Although we may sometimes abstractly acknowledge that our death will occur, we do not know when or how. The *when* and *how* of the patient's death become explicit issues when a potentially fatal disorder is diagnosed. Personal, cultural, and spiritual beliefs and experiences shape how we respond to the news about our impending death. After the initial diagnosis, there is often a progressive series of losses in the dying process, each punctuated by the clinician delivering additional bad news. Each step of this process can evoke strong emotional and cognitive reactions. It may elicit overwhelming fear and anxiety, or it may be met with outward equanimity.

NONABANDONMENT OF THE DYING PATIENT

When a patient is informed of a life-threatening illness, a wide spectrum of feelings may emerge: denial, intense anxiety, fear, sadness, anger. If the practitioner is inexperienced in palliative care or is extremely discomfited by death, there may be a tendency to withdraw from the patient's care. The commitment not to abandon the patient requires that clinicians learn to work through their own feelings, become knowledgeable about palliative care, and recognize that the process of dying can be a unique spiritual and personal experience for both doctor and patient. The goal is to form a partnership that will help the patient face the future with courage and dignity.

The goals of partnership and shared decision making are sometimes limited by strong emotional reactions as well as long-standing personality traits that can isolate the patient from the clinician, friends, and family. In addition, physicians may be unable to commit the time and energy to help develop close personal contact with the dying patient. Clinicians need to realize that extraordinary effort is sometimes required to be a partner with the patient for a "good" death.

The Difficult Patient

Case illustration 2: At 68 years old, Albert has severe end-stage emphysema, complicated by mitral regurgitation, congestive heart failure, cardiac arrhythmias, alcoholism, and years of smoking. He lives with his wife, whom he has bullied and dominated throughout their 40-year marriage. He has been on home oxygen and has had multiple hospital admissions for shortness of breath.

Admitted to the emergency room with severe shortness of breath, Albert is found to have pneumonia and heart failure. He had previously decided not to have cardiopulmonary resuscitation and wanted "no part of any of those damned machines." He is admitted to the hospital and treated with aggressive medical means but is not put on a respirator. Albert regularly yells and curses at the respiratory therapists, nursing staff, physicians, and his family for not taking care of him; for making him suffer; and for not being prompt enough with meals, medicines, and treatments. He insists that nothing is wrong with him except that the medicines are making him sick.

Efforts to engage Albert in a dialogue that explores his feelings meet first with an unwillingness to talk and then a life history of feeling abandoned, powerless, betrayed by employers, and subject to bad luck. He describes himself as an "ornery son of a bitch." He fears lingering and suffering in the hospital, and although he hopes he will die quickly, he is also afraid to die. One of Albert's fears is of being buried alive, a phobia fed by a television program he had seen about the difficulty of determining when someone was dead and the possibility of being sent to the undertaker while still alive. The anxiety of being trapped in a "tight" place is overwhelming to him.

Albert's physicians have resisted placing him on anxiolytic drugs or narcotics out of fear they would compromise his breathing. The issue of comfort care is discussed with him and his wife, and the primary goal of relieving his suffering, rather than prolonging his life, is affirmed. Anxiolytic drugs are started. Placed in a room with a large picture window to the outside, he spends long periods of time staring out the window. His complaints diminish and he seems more relaxed, finally telling his wife he has suffered enough and does not want to live any longer. He gradually becomes more confused as a result of the rising carbon dioxide levels and dies several nights later.

It is unusual for a life-long pattern of behavior to be altered by the dying process. Although for some people dying may be a time for personal growth, reflection, and meaning, for others, personal factors and emotional reactions block an acceptance of death. The most frequently encountered of these reactions are denial, anger, depression, fear, and anxiety. These reactions may be present in different degrees and at different times in the dying process. Clinicians need to acknowledge, explore, and eventually understand what function the reaction is serving for the patient. Empathy, rather than withdrawal, is the way to deepen the patient-clinician relationship (see Chapter 2).

The Abandoned Patient

Case illustration 3: Max, a 63-year-old, recently retired, and previously healthy man, develops abdominal pains and is found to have widely metastasized colon cancer. He goes to a physician and is advised that no treatment would be beneficial and that he has approximately 6–12 months to live. He is given acetaminophen and codeine for pain and told to come back when the combination no longer relieves the discomfort. Max and his wife cannot bear the thought of just waiting for him to die and decide to seek a cure—or at least some kind of treatment. They hear of a cancer-treatment clinic out of the country and go there for a 6-week program of intensive vitamin and herbal treatments, coffee enemas, a variety of teas, and dietary supplements and modifications. Max is also given a long list of treatments to follow when they return home; this keeps them busy trying to beat the cancer. The clinic is supposed to provide follow-up by mail or telephone; however, several months go by and they do not hear from the clinic.

Discouraged, Max and his wife go to another physician in their home town when the pains in his liver intensify and ascites and jaundice set in. After the physician and the couple discuss the available options, comfort-care measures are agreed on; Max dies 4 weeks later, approximately 9 months from the time of diagnosis. His wife never receives any follow-up information from the overseas clinic, nor does anyone from the original physician's office call to offer condolences on her husband's death.

This patient has been abandoned twice. The first treating physician failed to explore all treatment alternatives and then offered inadequate follow-up. The alternative clinic offered the patient an active treatment approach, which he and his wife needed—but then deserted him by failing to follow through when the treatment did not work (see further discussion, later in this chapter in 'Hope and Meaning').

Nonabandonment is a key element in the care of the dying patient.

Dealing With Grief

At times it may be difficult to distinguish normal grief reactions to the dying process from pathological states that may need consultation and special treatment. There is a natural sadness that human beings experience in regard to death. This sadness may be a way of preparing for death, and has been called **preparatory** or **anticipatory grief.** Grieving over the loss of physical abilities, social position, and contact with pleasurable routines—whether one's own or those of a loved one—is a natural reaction. The absence of grief over these losses may indicate denial and emotional numbing. Sharing and exploring the grief helps both patient and clinician enter a relationship that acknowledges one another's humanity. Having the courage to explore these feelings assists the patient in coming to terms with death and may avoid the clinical depression to which some patients are prone.

Distinguishing clinical depression from the natural grieving process that accompanies a terminal illness may be difficult, as they share many common symptoms. The vegetative symptoms of depression—fatigue, appetite changes, sleep disorders, decreased sexual drive—are all common in serious illness. The affective and cognitive signs of depression, such as loss of interest, withdrawal, hopelessness, shame, guilt, sadness, inability to concentrate, and suicidal ideation, may be realistic assessments in the face of severe suffering, fear of a loss of dignity, and the expectation of death. When the cognitive symptoms, dysphoria, or isolation seem out of proportion to the patient's situation, a major depression should be considered and the physician might refer the patient (and the family) to a mental health professional. Psycho-

therapists who are familiar with the dying process and are experienced with medically ill patients provide an invaluable resource, both diagnostically and therapeutically, in the care of the terminally ill.

TRANSITIONS

Each transition—each diminishment of health—at the end of life includes loss, as well as the potential for personal growth and the acceptance of death. These transitions may initially be treated as another form of bad news, but they provide the opportunity for enhanced meaning and control in the dying process. Physicians caring for terminally ill patients must explore and work through these transitions with their patients. Questions that clinicians can ask their patients in exploring their views on end-of-life issues are listed in Table 35–1. These can be asked as hypothetical questions to explore the patient's beliefs about death and dying. In patients with more advanced illness, the questions and their answers may be highly relevant to immediate treatment decisions.

Education & Information

Clinicians need to provide the patient with information about the disease, the prognosis, the treatment options, and the anticipated course of the illness. Most patients and their families want to know how much time is left when a terminal diagnosis is made. Providing ranges of survival times, allowing for outliers on either end, is better than predicting an exact amount of time. Refusing to give time estimates entirely or withholding other grim information in order to protect the patient is usually not productive and may not allow the patient and family to prepare for death. The possibility of miracles or rare exceptions to the usual course of the illness allows a glimmer of

---

Table 35–1. End-of-life issues to be discussed with patients.

Life Support
- Do you have an advance directive (a living will or health-care proxy)?
- Do you know what CPR is? If you had a terminal illness would you want to undergo CPR?
- In the event an illness led to your being unable to eat or drink on a permanent basis, would you want to be fed with feeding tubes?
- Do you want your medical care geared to prolonging your life at all costs, or is improving or maintaining your quality of life more important?

Personal Beliefs
- What life experiences have you had around death and dying?
- How have these experiences affected your own attitudes about death?
- What are your worst fears about dying?
- What would be a good death for you?
- What do you believe happens to you when you die?

Long-Term Care and Support Systems
- If you become too ill to take care of yourself, who will take care of you?
- Who would you want to make health-care decisions for you if you became unable to do so?
- If you were dying, would you prefer to be at home or in an institution such as a hospital or nursing home?
- Do you know what hospice care is? Would you want that kind of care if you were terminally ill?
- Who would you want to be present at the time of your dying and death?
- Is there anything you need to get done before you die?

hope for some patients. In general, the physician should be guided by patients and their families in determining how detailed the information about the course of the illness should be (see Chapter 3).

Advance Directives

Advance directives are formal documents that direct health-care decisions if patients lose the capacity to speak for themselves. There are two types of advance directives: living wills and health-care proxies, or durable powers of attorney.

A living will allows a patient to direct the kinds of treatments wanted at the end of life. Some living wills focus on general goals, whereas others may specify exact treatments and explicit circumstances. Living wills become operative only when patients are unable to communicate for themselves.

A **health-care proxy,** or **durable power of attorney,** allows patients to designate a person to make decisions on their behalf should they become unable to do so. These directives allow more flexibility than do living wills, an important point, since it is difficult to anticipate all possible medical conditions and treatment options.

Many people complete both documents: a living will to present an overarching philosophy and a health-care proxy to designate a person to help interpret that philosophy when the patient can no longer do so. For healthy persons, discussing a living will or a health-care proxy may be the first time they have had to face their own mortality. For those with terminal illness, completing an advance directive may be seen as another indication of their inevitable deterioration.

Involving family members in the discussions of advance directives is useful. A proxy who is uninformed about the values and wishes of the patient has an arduous job when difficult care decisions must be made. Although they cannot cover every situation, living wills with clear statements about goals, values, and directions help the clinician and the designated proxy formulate a care plan. In addition, having a form to fill out helps many patients and their families discuss death-related issues. The advance directive decisions can provide a starting point for discussions about the limits of care and the burdens of suffering as well as orders not to resuscitate.

Do Not Resuscitate: The "do not resuscitate" (DNR) order refers to the withholding of cardiopulmonary resuscitation (CPR), specifically closed-chest cardiac massage, defibrillation, and artificially supplied respiratory support. For most patients with a terminal disease, CPR is at best ineffective and at worst a cruel and expensive technological death ritual. Many studies have shown that CPR provides no increase in out-of-hospital survival for patients with multisystem disease, particularly patients with advanced cancers and renal failure.

Unfortunately many patients and their families interpret a DNR order as an abandonment, or giving up,

and agonize over its issuance. This is in part due to the way medical personnel emphasize what will be withheld rather than what will be done. When alternative treatment strategies are not explained, patients and families think that a DNR order means nothing will be done to treat symptoms or to alleviate suffering. They sense that second-class treatment will be given—which may indeed happen if clinicians and the institutions they work in are not knowledgeable about palliative care. It should be understood that agreement to a DNR order in no way limits other treatment options.

DNR orders do, however, signal that things are different. The notion that being resuscitated from cardiopulmonary arrest will not add appreciably to the quality and or quantity of life is an open acknowledgment that death is near—and that reversing the dying process is not within medicine's power. Although some patients are initially frightened by this discussion, many feel relieved and appreciate the opportunity to avoid treatment they do not want.

Emergency rescue crews are obligated to attempt resuscitation unless they have specific instructions not to proceed. DNR orders that are valid in the inpatient setting may not be valid in the outpatient setting unless special forms, which vary by locality, are completed. These issues should be addressed with terminally ill patients who want to remain at home, since resuscitation may be carried out in times of crisis if the proper documentation is not on hand.

Comfort Care: Patients confronting a terminal illness may opt for all-out, aggressive, disease-oriented medical treatment, or a trial of aggressive medical care with set limits (such as a DNR order). When limited trials of aggressive care are undertaken, the patient has the experience to gauge whether or not the suffering engendered by the treatment is worth it, given the odds of success. When treatments begin to fail, or if supposedly curative treatments become too burdensome, the patient can stop at any time, and a transition to comfort care is considered. Relieving symptoms and alleviating suffering then take precedence over attempts to treat the underlying disease. Comfort care, hospice care, and palliative care are terms used to describe a treatment philosophy that is based on symptom control, an emphasis on quality of life, and relief of suffering. Frequently employed in hospice settings, but applicable to any level of treatment, palliative care methods put the care of the patient, and not cure of the disease, in the foreground of care. Comfort care emphasizes symptom relief, personal contact, and the search for hope and meaning, even in the face of seemingly overwhelming physical and psychological suffering.

Comfort care can be considered any time in the course of a serious illness, especially when the chances for recovery are slim or the burden of suffering is high. Some patients may want to continue to fight their disease until the bitter end, despite considerable suffering and poor odds, but others choose palliative care from the beginning. Clinicians should not withhold their own recommendations about how to proceed, but the choice of treatment philosophy should remain with the patient.

Hospice: Hospice programs provide comprehensive care to dying patients, with a multidisciplinary team of nurses, physicians, social workers, volunteers, and clergy. These programs accept only patients who have a life expectancy of less than 6 months. In the United States, only about 50,000 deaths annually (out of almost 2 million) occur in hospice programs. Unfortunately, many patients are referred too late in the course of their illness to take full advantage of the resources and supports available. The comfort care philosophy underlying hospice can be applied in a range of settings from acute-care hospitals to nursing homes to the patient's home. The advantage of hospice programs is the expertise brought to palliative care techniques by the multidisciplinary staff. In most outpatient programs, the primary care physician and the hospice team form a partnership to care for the patient. The primary care provider, with whom the patient may have a long-term relationship, should be intimately involved in both the decision for hospice referral and the patient's ongoing care. Once distressing symptoms are controlled, comfort care may then help the patient find avenues to hope, meaning, and ways of saying good-bye.

Case illustration 4: Carlos, a 70-year-old man, has been diagnosed with a hepatoma. In exploring the treatment options with his physician, he is clear about wanting only comfort care measures, and referral to a home hospice program is initiated. Carlos is not a verbal man, and discussions about death and dying meet with little response.

At first, periodic nursing visits are all that is needed. He has an antique tool collection and spends countless hours labeling and ordering the tools. His nurse talks to him about this process, which has come to symbolize his anticipatory grief. As he deteriorates, nursing visits become more frequent, and home health aides come to help with his personal care. Carlos gradually becomes bed-bound. Although his family initially feels uncomfortable with his dying at home, a family meeting with the physician and hospice nurse sets up a rotation of visits to provide for both company and supervision. Children who had been estranged are in the rotation, and it becomes a time of family healing. Though little is explicitly said about his approaching death, the presence of family and talk about the tools provide a vehicle for saying good-bye. Carlos dies quietly at home with his family present.

Hospice care, with its supportive team of physicians, nurses, and other caregivers, eases the patient's way to death by providing quality palliative care.

Terminal Care: An important goal in terminal care is to keep patients as pain-free as they choose. Long-acting opioid preparations, when given in sufficient quantity in a regular dosing schedule (not PRN) have proven effective in alleviating chronic pain with-

out significant sacrifice in quality of life. Knowing that they can control their own pain is reassuring to patients, especially those who have seen painful deaths. Unrealistic concerns about addiction from patients, families, and caregivers should be anticipated and addressed, since these worries often present a major obstacle to adequate pain relief. Withholding narcotics in the terminally ill because of fears about addiction is unwarranted—and cruel.

Delirium & Coma

Many patients die in profoundly altered states of sensorium. There is also an increasing number of patients with dementing illnesses in whom cognitive and affective life may have diminished significantly prior to the terminal episode. Terminally ill patients with delirium present the physician and the patient's family with a dilemma. The delirium may provide relief from the pain and grim reality of further physical decay, but it may also be due to reversible factors that, if treated, could extend life. The extent to which reversible causes of delirium are searched for and treated depends on the patient's current goals, previous directives, and concurrent discussions with the family. The prior degree of suffering and the patient's wishes should largely determine what should be done.

The internal, subjective experience of a person dying with altered mental status may vary significantly from the outside perception. Patients who recover from delirium and coma sometimes report nightmarish, terrifying visions; out-of-body travel; or visions of light and angelic beings, or they may not be able to remember anything about the experience. Occasionally the disorientation becomes profound and the sense of the world is lost.

Case illustration 5: Caleb is 101 years old, a rugged dairy farmer who has become partly deaf and then blind in the last 5 years of his life but remains alert and communicative. He develops a cough and fever, and despite treatment for pneumonia, becomes progressively more dyspneic. He tells his physician that he does not wish to be resuscitated. Because his elderly wife cannot care for him at home, Caleb is hospitalized. He becomes progressively more confused and withdrawn, and his deafness and blindness further confound communication. He lies still in bed for long periods of time. Efforts by physicians and nurses to engage him in conversation are usually met with short responses such as yes, no, or okay. His physician asks him one morning what experiences he is having, and he replies that he is flying over fields of golden wheat on a sunny day. Then, in a voice of wonderment, he asks if he is still alive, or if he has died already. His physician replies that he is still alive. Caleb dies later that day.

Patients who experience altered states at the end of life need supportive treatment. Once this stage has been reached, decisions about artificial hydration and feeding should have already been made and formalized through advance directives. If they have not (and frequently they have not) the designated health care agent or the family must make a substituted judgment as to what the patient would want if he could understand his condition and prognosis and speak for himself. Failing knowledge about this, the physician's decision should be based on what is in the best interest of the patient.

There is growing evidence that terminal dehydration and inanition may ease the dying process. Providing nutrition and hydration through feeding tubes and intravenous lines when the dying patient can no longer eat or drink may appear compassionate, but such practices may inadvertently prolong dying and aggravate suffering. The person with terminal illness is dying; our acceptance of this should guide all treatments in the direction of lessening the suffering, enhancing the quality of life left, and respecting the patient's dignity.

The Wish to Die

Sometimes, even with the best of palliative care methods, suffering cannot be alleviated to the patient's satisfaction. If this occurs, the patient may feel that dying is the only way out. The patient may no longer be able to tolerate the pain, humiliation, loss of control, increased dependency, or the burden the illness places on the family. Many such patients begin actively to contemplate ending their life.

Case illustration 6: Marvin is 63 years old; he has amyotrophic lateral sclerosis and has been on a respirator at home for a year. He has lost the ability to use his arms and legs and requires total care. He increasingly resents his life on the respirator and finally requests that it be removed and he be permitted to die. He makes this request repeatedly over the course of a month. His primary care physician sees him several times on home visits and discusses the request with Marvin's family. They agree that the respirator should be stopped. A psychiatrist visits the patient also and indicates that he finds Marvin competent, not depressed; he concurs with the patient, family, and primary care physician on removing the respirator. An attempt to remove the respirator without the sedative effects of morphine leads to air hunger and feelings of suffocation. A morphine drip is instituted and the respirator turned off. The patient dies comfortably several minutes later, attended by his family.

The **double effect** of giving medications that relieve suffering and yet may shorten the patient's life is an accepted part of medical practice and comfort care. Withdrawing life-sustaining but burdensome treatments, even though the withdrawal leads to death, is also an accepted part of practice. These practices have widespread legal, ethical, and medical acceptance and should not be confused with the controversy surrounding assisted suicide and voluntary euthanasia. In this case, the patient's wish to die can be acceded to, since a treatment that is life-sustaining but very burdensome could be removed with the assistance of a high-dose narcotic that is intended to lessen panic and suffering (Table 35–2). Patients, however, may ask the clinician, sometimes in an off-hand way, as if testing

Table 35–2. Euthanasia and assisted death: definitions.

Term	Definition	Legal Status in the United States
Physician-assisted death, physician aid in dying	These are general terms that include both physician-assisted suicide and voluntary active euthanasia. They emphasize the physician's intentional role as an assistant to an act initiated by the patient.	See Voluntary active euthanasia and Physician-assisted suicide.
Euthanasia	An "easy" death. Painlessly putting to death a person who is suffering from an incurable, painful disease.	Illegal under most circumstances
Voluntary active euthanasia	Intentionally intervening to cause the patient's death at the request of and with the informed consent of the competent patient.	Illegal
Nonvoluntary active euthanasia	Intentionally intervening to cause the patient's death without the explicit request of the patient.	Illegal
Passive euthanasia	Withholding or withdrawing life-sustaining care that results in the patient's death with the consent of the patient or surrogate.	Legal with the proper consent
Double effect	Administering drugs that are intended to relieve suffering but may shorten life.	Legal
Physician-assisted suicide	Physician provides, at the patient's request, the means for the patient to end his or her own life.	Illegal in most states, but recent federal appeals court rulings have declared bans on physician-assisted suicide unconstitutional.

the water, about help in dying (either assisted suicide or euthanasia). This subject has both ethical and legal repercussions, and patients are often as reluctant as their physicians to discuss it.

If the patient has terrible suffering but does not have a life-sustaining treatment that can be withdrawn (eg, respirator, dialysis) or the kind of pain that can justify high doses of narcotics, the request for help in dying would put the clinician in a more difficult legal and ethical position. Voluntary active euthanasia is the act of intentionally intervening to cause the patient's death, at the explicit request of, and with full informed consent of, the competent patient. The physician administers a lethal agent, with the intent of both alleviating suffering and causing death. Voluntary active euthanasia is illegal in the United States and would be prosecuted if discovered. In assisted suicide, the physician provides the means (such as a prescription for barbiturates) at the request of the patient, but the patient administers the lethal intervention. Assisted suicide is illegal in many states, but its legal status is currently in flux. A referendum legalizing assisted suicide at the request of a terminally ill patient was passed in Oregon, and both the 2nd and 9th Federal Circuit Courts recently found laws prohibiting physician-assisted suicide to be unconstitutional. These decisions are being appealed to the United States Supreme Court; the final outcome is uncertain.

Case illustration 7: Sara, a bedridden 84-year-old woman with end-stage congestive heart failure, is seen on rounds. She is on multiple medications, including morphine, to relieve her pulmonary edema. Despite intensive treatment, even eating causes her to be dyspneic. She looks up from her bed and asks to be given a lethal dose of medicine so that she can die. When asked why she wants to die now, Sara replies that she has lived long enough—through the deaths of her husband, two of her children, three of her brothers, and both her sisters. She has one son still living and he is dying of leukemia, with only weeks to live. She wants to die before him so she won't have to grieve his death. Her request for lethal medication is not granted. Sara leaves the hospital with public health nurses and family to look after her. Her physician agrees to make home visits as Sara is too weak to travel to the office. A few days later, she is found dead in bed by the visiting nurse. The physician is notified and comes to the house to pronounce the patient dead. She notices several empty pill bottles—including that from the morphine—at the bedside. The thought crosses her mind that this may have been a suicide, but she decides not to pursue it and simply completes the death certificate as for a natural death.

The patient's request to hasten death should be explored in detail. It may represent the wish to escape from depression, anxiety, uncontrolled physical pain, shame of dependency, and other psychosocial issues. Once the meaning of the request is understood, it can usually be ameliorated through appropriate palliative care techniques, and the request is frequently

withdrawn. If the request is ignored or belittled, the patient is left to deal with these feelings alone, and may, in fact, commit suicide because of suffering that might have been dealt with by other means.

There are times, however—as in our example—when protracted pain and other debilitating symptoms make death a desirable alternative to continued suffering. The relationship between the physician, patient, and family, as well as the physician's own values, determine the response to such requests. Clinicians who refuse to participate in assisted suicide, because of their own moral positions, should make this clear to the patient. In this event, they have an obligation to seek common ground with the patient and to continue to search for other avenues to relieve suffering. Those who are considering assisting the patient's suicide should fully explore the potential personal, professional, and legal consequences. Guidelines for assisted suicide have been published, and clinicians confronted with a reasonable request to end life should refer to these, as well as to colleagues experienced in terminal care, for help.

HOPE & MEANING

Throughout the dying process, the search for hope and meaning is always in the background. Hopelessness and despair are disturbing emotions. Hope helps patients and their loved ones endure suffering when faced with a terminal illness. It comes in many forms, not simply through cure or recovery. To hope for a peaceful death, to have a little more time in order to finish business, to find new meaning and the possibility of personal growth in our dying, or to become emotionally closer to loved ones or to God are all hopes and wishes not dependent on cure of the body.

Case illustration 8: Rhea, a 64-year-old woman with metastatic breast cancer, is on high-dose long-acting morphine because of bone pain. She has fractures of the clavicle and both femurs and has requested no resuscitation in the event of cardiac or pulmonary arrest. She hopes to be able to die at home, where she has very close family support, without more painful episodes or fractures.

Rhea now shows signs of increasing confusion and dehydration but wants to avoid hospitalization. She expresses the strong wish not to die yet because her children and their families are arriving in 2 weeks. She wants not only to see them, but to be as alert and pain-free as possible while they visit. Hypercalcemia is found on evaluation and hospitalization is advised. Because she wishes to die at home with only comfort measures taken, she remains at home for another day. She is torn by knowing that she could let herself die from the effects of the calcium, but that she then would not get to see her daughters. Despite attempts at oral treatment she becomes progressively less alert and is brought to the hospital by her family when her oral intake stops.

Treatment is initiated and the hypercalcemia corrected; her confusion clears, and she is able to go home after a week in the hospital. By the time her children arrive, Rhea is alert and able to communicate coherently. She is quite elated that she can have last words with them and her grandchildren. Despite the need for increased doses of morphine and multiple other medications to control her symptoms, she is not hospitalized again and dies at home several months later.

The hope for more time may be reasonable even if comfort care has been decided on. Relatively invasive interventions that extend meaningful life and are consistent with the patient's goals are sometimes appropriate. Remaining flexible in the face of changing, difficult situations and letting the patient's goals guide the treatment permit the clinician to hope, along with the patient, for a death with as little meaningless suffering as possible. When no hope is offered or found, the patient is left alone and isolated.

Case illustration 3 (the case of a patient who had been abandoned twice) is also germane here. The hopelessness engendered by the first clinician, who offered no hope and prescribed acetaminophen and codeine for metastatic cancer, led to feelings of despair. These were alleviated when the patient looked elsewhere for treatment and was given a complicated regimen to follow. By providing an activity on which to focus, the alternative clinic offered him hope, however false. In sum, the lack of continuity with the primary practitioner resulted in a desperate grasping at straws and left the patient and his wife open for exploitation.

The popularity of alternative healing methods offers hope to some patients when traditional methods are not working, have proven too burdensome, or are not consistent with the patient's preferences or beliefs about illness and healing. Patients who are interested in pursuing unproven remedies may be doing so because they have been told their case is hopeless and there is nothing left to be done. This sense of futility leaves them feeling abandoned, with nowhere to turn—except to alternative methods of treatment. The selection of such therapies out of desperation and abandonment is very different from choosing them because they are consistent with a person's goals and values. In order to explore these therapeutic alternatives, the clinician has to understand why the patient is turning to them. Hope that comes from long-shot aggressive medical therapies or unconventional therapies needs to be explored together. Examining the risks and benefits is frequently enough to begin the dialogue over what the possibilities and probabilities of improvement really are and to distinguish false hope from a meaningful alternative.

Trying to find and maintain hope when it becomes evident that recovery is hopeless calls for personal and spiritual exploration. The patient's feeling of hopelessness may need to be probed in depth before possible new avenues for hope and meaning can be explored. It is important not to provide false hope through simple or formulaic solutions to complex problems; hopeful solutions are often uniquely personal and may be discovered through continuing exploration by the patient with family, friends, health care providers, and clergy.

Some patients are not terrified to die and come to accept death as a natural step in completing the life cycle. Many such persons die with grace and ease, demonstrating that death does not always have to be feared or denied. Furthermore, some patients have profound experiences of personal growth in the dying process. For some highly independent persons, this becomes a time to be more accepting and appreciative of the love and care of others.

> *Case illustration 9:* A 64-year-old veterinarian, Richard, develops headaches so severe that he can no longer carry on his surgical practice. Within 3 months, he is diagnosed with an inoperable brain tumor. Over the ensuing 6 months, he loses the ability to walk and swallow. Because of recurrent aspiration, he is placed on a home ventilator and fed through a gastrostomy tube. In the face of his overwhelming losses, he decides he wants to tape a description of his life and journey to the point where he is now. Relatives, friends, colleagues, and members of his church come to his home, and joint recollections and reflections are taped. When this process is complete Richard says good-bye to his wife and family and requests that the respirator and fluids be withdrawn. With his physician's consent and instructions to family members, he is given regular doses of morphine and the respirator is turned off. He dies with his loved ones in attendance. His life and death leave a legacy of courage and an acquiescence to fate that touches the hearts of those he knew.

The search for love, connection to others, and a sense of meaning are essential in helping patients through the dying process. The ability to experience love and meaning can ameliorate considerable suffering. If love and purpose can be found, then fears usually lessen, and dying may be accepted as an adventure and entry into the next phase of existence.

CARE OF THE FAMILY

Terminal illness can help resolve or intensify family conflict. Issues of power, money, allegiances, previous losses, and grief may surface along with unforeseen courage and the noblest sacrifices that family members may ever have made on behalf of one another. Paradoxical feelings of anger and love, fear and bravery, anxiety and compassion, depression and transcendence never seem to be far removed on the part of the dying patient and his or her caregivers.

The physician can be a healing presence in this volatile mix by including the patient's family and other caregivers as part of the treatment team. Such collaboration broadens the patient's network of support, enlisting new allies, and more widely distributing the burden of care.

The clinician needs to communicate clearly with family members regarding care plans, prognosis, complications, and who will make decisions if the patient cannot. Addressing advance directives with the patient and the proxy is essential when it is likely the patient will lose capacity during the illness. The selection of a proxy forces the patient to choose among family members and may trigger old family wounds over who was favored and who has more power. The patient's wishes and choices should take precedence over what family members may want, although in actual practice this is sometimes difficult to achieve. When the patient loses mental capacity, the family becomes the focus of decision making, and processes are brought into play that may create conflict. Family pressures may influence even what the competent patient does in ways that go against his or her values. The clinician may need to remind family members that the patient's values, beliefs, and preferences need to be honored, whether or not the patient can speak for himself or herself.

When a family has many members, the clinician may want to meet regularly with a small group and at special times with more members. The family can be asked to designate representatives who can stay in close touch with the physician. If family members are in conflict about a certain plan, and the patient has lost the capacity to express his or her wishes, it is best to focus on what the patient would have wanted, applying the ethical principle of substituted judgment. If the patient's wishes are unknown, what is in the patient's best interest must be discussed. Views on what is truly in the patient's best interest may vary widely between family members and clinicians (see Chapter 9).

Unexpected Death: An unexpected death puts a particular strain on the family and the clinician. Sudden or traumatic death sends a shock through the family and, when it occurs in a medical facility, may elicit strong doubt about competence in clinicians. Meeting with the family, expressing sympathy, and answering questions in as straightforward a way as possible may be helpful. Family members should be allowed to view and stay with the deceased; when possible, the eyes and mouth should be closed and the limbs arranged peacefully. Strong emotional reactions should be anticipated and the tears of grief welcomed.

The clinician should recognize each family member present and solicit each person's reaction. Cultural norms may vary widely in the emotional behaviors displayed. The normal grief reactions in some cultures (screaming, yelling, falling to the ground) may seem inappropriate or embarrassing to a clinician from another, less demonstrative background. It is only through experience with these various manifestations of grief that the clinician can judge what "normal" grief should look like. Physicians and nurses may want to call in clergy and social workers; each may have something to offer a family that is trying to integrate the shock and loss.

When an unexpected death occurs in the context of ongoing medical care, the practitioner should critically examine what, if anything, could have been done to prevent its occurrence. Self-recrimination and blame may initially be part of this process for the clinician, especially if a medical misjudgment is involved. Learning from the experience, discussing it with trusted colleagues, and—if necessary—disclosing it to the family are often appropriate. It is important for clinicians not to bear the burdens of these experiences alone (see Chapter 32).

Unresolved Grief: Of all the causes of unremitting grief, one of the most overwhelmingly difficult for families and practitioners is the death of a child—especially when the death is unexpected. The parents' grief must be followed closely for signs of becoming pathological. The physician should not try to ameliorate the pain of the loss prematurely. Empathy may be the best initial approach. Follow-up visits to elicit stories and memories give the parents a chance to talk about the deceased if they choose. Discussing and expressing anger, guilt, and sadness can help the bereavement process. In many other cases, survivors are unable to deal with the loss of a parent, a sibling, a spouse or partner, or a long-time friend. Grief that is unresolved may lead to clinical depression, social isolation, and emotional numbing as well as multiple physical symptoms. Social problems of drug abuse, marital and work conflicts, and feelings of hopelessness and abandonment may also appear. If the clinician cannot help the family resolve the grief, referral should be made to an appropriate support group or a therapist for counseling.

SELF-CARE

How health-care workers take care of themselves when involved in death and dying work has not received a great deal of attention. Burnout is common among physicians and nurses who work with patients who are suffering a terminal illness. Having responsibility for dying patients' care and management, in a society that denies death, exacerbates the problem. From the initial delivery of bad news to decisions about whether to attend the funeral, clinicians are confronted with thoughts and feelings that enmesh them with the patient and the family. How closely the patient's family resembles their own may determine how emotionally involved they become. The grief that follows the death of a close patient may be quite profound and requires time and reflection to heal. Unfortunately, most institutions do not have an organized way for caregivers to get and give support during these times. The feelings of loss need to be recognized and discussed. Support or bereavement groups may help in this process. Hospital morbidity and mortality committees review the decedent's medical care, but they rarely reflect on how caregivers felt about the death, or what effect it has on the staff. Setting aside time to review the death from this perspective is likely to be helpful for staff morale, cohesiveness, and healing (see Chapter 8).

Since taking care of the dying patient brings us close to death itself, clinicians get to view this special time at very close range. Feelings of compassion and love as well as loneliness and vulnerability are frequently stirred up in providers. Healing responses may include turning to music, art, religion, literature, nature, humor, or psychotherapy for solace and understanding. Spiritual questions of purpose and meaning in life become more immediate in the face of impending death. Not only do workers in the death and dying realm midwife patients through the dying process, but the dying patient midwifes us into a fuller experience of life.

SUGGESTED READINGS

American Board of Internal Medicine, End of Life Care Project Committee: Caring for the dying: Identification and promotion of physician competency. 1996.

American Medical Association: Good care of the dying patient. JAMA 1996;275:474.

Block SD, Billings JA: Patient requests to hasten death. Arch Intern Med 1994;154:2039.

Clinical practice guideline: Management of cancer pain. Agency for Health Care Policy and Research. Publication No. 94-0592. Available through the National Cancer Institute.

Ebell MH: Prearrest predictors of survival following in-hospital cardiopulmonary resuscitation. J Fam Pract 1992; 34:551.

Quill TE: Doctor, I want to die. Will you help me? JAMA 1993;270:870.

Quill TE, Brody RV: Death and dying. In *Textbook of Primary Care Medicine*. Mosby-Year Book, 1996.

Quill TE, Cassel CK: Non-abandonment: A central obligation for physicians. Ann Intern Med 1995;122:368.

Quill TE: *Death and Dignity*. Norton, 1993.

Waisel DB, Truog RD: The cardiopulmonary-resuscitation-not-indicated order: Futility revisited. Ann Intern Med 1995;122:304.

Index

Note: Page numbers followed by *t* or *f* indicate tables or figures, respectively.

Psychosocial issues *(cont.)*
  chronic pelvic pain, 121, 122
  depression, 179
  gynecologic examinations, 118
  HIV (human immunodeficiency virus), 285–288
  hysterectomy, 123
  infertility, 122, 122*t*
  menopause, 123–124
  premenstrual syndrome, 120–121
  sleep disorders, 245–246
Psychostimulant treatment, 296
Psychotherapy
  depression, 184–185, 185*t*
  generalized anxiety disorder, 200–201
  personality disorders, 215
  stress, 273–274
  substance abuse, 172
Psychotic disorders *vs.* dementia, 231
Psychotropic medication
  dementia, 234–235
  insomnia, 241
Puberty, 82
Pulmonary system and stress, 270
Purging behavior, 158, 160

Quality of life, 139
Questions, asking
  anxiety, 193*t*
  behavioral change, 132–135
  children's interviews, 73–74, 76–77
  clarifying, 5
  demanding patients, 26
  domestic violence, 309
  global family function, 63–64
  HEADSS assessment format, 83–86
  HIV (human immunodeficiency virus), 296
  open-ended, 1–2
  pain, 278*t*
  safety net, creating a, 5
  self-report questionnaire, 271
  sexual problems, 249
  substance abuse, 166
  suicide, 180, 180*t*
  "yes, but . . ." patients, 27–28
Quetelet index, 150
Quinidine-like side effects of heterocyclic antidepressants, 187

Racism, 97
Rapid ejaculation, 257*t*, 260
Reactance, theory of, 126
Reactive depression, 178
Readiness-for-change model. *See* Behavioral change
Reality of symptoms and somatization, 208
Reassurance and giving bad news, 18
Reciprocal relationships, 57
Recommendations in brief advice interventions, 170
Redux, 154
Referral
  adherence to treatment problems, 140
  anxiety, 201–203
  childhood behavioral problems, 75–76
  chronic illness, 320
  difficult patients, 28–29
  domestic violence, 310
  gender identity disorders, 262
  HIV (human immunodeficiency virus), 297

  hypnosis and suggestions, 45
  lesbians and gay males, 114
  psychotherapeutic intervention, 70–71
  resistance to counseling, 67
  sexual problems, 255–256
  somatization, 210
  stress, 273–274
  substance abuse, 171–174
Reflection, empathic skill of, 11
Reframing attention to underlying family problems, 69–70
Rehabilitation of older adults with mental disorders, 94
Relapse-prevention techniques, 172
Relapse stage of change, 126*t*, 127*t*, 131, 134–135
Relational-based personal philosophy, 54, 54*t*
Relational basis of ethical/appropriate behavior, 33
Relational boundaries, 31
Relationships and chronic illness, 319–320
Relationship skills, 55
Relative weight (RW), 150
Relaxation and hypnosis, 43
Relaxation exercises, 201, 281*t*
REM-behavior disorder (RBD), 244
REM sleep, 179, 237
Reproductive system and stress, 270
Requests from patients, misguided, 48–49
Residential treatment programs, 173
Respect, empathic skill of, 12
Respiratory system and hypnosis, 44
Resting metabolic expenditure (RME), 151
Restless legs syndrome (RLS), 240
Restoril, 291
Rifampin, 289
Ritalin, 296
RLS Foundation, 246
Runaway teenagers, 86
Russians and cross-cultural communication, 106

Sadness and chronic illness, 318
Safety issues and dementia, 234
Safety nets, creating, 5
Sanorex, 154
Satisfaction, patient, 12
Schedule in SPEAK approach to counseling, 184, 190*t*
Schizoid personality disorder, 214–215*t*, 217–218
  diagnosis, 217
  management, 218
Screening methods. *See also* Ask, Assess, Advise, and Assist treatment model for substance abuse; Diagnosis
  anxiety, 193–194*t*
  Beck scale, 6
  breast cancer, 118*t*, 119
  CAGE questionnaire, 1, 2*t*
  childhood behavioral problems, 72–73, 73*t*
  depression, 181, 291
  domestic violence, 309
  family function, 63–65, 64–65*t*
  Hamilton scale, 6
  older patients and neurologic, 91
  Primary Care Screen for Mental Disorders, 7
  Symptom-Driven Diagnostic System for Primary Care, 7
  women's health, 118*t*, 118–119
  Zung scale, 6
Secondary CNS pathology, 288
Secondary orgasmic disorder, 261
Second-hand tobacco smoke, 142, 170
Sedative-hypnotic medications, 239, 239*t*, 241, 293
Seldane, 188